Introductory Textbook of

Psychiatry

SIXTH EDITION

INTRODUCTORY TEXTBOOK OF

Psychiatry

SIXTH EDITION

Donald W. Black, M.D.

Nancy C. Andreasen, M.D., Ph.D.

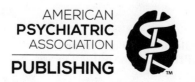

AMERICAN
PSYCHIATRIC
ASSOCIATION
PUBLISHING

Copyright © 2014 American Psychiatric Publishing
ALL RIGHTS RESERVED

Manufactured in the United States of America on acid-free paper
18 17 16   5 4 3 2
Sixth Edition

Typeset in Adobe's Palatino and Frutiger LT Std

American Psychiatric Publishing, Inc.
1000 Wilson Boulevard
Arlington, VA 22209-3901
www.appi.org

Bulk discounts of 20% are available on purchases of 25–99 copies of this or any other APP title; please contact APP Customer Service at appi@psych.org or 800-368-5777. To purchase 100 or more copies of the same title, e-mail bulksales@psych.org for a price quote.

Library of Congress Cataloging-in-Publication Data
Black, Donald W., 1956– author.
    Introductory textbook of psychiatry / Donald W. Black, Nancy C. Andreasen.— Sixth edition.
        p. ; cm.
    ISBN 978-1-58562-469-0 (hardcover : alk. paper)—ISBN 978-1-58562-470-6 (pbk. : alk. paper)
    I. Andreasen, Nancy C., author. II. Title.
    [DNLM: 1. Mental Disorders. 2. Psychiatry—methods. WM 100]
    RC454.4
    616.89--dc23
                                                    2013050017

British Library Cataloguing in Publication Data
A CIP record is available from the British Library.

CONTENTS

PART I
Background

PART II
Psychiatric Disorders

PART III
Special Topics

About the Authors

Donald W. Black, M.D., is Professor of Psychiatry at the University of Iowa Roy J. and Lucille A. Carver College of Medicine in Iowa City, Iowa. He is a graduate of Stanford University, where he received his undergraduate degree, and the University of Utah School of Medicine. He received his psychiatric training at the University of Iowa, where he now serves as Director of Residency Training and Vice Chair for Education in the Department of Psychiatry. Dr. Black is an authority on personality disorders and impulsive behavior. He has written several books, including *Bad Boys, Bad Men—Confronting Antisocial Personality Disorder (Sociopathy)* and *DSM-5 Guidebook* (with Jon E. Grant). He is a Distinguished Fellow of the American Psychiatric Association and Past President of the American Academy of Clinical Psychiatrists.

Nancy C. Andreasen, M.D., Ph.D., is the Andrew Woods Chair of Psychiatry at the University of Iowa Roy J. and Lucille A. Carver College of Medicine. She received a Ph.D. in English Literature from the University of Nebraska, and later, a medical degree from the University of Iowa, where she also trained in psychiatry. She is one of the world's leading authorities on schizophrenia and was a pioneer in the application of neuroimaging techniques to the study of major mental illnesses. She is the author of numerous books including *The Creating Brain: The Neuroscience of Genius, The Broken Brain: The Biological Revolution in Psychiatry,* and *Brave New Brain: Conquering Mental Illness in the Era of the Genome.* Dr. Andreasen received the National Medal of Science in 2000, America's highest award for scientific achievement. She is a member of the American Academy of Arts and Sciences and the Institute of Medicine of the National Academy of Science. She served as Editor-in-Chief of the *American Journal of Psychiatry* for 13 years.

Disclosures of Competing Interests

The authors of this book have indicated a financial interest in or other affiliation with a commercial supporter, a manufacturer of a commercial product, a provider of a commercial service, a nongovernmental organization, and/or a government agency, as listed below:

Nancy C. Andreasen, M.D., Ph.D.   *Research Support:* AstraZeneca, Genentech, Johnson & Johnson

Donald W. Black, M.D.   *Research Support:* AstraZeneca

Preface

Students sometimes begin working in psychiatry with a set of preconceptions about what it is—preconceptions shaped by the fact that information about psychiatry is omnipresent in popular culture. Taxi drivers, CEOs, teachers, and ministers often feel qualified to offer information and advice about how to handle "psychiatric problems" even though they may be unaware of distinctions as fundamental as the difference between psychiatry and psychology. These two disciplines are blurred together in the popular mind, and the term *psychiatry* evokes a potpourri of associations—Freud's couch, Jack Nicholson receiving electroconvulsive therapy in *One Flew Over the Cuckoo's Nest*, Dr. Drew discussing sexual adjustment on television. These images and associations tend to cloak psychiatry with an aura of vagueness, imprecision, muddle-headedness, and mindless coercion. It is unfortunate that such preconceptions are so pervasive, but fortunate that most of them are in error, as students who use this book in conjunction with studying psychiatry in a clinical setting will soon discover.

What is psychiatry? It is the branch of medicine that focuses on the diagnosis and treatment of mental illnesses. Some of these illnesses are very serious, such as schizophrenia, Alzheimer's disease, and the various mood disorders. Others may be less serious, but still very significant, such as anxiety disorders and personality disorders. Psychiatry differs from psychology by virtue of its medical orientation. Its primary focus is illness or abnormality, as opposed to normal psychological functioning; the latter is the primary focus of psychology. Of course, abnormal psychology is a small branch within psychology, just as understanding normality is necessary for the psychiatrist to recognize and treat abnormal functioning. The primary purposes of psychiatry as a discipline within medicine are to define and recognize illnesses, to identify methods for treating them, and ultimately to develop methods for discovering their causes and implementing preventive measures.

There are several reasons why psychiatry may be the most exciting discipline within medicine. First, psychiatrists are specialists who work with the most interesting organ within the body, the brain. The brain is intrinsically fascinating because it controls nearly all aspects of functioning within the rest of the body as well as the way people interact with and relate to one another. Psychiatry has rapidly advanced in recent years through the growth of neuroscience, which has provided the tools by which researchers have begun to decode brain anatomy, chemistry, and physiology. Understanding human emotion and behavior will ultimately lead to better and more effective treatments for mental illnesses.

Yet as psychiatry evolves into a relatively high-powered science, it remains a very clinical and human branch within medicine. It can be an especially rewarding field for students who have chosen medicine because they wish to have contact with patients. The clinician working in psychiatry must spend time with his or her patients and learn about them as human beings as well as individuals with distressing or impairing illnesses. Learning a person's life story is rewarding and interesting; as a colleague once said, "It amazed me when I realized that I would get paid for asking people things that everybody always wants to know about anyway!"

Finally, psychiatry has enormous breadth. As a scientific discipline, it ranges from the highly detailed facts of molecular biology to the abstract concepts of the mind. As a clinical discipline, it ranges from the absorbingly complex disturbances that characterize illnesses such as schizophrenia to the understandable fearfulness shown by young children when they must separate from their parents and attend school or be left with a babysitter. It can be very scientific and technical, as in the frontier-expanding research currently occurring in molecular genetics or neuroimaging; but it can also be very human and personal, as when a clinician listens to a patient's story and experiences the pleasure of being able to offer help by providing needed insights or even simple encouragement and support.

This book is intended as a tool to help you learn from your patients and from your teachers. We have tried to keep it simple, clear, and factual. References are provided for students who wish to further explore the topics covered in the various chapters. We have written this book primarily for medical students and residents in their first several years of training, although we anticipate that it may also be useful to individuals seeking psychiatric training from the perspectives of other disciplines such as nursing or social work. We hope that, using this book as a tool, students of all ages and types will learn to enjoy working with psychiatric patients and with the art and science of contemporary psychiatry as much as we do.

The current edition was prompted by the publication of DSM-5™, the diagnostic manual for the mental health field. We considered it essential that this book include the most current information on psychiatric diagnosis. The book has been reorganized along the lines of DSM-5, which now follows the developmental lifespan. This has involved moving several classes and categories, adding new diagnoses, consolidating others, and eliminating the multiaxial diagnostic system. We believe readers will agree that these are very positive changes.

We are grateful to the many readers who, over the years, have written to us with their useful suggestions. Medical students, psychiatry residents, and other trainees who have used the book have given us critical feedback that has helped shape this book. We thank our many colleagues who have provided help and guidance: Jennifer McWilliams, Linda Madson, Jon E. Grant, Jodi Tate, Jess Fiedorowicz, Robert Philibert, Laurie McCormick, Anthony Miller, Wayne Bowers, Mark Granner, Vicki Kijewski, Susan Schultz, Del Miller, Tracy Gunter, Russell Noyes, and Scott Temple.

We also thank the talented staff at American Psychiatric Publishing, including Editor-in-Chief Robert E. Hales, Rebecca Rinehart, John McDuffie, and others who shared our vision for the book and made it possible.

Introduction

You are not here merely to make a living.... You are here to enrich the world, and you impoverish yourself if you forget the errand.

Woodrow Wilson

Many of you reading this book will be getting your first introduction to psychiatry. You may not realize that, along with surgery, it is one of the oldest medical specialties. It emerged as a special branch of medicine in the eighteenth century, when a few general physicians decided to devote themselves exclusively to the care of the mentally ill. They were influenced by the humanistic and humane principles of the Enlightenment, which they shared with the American Founding Fathers who wrote the Declaration of Independence and the U.S. Constitution and with other great statesmen such as Woodrow Wilson.

Philippe Pinel, a leader of the French Revolution, is usually considered to be the founding father of modern psychiatry. In 1793, he was named director of the Bicêtre, the hospital in Paris for insane men. Soon afterward he instituted a grand, symbolic change by removing the chains that bound the patients to the walls at the Bicêtre and created a new type of treatment that he referred to as "moral treatment." (This meant treating patients in ways that were morally and ethically sensitive.) He was later made director of the corresponding hospital for women, the Salpêtrière. In addition to treating the mentally ill with kindness and decency, Pinel also tried to approach the study of mental illness scientifically. He described his efforts in his *Treatise on Insanity* (1806):

> I, therefore, resolved to adopt that method of investigation which has invariably succeeded in all the departments of natural history, viz. To notice successively every fact, without any other object than that of collecting materials for future use; and to endeavor, as far as possible, to divest myself of the influence, both of my own prepossessions and the authority of others. (p. 2)

Thus a new specialty within medicine was created, consisting of those doctors who chose to specialize in the care of the mentally ill. They became known as "psychiatrists," which means literally "physicians who heal the mind."

What does that mean? What does a psychiatrist actually do? Why do people choose to study psychiatry, and why do some choose to make this their specialty? People study psychiatry and become psychiatrists because they are interested in what makes human beings tick. Some of us have chosen to become psychiatrists because we want to understand the human mind and spirit as well as the human brain. We chose to join a very clinical specialty because we are interested in people, and we like to work with them as individuals. We like to think about people within the context of the social matrix in which they live, to skillfully elicit a "life narrative" that summarizes their past and current experiences, and to use that information to better understand how their symptoms arise and can be treated. Each person we encounter is a new adventure, a new voyage of discovery, and a new life story. Patterns tend to generalize across individuals, yet each patient is unique. This is what makes psychiatry challenging, intellectually rich, complex, and even enjoyable—despite the fact that we often care for people who suffer intensely and for whom we wish we could offer even more help. We are privileged to explore the most private and personal aspects of people's lives and to help them achieve more fulfilling lives.

Many people study psychiatry and become psychiatrists because they are fascinated by the human brain—the most complex and interesting organ in the human body. All of our emotions, thoughts, beliefs, and behaviors arise from the workings of that furrowed and folded chunk of tissue that is so carefully protected within our skulls. Modern neuroscience has begun to unlock the secrets of the human brain using a variety of tools that reach from the molecular to the systems level. What we contain within our memory stores forms the essence of our human individuality. We have already learned a great deal about how memories are stored and retained at the molecular and cellular level. We are also unlocking the mysteries of brain development and aging and the complex ways that human thoughts are created. Understanding these processes, as well as many others, offers the opportunity for understanding the mechanisms of mental illness, for finding better treatments, and perhaps even for preventing them. These are exciting times to be studying the human brain!

Last, people study psychiatry and become psychiatrists because mental illnesses are among the most clinically important diseases from which human beings suffer. In 1996 two investigators at Harvard University, working in collaboration with the World Health Organization, published a pivotal book titled *The Global Burden of Disease*. This book captured the attention of leaders in the medical community because it provided the first objective summary of the costs of various types of illness to society throughout the world. One head-turning fact is the cost exacted by mental illnesses. For example, unipolar major depression is the costliest illness in the world. Furthermore, four mental illnesses are among the top 10 diseases affecting people between ages 15 and 44 years: depression, alcohol use disorder, bipolar disorder, and schizophrenia. Because self-inflicted injuries are also a consequence of mental illness, 5 of the 10 leading causes of disability in the world are attributable to psychiatric disorders. The message is clear: doctors can no longer afford to ignore mental illnesses. Every physician must learn to identify and diagnose mental illnesses and either provide treatment or referral to a specialist. Some must pursue a deeper understanding by becoming psychiatrists.

The study of *psychiatry*, the branch of medicine devoted to the study of mental illnesses, is therefore a discipline dedicated to the investigation of abnormalities in brain function manifested in diseases that afflict individuals in interesting and important ways. The clinical appearance of these abnormalities may be obvious and severe, as in the case of schizophrenia, or subtle and mild, as in the case of an adjustment disorder. Ultimately the drive of modern psychiatry is to develop a comprehensive understanding of normal brain function at levels that range from mind to molecule and to determine how aberrations in these normal functions (produced either endogenously through genetic coding or exogenously through environmental influences) lead to the development of symptoms of mental illnesses.

About the DSM-5® criteria sets: The DSM-5 diagnostic criteria sets published in this book have been abridged to omit diagnostic codes and coding notes. Readers should consult DSM-5 for this information.

PART I

BACKGROUND

Chapter 1

Diagnosis and Classification

Knowledge keeps no better than fish.

Alfred North Whitehead

During the twenty-first century, all of medicine will experience a paradigm shift in the way that diseases are classified and defined. Our current diagnoses are primarily syndrome based. They rely heavily on clinical observations that signs and symptoms co-occur in groups of patients and also that they have a characteristic course and response to treatment. The twenty-first century will be the "era of the genome." Thanks to ongoing advances in genomics and molecular biology, we will begin to define diseases in terms of their etiologies rather than their signs and symptoms. Through this process, traditional medical classification—whether in pediatrics or psychiatry—will be challenged and revised over the ensuing decades. Today's medical students and residents will need to follow these advances carefully and to be prepared to revise the concepts that they are now being taught.

The fundamental purpose of diagnosis and classification is to isolate a group of discrete disease entities, each of which is characterized by a distinct pathophysiology and/or etiology. Ideally, all diseases in medicine would be defined in terms of etiology. For most illnesses, however, we do not know or understand the specific etiology. By and large, a full understanding of etiology is limited to the infectious diseases, in which the etiology is exposure to some infectious agent to a degree sufficient that the body's immune mechanisms are overwhelmed. Even in this instance, our knowledge of immune mechanisms is incomplete.

For most diseases, our understanding is at the level of pathophysiology rather than etiology. Diseases are defined in terms of the mechanisms that produce particular symptoms, such as infarction in the myocardium, inflammation in the joints, or abnormal regulation of insulin production.

In the areas of pathophysiology and etiology, psychiatry has more uncharted territory than the rest of medicine. Most of the disorders or diseases diagnosed in psychiatry are *syndromes:* collections of symptoms that tend to co-occur and appear to have a characteristic course and outcome. Much of the current research in psychiatry is directed toward the goal of identifying the pathophysiology and etiology of major mental illnesses, but this goal has been achieved for only a few, for example, Alzheimer's disease, vascular dementia, and Huntington's disease.

■ Why Diagnose Patients?

Diagnoses in psychiatry serve a variety of important purposes and are not just a "label." Making a careful diagnosis is as fundamental in psychiatry as it is in the remainder of medicine.

Diagnosis introduces order and structure to our thinking and reduces the complexity of clinical phenomena. Psychiatry is a diverse field, and symptoms of mental illness encompass a wide range of emotional, cognitive, and behavioral abnormalities. The use of diagnoses introduces order and structure to this complexity. Disorders are divided into broad classes based on common features (e.g., psychosis, substance abuse, dementia, anxiety). Within each major class, specific syndromes are then further delineated (e.g., dividing substance-related disorders according to the substance involved, or dividing the dementias by etiological subtype such as Alzheimer's disease and vascular dementia). The existence of broad groupings, subdivided into specific disorders, creates a structure within the apparent chaos of clinical phenomena and makes mental illnesses easier to learn about and understand. Although diagnoses are not necessarily defined in terms of etiology or pathophysiology, they are typically defined in terms of syndromal features.

Diagnoses facilitate communication among clinicians. When psychiatrists give a patient's symptoms a specific diagnosis, such as bipolar I disorder, they are making a specific statement about the clinical picture with which that particular patient presents. A diagnosis concisely summarizes information for all other clinicians who subsequently examine the patient's records or to whom the patient is referred. A diagnosis of bipolar I disorder, for example, indicates that

- The patient has had at least one episode of mania.
- During that episode of mania, the patient experienced a characteristic group of symptoms such as elated mood, increased energy, racing thoughts, rapid speech, grandiosity, and poor judgment.
- The patient probably has had episodes of depression as well, characterized by sadness, insomnia, decreased appetite, feelings of worthlessness, and other typical depressive symptoms.

The use of diagnostic categories gives clinicians a kind of "shorthand" through which they can summarize large quantities of information relatively easily.

Diagnoses help to predict outcome. Many psychiatric diagnoses are associated with a characteristic course and outcome. Bipolar I disorder, for instance, is usually episodic, with periods of relatively severe abnormalities in mood interspersed with periods of near normality or complete normality. Thus, patients with bipolar I disorder have a relatively good outcome. Some other types of disorders, such as schizophrenia or personality disorders, typically have a more chronic course. Diagnoses are a useful way of summarizing the clinician's expectations about the patient's future course of illness.

Diagnoses are often used to choose an appropriate treatment. As psychiatry has advanced clinically and scientifically, relatively specific treatments for particular disorders or groups of symptoms have been developed. For example, antipsychotic drugs are typically used to treat psychoses. They are used for disorders such as schizophrenia, in which psychosis is typically prominent, as well as for forms of mood disorder in which psychotic symptoms occur. A diagnosis of mania suggests the use of mood stabilizers such as lithium carbonate or valproate. Some relatively targeted medications are now available, such as the selective serotonin reuptake inhibitors for obsessive-compulsive disorder.

Diagnoses are used to assist in the search for pathophysiology and etiology. Clinical researchers use diagnoses to reduce heterogeneity in their samples and to separate groups of patients who may share a common mechanism or cause that produces their symptoms. Patients who share a relatively specific set of symptoms, such as severe schizophrenia characterized by negative symptoms, are often hypothesized to have a disorder that is mechanistically or etiologically distinct. Knowledge about specific groupings of clinical symptoms can be related to knowledge about brain specialization and function in order to formulate hypotheses about the neurochemical or anatomical substrates of a particular disorder. Ideally, the use of diagnoses defined on the basis of the clinical picture will lead ultimately to diagnoses that serve the fundamental purpose of identifying causes.

■ Other Purposes of Diagnosis

Beyond these clinical uses, diagnostic systems also have other purposes. Although physicians prefer to conceptualize their relationships with patients in terms of care and treatment, diagnoses are used by other health care providers, attorneys, epidemiologists, and insurance companies. Each time a clinician makes a diagnosis and records it, he or she must do so with an awareness of the nonclinical uses to which it may be put. Because mental illnesses may be subject to discrimination and misunderstanding, these diagnoses involve a particular risk. The clinician obviously must walk a fine line—perhaps impossibly fine.

Diagnoses are used to monitor treatment and to make decisions about reimbursement. As health care has become increasingly managed, diagnoses are often used to determine the length of a hospital stay or the choice of a treatment course for a specific condition. Physicians or their assistants sometimes must spend hours speaking on the telephone with insurers to request additional days, or in writing letters appealing their decisions for denial of care if the patient's course of treatment appears to exceed the preset guidelines. Depending on the insurer, some diagnoses may not be covered at all—for example, substance-related disorders. The range of diagnoses covered by insurers continues to change rapidly and, particularly in response to the 2010 Affordable Care Act, medical students and residents will need to carefully follow these changes and learn how this new law will affect patient care.

Diagnoses are used by attorneys in malpractice suits and in other litigation. Even though psychiatrists are the least frequently sued among medical specialists, lawsuits are of concern to all physicians in our litigious society. Some mental illnesses, such as major depression, carry with them a clear set of risks, including suicide. Clinicians must be aware of those risks and carefully document that they have provided appropriate care. As the *Diagnostic and Statistical Manual of Mental Disorders* (DSM) has made the diagnostic system of psychiatry more open and available, both lawyers and patients have learned much more about psychiatric classification. A physician called into court must expect to defend a recorded diagnosis with appropriate documentation that the various criteria have been assessed and are met.

Diagnoses are used by health care epidemiologists to determine the incidence and prevalence of various diseases throughout the world. Diagnoses recorded in hospital or clinic charts are translated into a standard system established by the World Health Organization (WHO), the *International Classification of Diseases* (ICD). This system is used to track regional differences in disease patterns as well as changes over time.

Diagnoses are used to make decisions about insurance coverage. A carelessly made diagnosis, be it of hypertension or major depression, may make it difficult for a patient to obtain life insurance or future health care insurance. Diagnoses also are sometimes used to make decisions about employment, admission to college, and other important opportunities.

■ The History Behind DSM

The process of diagnosis in psychiatry has been simplified by the fact that the national professional organization to which most psychiatrists in the United States belong, the American Psychiatric Association, has formulated a manual that summarizes all of the diagnoses used in psychiatry. The manual specifies symptoms that must be present to make a given diagnosis, and organizes these diagnoses together into a classification system. This manual is titled the *Diagnostic and Statistical Manual of Mental Disorders* (DSM).

The impetus to organize a DSM began during World War II. For the first time, psychiatrists from all over the United States were brought together in clinical settings that required them to communicate clearly with one another. It became apparent that diagnostic practices varied widely in the United States, no doubt reflecting a diversity of training. Shortly thereafter, the American Psychiatric Association convened a task force to develop a diagnostic manual. The first DSM (now referred to as DSM-I) was published in 1952. Over the years, the DSM has undergone four major revisions (DSM-II, DSM-III, DSM-IV, and DSM-5). Currently, diagnoses in psychiatry are based on DSM-5, which was published in 2013.

Compared with later editions, DSM-I and DSM-II were relatively simple. For example, the definition of manic-depressive illness in DSM-II was as follows:

Manic-Depressive Illnesses (Manic-Depressive Psychoses)
These disorders are marked by severe mood swings and a tendency to remission and recurrence. Patients may be given this diagnosis in the absence of a previous history of affective psychosis if there is no obvious precipitating event. This disorder is divided into three major subtypes: manic type, depressed type, and circular type. (p. 8)

These early handbooks were relatively short. DSM-I contained 132 pages, and DSM-II contained 134 pages. DSM-III, which came out in 1980, was the first effort by a medical specialty to provide a comprehensive and detailed diagnostic manual in which all disorders were defined by specific criteria.

DSM-III was not only significantly larger than its predecessors (494 pages) but its use of diagnostic criteria helped change the way psychiatrists and other mental health professionals go about the diagnostic process. Because of their vagueness and imprecision, the definitions in DSM-I and DSM-II did not adequately fulfill many of the purposes for making a diagnosis. In particular, the descriptions were not specific enough to facilitate communication among clinicians and to delineate one disorder from another. Research investigations made it clear that different clinicians using DSM-I or DSM-II guidelines would give different diagnoses to the same patient. The authors of DSM-III agreed to formulate diagnostic criteria that would be as objective as possible to define each of the disorders, and would make their decisions about defining criteria and overall organizational structure on the basis of existing research data whenever possible. They largely achieved their aim, and helped to change what had been an often arbitrary (and ridiculed) practice of psychiatric diagnosis. The successor manuals, DSM-IV and DSM-5, have continued the practice of including objective and reliable diagnostic criteria. (Note that with DSM-5, the American Psychiatric Association decided to designate the manual with an Arabic numeral, anticipating future revisions or editions as DSM-5.1, DSM-5.2, and so on.)

Psychiatry is the only specialty in medicine that has so consistently and comprehensively formalized the diagnostic processes for the disorders within its domain. This precision and structure are particularly important in psychiatry because there are no specific laboratory diagnostic tests and confirmed etiologies for most disorders. Consequently, a DSM diagnosis relies largely on the patient's presenting symptoms and history. Without the structure provided by diagnostic criteria, the diagnostic process could become imprecise and unreliable. Yet the DSM system has not been without controversy or untoward side effects.

■ Advantages and Disadvantages of the DSM System

Advantages

The advantages of the DSM system can be summarized as follows:

The DSM system has substantially improved the reliability of diagnosis. *Reliability,* a biometric concept, refers to the ability of two observers to agree on what they see. Thus, psychiatrists working in different cities (or countries), and seeing the same patient, will arrive at the same diagnosis. Reliability is measured by a variety of statistical methods, such as percent agreement, correlation coefficients, and the kappa statistic, which corrects for chance agreement. The reliability of psychiatric diagnosis has been assessed in extensive field trials organized for each revision and has been found to range from good to excellent for most of the major categories.

The DSM system has clarified the diagnostic process and facilitated history taking. Because DSM-5 specifies exactly which symptoms must be present to make a diagnosis, as well as the characteristic course of disorders whenever this is appropriate, it is highly objective. During the 1970s, many psychiatrists received predominantly psychodynamic training that deemphasized a medical approach to diagnosis. This approach stressed the importance of recognizing underlying psychological processes rather than objective signs and symptoms. Although clinically useful, this approach was often subjective, was difficult to teach to beginners, and required substantial training. The DSM system provided a simpler approach that brought signs and symptoms back to the forefront of evaluation. Its criteria specify which signs must be observed and which symptoms must be inquired about. This structured approach also makes it an excellent teaching tool for medical students and residents.

The DSM system has clarified and facilitated the process of differential diagnosis. Because it is so explicit, DSM helps clinicians decide which symptoms must be present to rule in or to rule out a particular diagnosis. For example, it specifies that a diagnosis of schizophrenia cannot be made if mood episodes have been present for a majority of the total duration of the illness. Likewise, a diagnosis cannot be made if some type of drug of abuse, such as amphetamine, has led to the presence of psychotic symptoms. Not only are differential diagnostic issues embedded in the criteria, but the text of each DSM also contains a relatively detailed discussion of the differential diagnosis for each disorder.

Disadvantages

Every paradise has its serpent and poisoned apple. Every treatment has its unwanted side effects. Thus, the DSM system also has certain problems and disadvantages:

The increased precision sometimes gives clinicians and researchers a false sense of certainty about what they are doing. The DSM criteria are simple provisional agreements, arrived at by a group of experts, on what characteristic features must be present to make a diagnosis. Although diagnostic criteria are based on data whenever possible, the available data are often inadequate or incomplete. Thus, the selection of signs and symptoms is sometimes arbitrary. The diagnoses themselves are certainly arbitrary. They will remain arbitrary as long as we are ignorant about pathophysiology and etiology. Medical students and residents tend to crave certainty (as do many physicians long out of training), so they want very much to believe that a given DSM diagnosis refers to some "real thing." Thus, the DSM system sometimes leads clinicians to lapse into petty and pointless debates about whether a patient "really" is depressed if he or she does or does not meet the DSM criteria. The criteria should be seen for what they are: useful tools that introduce structure but often require a healthy amount of skepticism.

The DSM system may sacrifice validity for reliability. *Reliability* refers to the capacity of individuals to agree on what they see, whereas *validity* refers to the capacity to predict prognosis and outcome, response to treatment, and ultimately etiology. Psychodynamically oriented clinicians have objected that the DSM system has sacrificed some of psychiatry's most clinically important concepts because psychodynamic explanations and descriptions are generally excluded. Biologically oriented psychiatrists have objected to the lack of validity in DSM as well. In this instance, they point to the arbitrary nature of the definitions, which are not rooted in information about biological causes.

The DSM system may encourage clinicians to treat diagnosis as no more than a checklist and forget about the patient as a person. DSM-5 can be used to streamline clinical interviews because it encourages the use of a checklist of symptoms in making a diagnosis. There is nothing wrong with the checklist approach, but the initial diagnostic interview should include many more aspects of the patient's life as well. Perhaps the most important contribution that psychiatry makes to medicine in general is that it emphasizes the importance of establishing rapport with patients and knowing each patient as a unique person. The opportunity to establish a close doctor–patient relationship, based on asking about many facts of a person's life, makes psychiatry a particularly interesting and enjoyable specialty in medicine—at least for those physicians who are interested in having a caring and human relationship with their patients. This emphasis on care and compassion in addition to "cure" has been the essence of medical care since the time of Hippocrates.

■ Learning to Use DSM-5

DSM-5 is large (947 pages) and complex, but beginners should not allow these features to intimidate them. Rather than attempt to master everything at once, they should focus on the major classes and categories seen either in psychiatric practice or in primary care settings, such as schizophrenia, major depression, or the addictions. (Table 1–1 lists the major diagnostic classes in DSM-5.) One innovation is that chapters are organized along the developmental lifespan. DSM-5 begins with the neurodevelopmental disorders, often diagnosed in infancy and early childhood, and progresses through diagnostic areas more commonly diagnosed in adulthood, such as sleep-wake disorders.

A few sets of symptom criteria (e.g., major depression) should be committed to memory, simply because they are used so often in so many different settings. Learners may wish to carry the pocket edition of DSM-5 (*Desk Reference to the Diagnostic Criteria From DSM-5*) or use its online counterpart from which they can easily download needed criteria sets. The system is too vast to commit all of it to memory, however, and learners should not feel reluctant to refer back to the criteria when evaluating a patient's symptoms and making a diagnosis.

■ Recording the Diagnosis

Those new to the diagnostic process sometimes ask how they should make and record a psychiatric diagnosis. As will become clear in the following chapter ("Interviewing and Assessment"), the diagnostic process is complex and typically follows an intensive data-gathering

---

TABLE 1–1.   DSM-5 diagnostic classes

Neurodevelopmental disorders

Schizophrenia spectrum and other psychotic disorders

Bipolar and related disorders

Depressive disorders

Anxiety disorders

Obsessive-compulsive and related disorders

Trauma- and stressor-related disorders

Dissociative disorders

Somatic symptom and related disorders

Feeding and eating disorders

Elimination disorders

Sleep-wake disorders

Sexual dysfunctions

Gender dysphoria

Disruptive, impulse-control, and conduct disorders

Substance-related and addictive disorders

Neurocognitive disorders

Personality disorders

Paraphilic disorders

Other mental disorders

---

process that includes recording the patient's history, performing a mental status examination, gathering collateral information from the patient's family members or friends (whenever possible), and conducting appropriate laboratory tests. At that point, the process of circling in on a diagnosis begins, typically by rank ordering the various possibilities and discarding or ruling out diagnoses that are less likely. This is the process of *differential diagnosis*. It is not unusual for the diagnostic process to continue as additional information is gathered, and for the clinician to revise his or her initial impression.

Once the diagnostic possibilities have been whittled down, the next question is how they are to be recorded. With only a few exceptions, DSM-5 encourages clinicians to make multiple diagnoses when necessary to fully describe the patient's condition. In DSM-III and DSM-IV, diagnoses were recorded using a multiaxial system in which major diagnoses were coded on Axis I, personality disorders and mental retardation on Axis II, medical disorders on Axis III, stressors on Axis IV, and current global functioning on Axis V. For various reasons, including the fact that no other diagnostic system uses a multiaxial system—thus placing DSM in conflict with the rest of medicine—the authors of DSM-5 chose to scrap the system that had been in place since 1980.

In DSM-5, diagnoses are ranked in order of their focus of attention or treatment, listing the condition chiefly responsible for a patient's hospital stay (or outpatient clinic visit) as the *principal diagnosis* (or *reason for visit*), which may be written parenthetically after the diagnosis—e.g., "(principal diagnosis)." The only exception is that—according to the arcane coding rules in the ICD system—if the mental disorder results from a medical condition, *that* medical condition is listed first. For example, if an outpatient with HIV disease seeks care for symptoms related to a mild neurocognitive disorder caused by the HIV, "HIV infection" is listed first, followed by "mild neurocognitive disorder due to HIV infection (reason for visit)."

If the clinician does not have sufficient information to allow a firm diagnosis, the clinician may indicate this uncertainty by recording "(provisional)" following the diagnosis. For example, the clinical presentation may strongly suggest schizophrenia, but the patient is unable to provide sufficient history to confirm the diagnosis. Sometimes it is difficult to determine the patient's principal diagnosis or reason for visit, particularly when multiple conditions are present (e.g., is the patient's schizophrenia or his alcohol use disorder the main problem?). Any diagnostic list will appear arbitrary to a certain extent, and while we all crave certainty, that may not be possible.

Several examples follow of how a clinician might record a diagnosis (or diagnoses) following an evaluation:

Example 1: A 25-year-old man is brought to the emergency room by family members for bizarre behavior including making threats of harm, muttering obscenities, and talking to himself. His bizarre behavior appears motivated by paranoid delusions. Family members report that he drinks nearly daily to intoxication and that he smokes cigarettes nearly nonstop. He has had several prior hospitalizations for similar reasons and has been diagnosed with schizophrenia. His DSM-5 diagnoses are:

- Schizophrenia (principal diagnosis)
- Alcohol use disorder, moderate
- Tobacco use disorder, severe

Example 2: A 65-year-old man is brought to the clinic by his worried spouse. She reports that he has been diagnosed with lung cancer, which his doctors believe has metastasized to his brain. He hears "voices" that tell him not to trust family members. He has become very suspicious and has threatened family members who he believes are planning to kill him. There is no psychiatric history. His DSM-5 diagnoses are:

- Malignant lung neoplasm
- Psychosis due to malignant lung neoplasm (provisional)

Example 3: A 27-year-old woman presents to the clinic for treatment of intrusive thoughts about a recent rape and recurrent nightmares. Prior to her recent symptoms, she reports having experienced overwhelming anxiety in social situations. She also reports a history of deliberate self-harm by cutting, relationship difficulties, and abandonment fears. Her DSM-5 diagnoses are:

- Posttraumatic stress disorder (reason for visit)
- Social anxiety disorder
- Borderline personality disorder

DSM-5 does *not* include treatment guidelines. Nonetheless, accurate diagnosis is the first step in providing appropriate treatment for any medical condition, and mental disorders are no exception. For that reason, DSM-5 will be the starting point for clinicians as they begin by conducting a comprehensive assessment of their patient. Despite the absence of treatment information, DSM-5 provides a wealth of information about diagnostic classes and disorders that learners from all backgrounds will find useful. These resources are detailed in Table 1–2.

Students should understand that the diagnosis of a mental disorder is not equivalent to a need for treatment. Decisions regarding treatment involve consideration of the patient's symptom severity, subjective distress and disability associated with the symptoms, and other factors (e.g., psychiatric symptoms complicating medical conditions). Importantly, clinicians may encounter individuals who do not meet full criteria for a mental disorder but have a clear need for treatment or care. *Access to care should not be limited just because a person does not show all symptoms of a diagnosis.*

TABLE 1–2.	Useful information in DSM-5 regarding each diagnosis

Recording procedures (where applicable)

Subtypes and/or specifiers (where applicable)

Diagnostic features

Associated features supporting diagnosis

Prevalence

Development and course

Risk and prognostic factors

Culture-related diagnostic issues

Gender-related diagnostic issues

Diagnostic markers

Suicide risk

Functional consequences

Differential diagnosis

Comorbidity

■ Self-Assessment Questions

1. What is the overall purpose of diagnosis and classification in medicine? Describe the extent to which it has been achieved in psychiatry.
2. Describe some of the specific purposes of psychiatric diagnosis.
3. Describe some of the changes introduced by DSM-III and carried forth to the present.
4. Define the concepts of reliability and validity. How is reliability measured?
5. Describe the advantages of the DSM approach. What are some of its disadvantages?
6. If the patient has several psychiatric diagnoses, how are they listed according to DSM-5? When is the term *provisional* used?

Chapter 2

Interviewing and Assessment

Festina lente.

(Make haste slowly.)

A Latin proverb

The first encounter with a patient begins with taking a clinical history, just as in other specialties. The novice may feel some anxiety about approaching and interviewing people with mental illnesses, but largely because they have been portrayed in the media in such disturbing ways. Think of Randle Patrick McMurphy in *One Flew Over the Cuckoo's Nest*, or John Nash in *A Beautiful Mind*. Furthermore, psychiatric history-taking requires the interviewer to ask uncomfortable questions such as "Do you hear voices when no one is around?" or to ask about areas of life that are especially private and intimate, such as sexual preferences and practices. However, it is a bit like learning to ski or swim. Once you head down the mountain (or get in the water), you will find history-taking to be surprisingly easy, interesting, and even fun. Demands placed on the interviewer will vary, of course, depending on the type of illness the patient has and its severity. Patients with milder syndromes, such as anxiety disorders or personality disorders, are usually more capable of describing their symptoms and history clearly and articulately. The severely ill depressed, manic, or psychotic patient presents a real challenge, and clinicians may have to depend on informants, such as family members or friends, in addition to the patient.

■ The Psychiatric Interview

An initial psychiatric evaluation serves several purposes. One is to formulate an impression as to the patient's diagnosis or differential diagnosis and to begin to generate a treatment plan. The second purpose is to produce a document for the patient's record that contains information organized in a standard, readable, and easily interpretable way. The initial interview is often therapeutic as well, in that it permits the clinician to establish a relationship with the patient and to reassure him or her that help will be provided.

The outline of that written record is summarized in Table 2–1. As the table indicates, a standard psychiatric evaluation is very similar to the evaluations used in the rest of medicine, with some minor modifications. The content of the present illness and past history is focused primarily on psychiatric symptoms, and the family history includes more information about psychiatric illnesses in family members. Family history and social history also include more social and personal information than is recorded in the standard medical history. An important part of the interview—the mental status examination—is typically included only in psychiatric and neurological evaluations.

TABLE 2–1.   Outline of the psychiatric evaluation

Identification of patient and informants

Chief complaint

History of present illness

Past psychiatric history

Family history

Social history

General medical history

Mental status examination

General physical examination

Neurological examination

Diagnostic impression

Treatment and management plan

Identification of Patient and Informants

Identify the patient by stating his or her age, race, gender, marital status, and occupational status. Indicate whether the patient was the sole informant or whether additional history was obtained from family members or previous psychiatric records. Indicate whether the patient was self-referred, was brought in at the request of family members, or was referred by a physician; if either of the latter two, specify which family members or physician. In addition, indicate how reliable the informant appears to be.

Chief Complaint

Begin by stating the patient's chief complaint in his or her own words, using quotation marks (e.g., "I'm thinking of killing myself" or "The voices tell me to hurt people"). An additional sentence or two of amplifying information also may be provided, particularly if the patient's chief complaint is relatively vague.

History of Present Illness

Provide a concise history of the illness or problem that brought the patient in for treatment. Begin by describing the onset of the symptoms. If this is the patient's first episode, first psychiatric evaluation, or first hospital admission, that should be stated early in the history of the present illness. Indicate how long ago the first symptoms began, the nature of their onset (e.g., acute, insidious), and whether the onset was precipitated by any particular life events or problems. If the latter, describe these events or problems in some detail. Likewise, medical conditions that may have served as precipitants should be described. If drug or alcohol abuse was a potential precipitant, that also should be noted.

The evolution of the patient's various symptoms should be described. A systematic summary of all symptoms present, in a form useful for making a differential diagnosis of the present illness, should be provided. This listing of symptoms should reflect the criteria included in DSM-5 and should specify both which symptoms are present and which symptoms are absent. The description of symptoms should not be limited to those included in the DSM-5 diagnostic criteria, however, because these typically do not provide a full description of the range of symptoms that patients have (i.e., they are minimal, not comprehensively descriptive). The description of the present illness also should indicate the degree of incapacity that the patient is experiencing as a consequence of the symptoms, as well as the influence of the symptoms on personal and family life. Any treatments the patient has received for the present illness should be noted, including dosages, duration of treatment, and effectiveness of the specific medications, because these will often dictate the next step.

Past Psychiatric History

The past psychiatric history provides a summary of past illnesses, problems, and their treatment. In patients with complex histories and chronic psychiatric illnesses, this portion of the history will be quite extensive. It should begin by noting the age at which the patient was first seen for psychiatric evaluation and the number of past hospitalizations or episodes. Thereafter, past episodes should be described in chronological order, with some information about duration of episodes, types of symptoms present, severity of symptoms, treatments received, and response to treatment. If a characteristic pattern is present (e.g., episodes of mania are always followed by episodes of depression, or past depressive episodes have consistently responded to a particular medication), this should be noted because it provides useful prognostic treatment information. If the patient's memory for past symptoms is relatively poor, or the bulk of the past history is obtained from old records rather than from the patient himself or herself, this also should be recorded. Confirmation by family members of types and patterns of symptoms and number of episodes also should be noted.

Family History

The age and occupation of both parents and all siblings should be noted, as should the age and education or occupation of all children (if applicable). If any of these first-degree relatives (parents, siblings, children) has a history of any mental illness, the specific illness should be mentioned, along with information about treatment, hospitalization, and long-term course and outcome. It may be necessary to describe specific disorders because many patients will not recognize alcoholism or criminality, for example, as relevant problems: "Do any blood relatives have a history of alcoholism, criminality, drug abuse, severe depression, suicide attempts, or suicide? Have any ever been psychiatrically hospitalized or institutionalized? Have any ever taken 'nerve pills' or seen psychiatrists, psychologists, or counselors?" The interviewer should obtain as much information as possible about mental illness in the extended family as well. Any relevant information about the family's social, cultural, or educational background also may be included in this section of the interview. It is often helpful to draw pedigrees in complicated cases.

Social History

The social history provides a concise narrative description of the patient's life history. It includes information about where the patient was born, where he or she grew up, and the nature of his or her early life adjustment. Any problems during childhood, such as temper tantrums, school phobia, or delinquency, should be noted. The patient's relationships with his or her parents and siblings should be described. Psychosexual development, such as age at first sexual experience, also should be described. Information about familial religious or cultural attitudes that is relevant to the patient's condition should be noted. Educational history should be summarized, including information about how many years of school the patient completed, quality of school performance, and nature of academic interests. Some description should be provided of the patient's interest and participation in extracurricular activities and interpersonal relationships during adolescence and early adulthood. Work history and military history also should be summarized. Certain areas may need more emphasis and detail, depending on the chief complaint and diagnostic formulation.

This section also contains a summary of the patient's current social situation, including marital status, occupation, and income. With patients who are unemployed or disabled, it may be helpful to ask, "What was your usual (or past) occupation?" The location of the patient's residence should be described, as well as the specific family members who live with the patient. This section of the history should provide information about the various social supports currently available to the patient. Habits (e.g., cigarette smoking, alcohol use) should be recorded.

General Medical History

The patient's current and past state of health should be summarized. Any existing medical illness for which the patient is currently receiving treatment should be noted, as well as the types of treatments, medications, and their dosages. Include vitamins, supplements, herbals, or other alternative or complementary treatments (e.g., acupuncture, chiropractic, dietary supplements). Allergies, past surgeries, traumatic injuries, or other serious medical illnesses should be summarized. Head injuries, headaches, seizures, and other problems involving the central nervous system are particularly relevant.

Mental Status Examination

The mental status examination is the psychiatric equivalent of the physical examination in medicine. It includes a comprehensive evaluation of the patient's appearance, thinking and speech patterns, memory, and judgment.

The components of the mental status examination are summarized in Table 2–2. Some domains are determined simply by observing the patient (e.g., appearance, affect). Other portions are determined by asking the patient relatively specific questions (e.g., mood, abnormalities in perception). Still others are assessed by asking the patient a specified set of questions (e.g., memory, general information). The interviewer should develop his or her own repertoire of techniques to assess functions such as memory, general information, and calculation. This repertoire should be consistently used for all patients so that he or she develops a good sense of the range of normal and abnormal responses in individuals of various ages, educational levels, and diagnoses.

Appearance and Attitude

Describe the patient's general appearance, including grooming, hygiene, and facial expression. Note whether the patient looks his or her stated age, younger, or older. Note type and appropriateness of dress. Describe whether the patient's attitude is cooperative, guarded, angry, or suspicious.

TABLE 2–2.   Outline of the mental status examination

Appearance and attitude	General information
Motor activity	Calculations
Thought and speech	Capacity to read and write
Mood and affect	Visuospatial ability
Perception	Attention
Orientation	Abstraction
Memory	Judgment and insight

Motor Activity

Note the patient's level of motor activity. Does he or she sit quietly, or is he or she physically agitated? Note any abnormal movements, tics, or mannerisms. If relevant, evaluate for and note any indications of catatonia, such as waxy flexibility (described later in the chapter under "Catatonic Motor Behavior"). Determine whether any indications of abnormal movements are present, such as the oral-buccal movements seen in persons with tardive dyskinesia.

Thought and Speech

Psychiatrists often speak about "thought disorder" or "formal thought disorder." This concept refers to the patient's pattern of speech, from which abnormal patterns of thought are inferred. It is, of course, not possible to evaluate thought directly. Note the rate of the patient's speech—whether it is normal, slowed, or pressured. Note whether the patient's speech indicates a pattern of thought that is logical and goal directed or whether any of a variety of abnormalities in form of thought is present (e.g., derailment, incoherence, poverty of content of speech). Summarize the content of the thought, noting in particular any delusional thinking that is present. Delusions, when present, should be described in detail. (If already noted in the history of the present illness, this can be indicated with a simple statement such as "Delusions were present as described above.")

Mood and Affect

The term *mood* refers to an emotional attitude that is relatively sustained; it is typically determined through the patient's own self-report, although some inferences can be made from the patient's facial expression. Note whether the patient's mood is neutral, euphoric, depressed, anxious, or irritable.

Affect is inferred from emotional responses that are usually triggered by some stimulus. Affect refers to the way that a patient conveys his or her emotional state, as perceived by others. The examiner watches the response of the patient's face to a joke or a smile, determines whether the patient shows appropriate or inappropriate emotional reactions, and notes the degree of reactivity of emotion. Affect is typically described as full, flat, blunted, or inappropriate. *Flat* or *blunted affect* is inferred when the patient shows very little emotional response and seems emotionally dulled, whereas *inappropriate affect* refers to emotional responses that are not appropriate to the content of the discussion, such as silly laughter for no apparent reason.

Perception

Note any abnormalities in perception. The most common perceptual abnormalities are hallucinations: abnormal sensory perceptions in the absence of an actual stimulus. Hallucinations may be auditory, visual, tactile, or olfactory. Sometimes hypnagogic or hypnopompic hallucinations occur when the patient is falling asleep or waking from sleep; these are not considered true hallucinations. An *illusion* is a misinterpretation of an actual stimulus—for example, seeing a shadow and believing it is a man.

Orientation

Describe the patient's level of orientation. Normally, this includes orientation to time, place, and person. Orientation is assessed by asking the patient to describe the day, date, year, time, place where he or she is currently residing, his or her name and identity, and why he or she is in the hospital (or clinic).

Memory

Memory is divided into very short term, short term, and long term. All three types should be described. Very-short-term memory involves the immediate registration of information, which is usually assessed by having the patient repeat back immediately a series of digits or three pieces of information (e.g., the color green, the name Mr. Williams, and the address 1915 High Street). The examiner determines whether the patient can recall these items immediately after he or she is told them. If the patient has difficulty, he or she should be given the items repeatedly until he or she is able to register them. If he or she is unable to register them after three or four trials, this should be noted. The patient should then be warned that he or she will be asked to recall these items in 3–5 minutes. His or her ability to remember them after that time interval is an indication of his or her short-term memory. Long-term memory is assessed by asking the patient to recall events that occurred in the past several days, as well as events that occurred in the more remote past, such as months or years ago.

General Information

General information is assessed by asking the patient a specific set of questions covering topics such as the names of the last five presidents, current events, or information about history or geography (e.g., "Can you tell me what happened on September 11, 2001?"; "Who is our president?"). The patient's fund of general information should be noted in relation to his or her level of educational achievement. This is particularly important in assessing the possibility of dementia.

Calculations

The standard test of calculations is serial 7s. This test involves having the patient subtract 7 from 100, then 7 from that product, and so on for at least five subtractions. Some chronic patients become relatively well trained in this exercise, so it is a good idea to have other tools in one's repertoire. One that is quite useful involves asking the patient to make calculations necessary in daily living (e.g., "If I went to the store and bought six oranges, priced at three for a dollar, and gave the clerk a $10 bill, how much change would I get back?"). Calculations can be modified for the patient's educational level. Poorly educated patients may need to calculate serial 3s. Likewise, real-life calculations can be simplified or made more complex.

Capacity to Read and Write

The patient should be given a simple text and asked to read it aloud. He or she also should be asked to write down a specific sentence, either of the examiner's choice or of his or her own choice. The patient's ability to read and write should be assessed relative to his or her level of education.

Visuospatial Ability

The patient should be asked to copy a figure. This figure can be quite simple, such as a square inside a circle. An alternative task is to ask the patient to draw a clock face and set the hands at some specified time, such as 10 minutes past 11 o'clock.

Attention

Attention is assessed in part by several of the tasks just described, such as calculations or clock setting. Additional tests of attention can be used, such as asking the patient to spell a word backward (e.g., "world"). The patient also can be asked to name five things that start with a specific letter, such as *d*. The latter is a good test of cognitive and verbal fluency.

Abstraction

The patient's capacity to think abstractly can be assessed in a variety of ways. One favorite method is asking the patient to interpret proverbs, such as "A rolling stone gathers no moss" or "Don't cry over spilled milk." Alternatively, the patient can be asked to identify commonalities between two items (e.g., "How are an apple and an orange alike?"; "How are a fly and a tree alike?").

Judgment and Insight

Assess overall judgment and insight by noting how realistically the patient has appraised his or her illness and various life problems. Insight can be ascertained relatively directly—for example, by asking "Do you believe you are mentally ill?" or "Do you believe you need treatment?" Judgment may not be as easily assessed, but the patient's recent choices and decisions will help in its determination. Sometimes simple questions may be helpful. The following examples are often used: "If you found a stamped, addressed envelope, what would you do?" and "If you were in a movie theater and smelled smoke, what would you do?"

General Physical Examination

The general physical examination should follow the standard format used in the rest of medicine, covering organ systems of the body from head to foot. Examinations of patients of the opposite sex (e.g., male physician examining a female patient) should always be chaperoned.

Neurological Examination

A standard neurological examination should be performed. A detailed neurological evaluation is particularly important in psychiatric patients to rule out focal signs that might help to explain the patient's symptoms.

Diagnostic Impression

The clinician should note his or her diagnostic impression based on DSM-5 classes and categories. If appropriate, more than one diagnosis should be made. With DSM-5, the diagnoses are rank ordered in terms of importance or relevance to the situation. Not infrequently, it is difficult to make a definitive diagnosis at the time of the index evaluation. When this situation occurs, differential diagnostic possibilities should be listed.

Treatment and Management Plan

The treatment and management section will vary, depending on the level of diagnostic certainty. If the diagnosis is quite uncertain, the first step in treatment and management will involve additional assessments to determine the diagnosis with more certainty. Thus the treatment and management plan may include a list of laboratory tests appropriate to assist in the differential diagnosis listed above. Alternatively, when the diagnosis is straightforward, a specific treatment plan can be outlined, including a proposed medication regimen, plans for vocational rehabilitation, a program for social skills training, occupational therapy, marital counseling, or other ancillary treatments appropriate to the patient's specific problems.

■ Interviewing Techniques

Although the demands of the interview may vary depending on the patient and his or her illness, some techniques are common to most interviewing situations.

Establish rapport as early in the interview as possible. It is often best to begin by asking the patient about himself or herself (e.g., What kind of work do you do? What do you do for fun? How old are you?). Questions about these topics should not be asked in a manner that seems to "grill" the patient but rather in a way that indicates that the interviewer is genuinely interested in getting to know the patient. Interest can be indicated through follow-up questions. The overall tone of the opening of the interview should convey warmth and friendliness. Once rapport has been established, the interviewer should then inquire about what kind of problem the patient has been having, and what brought him or her to the clinic or hospital.

Determine the patient's chief complaint. Sometimes this complaint will be helpful and explicit (e.g., "I've been feeling very depressed," or "I've been having a pain in my head that other doctors can't explain"). At other times, the chief complaint may be relatively vague (e.g., "I don't know why I'm here—my family brought me," or "I've been having trouble at work"). When the replies are not particularly explicit, the interviewer will need to follow up his or her initial questions with others that will help determine the nature of the patient's problem (e.g., "What kinds of things have been bothering your family?" "What kind of trouble at work?"). The initial portion of the interview, devoted to eliciting the chief complaint, should take as long as is necessary to determine the patient's primary problem. When the patient is a clear, logical informant, he or she should be allowed to tell his or her story as freely as possible without interruption. When he or she is a relatively poor informant, the interviewer will need to be active and directive.

Use the chief complaint to develop a provisional differential diagnosis. As in the rest of medicine, once the patient's primary problem has been determined, the interviewer begins to construct in his or her mind a range of explanations as to the specific diagnosis that might lead to that particular problem. For example, if the patient indicates that he or she has been hearing voices, the differential diagnosis includes a variety of disorders that produce this type of psychotic symptom, such as schizophrenia, schizophreniform disorder, psychotic mania, substance misuse involving hallucinogens, or alcoholic hallucinosis. It may be comforting to realize that the fundamental process of interviewing and diagnosing is the same in psychiatry as it is in internal medicine or neurology.

Rule the various diagnostic possibilities in or out by using more focused and detailed questions. DSM-5 is particularly helpful in this regard. If the patient's chief complaint has suggested three or four different possible diagnoses, the interviewer can determine which is most relevant by referring to the diagnostic criteria for those disorders. Thus the interviewer elicits additional symptoms beyond those already enumerated when discussing the chief complaint. The interviewer inquires about the course and onset of the symptoms and about the presence of physical or psychological precipitants, such as drugs, alcohol, or personal losses.

Follow up vague or obscure replies with enough persistence to accurately determine the answer to the question. Some patients, particularly psychotic patients, have great difficulty answering questions clearly and concisely. They may say "yes" or "no" to every question asked. When a pattern of this sort is observed, the patient should be repeatedly asked to describe his or her experiences as explicitly as possible. For example, if the patient says that he or she hears voices, he or she should be asked to describe them in more detail—whether they are male or female, what they say, and how often they occur. The greater the level of detail the patient is able to provide, the more confident the clinician can feel that the symptom is truly present. Because making a diagnosis of schizophrenia or another major psychiatric disorder has important prognostic implications, the clinician should not hastily accept an answer that suggests vaguely that the patient may have a particular symptom of a disorder.

Let the patient talk freely enough to observe how tightly his or her thoughts are connected. Most patients should be allowed to talk for at least 3 or 4 minutes without interruption in the course of any psychiatric interview. The very laconic patient, of course, will not be able to do this, but most can. The coherence of the pattern in which the patient's thoughts are presented may provide major clues to the type of problem that he or she is experiencing. For example, patients with schizophrenia, mania, or depression may have any one of a variety of types of "formal thought disorder" (see section "Definitions of Common Signs and Symptoms and Methods for Eliciting Them" later in this chapter). Coherence of thought also may be helpful in making a differential diagnosis between dementia and depression.

Use a mixture of open and closed questions. Interviewers can learn a great deal about patients by mixing up their types of questions, just as a good pitcher mixes up his or her pitches. Open-ended questions permit the patient to ramble and become disorganized, whereas closed questions determine whether the patient can come up with the specifics when pressed. These are important indicators as to whether the patient is conceptually disorganized or confused, whether he or she is being evasive, or whether he or she is answering randomly or falsely. The content of the questions should be mixed as well. For example, at some point in the interview, the interviewer will probably want to drop his or her objective style of interviewing and focus on some personal topic that is affect laden, such as sexual or interpersonal relationships (e.g., "Can you tell me about your relationship with your mother?" or "Tell me about your marriage"). These questions will give the interviewer important clues about the patient's capacity to show emotional responsiveness. Evaluating the patient's mood and affect is a fundamental aspect of the psychiatric evaluation, just as is evaluating the coherence of his or her thinking and communication.

Do not be afraid to ask about topics that you or the patient might find difficult or embarrassing. Beginning interviewers sometimes find it difficult to ask about topics such as sexual relationships, sexual experiences, or even use of alcohol or drugs. Yet all this information is part of a complete psychiatric interview and must be included. Nearly all patients expect doctors to ask these questions and are not offended. Likewise, beginning interviewers are sometimes embarrassed to ask about symptoms of psychosis, such as hearing voices. To the interviewer, these symptoms seem so "crazy" that the patient might be insulted by being asked about them. Again, however, information of this type is basic and cannot be avoided. If the patient seems "obviously" not psychotic, questions about psychotic symptoms still should be asked—and in an unapologetic manner. If the patient seems amused or annoyed, then the interviewer can explain that it is necessary to cover all kinds of questions to provide a comprehensive evaluation of each patient.

Do not forget to ask about suicidal thoughts. This is another topic that may seem to fall into the "embarrassing" category. Nevertheless, suicide is a common outcome of many psychiatric illnesses, and it is incumbent on the interviewer to ask about it. The subject can be broached quite tactfully by a question such as "Have you ever felt life isn't worth living?" The topic of suicide can then be broached, leading to questions such as "Have you ever thought about taking your life?" Further tips on interviewing the suicidal patient are provided in Chapter 18, "Psychiatric Emergencies."

Give the patient a chance to ask questions at the end. From the patient's point of view, there is nothing more frustrating than being interviewed for an hour and then ushered out of the office or examining room with his or her own questions unanswered. The questions that patients ask often tell a great deal about what is on their mind. A patient might be prompted by asking, "Is there anything you feel is important that we haven't talked about?" Even if their questions are not helpful to the diagnostic process, they are significant to the patient and therefore intrinsically important.

Conclude the initial interview by conveying a sense of confidence and, if possible, of hope. Thank the patient for providing so much information. Compliment him or her, in whatever way it can be done sincerely, on having told his or her story well. Indicate that you now have a much better understanding of his or her problems, and conclude by stating that you will do what you can to help him or her. If you already have a relatively good idea that his or her problem is one that is amenable to treatment, explain that to the patient. At the end of the initial interview, if you are uncertain about diagnosis or treatment, indicate that you have learned a great deal but that you need to think about the problem some more and perhaps gather more information before arriving at a recommendation.

■ Definitions of Common Signs and Symptoms and Methods for Eliciting Them

A vast panoply of signs and symptoms characterizes major mental illnesses. The following are some of the more common ones seen in psychiatric patients. Where appropriate, some suggested questions are provided that can be used to probe for these symptoms. Follow-up questions appear in parentheses.

Symptoms That Frequently Occur in Psychotic Disorders

The term *psychosis* has several different meanings, which may be especially confusing to beginning students. In the broadest sense, the term refers to the group of symptoms that characterize the most severe mental illnesses, such as schizophrenia or mania, and that involve impairment in the ability to make judgments about the boundaries between what is real and unreal (sometimes called "impaired reality testing"). At a more operational level, *psychosis* refers to a specific group of symptoms that are common in these severe disorders. In the narrowest sense, psychosis is synonymous with having delusions and hallucinations. A somewhat broader operational definition also includes bizarre behavior, disorganized speech ("positive formal thought disorder"), and inappropriate affect. This group of symptoms is also known as *positive symptoms;* they may occur in any psychotic disorder, but are most common in schizophrenia. A second group of symptoms, referred to as *negative symptoms,* occur primarily in schizophrenia; they include alogia, affective blunting, avolition-apathy, anhedonia-asociality, and attentional impairment.

Delusions

Delusions represent an abnormality in content of thought. They are false beliefs that cannot be explained on the basis of the patient's cultural background. Sometimes defined as *fixed false beliefs,* in their mildest form delusions may persist for only weeks to months, and the patient may question his or her beliefs or doubt them. The patient's behavior may or may not be influenced by the specific delusions. The assessment of the severity of delusions and of the global severity of delusional thinking should take into account their persistence, their complexity, the extent to which the patient acts on them, the extent to which the patient doubts them, and the extent to which the beliefs deviate from those that nonpsychotic people might have. Beliefs held with less than a delusional intensity are considered *overvalued ideas.*

Persecutory delusions. People with persecutory delusions believe that they are being conspired against or persecuted in some way. Common manifestations include the belief that one is being followed, that one's mail is being opened, that one's room or office is bugged, that the telephone is tapped, or that one is being harassed by police, government officials, neighbors, or fellow workers. Persecutory delusions are sometimes relatively isolated or fragmented, but in some cases the person has a complex system of delusions involving both a wide range of forms of persecution and a belief that there is a well-planned conspiracy behind them: for example, that the patient's house is bugged and that he or she is being followed because the government wrongly considers him or her a secret agent of a foreign government. This delusion may be so complex that at least to the patient, it explains almost everything that happens to him or her.

- Have you had trouble getting along with people?
- Have you felt that people are against you?
- Has anyone been trying to harm you in any way?
- (Do you think people have been conspiring or plotting against you? Who?)

Delusions of jealousy. The patient believes that his or her spouse or partner is having an affair with someone. Random bits of information are construed as "evidence." The person usually goes to great effort to prove the existence of the affair, searching for hair in the bedclothes, the odor of shaving lotion or smoke on clothing, or receipts or checks indicating that a gift has been bought for the lover. Elaborate plans are often made to trap the two together.

- Have you worried that your (husband, wife, boyfriend, girlfriend) might be unfaithful to you?
- (What evidence do you have?)

Delusions of sin or guilt. The patient believes that he or she has committed some terrible sin or done something unforgivable. Sometimes the patient is excessively or inappropriately preoccupied with things he or she did as a child that were wrong, such as stealing candy from a store. Sometimes the patient feels responsible for causing some disastrous event, such as a fire or an accident, with which he or she in fact has no connection. Sometimes these delusions have a religious flavor, involving the belief that the sin is unpardonable and that the patient will suffer eternal punishment from God. Sometimes the patient simply believes that he or she deserves punishment by society. The patient may spend a good deal of time confessing these sins to whoever will listen.

- Have you felt that you have done some terrible thing?
- Is there anything that is bothering your conscience?
- (What is it?)
- (Do you feel you deserve to be punished for it?)

Grandiose delusions.   The patient believes that he or she has special powers or abilities or is a famous person, such as a rock star, Napoleon, or Christ. The patient may believe he or she is writing some definitive book, composing a great piece of music, or developing some wonderful new invention. The patient is often suspicious that someone is trying to steal his or her ideas and may become quite irritated if his or her abilities are doubted.

- Do you have any special powers, talents, or abilities? Great wealth?
- Do you feel you are going to achieve great things?

Religious delusions.   The patient is preoccupied with false beliefs of a religious nature. Sometimes these exist within the context of a conventional religious system, such as beliefs about the Second Coming, the Antichrist, or possession by the Devil. At other times, they may involve an entirely new religious system or a pastiche of beliefs from a variety of religions, particularly Eastern religions, such as ideas about reincarnation. Religious delusions may be combined with grandiose delusions (if the patient considers himself or herself a religious leader), delusions of guilt, or delusions of being controlled. Religious delusions must be outside the range of beliefs considered normal for the patient's cultural and religious background.

- Are you a religious person?
- Have you had any unusual religious experiences?
- Have you become closer to God?

Somatic delusions.   The patient believes that somehow his or her body is diseased, abnormal, or changed. For example, the patient may believe that his or her stomach or brain is rotting, that his or her hands have become enlarged, or that his or her facial features are ugly or misshapen. Sometimes somatic delusions are accompanied by tactile or other hallucinations, and when this occurs, both should be considered to be present. For example, a patient believes that he has ball bearings rolling about in his head, placed there by a dentist who filled his teeth, and can actually hear them clanking against one another!

- Is there anything wrong with the way your body is working?
- Have you noticed any change in your appearance?

Ideas and delusions of reference.   The patient believes that insignificant remarks, statements, or events have some special meaning for him or her. For example, the patient walks into a room, sees people laughing, and suspects that they were just talking about him or her. Sometimes items read in the newspaper, seen on television, or transmitted over the Internet are considered special messages to the person. In the case of *ideas of reference*, the patient is suspicious but recognizes that his or her idea may be erroneous. When the patient actually believes that the statements or events refer to him or her, then this is considered a delusion of reference.

- Have you walked into a room and thought that people were talking about you or laughing at you?
- Have you seen things in magazines or on TV that seem to refer to you or contain a special message for you?
- Have you received special messages in any other ways?

Delusions of passivity (being controlled).   The patient has a subjective experience that his or her feelings or actions are controlled by some outside force. The central requirement for this type of delusion is an actual strong subjective experience of being controlled. It does not include simple beliefs or ideas, such as that the patient is acting as an agent of God or that friends or parents are trying to coerce him or her into doing something. Rather, the patient must describe, for example, that his or her body has been occupied by some alien force that is making it move in peculiar ways, or that messages are being sent to his or her brain by radio waves and causing him or her to experience particular feelings that the person recognizes are not his or her own.

- Have you felt that you were being controlled by some outside person or force?
- (Do you feel like a puppet on a string?)

Delusions of mind reading.   The patient believes that people can read his or her mind or know his or her thoughts—that is, the patient subjectively experiences and recognizes that others know his or her thoughts, but he or she does not think that they can be heard out loud.

- Have you had the feeling that people could read your mind or know what you are thinking?

Thought broadcasting/Audible thoughts.   The patient believes that his or her thoughts are broadcast so that he or she or others can hear them. Sometimes the patient experiences his or her thoughts as a voice outside his or her head; this is an auditory hallucination as well as a delusion. Sometimes the patient feels that his or her thoughts are being broadcast, although he or she cannot hear them. Sometimes he or she believes that his or her thoughts are picked up by a microphone and broadcast on the radio, the television, or through the Internet.

- Have you heard your own thoughts out loud, as if they were a voice outside your head?
- Have you felt that your thoughts were broadcast so that other people could hear them?

Thought insertion.   The patient believes that thoughts that are not his or her own have been inserted into his or her mind. For example, the patient may believe that a neighbor is practicing voodoo and planting alien sexual thoughts into his or her mind. This symptom should not be confused with experiencing unpleasant thoughts that the patient recognizes as his or her own, such as delusions of persecution or guilt.

- Have you felt that thoughts were being placed into your head by some outside person or force?

Thought withdrawal.   The patient believes that thoughts have been taken away from his or her mind. He or she is able to describe a subjective experience of beginning a thought and then suddenly having it removed by some alien force. This symptom does not include the mere subjective recognition of alogia.

- Have you felt that your thoughts were taken away by some outside person or force?

Hallucinations

Hallucinations represent an abnormality in perception. They are false perceptions occurring in the absence of an identifiable external stimulus. They may be experienced in any of the sensory modalities, including hearing, touch, taste, smell, and vision. True hallucinations should be distinguished from illusions (which involve a misperception of an external stimulus), hypnagogic and hypnopompic experiences (which occur when a patient is falling asleep and waking up, respectively), or normal thought processes that are exceptionally vivid. If the hallucinations have a religious quality, then they should be judged within the context of what is normal for the patient's social and cultural background.

Auditory hallucinations.   The patient reports hearing voices, noises, or sounds. The most common auditory hallucinations involve hearing voices speaking to the patient or calling his or her name. The voices may be male or female, familiar or unfamiliar, and critical or complimentary. Typically, patients with schizophrenia experience the voices as unpleasant and negative. Less frequently patients report that the voices are comforting or provide companionship. Hallucinations involving sounds other than voices, such as noises or music, should be considered less characteristic and less severe.

- Have you heard voices or other sounds when no one was around or when you could not account for them?
- (What did they say?)

Voices commenting.   These hallucinations involve hearing a voice that makes a running commentary on the patient's behavior or thought as it occurs (e.g., "Carl is brushing his teeth. Carl is about to eat breakfast").

- Have you heard voices commenting on what you are thinking or doing?
- (What do they say?)

Voices conversing.   These hallucinations involve hearing two or more voices talking with each other, usually discussing something about the patient.

- Have you heard two or more voices talking with each other?
- (What do they say?)

Somatic or tactile hallucinations.   Somatic or tactile hallucinations involve experiencing peculiar physical sensations in the body. They include burning, itching sensations, or tingling sensations or the perception that the body has changed in shape or size.

- Have you had burning sensations or other strange sensations in your body?
- (What were they?)

Olfactory hallucinations. The patient experiences unusual odors that are typically quite unpleasant. Sometimes the patient may believe that he or she smells bad. This belief should be considered a hallucination if the patient can actually smell the odor but should be considered a delusion if he or she believes that only others can smell the odor.

- Have you experienced any unusual smells or smells that others do not notice?
- (What were they?)

Visual hallucinations. The patient sees shapes or people that are not actually present. Sometimes these are shapes or colors, but most typically they are figures of people or humanlike objects. They also may be characters of a religious nature, such as the Devil or Christ. As always, visual hallucinations involving religious themes should be judged within the context of the patient's cultural background.

- Have you had visions or seen things that other people cannot?
- (What did you see?)

Bizarre or Disorganized Behavior

The patient's behavior is unusual, bizarre, or fantastic. The information for this symptom will sometimes come from the patient, sometimes come from other sources, and sometimes come from direct observation. Bizarre behavior due to the immediate effects of intoxication with alcohol or drugs should not be considered a symptom of psychosis. Social and cultural norms must be considered in making the determination of bizarre behavior, and detailed examples should be elicited and noted.

Clothing and appearance. The patient dresses in an unusual manner or does other strange things to alter his or her appearance. For example, the patient may shave off all his or her hair or paint various body parts different colors. The patient's clothing may be quite unusual; for example, he or she may choose to wear an outfit that appears generally inappropriate and unacceptable, such as a baseball cap backward with rubber galoshes and long underwear covered by denim overalls. The patient may dress in a fantastic costume representing some historical personage or a person from outer space. He or she may wear clothing completely inappropriate to the climatic conditions, such as heavy wools in summer.

- Has anyone made comments about the way you dress?
- (What did they say?)

Social and sexual behavior.   The patient may do things that are considered inappropriate according to usual social norms. For example, he or she may urinate or defecate in inappropriate receptacles, walk along the street muttering to himself or herself, or begin talking to people whom he or she has never before met about intimate personal matters (as when riding on a subway or standing in some public place). He or she may drop to his or her knees praying and shouting or suddenly assume a fetal position when in the midst of a crowd. He or she may make inappropriate sexual overtures or remarks to strangers.

- Have you done anything that others might think is unusual or that has called attention to yourself?
- Has anyone complained or commented about your behavior?
- (What were you doing at the time?)

Aggressive and agitated behavior.   The patient may behave in an aggressive, agitated manner, often quite unpredictably. He or she may start arguments inappropriately with friends or members of his or her family or accost strangers on the street and begin haranguing them angrily. He or she may write letters or send e-mails of a threatening or angry nature to government officials or others with whom he or she has some quarrel. Occasionally, patients may perform violent acts, such as injuring or tormenting animals or attempting to injure or kill human beings.

- Have you been unusually angry or irritable with anyone?
- (How did you express your anger?)
- Have you done anything to try to harm animals or people?

Ritualistic or stereotyped behavior.   The patient may develop a set of repetitive actions or rituals that he or she must perform over and over. Sometimes he or she will attribute some symbolic significance to these actions and believe that they are either influencing others or preventing himself or herself from being influenced. For example, he or she may eat jelly beans every night for dessert, assuming that different consequences will occur depending on the color of the jelly beans. He or she may have to eat foods in a particular order, wear particular clothes, or get dressed in a certain order. He or she may have to write messages to himself or herself or to others over and over, sometimes in an unusual or occult language.

- Are there any things that you do over and over?
- Are there any things that you have to do in a certain way or in a particular order?
- (Why do you do it?)
- (Does it have any special meaning or significance to you?)

Disorganized Speech (Positive Formal Thought Disorder)

Disorganized speech, which is also referred to as *positive formal thought disorder,* is fluent speech that tends to communicate poorly for a variety of reasons. The patient tends to skip from topic to topic without warning; is distracted by events in the nearby environment; joins words together because they are semantically or phonologically alike, even though they make no sense; or ignores the question asked and answers another. This type of speech may be rapid, and it frequently seems quite disjointed. Unlike alogia (negative formal thought disorder; see subsection "Alogia" later in this chapter), a wealth of detail is provided, and the flow of speech tends to have an energetic rather than an apathetic quality to it.

To evaluate thought disorder, the patient should be permitted to talk without interruption for as long as 5 minutes. The interviewer should observe closely the extent to which the patient's sequencing of ideas is well connected. Close attention should also be paid to how well the patient can reply to various types of questions, ranging from simple ("When were you born?") to more complicated ("Why did you come to the hospital?"). If the ideas seem vague or incomprehensible, the interviewer should prompt the patient to clarify or elaborate.

Derailment (loose associations).   The patient has a pattern of spontaneous speech in which the ideas slip off the track onto another that is clearly but obliquely related or onto one completely unrelated. Things may be said in juxtaposition that lack a meaningful relationship, or the patient may shift idiosyncratically from one frame of reference to another. At times, there may be a vague connection between the ideas, and at other times, none will be apparent. This pattern of speech is often characterized as sounding "disjointed." Perhaps the most common manifestation of this disorder is a slow, steady slippage, with no single derailment being particularly severe, so that the speaker gets farther and farther off the track with each derailment without showing any awareness that his or her reply no longer has any connection with the question that was asked. This abnormality is often characterized by lack of cohesion between clauses and sentences and by unclear pronoun references.

Interviewer: Did you enjoy college?

Subject: Um-hm. Oh hey well I, I oh, I really enjoyed some communities. I tried it, and the, and the next day when I'd be going out, you know, um, I took control, like, uh, I put, um, bleach on my hair in, in California. My roommate was from Chicago and she was going to the junior college. And we lived in the Y.W.C.A., so she wanted to put it, um, peroxide on my hair, and she did, and I got up and I looked at the mirror and tears came to my eyes. Now do you understand it—I was fully aware of what was going on but why couldn't I, I...why the tears? I can't understand that, can you?

Tangentiality. The patient replies to a question in an oblique, tangential, or even irrelevant manner. The reply may be related to the question in some distant way, or the reply may be unrelated and seem totally irrelevant.

Interviewer: What city are you from?

Subject: Well, that's a hard question to answer because my parents... I was born in Iowa, but I know that I'm white instead of black, so apparently I came from the North somewhere and I don't know where, you know, I really don't know whether I'm Irish or Scandinavian, or I don't, I don't believe I'm Polish, but I think I'm, I think I might be German or Welsh.

Incoherence (word salad, schizophasia). The patient has a pattern of speech that is essentially incomprehensible at times. Incoherence is often accompanied by derailment. It differs from derailment in that with incoherence the abnormality occurs at the level of the sentence or clause, which contains words or phrases that are joined incoherently. The abnormality in derailment involves unclear or confusing connections between larger units, such as sentences or clauses. This type of language disorder is relatively rare. When it occurs, it tends to be severe or extreme, and mild forms are quite uncommon. It may sound quite similar to Wernicke's aphasia or jargon aphasia, and in these cases the disorder should only be called incoherence definitively when history and laboratory data exclude the possibility of a past stroke and clinical testing for aphasia has negative results.

Interviewer: What do you think about current political issues like the energy crisis?

Subject: They're destroying too many cattle and oil just to make soap. If we need soap when you can jump into a pool of water, and then when you go to buy your gasoline, my folks always thought they should, get pop but the best thing to get, is motor oil, and, money. May, may as, well go there and, trade in some, pop caps and, uh, tires, and tractors to grup, car garages, so they can pull cars away from wrecks, is what I believed in.

Illogicality. The patient has a pattern of speech in which conclusions are reached that do not follow logically. Illogicality may take the form of non sequiturs (meaning "it does not follow"), in which the patient makes a logical inference between two clauses that is unwarranted or illogical. It may take the form of faulty inductive inferences. It may also take the form of reaching conclusions based on faulty premises without any actual delusional thinking.

> Subject: Parents are the people that raise you. Anything that raises you can be a parent. Parents can be anything—material, vegetable, or mineral—that has taught you something. Parents would be the world of things that are alive, that are there. Rocks—a person can look at a rock and learn something from it, so that would be a parent.

Circumstantiality. The patient has a pattern of speech that is very indirect and delayed in reaching its goal ideas. In the process of explaining something, the speaker brings in many tedious details and sometimes makes parenthetical remarks. Circumstantial replies or statements may last for many minutes if the speaker is not interrupted and urged to get to the point. Interviewers will often recognize circumstantiality on the basis of needing to interrupt the speaker to complete the process of history taking within an allotted time. When not called circumstantial, these people are often referred to as long-winded.

Although it may coexist with instances of poverty of content of speech or loss of goal, circumstantiality differs from poverty of content of speech in containing excessive amplifying or illustrative detail and from loss of goal in that the goal is eventually reached if the person is allowed to talk long enough. It differs from derailment in that the details presented are closely related to some particular goal or idea and that the particular goal or idea must, by definition, eventually be reached (unless the patient is interrupted by an impatient interviewer).

Pressure of speech. The patient has an increase in the amount of spontaneous speech as compared with what is considered ordinary or socially customary. The patient talks rapidly and is difficult to interrupt. Pressured speech is often seen in mania but can be found in other syndromes as well. Some sentences may be left uncompleted because of eagerness to get on to a new idea. Simple questions that could be answered in only a few words or sentences are answered at great length so that the answer takes minutes rather than seconds and indeed may not stop at all if the speaker is not interrupted. Even when interrupted, the speaker often continues to talk. Speech tends to be loud and emphatic. Sometimes speakers with severe pressure will talk without any social stimulation and talk even though no one is listening. When patients are receiving antipsychotics or mood stabilizers, their speech is often slowed down by medication, and then it can be judged only on the basis of amount, volume, and social appropriateness. If a quantitative measure is applied to the rate of speech, then a rate greater than 150 words per minute is usually considered rapid or pressured. This disorder may be accompanied by derailment, tangentiality, or incoherence, but it is distinct from them.

Distractible speech.   During the course of a discussion or an interview, the patient stops talking in the middle of a sentence or idea and changes the subject in response to a nearby stimulus, such as an object on a desk, the interviewer's clothing or appearance, and so forth.

> **Subject:** Then I left San Francisco and moved to…where did you get that tie? It looks like it's left over from the '50s. I like the warm weather in San Diego. Is that a conch shell on your desk? Have you ever gone scuba diving?

Clanging.   The patient has a pattern of speech in which sounds rather than meaningful relations appear to govern word choice, so that the intelligibility of the speech is impaired and redundant words are introduced in addition to rhyming relationships. This pattern of speech also may include punning associations, so that a word similar in sound brings in a new thought.

> **Subject:** I'm not trying to make a noise. I'm trying to make sense. If you can make sense out of nonsense, well, have fun. I'm trying to make sense out of sense. I'm not making sense [cents] anymore. I have to make dollars.

Catatonic Motor Behavior

Catatonic motor symptoms are not common and should only be considered present when they are obvious and have been directly observed by the clinician or some other professional.

Stupor.   The patient has a marked decrease in reactivity to the environment and reduction of spontaneous movements and activity. The patient may appear to be aware of the nature of his or her surroundings.

Rigidity.   The patient shows signs of motor rigidity, such as resistance to passive movement.

Waxy flexibility (catalepsy).   The patient maintains postures into which he or she is placed for at least 15 seconds.

Excitement.   The patient has apparently purposeless and stereotyped excited motor activity not influenced by external stimuli.

Posturing and mannerisms.   The patient voluntarily assumes an inappropriate or a bizarre posture. Manneristic gestures or tics also may be observed. These involve movements or gestures that appear artificial or contrived, are not appropriate to the situation, or are stereotyped and repetitive. (Patients with tardive dyskinesia may have manneristic gestures or tics, but these should not be considered manifestations of catatonia.)

Inappropriate Affect

The patient's affect expressed is inappropriate or incongruous, not simply flat or blunted. Most typically, this manifestation of affective disturbance takes the form of smiling or assuming a silly facial expression while talking about a serious or sad subject. For example, the patient may laugh inappropriately when talking about thoughts of harming another person. (Occasionally, patients may smile or laugh when talking about a serious subject that they find uncomfortable or embarrassing. Although their smiling may seem inappropriate, it is due to anxiety and therefore should not be rated as inappropriate affect.)

Alogia

Alogia is a general term coined to refer to the impoverished thinking and cognition that often occur in patients with schizophrenia (from the Greek *a*, "no"; *logos,* "mind, thought"). Patients with alogia have thinking processes that seem empty, turgid, or slow. Because thinking cannot be observed directly, it is inferred from the patient's speech. The two major manifestations of alogia are nonfluent empty speech (poverty of speech) and fluent empty speech (poverty of content of speech). Blocking and increased latency of response also may reflect alogia.

Poverty of speech.   The patient has a restricted *amount* of spontaneous speech, so that replies to questions tend to be brief, concrete, and unelaborated. Unprompted additional information is rarely provided. Replies may be monosyllabic, and some questions may be left unanswered altogether. When confronted with this speech pattern, the interviewer may find himself or herself frequently prompting the patient, to encourage elaboration of replies. To elicit this finding, the examiner must allow the patient adequate time to answer and to elaborate his or her answer.

> **Interviewer:** Can you tell me something about what brought you to the hospital?
> **Subject:** A car.
> **Interviewer:** I was wondering about what kinds of problems you've been having. Can you tell me something about them?
> **Subject:** I dunno.

Poverty of content of speech.   Although the patient's replies are long enough so that speech is adequate in amount, it conveys little information. Language tends to be vague, often overabstract or overconcrete, repetitive, and stereotyped. The interviewer may recognize this finding by observing that the patient has spoken at some length but has not given adequate information to answer the question. Alternatively, the patient may provide enough information but require many words to do so, so that a lengthy reply can be summarized in a sentence or two. This abnormality differs from circumstantiality in that the circumstantial patient tends to provide a wealth of detail.

> **Interviewer:** Why is it, do you think, that people believe in God?
> **Subject:** Well, first of all because He, uh, He are the person that is their personal savior. He walks with me and talks with me. And, uh, the understanding that I have, um, a lot of people, they don't readily, uh, know their own personal self. Because, uh, they ain't, they all, just don't know their personal self. They don't, know that He, uh—seemed like to me, a lot of 'em don't understand that He walks and talks with 'em.

Blocking.   The patient's train of speech is interrupted before a thought or an idea has been completed. After a period of silence, which may last from a few seconds to minutes, the person indicates that he or she cannot recall what he or she has been saying or meant to say. Blocking should be judged to be present only if a person voluntarily describes losing his or her thought or if, on questioning by the interviewer, the person indicates that that was his or her reason for pausing.

> **Subject:** So I didn't want to go back to school so I…(1-minute silence while the patient stares blankly)
> **Interviewer:** What about going back to school? What happened?
> **Subject:** I dunno. I forgot what I was going to say.

Increased latency of response.   The patient takes a longer time to reply to questions than is usually considered normal. He or she may seem distant, and sometimes the examiner may wonder whether he or she has heard the question. Prompting usually indicates that the patient is aware of the question but has been having difficulty formulating his or her thoughts to make an appropriate reply.

> **Interviewer:** When were you last in the hospital?
> **Subject:** (30-second pause) A year ago.
> **Interviewer:** Which hospital was it?
> **Subject:** (30-second pause) This one.

Perseveration.   The patient persistently repeats words, ideas, or phrases so that once a patient begins to use a particular word, he or she continually returns to it in the process of speaking. Perseveration differs from "stock words" in that the repeated words are used in ways inappropriate to their usual meaning. Some words or phrases are commonly used as pause-fillers, such as "you know" or "like," and these should not be considered perseverations.

> **Interviewer:** Tell me what you are like—what kind of person you are.
> **Subject:** I'm from Marshalltown, Iowa. That's 60 miles northwest, northeast of Des Moines, Iowa. And I'm married at the present time. I'm 36 years old; my wife is 35. She lives in Garwin, Iowa. That's 15 miles southeast of Marshalltown, Iowa. I'm getting a divorce at the present time. And I am at present in a mental institution in Iowa City, Iowa, which is 100 miles southeast of Marshalltown, Iowa.

Affective Flattening or Blunting

Affective flattening or blunting manifests itself as a characteristic impoverishment of emotional expression, reactivity, and feeling. Affective flattening can be evaluated by observation of the patient's behavior and responsiveness during a routine interview. The evaluation of affective expression may be influenced by the patient's use of prescription drugs, because the parkinsonian side effects of antipsychotics may lead to mask-like facies and diminished associated movements. Other aspects of affect, such as responsivity or appropriateness, will not be affected, however.

Unchanging facial expression.   The patient's face does not change expression, or changes less than normally expected, as the emotional content of the discourse changes. His or her face appears wooden, mechanical, and frozen. Because antipsychotics may partially mimic this effect, the interviewer should be careful to note whether the patient is taking medication.

Decreased spontaneous movements.   The patient sits quietly throughout the interview and shows few or no spontaneous movements. He or she does not shift position, move his or her legs, or move his or her hands or does so less than normally expected.

Paucity of expressive gestures.   The patient does not use his or her body as an aid in expressing his or her ideas through means such as hand gestures, sitting forward in his or her chair when intent on a subject, or leaning back when relaxed. Paucity of expressive gestures may occur in addition to decreased spontaneous movements.

Poor eye contact.   The patient avoids looking at others or using his or her eyes as an aid in expression. He or she appears to be staring into space even when he or she is talking. The interviewer should consider the quality as well as the quantity of eye contact.

Affective nonresponsivity.   The patient fails to smile or laugh when prompted. This function may be tested by smiling or joking in a way that would usually elicit a smile from a psychiatrically normal individual.

Lack of vocal inflections.   While speaking, the patient fails to show normal vocal emphasis patterns. Speech has a monotonic quality, and important words are not emphasized through changes in pitch or volume. The patient also may fail to change volume with changes of content, so that he or she does not drop his or her voice when discussing private topics or raise it as he or she discusses things that are exciting or for which louder speech might be appropriate.

Avolition-Apathy

Avolition-apathy manifests itself as a characteristic lack of energy and drive. Patients become inert and are unable to mobilize themselves to initiate or persist in completing many different kinds of tasks. Unlike the diminished energy or interest of depression, the avolitional symptom complex in schizophrenia usually is not accompanied by saddened or depressed affect. The avolitional symptom complex often leads to severe social and economic impairment.

Grooming and hygiene.   The patient pays less attention to grooming and hygiene than is normal. Clothing may appear sloppy, outdated, or soiled. He or she may bathe infrequently and not care for his or her hair, nails, or teeth—leading to manifestations such as greasy or uncombed hair, dirty hands, body odor, or unclean teeth and bad breath. Overall, the appearance is dilapidated and disheveled. In extreme cases, the patient may even have poor toilet habits.

Impersistence at work or school. The patient has difficulty in seeking or maintaining employment (or doing schoolwork) as appropriate for his or her age and gender. If a student, he or she does not do homework and may even fail to attend class. Grades will tend to reflect this. If a college student, he or she may have registered for courses but dropped several or all of them. If of working age, the patient may have found it difficult to work at a job because of an inability to persist in completing tasks and apparent irresponsibility. He or she may go to work irregularly, wander away early, fail to complete expected assignments, or complete them in a disorganized manner. He or she may simply sit around the house and not seek any employment or seek it only in an infrequent or desultory manner. If a homemaker or a retired person, the patient may fail to complete chores, such as shopping or cleaning, or complete them in a careless and half-hearted way. If in a hospital or an institution, he or she does not attend or persist in vocational or rehabilitative programs effectively.

- Have you been able to (work, go to school) during the past month?
- Have you been attending vocational rehabilitation or occupational therapy sessions (in the hospital)?
- What have you been able to do?
- (Do you have trouble finishing what you start?)
- (What kinds of problems have you had?)

Physical anergia. The patient tends to be physically inert; he or she may sit in a chair for hours at a time and not initiate any spontaneous activity. If encouraged to become involved in an activity, he or she may participate only briefly and then wander away or disengage himself or herself and return to sitting alone. He or she may spend large amounts of time in some relatively mindless and physically inactive task such as watching television or playing solitaire. Family members may report that the patient spends most of his or her time at home "doing nothing except sitting around." Either at home or in an inpatient setting, he or she may spend much of his or her time sitting unoccupied.

- How have you been spending your time?
- Do you have any trouble getting yourself going?

Anhedonia-Asociality

Anhedonia-asociality encompasses the patient's difficulties in experiencing interest or pleasure. It may express itself as a loss of interest in pleasurable activities, an inability to experience pleasure when participating in activities normally considered pleasurable, or a lack of involvement in social relationships of various kinds.

Recreational interests and activities.   The patient may have few or no interests, activities, or hobbies. Although this symptom may begin insidiously or slowly, there will usually be some obvious decline from an earlier level of interest and activity. Patients with relatively milder loss of interest will engage in some activities that are passive or nondemanding, such as watching television, or will show only occasional or sporadic interest. Patients with the most extreme loss will appear to have a complete and intractable inability to become involved in or enjoy activities. The evaluation in this area should take both the quality and the quantity of recreational interests into account.

- What do you do for enjoyment?
- (How often do you do those things?)
- Have you been attending recreational therapy?
- (What have you been doing?)
- (Do you enjoy it?)

Sexual interest and activity.   The patient may show a decrement in sexual interest and activity or enjoyment as compared to what would be judged healthy for the patient's age and marital status. Individuals who are married may manifest disinterest in sex or may engage in intercourse only at the partner's request. In extreme cases, the patient may not engage in sex at all. Single patients may go for long periods without sexual involvement and make no effort to satisfy this drive. Whether married or single, patients may report that they subjectively feel only minimal sex drive or that they take little enjoyment in sexual intercourse or in masturbatory activity even when they engage in it.

- What has your sex drive been like?
- Have you been able to enjoy sex lately?
- (What is your usual sexual outlet?)
- (When was the last time you engaged in sexual activity?)

Ability to feel intimacy and closeness.   The patient may be unable to form intimate and close relationships of a type appropriate for his or her age, gender, and family status. In the case of a younger person, this area should be evaluated in terms of relationships with the opposite sex and with parents and siblings. In the case of an older person who is married, the relationship with the spouse and with children should be evaluated, whereas unmarried individuals should be judged in terms of opposite- or same-sex relationships or relationships with family members who live nearby. Patients may show few or no feelings of affection to available family members, or they may have arranged their lives so that they are completely isolated from any intimate relationships, live alone, and make no effort to initiate contacts with family or others.

- Do you feel close to your family (husband, wife, partner, children)?
- Is there anyone outside your family to whom you feel especially close?
- (How often do you see [them, him, her]?)

Relationships with friends and peers.   Patients also may be relatively restricted in their relationships with friends and peers of either gender. They may have few or no friends, make little or no effort to develop such relationships, and choose to spend all or most of their time alone.

- Do you have many friends?
- (Are you very close to them?)
- (How often do you see them?)
- (What do you do together?)
- Have you gotten to know any patients in the hospital?

Attention

Attention is often poor in patients with severe mental illnesses. The patient may have trouble focusing his or her attention or may be able to focus only sporadically and erratically. He or she may ignore attempts to converse with him or her, wander away while in the middle of an activity or a task, or appear to be inattentive when engaged in formal testing or interviewing. He or she may or may not be aware of the difficulty in focusing attention.

Social inattentiveness.   While involved in social situations or activities, the patient appears inattentive. He or she looks away during conversations, does not pick up the topic during a discussion, or appears uninvolved or disengaged. He or she may abruptly terminate a discussion or a task without any apparent reason. He or she may seem "spacey" or "out of it." He or she may seem to have poor concentration when playing games, reading, or watching television.

Inattentiveness during mental status testing. The patient may perform poorly on simple tests of intellectual functioning despite adequate education and intellectual ability. Inattentiveness should be assessed by having the patient spell *world* (or some equivalent five-letter word) backward and by serial 7s (at least a 10th-grade education) or serial 3s (at least a 6th-grade education) for a series of five subtractions.

Manic Symptoms

Euphoric mood. The patient has had one or more distinct periods of euphoric, irritable, or expansive mood not due to alcohol or drug intoxication.

- Have you been feeling too good or even high—clearly different from your normal self?
- (Do your friends or family think this is more than just feeling good?)
- Have you felt irritable and easily annoyed?
- (How long has this mood lasted?)

Increase in activity. The patient shows an increase in involvement or activity level associated with work, family, friends, sex drive, new projects, interests, or activities (e.g., telephone calls, letter writing).

- Are you more active or involved in things compared with the way you usually are?
- (How about at work, at home, with your friends, or with your family?)
- (What about your involvement in hobbies or other interests?)
- Have you been unable to sit still, or have you had to be moving or pacing back and forth?

Racing thoughts/Flight of ideas. The patient has the subjective experience that his or her thinking is markedly accelerated. For example, "My thoughts are ahead of my speech."

- Have your thoughts been racing through your mind?
- Do you have more ideas than usual?

Inflated self-esteem. The patient has increased self-esteem and appraisal of his or her worth, contacts, influence, power, or knowledge (may be delusional) as compared with his or her usual level. Persecutory delusions should not be considered evidence of grandiosity unless the patient feels persecution is due to some special attributes (e.g., power, knowledge, or contacts).

- Do you feel more self-confident than usual?
- Do you feel that you are a particularly important person or that you have special talents or abilities?

Decreased need for sleep. The patient needs less sleep than usual to feel rested. (This rating should be based on the average of several days rather than a single severe night.)

- Do you need less sleep than usual to feel rested?
- (How much sleep do you ordinarily need?)
- (How much sleep do you need now?)

Distractibility. The patient's attention is too easily drawn to unimportant or irrelevant external stimuli. For example, the patient gets up and inspects some item in the room while talking or listening, shifts his or her topic of speech, and so forth.

- Are you easily distracted by things around you?

Poor judgment. The patient shows excessive involvement in activities that have a high potential for painful consequences that are not recognized (e.g., buying sprees, sexual indiscretions, foolish business investments, reckless giving).

- Have you done anything that caused trouble for you or your family or friends?
- Looking back now, have you done anything that showed poor judgment?
- Have you done anything foolish with money?
- Have you done anything sexually that was unusual for you?

Depressive Symptoms

Dysphoric mood. The patient feels sad, despondent, discouraged, or unhappy; significant anxiety or tense irritability also should be rated as a dysphoric mood. The evaluation should be made irrespective of length of mood.

- Have you been having periods of feeling depressed, sad, or hopeless? When you didn't care about anything or couldn't enjoy anything?
- Have you felt tense, anxious, or irritable?
- (How long did this last?)

Change in appetite or weight.   The patient has had significant weight change. This should not include change due to dieting, unless the dieting is associated with some depressive belief that approaches delusional proportions.

- Have you had any changes in your appetite—either increased or decreased?
- Have you lost or gained much more weight than is usual for you?

Insomnia or hypersomnia.   Insomnia may include waking up after only a few hours of sleep as well as difficulty in getting to sleep. Patterns of insomnia include *initial* (trouble going to sleep), *middle* (waking in the middle of the night but eventually falling asleep again), and *terminal* (waking early—e.g., 2:00 A.M. to 5:00 A.M.—and remaining awake).

- Have you had trouble sleeping?
- (What was it like?)
- (Do you have trouble falling asleep?)
- (Do you wake up too early in the morning?)
- Have you been sleeping more than usual?
- How much sleep do you get in a typical 24-hour period?

Psychomotor agitation.   The patient is unable to sit still, with a need to keep moving. (Do not include mere subjective feelings of restlessness.) Objective evidence (e.g., hand wringing, fidgeting, pacing) should be present.

- Have you felt restless or agitated?
- Do you have trouble sitting still?

Psychomotor retardation.   The patient feels slowed down and experiences great difficulty moving. (Do not include mere subjective feelings of being slowed down.) Objective evidence (e.g., slowed speech) should be present.

- Have you been feeling slowed down?

Loss of interest or pleasure.   The patient has loss of interest or pleasure in usual activities or a decrease in sexual drive. This may be similar to the anhedonia seen in psychosis. In the depressive syndrome, loss of interest or pleasure is invariably accompanied by intense, painful affect, whereas in psychosis, the affect is often blunted.

- Have you noticed a change in your interest in things you normally enjoy?
- (What have you been less interested in?)

Loss of energy.   The patient has a loss of energy, becomes easily fatigued, or feels tired. These energy comparisons should be based on the person's usual activity level whenever possible.

- Have you had a tendency to feel more tired than usual?
- (Have you been feeling as if all your energy is drained?)

Feelings of worthlessness.   In addition to feelings of worthlessness, the patient may report feelings of self-reproach or excessive or inappropriate guilt. (Either may be delusional.)

- Have you been feeling down on yourself?
- Have you been feeling guilty about anything?
- (Could you tell me about some of the things for which you feel guilty?)

Diminished ability to think or concentrate.   The patient complains of diminished ability to think or concentrate, such as slowed thinking or indecisiveness, not associated with marked derailment or incoherence.

- Have you had trouble thinking?
- What about your concentration?
- Have you had trouble making decisions?

Recurrent thoughts of death/suicide.   The patient has thoughts about death and dying, plus possible wishes to be dead or to take his or her life.

- Have you been thinking about death or about taking your own life?
- (How often have these thoughts occurred?)
- (What were you thinking of doing?)

Distinct quality to mood.   The patient's depressed mood is experienced as distinctly different from the kind of feelings experienced after the death of a loved one. If the patient has not lost a loved one, ask him or her to compare the feelings with those after some significant personal loss appropriate to his or her age and experience.

- The feelings of (sadness) you are having now—are they the same as the feelings you would have had when someone close to you died, or are they different?
- (How are they similar or different?)

Nonreactivity of mood.   The patient does not feel much better, even temporarily, when something good happens.

- Do your feelings of depression go away or get better when you do something you enjoy, such as talking with friends, visiting your family, or playing with a pet (engaging in some other favorite activity)?

Diurnal variation.   The patient's mood shifts during the course of the day. Some patients feel terrible in the morning but feel steadily better as the day goes on and even near normal in the evening. Others feel good in the morning and worse as the day progresses.

- Is there any time of the day that is especially bad for you?
- (Do you feel worse in the morning? In the evening? Or is it about the same all the time?)

Anxiety Symptoms

Panic attacks.   The patient has discrete episodes of intense fear or discomfort in which a variety of symptoms occur, such as shortness of breath, dizziness, palpitations, or shaking.

- Have you ever experienced a sudden attack of panic or fear, in which you felt extremely uncomfortable?
- (How long did it last?)
- (Did you notice any other symptoms occurring at the same time?)
- (Did you feel as if you were going to die or go crazy?)

Agoraphobia.   The patient has a fear of going outside (literally "a fear of the marketplace"). In many patients, however, the fear is more generalized and involves being afraid of being in a place or situation from which escape might be difficult.

- Have you ever been afraid of going outside, so that you tended to just stay home all the time?
- Have you been afraid of getting caught or trapped somewhere so that you would be unable to escape?

Social phobia.   The patient has a fear of being in some social situation in which he or she will be seen by others and may do something that he or she might find to be humiliating or embarrassing. Some common social phobias include fear of public speaking, fear of eating in front of others, and fear of using public bathrooms.

- Do you have any special fears, such as a fear of public speaking?
- Of eating in front of others?

Specific phobia.   The patient is afraid of some specific circumscribed stimulus, such as animals (e.g., snakes, insects), seeing blood, being at high places, or being afraid to fly on airplanes.

- Are you afraid of snakes?
- The sight of blood?
- Air travel?
- Do you have any other specific fears?

Obsessions.   The patient experiences persistent ideas, thoughts, or impulses that are unwanted and experienced as unpleasant. The patient tends to ruminate and worry about them. The patient may try to ignore or suppress them but typically finds this difficult. Some common obsessions include repetitive thoughts of performing a violent act or becoming contaminated by touching other people or inanimate objects, such as a doorknob.

- Are you ever bothered by persistent ideas that you can't get out of your head, such as being dirty or contaminated?
- (Can you give me some specific examples?)

Compulsions.   The patient has to perform specific acts over and over in a way that he or she recognizes to be senseless or inappropriate. The compulsions are usually performed to ease some worry or obsession or to prevent some feared event from occurring. For example, a patient may have the worry that he or she has left the door unlocked and must return to check it repeatedly. Obsessions about contamination may lead to repetitive hand washing. Obsessions about thoughts of violence may lead to ritualistic behavior designed to prevent injury to the person about whom violence has been imagined.

- Are there any types of actions that you have to perform over and over, such as washing your hands or checking the stove?
- (Can you give me some examples?)

■ Self-Assessment Questions

1. Describe the way in which the patient's chief complaint can be used to take a history and to develop a differential diagnosis.
2. Describe several techniques that are important for concluding the initial interview with a patient.
3. Enumerate the components of a standard psychiatric history, giving each of the main headings of the overall outline.
4. Summarize the major components of the mental status examination.
5. List and describe at least four of the positive symptoms of psychosis. Give examples of several typical kinds of delusions and hallucinations.
6. List and describe at least four negative symptoms.
7. List and define some of the symptoms observed in depression.
8. List and define some of the symptoms observed in mania.
9. List and define some of the symptoms observed in anxiety and phobic disorders.

Chapter 3

The Neurobiology and Genetics of Mental Illness

Men ought to know that from the brain, and from the brain only, arise our pleasures, joys, laughter, and jests, as well as our sorrows, pains, griefs, and fears. Through it, in particular, we think, see, hear....

Hippocrates

Students of psychiatry are privileged to study diseases that affect the most interesting and important organ in the body: the miraculous human brain. The human brain has created and invented the myriad achievements that surround us every day—skyscrapers, computers, complex economic markets, advances in medical science ranging from vaccines to antibiotics to magnetic resonance scanners, an understanding of quantum mechanics and chaos theory, and art, music, and literature. These achievements have been accomplished because the human brain is one of the most complex systems in the universe. Composed of more than 100 billion neurons (more nerve cells than the stars in the Milky Way), the brain expands its communicating and thinking power by multiplying connectivity through an average of 1,000–10,000 synapses per nerve cell. The synapses are "plastic" in that they remodel themselves continuously in response to changes in their environment and the inputs that they receive. The whole human brain system is composed of feedback loops and circuits composed of multiple neurons, further expanding the fine-tuning and thinking capacities. The abilities that we all have to think, feel emotions, and relate to other people in normal ways depend on the activity of this complex organ. The disturbances in thought, emotion, and behavior that we observe in the

57

mentally ill also are ultimately due to aberrations in the brain. Understanding those brain aberrations—and correcting them—is our ultimate
challenge.

Modern psychiatry stretches from mind to molecule and from clinical neuroscience to molecular biology as it attempts to understand how
aberrations in thinking and behavior are rooted in underlying biological mechanisms. During the past several decades neuroscience has
grown to become one of the largest domains of scientific research. This
chapter provides a selective overview of a few topics from neurobiology that are relevant to understanding either the symptoms or treatment of mental illnesses.

■ Anatomical and Functional Brain Systems

The human brain may be divided into a variety of systems that mediate
many different cognitive, emotional, and perceptual functions, such as
the motor system, the visual system, the auditory system, and the somatosensory system. The systems that are of special interest to psychiatry are those that represent circuitry or functions that are particularly
disturbed in mental illnesses. These systems represent some of the "last
frontiers" in the study of the human brain. Three important anatomical
systems are the prefrontal system, the limbic system, and the basal ganglia system. Important functional systems include the executive function, memory, language, attention, and reward systems.

Any method for dividing the brain into parts or systems is somewhat
arbitrary because the three anatomical systems are all interconnected with
one another and work interactively. The functional systems are also highly
interdependent with one another and with the prefrontal, limbic, and basal
ganglia systems as well. Furthermore, the division of the brain into "functional and anatomical systems" and "neurochemical systems" is also arbitrary. These oversimplifications are introduced purely for conceptual
convenience, providing a strategy for reducing the overwhelming complexity of the central nervous system (CNS) to a level that permits discussion and analysis. Ultimately, however, a full understanding of the brain
can only occur by an ongoing process of analysis (or breakdown and sim-
plification) as well as synthesis (or rebuilding and unifying).

One must add a word of caution about our existing level of igno-
rance. We do not as yet have a complete map of the human brain, sum-

marizing accurately its various neural circuits and chemical anatomy. This process is ongoing and becoming much more sophisticated, particularly with the aid of neuroimaging techniques such as structural and functional magnetic resonance imaging (sMRI and fMRI), diffusion tensor imaging (DTI), magnetic resonance spectroscopy (MRS), magnetoencephalography (MEG), and positron emission tomography (PET). These technologies permit researchers to study the anatomy and physiology of the human brain in ways that were previously impossible. Prior to the availability of neuroimaging, our knowledge about circuitry and functional systems was based primarily on lesion and postmortem studies. Directly visualizing how the brain performs mental work with fMRI or PET imaging is clearly more accurate than trying to infer indirectly how it works by observing what it cannot do when parts are missing.

The Prefrontal System and Executive Functions

The prefrontal system, or prefrontal cortex, is one of the largest cortical subregions in the human brain. It constitutes 29% of the cortex in human beings, compared with 17% in chimpanzees, 7% in dogs, and 3.5% in cats. The relative development of the prefrontal cortex in various animal species is shown in Figure 3–1.

This huge association region in the brain integrates input from much of the neocortex, limbic regions, hypothalamic and brainstem regions, and (via the thalamus) most of the rest of the brain. Its high degree of development in human beings suggests that it may mediate a variety of specifically human functions often referred to as *executive functions*, such as high-order abstract thought, creative problem solving, and the temporal sequencing of behavior. Lesion and trauma studies, supplemented by experimental studies in nonhuman primates, have substantially added to this view of the functions of the prefrontal cortex. It is now clear that the prefrontal cortex mediates a large variety of functions, including attention and perception, moral judgment, temporal integration, and affect and emotion.

The intactness of the prefrontal cortex can be assessed by a variety of cognitive tasks, and it has been explored through neuroimaging as well. The Wisconsin Card Sorting Test, the Continuous Performance Test, the Sternberg Working Memory Task, and the Tower of London are standard "frontal lobe" tests in neuropsychology. Several of these tests have been explored using fMRI and PET and have been shown to pro-

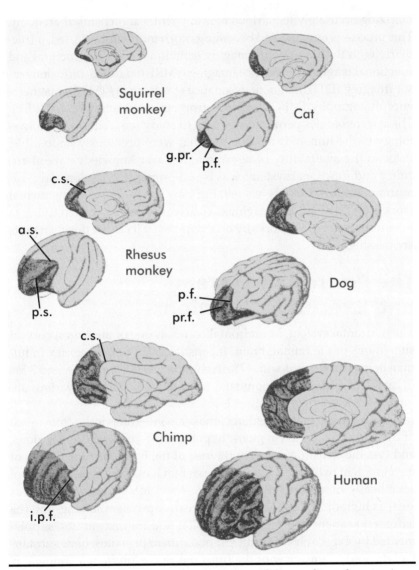

FIGURE 3–1.   Phylogenetic development of the prefrontal cortex.

a.s.=arcuate sulcus; c.s.=cingulate sulcus; g.pr.=gyrus proreus; i.p.f.=inferior precentral fissure; p.f.=presylvian fissure; pr.f.=proreal fissure; p.s.=principal sulcus.

Source.   Reprinted from Fuster JM: *The Prefrontal Cortex: Anatomy, Physiology, and Neuropsychology of the Frontal Lobe,* 2nd Edition. New York, Raven Press, 1989. © Lippincott Williams & Wilkins (www.lww.com). Used with permission.

duce frontal lobe activation. Because the negative symptoms of schizophrenia reflect impairment in many frontally mediated functions, researchers have proposed that some patients with schizophrenia might have frontal lobe abnormalities, a finding now supported in numerous anatomical and functional neuroimaging studies. Abnormalities in frontal lobe structure and function have also been observed in many other disorders, such as mood disorders, obsessive-compulsive disorder, and autism spectrum disorders.

The Limbic System

The word *limbic* means "border" in Latin. This term was first used by Paul Broca, a French neurologist, to refer to the circular ring of tissue that appears to "hem" the prefrontal, parietal, and occipital neocortex when the brain is viewed from a midsagittal perspective. There is still no consensus as to what constitutes a clear definition of the limbic system or its components. As in other brain systems, boundaries can be defined on the basis of cytoarchitectonics, interconnections, or inputs. Walle Nauta later proposed, as a unifying concept, that the various structures in the limbic system share circuitry that connects them to the hypothalamus. He pointed out that the interconnections between the hypothalamus (via the mamillary bodies), the amygdala, the hippocampus, and cingulate gyrus are reciprocal. The hypothalamus collects visceral sensory signals from the spinal cord and brainstem, while input also comes to this circuit through two major neocortical association regions, the prefrontal cortex and the inferior temporal association cortex.

The functions of the limbic system are of great importance to the understanding of human emotion. The various interconnections suggest functions related to integrating visceral sensation and the experience of the external environment through multiple modalities (e.g., visual, sensory, auditory). Lesion, animal, and neuroimaging studies have shown that the amygdala and hippocampus mediate aspects of learning and memory. The amygdala is known as "the hub in the wheel of fear" and is implicated in the neurobiology of a variety of anxiety disorders.

The Basal Ganglia

The major structures of the basal ganglia include the caudate, putamen, and globus pallidus, which are shown schematically in Figure 3–2. A triplanar view of the caudate and other basal ganglia structures as seen with sMRI is shown in Figure 3–3. The substantia nigra, located in the midbrain, is not visualized. The caudate is a C-shaped mass of gray

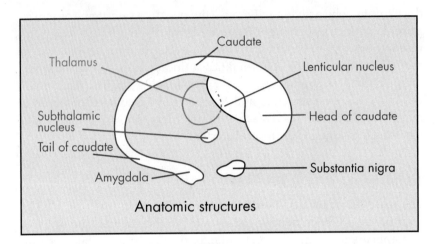

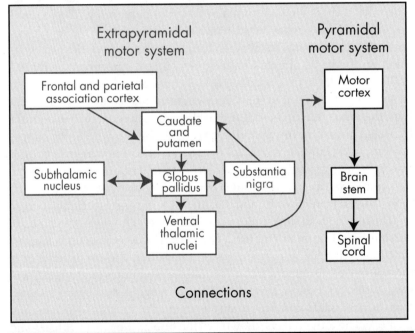

FIGURE 3–2. Interconnections of the basal ganglia.

Source. Reprinted from Andreasen NC: *The Broken Brain: The Biological Revolution in Psychiatry.* New York, Harper & Row, 1984, p. 105. Copyright © 1984 Nancy C. Andreasen.

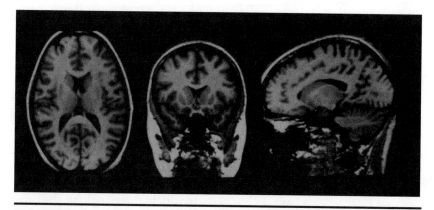

FIGURE 3-3.   The basal ganglia as seen with magnetic resonance imaging.

The triplanar resampling and visualization, achieved through locally developed software for image analysis (BRAINS, or Brain Research: Analysis of Images, Networks, and Systems), permits viewing of structures with a complex shape such as the caudate from three different angles, thus enhancing our capacity to understand brain anatomy three-dimensionally.

Source.   Copyright © 1993 Nancy C. Andreasen.

matter tissue that has its head at the lateral anterior borders of the frontal horns of the ventricles. It arches back posteriorly in a circular fashion and then curls forward again, ending in the amygdala bilaterally. Separated from it, and lateral to it, is the lentiform nucleus, so called because it is shaped like a lens. The medial portion of the lentiform nucleus, which is darker and more densely full of gray matter, is the putamen, whereas the globus pallidus is lateral to it. The caudate is separated from the lentiform nucleus by the anterior limb of the internal capsule, but the sMRI scan shows clearly that bands of gray matter interconnect these two nuclei; posteriorly the lentiform nucleus is separated from the thalamus by the posterior limb of the internal capsule. Because these structures contain a combination of gray and white matter, they have a striped appearance in postmortem brains and on sMRI scans, causing them to be referred to as the "corpus striatum" (striped body).

This brain region is of importance to the understanding of mental illness for several reasons. First, there are several major syndromes involving abnormalities in these regions that manifest psychiatric symptoms. Huntington's disease, characterized by severe atrophy in the caudate nucleus, typically presents with a variety of delusional and depressive symptoms. Severe dementia may also develop. Parkinson's disease is another syndrome affecting the basal ganglia; it is due to neuronal loss in the substantia nigra, which uses dopamine as its primary neurotransmitter. Loss of pigmented neurons and a decrease in dopaminergic activity produce a variety of symptoms similar to the negative symptoms of schizophrenia, including affective blunting and loss of volition.

The basal ganglia are also relevant to psychiatry because of their chemical anatomy. The caudate and putamen contain a very high concentration of dopamine receptors, particularly D_2 receptors. The efficacy of antipsychotic medications is highly correlated with their ability to block D_2 receptors (see "Neurochemical Systems" later in the chapter). Because D_2 receptors have a very high density in these regions, the caudate and putamen may be important sites for antipsychotic drug action.

The Memory System

The memory system is a major functional brain system that may be impaired in some mentally ill patients. Deficits in learning and memory are the hallmark of the dementias. Although patients with psychotic disorders do not typically have severe memory deficits, some investigators have speculated that the neural mechanisms of delusions and hallucinations might be based on either abnormal excitability or abnormal connectivity in the neural circuitry used for the encoding, retrieval, and interpretation of memories. Within psychoanalytic theory, it has long been believed that the various "neuroses," such as anxiety disorders or hysteria (i.e., somatic symptom disorder), might represent the painful stimulus of repressed memories that have not been psychologically integrated. The process of psychotherapy involves the process of learning, which is based in turn on memory; patients who successfully complete a course of psychotherapy have learned new ways of understanding their past experiences and relating to other people.

Memory is in fact a diverse set of functions that are mediated in different ways. Typically, memory is now thought of as a two-stage process. The first stage involves working memory; this is the form we use when we "learn" a telephone number long enough to dial it or a driver's license number long enough to write it down. This type of memory is accessible in short-term storage and is used as a mental scratchpad that we call on when we perform mental operations such as arithmetic calculations from numbers that have been quoted to us. Long-term memory, on the other hand, consists of information that we have learned and retained for periods of time greater than a few minutes. This type of memory is sometimes referred to as "consolidated" memory and is currently being employed by the students reading this textbook.

Normal human experience, as well as research in neuroscience, indicates that a variety of techniques can be used to facilitate learning, or consolidation of memory. These include such things as repetition, rehearsal, or mnemonic devices. This type of memory is mediated by a different set of mechanisms that lead to long-term storage of information. The work of Eric Kandel, using the gill withdrawal reflex in the snail *Aplysia* as a model, has shown that long-term memory depends on the synthesis of proteins in neurons that are synaptically connected during the time that short-term learning has been occurring; this process creates a molecular consolidation of memory that is more permanently stored. Kandel, a psychiatrist, received the Nobel Prize in Physiology or Medicine in 2000 for this work, which explains the extraordinary capacity of the human brain for neuroplastic remodeling throughout the life span.

The Language System

As far as we know, the capacity to communicate in a highly developed and complex language is limited to human beings. Although porpoises, dolphins, and a few other creatures are believed to communicate specific messages to one another, human beings alone appear to have a syntactically complex language that exists in both oral and written forms. The ability to record our history and to communicate scientifically and culturally has permitted us to repeatedly build complex civilizations and social systems, and to destroy them as well.

The capacity to communicate in oral and written language is facilitated by dedicated brain regions that probably occur only in human beings. These language systems are localized in the neocortex. A simplified schematic diagram of the human brain circuitry traditionally considered to mediate language functions appears in Figure 3–4. Lesion studies suggest that this system is located primarily in the left hemisphere in most individuals, although functional imaging studies have revealed some bilaterality. About one-third of left-handers use either their right hemisphere or both hemispheres to perform language functions.

Within the left hemisphere there are two major language regions as well as some subsidiary ones. Broca's area is the region dedicated to the production of speech. It contains information about the syntactical structure of language, provides the "little words" such as prepositions that tie the fabric of language together, and is the generator for fluent

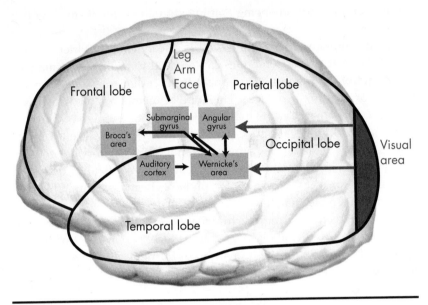

FIGURE 3–4. Interconnections of the language system.
Source. Andreasen 2001. Copyright © 1984 Nancy C. Andreasen.

speech. Lesions to Broca's area, which occur in stroke victims (often with an accompanying right hemiparesis), lead to halting, stammering, and ungrammatical speech. Wernicke's area is often referred to as the "auditory association cortex." It encodes the information that permits us to "understand" the sounds expressed in speech. The perception of sound waves, which encode speech, occurs through transducers in the ear that convert the information to neural signals. The signals are received in the auditory cortex, but the meaning of the specific signals cannot be understood (i.e., perceived as constituting words with specific meanings—as opposed, for example, to the wordless music of a symphony) without being compared to "templates" in Wernicke's area. An analogous process occurs when we understand written language. In this case the information is collected through our eyes, relayed via the optic tracts back to the primary visual cortex in the occipital lobe, and then forwarded on to the angular gyrus, a visual association cortex that contains the information or templates that permit us to recognize language presented in visual form.

Patients with major mental illnesses have a variety of disruptions in their capacity to communicate in language. Some of these incapacities are similar to those observed in the aphasias, but none is precisely identical. Some patients with schizophrenia have impoverished speech reminiscent of Broca's aphasia but lacking its halting, agrammatical quality.

Likewise, some patients with schizophrenia or mania produce very disorganized, abundant speech similar to Wernicke's aphasia, but (unlike the patient with Wernicke's aphasia) they appear to have intact comprehension. Auditory hallucinations ("voices") are abnormal auditory perceptions of language—that is, the individual perceives auditory speech when none is present. The reasons for these various disruptions and aberrations in language function in psychosis (and in many of the dementias as well) are still not clear. They may represent specific abnormalities in specialized language regions in the brain, but more likely they represent a disorganization at some higher integrative level.

The Attention System

Attention is the cognitive process through which the brain identifies stimuli within the context of time and space and selects what is relevant for both input and output. We are bombarded continually with sensory information in multiple modalities as well as with the information within our internal cognitive repertoire. A person driving a car on a busy highway is receiving information about other cars, the road, and the surrounding terrain from the visual system and auditory input from the car motor or the sound of other vehicles as they pass; there is also tactile input from hands on the steering wheel and the foot on the gas pedal and the physical sensations experienced by the rest of the body as the car grips the road or bounces and sways. The person may also be talking on a cell phone, listening to music, or thinking about a recent conversation. Attention is the cognitive process that permits the person to suppress irrelevant stimuli (e.g., to ignore most of the landscape), to notice important stimuli (e.g., that the car in front is putting on the brakes and slowing down suddenly), and to shift from one stimulus to another (e.g., from thoughts about the recent conversation to the traffic). If we lacked this capacity, we would be overwhelmed with stimuli. Attention is sometimes compared to a spotlight that the brain uses to highlight what is important.

Attention is mediated through multiple brain systems. Input to the brain is first provided by the reticular activating system, which arises in the brainstem. Midline circuitry passes this information through the thalamus, which plays a major role in "gating" or "filtering." Many other brain regions also play a major role in attention, including the cingulate gyrus, the hypothalamus, the hippocampus and amygdala, and the prefrontal, temporal, parietal, and occipital cortices. Neuroimaging studies using both fMRI and PET have demonstrated that the cingulate gyrus shows increases in activity during tasks that place heavy demands on the attentional system, such as those that involve competition and interference between stimuli. Attention is impaired in many mental illnesses, ranging from schizophrenia to attention-deficit/hyperactivity disorder (ADHD) to the mood disorders.

The Reward System

As behaviorists have noted for many years, human beings are strongly motivated by positive reinforcement. Put more simply, they are prone to seek pleasure and to avoid pain. Therefore, it is not surprising that the brain also possesses a reward system—a network that is used for the experience of pleasure. Its major components are the ventral tegmental area, the nucleus accumbens, the prefrontal cortex (particularly the anterior cingulate and ventral frontal cortex), the amygdala, and the hippocampus.

The reward system is relevant to many types of psychiatric disorders. It is often said that substance abuse develops when exposure to a drug such as cocaine "hijacks the brain reward system" by inducing an intense experience of pleasure that stimulates craving and repeated drug-seeking behavior. This system has been implicated in the use of all types of illegal (e.g., amphetamines, opiates) and legal (e.g., nicotine, alcohol) substances. It is also thought to provide the basis for other types of pleasure-seeking or addictive behaviors and their consequences, such as gambling disorder or compulsive overeating.

■ Neurochemical Systems

In addition to the functional and anatomical systems described earlier, the brain also consists of a grouping of neurochemical systems. These systems provide the "fuel" that permits the functional and anatomical systems to run (or run poorly, when an abnormality occurs). The neurochemical systems are interwoven and interdependent with the anatomical and functional systems. Any anatomic subsystem within the brain usually runs on multiple classes of neurotransmitters. Clearly, this complexity of anatomic and neurochemical organization permits much greater fine tuning of the entire system.

The Dopamine System

Dopamine, a catecholamine neurotransmitter, is the first product synthesized from tyrosine through the enzymatic activity of tyrosine hy-

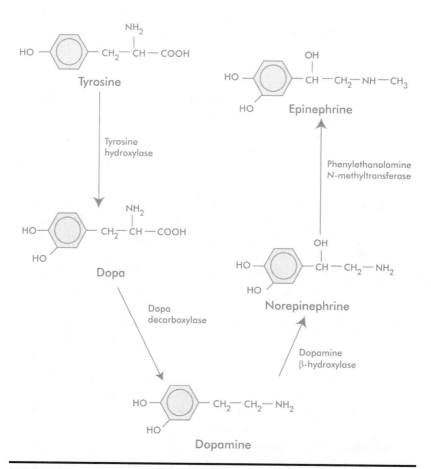

FIGURE 3–5. Synthetic pathway of dopamine.

droxylase. Its synthetic pathway, as well as the subsequent ones of norepinephrine and epinephrine, is shown in Figure 3–5.

There are three subsystems within the brain that use dopamine as their primary neurotransmitter. These all arise in the ventral tegmental area. One group, arising in the substantia nigra, projects to the caudate and putamen and is referred to as the nigrostriatal pathway. Its terminations appear to be rich in both D_1 and D_2 receptors. A second major tract, called the mesocortical or mesolimbic (or mesocorticolimbic), arises in the ventral tegmental area and projects to the prefrontal cortex and temporolimbic regions such as the amygdala and hippocampus. The concentration of D_2 receptors in these regions is minimal, whereas D_1 receptors predominate. The third component of the dopamine system originates in the arcuate nucleus of the hypothalamus and projects to the pituitary. The first two of these dopamine subsystems are summarized in Figure 3–6. As the figure indicates, the dopamine system is fairly specifically localized in the human brain. Because its projections include only a limited part of the cortex and focus primarily on brain regions important to cognition and emotion, it is considered to be one of the most important neurotransmitter systems for the understanding of these functions and potentially for the understanding of their disturbances in many types of mental illnesses.

For many years schizophrenia, the most important among the various psychotic disorders, was explained by the *dopamine hypothesis,* which proposed that the symptoms of this illness were due to a functional excess of dopamine. Because the efficacy of many of the antipsychotic drugs used to treat psychosis is highly correlated with their ability to block D_2 receptors, the dopamine hypothesis also suggested that the abnormality in this illness might specifically lie with D_2 receptors. There is a modest but much weaker correlation with their ability to block D_1 receptors. The dopamine hypothesis is being reappraised, however, in the light of several new lines of evidence that have emerged. First, the distribution of D_1 and D_2 receptors has been more specifically mapped, and there appears to be a rather sparse density of D_2 receptors in critical brain regions that mediate cognition and emotion, such as the prefrontal cortex, amygdala, and hippocampus. These regions are, however, high in D_1 and serotonin type 2 receptors (5-HT$_2$). These observations, coupled with the prominent effects on serotonin and D_1 by the new second-generation antipsychotics, suggest that the traditional dopamine hypothesis needs revision.

Understanding the projections of the dopamine system, as well as the differential localization of D_1 and D_2 receptors, clarifies some of the other effects of antipsychotic drugs. Some of these drugs have potent extrapyramidal side effects as a consequence of blocking D_2 receptors in the nigrostriatal pathway. Drugs that have a weak D_2 effect (of which clozapine and quetiapine are examples) thus are more likely to have fewer extrapyramidal ("parkinsonian") side effects.

Dopamine is sometimes called the "pleasure neurotransmitter," because it is the primary neurotransmitter in the brain reward system and is associated with adventuresome and exploratory behaviors. Many drugs of abuse (e.g., amphetamines, cocaine) exert their psychoactive effects by increasing dopaminergic tone.

The Norepinephrine System

The norepinephrine system arises in the locus coeruleus and sends projections diffusely throughout the entire brain. These projections are

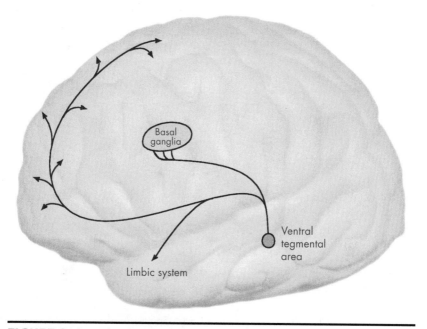

FIGURE 3–6.   The dopamine system.

Source.   Andreasen 2001. Copyright © 1984 Nancy C. Andreasen.

summarized in Figure 3–7. As that figure illustrates, norepinephrine appears to exert effects on almost every brain region in the human brain, including the entire cortex, the hypothalamus, the cerebellum, and the brainstem. This distribution suggests that it may have a diffuse modulatory or regulatory effect within the CNS.

There is some evidence that norepinephrine may play a major role in mediating symptoms of major mental illnesses, especially mood disorders. Soon after they were developed, it was demonstrated that tricyclic antidepressants inhibit norepinephrine reuptake, thereby enhancing the amount of norepinephrine available to stimulate postsynaptic receptors. Likewise, monoamine oxidase inhibitor antidepressants also enhance noradrenergic transmission by inhibiting neurotransmitter breakdown. However, it is also clear that many antidepressants have mixed noradrenergic and serotonergic activities or purely serotonergic effects (i.e., the selective serotonin reuptake inhibitors [SSRIs]). Thus, the original catecholamine hypothesis of mood disorders, which suggested that depression was due to a functional deficit of norepinephrine at crucial nerve terminals, whereas mania was due to a functional excess, was clearly an oversimplification.

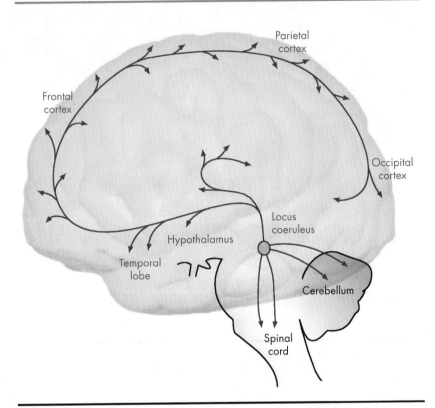

FIGURE 3–7. The norepinephrine system.
Source. Andreasen 2001. Copyright © 1984 Nancy C. Andreasen.

The Serotonin System

Serotonergic neurons have a distribution strikingly similar to that of norepinephrine neurons. This is summarized in Figure 3–8. Serotonergic neurons arise in the raphe nuclei, localized around the aqueduct in the midbrain. They project to a similarly wide range of CNS regions, including the entire neocortex, the basal ganglia, temporolimbic regions, the hypothalamus, the cerebellum, and the brainstem. As is the case with the norepinephrine system, the serotonin system appears to be a general modulator.

Serotonin plays a role in modulating mood, anxiety, and aggressive or violent behavior. A serotonin hypothesis of depression has been proposed, largely because many antidepressant medications (e.g., fluoxetine) facilitate serotonergic transmission by blocking reuptake. These medications are also used in the treatment of anxiety disorders. A high serotonergic tone has been shown to be associated with impulsive, vio-

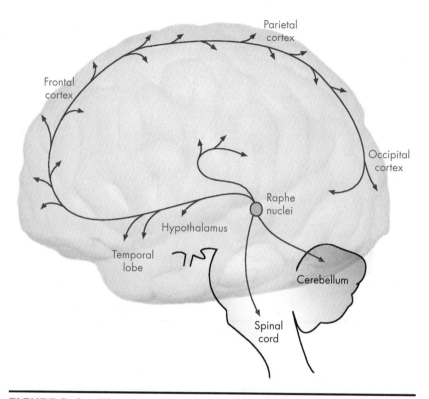

FIGURE 3–8. The serotonin system.
Source. Andreasen 2001. Copyright © 1984 Nancy C. Andreasen.

lent, or suicidal behavior. Serotonin is probably also involved in schizophrenia and other psychotic disorders, because clozapine and the newer second-generation antipsychotics (e.g., olanzapine) have significant effects on the serotonin system. As these examples indicate, there are no simple single-neurotransmitter to single-illness relationships.

The Cholinergic System

Like dopamine, acetylcholine has a relatively more specific localization in the human brain, as shown schematically in Figure 3–9. The cell bodies of a major group of acetylcholine neurons are located in the nucleus basalis of Meynert, which lies in the ventral and medial regions of the globus pallidus. Neurons from the nucleus basalis of Meynert project throughout the cortex. The second group of acetylcholine projections originating in the diagonal band of Broca and the septal nucleus project to the hippocampus and cingulate gyrus. A third group of cholinergic neurons are local circuit neurons that enter main structures within the basal ganglia.

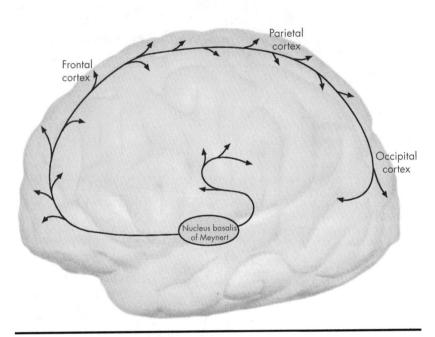

FIGURE 3–9.   The acetylcholine system.
Source.   Andreasen 2001. Copyright © 1984 Nancy C. Andreasen.

The acetylcholine system plays a major role in the encoding of memory, although the precise mechanisms are not understood. Patients with Alzheimer's disease show losses of acetylcholine projections both to the cortex and to the hippocampus, and blockade of muscarinic receptors produces memory impairment. Dopamine and acetylcholine share heavy concentrations of activity within the basal ganglia, and the drugs used to block the extrapyramidal side effects of antipsychotics are cholinergic agonists; this suggests a possible reciprocal relationship between dopamine and acetylcholine in the modulation of motor activity and possibly of psychosis as well. Cholinergic agonists also may impair cognitive functions such as learning and memory in individuals for whom they are prescribed.

The GABA System

γ-Aminobutyric acid (GABA) is an amino acid neurotransmitter, as is glutamate. These two major amino acid neurotransmitters serve complementary functions, with GABA playing an inhibitory role and glutamate playing an excitatory role.

GABAergic neurons are a mix of local circuit and long-tract systems. Within the cerebral cortex and the limbic system, GABAergic neurons are predominately local circuit. The cell bodies of GABAergic neurons in the caudate and putamen project to the globus pallidus and substantia nigra, making them relatively long tract, and long-tract GABA neurons also occur in the cerebellum.

The GABA system has substantial importance for the understanding of the neurochemistry of mental illness. Many of the anxiolytic drugs (e.g., diazepam) act as GABA agonists, thereby increasing the inhibitory tone within the CNS. Loss of the long-tract GABA neurons connecting the caudate to the globus pallidus releases the later structure from inhibitory control, thereby permitting the globus pallidus to "run free" and produce the choreiform movements that characterize Huntington's disease.

The Glutamate System

Glutamate, an excitatory amino acid neurotransmitter, is produced by pyramidal cells throughout the cerebral cortex and hippocampus. For example, the projections from the prefrontal cortex to the basal ganglia are glutamatergic.

The glutamate system is very complex and has many functions. It plays a role in synapse formation and stabilization, long-term potentiation (LTP), and learning and memory. Maintaining an adequate balance between excessive and inadequate levels of glutamate tone is crucial for CNS function. At high levels it is neurotoxic (as occurs in stroke). On the other hand, a hypoactive glutamate system leads to impaired LTP, synaptic plasticity, and cognitive performance. Two drugs that block N-methyl-D-aspartate (NMDA) receptors within the glutamate system, phencyclidine (PCP) and ketamine, produce a syndrome that closely resembles schizophrenia. Both can cause a psychosis characterized by withdrawal, stupor, disorganized thinking and speech, and hallucinations. This has suggested an alternative to the dopamine hypothesis, the *NMDA receptor hypofunction hypothesis*, and that the NMDA receptor could be a potential target for antipsychotic drug development. Some potential agents that modulate NMDA receptor function are currently under development.

■ The Genetics of Mental Illnesses

Thanks to the completion of the mapping of the human genome, we now know that it is composed of approximately 30,000 genes, about 70,000 fewer than the number that appeared in textbooks just a few years ago. More than half of these genes are expressed in the brain. During the next several decades, all physicians will be living in the "Era of the Genome"—a time when we will begin to discover the mechanisms of major mental disorders at the molecular level. Increasingly, we will begin to understand how gene expression and gene products produce the manifestations of a variety of diseases. We also will increasingly recognize that most major medical disorders are complex—that is, that very few illnesses are simple Mendelian disorders. The opportunity to understand illnesses at the genetic and genomic levels offers great promise for the future. Understanding mechanisms offers the opportunity to intervene early and perhaps ultimately implement preventive measures by modifying gene expression and gene products. This is the "holy grail" of psychiatric genetics.

Epidemiological Approaches

It has been recognized for many years that mental illnesses have a significant genetic component. A variety of studies have used the tools of psychiatric epidemiology and demonstrated that mental illnesses tend to run in families. Such studies are usually divided into three broad groups: family studies, twin studies, and adoption studies. Each of these types of studies offers different perspectives on the genetics of disorders.

Family Studies

Family studies examine the pattern of aggregation within a family, beginning with the identification of a proband (or index case) who has a particular disorder of interest, such as bipolar disorder or schizophrenia. Thereafter, all available first-degree relatives (parents, siblings, children) are also evaluated. The prevalence of the specific disorder under investigation is compared with the prevalence in a carefully selected control group. If an increased rate of the specific mental illness under study is observed in the relatives of the probands as compared with the relatives of the control subjects, then these results suggest that a disorder is familial and possibly genetic. These studies cannot exclude the possibility that the disorder has prominent nongenetic causes. Disorders can also run in families because of learned behavior, role modeling, or predisposing social environments. The following mental illnesses have been found to "run in families": major depression, bipolar disorder, schizophrenia, panic disorder, social phobia, obsessive-compulsive disorder, antisocial personality disorder, borderline personality disorder, autism spectrum disorder, ADHD, and even gambling disorder. Family studies have also led to the understanding that a spectrum of disorders is related to schizophrenia, including schizotypal personality disorder.

Twin Studies

Twin studies offer a better perspective on the extent to which a disorder is actually genetic. Twin studies typically compare the rate of a specific disorder in monozygotic (identical) versus dizygotic (nonidentical) twins. The rationale behind twin studies is that monozygotic twins have identical genetic material, whereas dizygotic twins share an average of 50% of their genetic material. The higher the rate of concordance in monozygotic twins, as compared with dizygotic twins, the greater the degree of genetic influence. Thus if a disorder were totally genetic and fully penetrant, the concordance rate in monozygotic twins would theoretically be 100%, whereas in dizygotic twins it would be 50%. In fact, actual rates for both groups are lower for most major mental illnesses. Table 3–1 shows the concordance rates for a variety of medical conditions that have been evaluated through twin studies. It is noteworthy that mental illnesses appear to be more highly genetic, as indicated by the twin method, than other medical disorders.

Although powerful, twin studies are not a perfect method for studying the genetics of major mental illnesses, because nongenetic psychological factors may play a significant role. Because twins are reared together, role modeling can be an influential factor. Furthermore, this factor is likely to be greater in monozygotic than in dizygotic twins because monozygotic twins are often treated as identical by their parents and peers, even being given the same toys and being dressed in the same clothing.

TABLE 3–1.   **Concordance rates in identical and nonidentical twins for various psychiatric conditions, coronary heart disease, and breast cancer**

Type of illness	Identical twins	Nonidentical twins
Autism, schizophrenia, bipolar disorder	60%	5%
Coronary artery disease	40%	10%
Depression	50%	15%
Breast cancer	30%	10%

Adoption Studies

Adoption studies are the most refined technique for disentangling environmental and genetic influences. In adoption studies, the focus is on children born to parents with a major mental illness and then adopted at birth and reared by parents without the disorder. These children are compared with a control group consisting of children born to psychiatrically well mothers, similarly adopted at birth, and reared by psychiatrically well parents. To whatever extent the rate of illness is higher in the adopted children of the mothers with a specific mental illness, that mental illness can be considered to be transmitted genetically rather than environmentally. In this model, learned behavior and role modeling of parents with mental illness are excluded, because the child is reared apart from the ill parent. Adoption studies have been conducted for schizophrenia and mood disorders and clearly demonstrate a significant genetic component.

Simple Versus "Complex" Illnesses

Researchers "gene hunting" for brain diseases were overly optimistic during its early era because of the success in finding the gene for Huntington's disease, a Mendelian autosomal dominant disorder caused by a single gene that is highly penetrant. Using classic positional cloning techniques, linkage was relatively quickly established on chromosome 4 through the study of a large Venezuelan pedigree. This quickly led to the development of a premorbid test for the disease. Thus individuals from families with Huntington's disease could determine if they possessed the disease-causing gene, refrain from having children at risk if they chose, and plan their lives for an unfortunate outcome. We also know that the gene causes trinucleotide repeats, that 40 or more repeats result in disease occurrence, and that a greater number of repeats leads to an earlier age at onset. Nevertheless, illustrating the intransigent puzzles inherent in human biology, we still do not know what the abnormal structural or regulatory protein is that produces this illness, and we still are unable to either treat or prevent the illness. Even with a clear, relatively simple autosomal dominant disease for which the genetic abnormality has been identified, the final answer that we seek has not come easily.

Most mental illnesses, like other common disorders in medicine such as hypertension or diabetes, are complex illnesses. They are clearly non-Mendelian and are generally considered to be due to multiple genes of small effect that interact with multiple nongenetic factors, causing the disease to emerge if enough cumulative genetic and nongenetic risk factors co-occur. Further complicating the search for these genes, mental illnesses are relatively common in the general population, making it difficult to find families in which a specific disease breeds true.

Finding the Genes

Several approaches have been used to locate genes for mental illnesses and identify their functions.

Linkage Studies

Linkage studies were among the earliest approaches used in the search for genes. Although linkage studies have yielded significant results for a few disorders (e.g., Huntington's disease), they have been considerably less successful for other types of mental illness, which are most likely to be genetically complex. Linkage studies of mental illnesses have sometimes been said to have a "manic-depressive history." Early reports identify a linkage between a site on a given chromosome and a specific illness, leading to enthusiasm and excitement, followed by replication studies that are unable to reproduce the initial finding in a different population of subjects, leading to depression. Examples are the initial reports of linkage for bipolar illness on chromosome 11 or the X chromosome, or linkages between schizophrenia and sites on chromosomes 6, 8, and 22. Linkage studies have largely been supplanted by other methods.

Candidate Gene Studies

Candidate gene studies typically begin with hypothesis-driven selection of a candidate gene. Candidate genes are chosen because they have single nucleotide polymorphisms (SNPs) and because they code for a protein that could have some effect leading to a specific mental illness. Examples of candidate genes include proteins regulating brain development such as brain-derived neurotrophic factor (*BDNF*), enzymes that affect neurotransmitter synthesis such as catechol-*O*-methyltransferase (*COMT*), or hormones that regulate brain activity such as neuropeptide Y. The strength of the candidate gene approach is that it directly permits investigators to determine whether a particular protein has any relevance to a specific mental illness. With this approach, a group of patients with the specific disorder is usually compared with a group of normal controls to determine whether a specific allele occurs more frequently in the patients.

Candidate gene studies have some of the same limitations as the linkage studies. They may yield false-positive results, particularly if samples are not carefully chosen, and like linkage studies, their credibility depends on repeated replications. Despite these disclaimers, several candidate genes have been identified and replicated as potential vulnerability genes for schizophrenia. These include *BDNF, COMT,* dysbindin, Disrupted-in-Schizophrenia (*DISC*), and neuregulin 1. Several candidate genes that confer vulnerability to autism spectrum disorders also have been identified, such as neurexin and ubiquitin, and the serotonin transporter gene has been implicated in mood disorders. In addition to examining disease association, investigators also have begun to do "deep phenotyping" of some genes using a variety of techniques such as animal models or neuroimaging. The *Met* allele in the *BDNF* promoter region is associated with schizophrenia, and individuals with this particular genotype also show decreased hippocampal activity during fMRI studies, smaller volume of frontal gray matter and hippocampus as measured with sMRI, progressive gray matter loss over the course of the disease, and poorer episodic memory than normal control subjects.

Copy Number Variants

Until relatively recently, it was assumed that all autosomal genes are present in two faithfully duplicated copies, with one allele inherited from each parent. We now know that large-scale variations in copy number are common and have the potential to confer disease liability. Copy number variants (CNVs) are mutations in DNA that are large (1 kilobase or larger) and can include deletions, insertions, and duplications. It is estimated that there are an average of 12 CNVs per individual, that they cover approximately 12% of the human genome, and that at least half occur in protein-coding regions. This finding has launched a search for their possible relationship to a variety of diseases, including mental illnesses. They have now been found to be associated with rare disorders such as Prader-Willi and Angelman syndromes, but also with Alzheimer's disease and schizophrenia.

Genome-Wide Association Studies

Genome-wide association studies are another approach to finding genes for mental illnesses, made possible through advances such as the haplotype map of the entire human genome and the assembly of large databases containing DNA from thousands of individuals who suffer from specific disorders. To date, none of these genome-wide surveys has produced robust results. They have generated some evidence for genes on chromosomes 9, 10, and 12 for the dementias and chromosomes 1, 6, 8, 10, 11, 13, and 22 for the psychoses. However, evidence for linkage is often across a broad region, with different groups mapping to nonoverlapping areas of the same chromosome arm. Nonetheless, as statistical methods improve, and as haplotype map data are integrated with the method, genome-wide association studies may provide significant additional information about the location of the various genes over the next decade.

■ Self-Assessment Questions

1. Describe the functions performed by the prefrontal cortex.
2. Describe the locations and functions of the two major language regions in the brain.
3. Identify the anatomic components of the reward system and discuss its relationship to at least two psychiatric disorders.
4. Discuss the role of serotonin in modulating behavior and the ways that this role is associated with mental illnesses.
5. Describe the location and function of the dopamine system and discuss its relationship to at least two mental illnesses.
6. Describe the functions of glutamate and its possible relation to the symptoms of psychosis.
7. Describe the relative strengths of family studies, twin studies, and adoption studies as methods for determining the familiality of mental illnesses and the degree to which purely genetic factors play a causal role.
8. Discuss the possible interaction between genes and environmental factors in producing mental illness.
9. What are single nucleotide polymorphisms? Copy number variants? Genome-wide association studies? What have we learned from them about genetic mechanisms of mental illnesses?

PART II

PSYCHIATRIC DISORDERS

Chapter 4

Neurodevelopmental (Child) Disorders

Children sweeten labors, but they make misfortunes more bitter. They increase the cares of life, but they mitigate the remembrance of death.

Francis Bacon

As any **17-year-old** will testify, the distinction between childhood and adulthood is arbitrary and frequently fluctuates in response to the needs of the person invoking the distinction. Psychiatric classification is no exception, and many of the disorders described in other chapters occur frequently in children, such as the mood and anxiety disorders. Schizophrenia often arises during adolescence and occasionally during childhood. Furthermore, "childhood" disorders such as intellectual disability or autism spectrum disorder may be diagnosed in adults. Nevertheless, DSM-5 has specified a group of disorders that are considered to be relatively specific to children and adolescents, in that these disorders typically *arise* during that period of life rather than simply *occur* during childhood and adolescence. These are the *neurodevelopmental disorders,* and they are listed in Table 4–1.

Estimates of prevalence of childhood mental disorders vary depending on breadth or narrowness of definition, but it is probably a reasonable estimate that 5%–15% of children will experience a psychiatric disturbance that is sufficiently severe to require treatment or to impair their functioning during the course of a year. Unfortunately, many childhood disorders will go unrecognized and untreated.

To permit more complete coverage of the most important disorders, we selectively review only some of them in this chapter, focusing on those that are most frequently seen in child psychiatry clinics or in a family practice setting. These include intellectual disability, commu-

---

TABLE 4–1.   DSM-5 neurodevelopmental disorders

Intellectual disabilities
   Intellectual disability (intellectual developmental disorder)
   Global developmental delay
   Unspecified intellectual disability

Communication disorders
   Language disorder
   Speech sound disorder
   Childhood-onset fluency disorder (stuttering)
   Social (pragmatic) communication disorder
   Unspecified communication disorder

Autism spectrum disorder

Attention-deficit/hyperactivity disorder
   Attention-deficit/hyperactivity disorder
   Other specified attention-deficit hyperactivity disorder
   Unspecified attention-deficit hyperactivity disorder

Specific learning disorder

Motor disorders
   Developmental coordination disorder
   Stereotypic movement disorder
   Tic disorders
      Tourette's disorder
      Persistent (chronic) motor or vocal tic disorder
      Provisional tic disorder
      Other specified tic disorder
      Unspecified tic disorder

Other neurodevelopmental disorders
   Other specified neurodevelopmental disorder
   Unspecified neurodevelopmental disorder

---

nication disorders, autism spectrum disorder, attention-deficit/hyper-activity disorder (ADHD), specific learning disorder, and motor disorders (including tic disorders). In addition, a brief overview is provided of those adult disorders that are commonly seen in children, including major depression, bipolar disorder, and schizophrenia. Several other disorders associated with childhood are included in other chapters, such as disruptive mood dysregulation disorder (see Chapter 6, "Mood Disorders"), and oppositional defiant disorder and conduct disorder (see Chapter 14, "Disruptive, Impulse-Control, and Conduct Disorders").

Child psychiatry is one of the most challenging and interesting areas of specialization within psychiatry. Because the child psychiatrist must know a great deal about other childhood illnesses, maturational processes, and developmental disorders, the field is closely allied with pediatrics and requires a good knowledge of general medicine. Furthermore, the clinician working in child psychiatry has an opportunity to catch disorders at their earliest; because children are adaptable, fresh in outlook, and pleasantly unpredictable, working with them and helping them overcome their problems can be particularly rewarding.

■ Special Aspects of the Assessment of Children

There are many continuities between adult and child psychiatry, but there are also important differences in emphasis and approach. These differences include techniques of assessment, the importance of flexible norms or criteria, an involvement of family or significant others, an increased role of nonphysicians in the health care team, and the frequent occurrence of psychiatric comorbidity.

Trajectories of Development

The pace of growth and development and the effect of life events is much greater in children than in adults. For that reason, when working with children it is important to emphasize a longitudinal and developmental approach. This approach must take into account the growth and maturational processes that all children undergo, assessing them in the light of each particular child's life situation and strengths and weaknesses. Children have a natural trajectory of development that will be completed through the process of passing from infancy to adulthood. As each child is evaluated, the clinician must ask himself or herself the following questions:

- What level of emotional and intellectual maturity does this child have?
- What are his or her particular strengths?
- How do they provide a protective and healing element?
- What particular weaknesses are present?
- What stresses are affecting the child?
- How do those stresses affect him or her at this particular stage of life?
- How do gender-specific challenges affect the expression of illness and its treatment?

For example, maternal death would have a very different effect on each child in a family of five children, the oldest of whom is a 16-year-old girl (who is likely to assume the maternal role) and the youngest of whom is 2 years old. The effect would be different for the children whose surviving father is unemployed and alcoholic than it would be for the children whose surviving father is a high-functioning blue- or white-collar worker. The effect also would be different depending on whether the eldest child is herself highly functional or has some mental illness, such as autism or conduct disorder. The effect on each child would vary depending on the availability of other social supports, such as an extended family with grandparents, a good or a weak school system, and a safe environment or one characterized by crime, violence, and drug use. All things being constant, a 2-year-old will have a very different understanding of parental loss or abandonment than will an older child, because the younger child will have had little time to build either a self-image incorporating that parent or a conceptual structure that can be used to comprehend parental loss.

Who Is the Patient?

Children rarely pick up the telephone or go online to make an appointment to see a child psychiatrist. Usually they are brought in at someone else's request. The child may be unwilling, noncompliant, distrusting, or resentful. In this instance, the assessment is likely to be particularly challenging because the clinician must win the child's trust. Even when the child is the identified patient, the parents usually are interviewed and evaluated as well. Not infrequently, it becomes clear that the parents themselves have serious problems that can complicate the situation further. In this instance, it may be necessary to reassess and to suggest treatment of the parents in addition to (or even instead of) the child. This can be especially challenging, because such recommendations need to be made in a tactful and noncritical manner to avoid alienating the parents. Furthermore, in child psychiatry, as in few other medical specialties, the clinician is likely to feel ambivalent and confused from time to time about the appropriate role to play. The child usually will be the identified patient, even though others may be in greater need of intervention and yet do not seek or accept it.

Assessment of the Child

Childhood disorders can be diagnosed in individuals ranging from infants through people in their late teens or early 20s. Obviously, standard approaches to interviewing and assessment, described in Chapter 2 ("Interviewing and Assessment"), do not apply well to infants, children, or young teenagers. Standard techniques for the psychiatric assessment of adults, which may be applicable to patients in their late teens and are applicable to patients in their early 20s, require verbal and cognitive skills not yet achieved in the maturational process of children. For example, young children may not be able to respond to questions about concepts such as depression, loneliness, or anger. The interviewer often needs to talk to children at a much more concrete level, asking questions such as

- Do you feel like crying?
- What kinds of things make you feel like crying?
- Do you ever want to hit people?
- Whom do you feel like hitting?
- Who are your best friends?
- How often do you see them?
- What kinds of things do you do together?
- Do they like you?

In addition to interviewing, playing games with the child often gives the clinician some insight into the child's ability to function interpersonally, to tolerate frustration, or to focus his or her attention. Imaginative play, using dolls that can represent important figures in the child's life, also may give some sense as to his or her feelings toward and relationships with others. Taking turns in telling stories also may elicit interesting information. For example, if the clinician suspects that the child may be feeling anxious about something, he or she may tell a story about "how Jimmy is afraid of going to school because the other children make fun of him." When the child then tells his or her own story, he or she may be able to describe his or her own fears in this indirect manner. Direct observation of activity level, motor skills, verbal expression, and vocabulary is also a fundamental component of assessment. Observing the child's behavior may help compensate for the limited reliability of any symptom reporting in very young children. For that reason, it is important to interview parents to fill in historical details and to elicit their observations of their child. Schoolteachers also are in a unique position to provide additional behavioral observations about the child.

Application of Norms and Criteria

When assessing children, the clinician must have a good sense of what is normal for a given child at a given age, as well as an awareness that norms may vary widely. Younger clinicians who are completing medical school or a residency usually have not had the experience of rearing their own children or of watching a large number of younger siblings develop. Thus they must get their sense of norms from reading textbooks, from observing large numbers of children, or from recalling their own experiences in the process of growing up.

Having a sense of what is normal or abnormal for a given child, in a given family, and in a given social and intellectual environment can be extremely difficult. For example, a typical normal 10-year-old has an IQ of 100, is able to read at a fourth-grade level, is able to perform addition and subtraction and some multiplication, and is able to throw, catch, and kick a ball with at least some accuracy. Some normal children have an IQ of only 85, however, whereas some have an IQ of 160. These children will clearly differ from one another a great deal in their school performance. Boys and girls also have quite different levels of maturation both physically and mentally, and these differences are especially pronounced in younger children. Boys and girls also have different maturational tasks as they go through puberty and enter adolescence, and consequently they experience different stresses. Success and failure also mean different things to an inner-city child than to a child from an affluent background.

Involvement of Family and Significant Others

Clinicians who work with children usually need to work with their families and significant others as well. The degree of family involvement varies, of course, depending on the age of the child. In the case of very young children, the parents are likely to be the primary informants and important recipients of treatment as well because they will probably need both psychological support and assistance in learning behavioral techniques to manage their child's behavior. For grade school children, involvement of family members is essential, but the child becomes an increasingly important protagonist in both assessment and treatment. Teenagers, who are going through important maturational changes as they move into adulthood, usually are brought to the forefront of the assessment and treatment process, although the family also will provide resources much of the time.

Deciding whether to maintain complete confidentiality or to share information becomes a critical issue in the assessment of teenagers. In general, teenagers should be assured that what they tell the clinician will end there, unless the teenager gives permission to share the information or can be encouraged to bring it out in a family or group setting. The assurance of confidentiality is important in establishing a bond of trust between teenager and clinician, because the patient otherwise is likely to see the therapist as a potentially antagonistic authority figure.

Only in situations dangerous to the child, such as a clear risk of suicide, should confidentiality be breached. This rule should be tactfully explained to the parents so that they do not feel excluded. Depending on circumstances, the clinician also may choose to see the parents independently. Alternatively, he or she may refer the parents to another psychiatrist, psychologist, or social worker with whom he or she has a good working relationship.

Involvement of Nonphysicians in the Health Care Team

Because of the diversity of the domains involved, many clinicians working in the area of child psychiatry like to operate within the context of a health care team. This team may be relatively small, involving a psychologist or social worker in addition to the psychiatrist. In larger settings, however, it includes a psychiatrist (who works primarily with the child in psychotherapy and the prescription of medication), a social worker (who works primarily with the family), an educational specialist (who assesses the child's educational achievement and assists in designing remediation programs as needed), and a psychologist (who develops programs for behavioral management, may do psychotherapy, and may work with child, family, and school system).

Psychological and Educational Testing in Child Psychiatry

Psychological and educational testing often plays a central role in the evaluation of children. Several tests that are commonly used in child psychiatry are listed in Table 4–2.

General Intelligence

General intelligence may be assessed with the Stanford-Binet Intelligence Scale, the fourth edition of the Wechsler Intelligence Scale for Children (WISC-IV), and other well-validated instruments. The Stanford-Binet Intelligence Scale was one of the earliest IQ tests to be developed, and it is

TABLE 4–2. Cognitive, psychological, and educational tests used in child psychiatry

Factor	Test
Intelligence	Stanford-Binet Intelligence Scale, Wechsler Intelligence Scale for Children (WISC-IV), Peabody Picture Vocabulary Test, Kaufman ABC, Wechsler Preschool and Primary Scale of Intelligence (WPPSI)
Educational achievement	Iowa Test of Basic Skills (ITBS), Iowa Test of Educational Development (ITED), Wide Range Achievement Test—Revised (WRAT-R)
Adaptive behavior	Vineland Adaptive Behavior Scales, Conners' Teacher Rating Scale—Revised
Perceptual-motor abilities	Draw-a-Person Test, Bender-Gestalt, Benton Visual Retention Test, Purdue Pegboard Test, Beery Developmental Test of Visual-Motor Integration
Personality	Thematic Apperception Test, Rorschach Test

still appropriate for relatively young children because its bottom threshold is lower and does not require extensive acquisition of knowledge. The Kaufman ABC and the Wechsler Preschool and Primary Scale of Intelligence are appropriate for assessing young children.

The WISC-IV is the standard test for assessing the intelligence of school-age children between the ages of 6 and 16 years. (The Wechsler Adult Intelligence Scale—IV [WAIS-IV] is used for children older than 16 years.) The WISC-IV consists of a group of ten core subtests that assess a variety of cognitive functions (e.g., vocabulary, comprehension, block design, matrix reasoning, digit span, symbol search). These are used to generate a full-scale IQ, verbal and performance IQs, and four composite scores known as indices (verbal comprehension, perceptual organization, processing speed, and working memory).

Examining the scores on individual WISC-IV subtests gives clinicians a sense of the child's overall intellectual skills and weaknesses. The test is scaled to have a mean of 100 and a standard deviation of 15. Sixty-seven percent of children have IQs that fall between 85 and 115, whereas 95% have IQs that fall between 70 and 130. Children from middle-class and culturally advantaged backgrounds tend to perform better on these tests. In such instances, the performance scales of the test may give a somewhat better indication of the child's "culture-free intelligence," although this clearly will not be helpful for those children who have performance deficits for some reason (e.g., visual-motor and/or perception difficulties).

Interpretation of the WISC-IV must be made within the context of each child's social background and educational opportunities.

Other briefer and simpler tests are also sometimes used to obtain an approximate estimate of intelligence. For example, the Peabody Picture Vocabulary Test is sometimes used to give a global measure of intelligence. The test uses pictures to provide a measure of oral language comprehension, from which verbal intelligence can be inferred. In general, IQ based on the Peabody or other similar tests tends to be an overestimate.

Educational Achievement

Standardized educational achievement tests are often used in the public school systems. Two widely used tests are the Iowa Test of Basic Skills (ITBS) and the Iowa Test of Educational Development (ITED); these are representative of the type of standardized tests now used throughout most of the United States. The former is typically used for younger children, whereas versions of the latter are available for assessment of patients up to completion of high school. For the ITBS and the ITED, national, state, and school-specific norms are available, so that the child's achievement can be assessed within his or her specific environmental context. Achievement tests provide scores for specific areas such as reading, language arts, study skills, arithmetic, and social studies. Evaluating the pattern of achievement can provide some index as to whether the child has a learning disorder.

Adaptive Behavior

Various standard questionnaires can be used to assess adaptive behavior. The Vineland Adaptive Behavior Scales were originally developed to evaluate children with mental retardation but are also used to provide a standardized measure of adaptive skills for children with a broader range of problems, including those with normal intelligence. The Conners' Teacher Rating Scale—Revised was developed to assess the child's behavior in the classroom. It is a pencil-and-paper test specifically targeted to assess behavior associated with ADHD, such as impulsivity, physical activity, or impaired attention. It also has subscales to assess social withdrawal and aggressive behavior. A complementary rating scale to be completed by parents is also available.

Perceptual-Motor Skills

Various standardized tests are used to assess perceptual-motor skills. In the assessment of young children, the Draw-a-Person Test is one of the most popular. The complexity and detail of the person drawn give a crude indication of the child's maturity, whereas the drawing skills shown allow assessment of the child's ability to translate his or her thoughts into a visual representation. The Bender-Gestalt and Benton Visual Retention Test assess the ability to copy a design and to recall it later, which are also fundamental aspects of perceptual-motor skills. The Purdue Pegboard Test is a somewhat pure test of manual dexterity, assessing the child's ability to place pegs in appropriate slots. The Beery Developmental Test of Visual-Motor Integration is popular with school systems.

Personality Style and Social Adjustment

Personality style and social adjustment are typically evaluated in children through projective tests. The Thematic Apperception Test uses a series of cards depicting obscure figures in ambiguous situations; the child is asked to describe what is happening and tell a story about it. The Rorschach Test is the famous inkblot test. In this test, the child is shown cards containing inkblots that have ambiguous and suggestive shapes. The child is asked to identify and label what he or she sees (e.g., two men dancing) and to indicate the basis for his or her perception. Although semistandardized scores can be applied, one of the most common applications of these tests is to provide a standardized structured stimulus to the child, using his or her response as an indication of interpersonal experiences, anxieties, fears, and drives.

Physical Examination

The physical examination is an important part of the child's evaluation. In addition to the standard physical examination, the clinician should inspect the child for indications of congenital anomalies, such as a high-arched palate, low-set ears, single palmar creases, unusual carrying angle, webbing, abnormalities of the genitalia, and neuroectodermal anomalies. Congenital anomalies tend to occur together, and midline or neuroectodermal anomalies are more likely to be associated with central nervous system anomalies. The observation of such anomalies is an indication for magnetic resonance imaging (MRI) scan to assess for the presence of structural brain abnormalities, particularly in the midline.

The clinician should be attentive to assessment of neurological soft signs in children as well. A standardized repertoire should be developed for assessing graphesthesia, left-right discrimination, motor coordination, and simple perceptual-motor skills that can be evaluated at the bedside. For example, left-right discrimination can be examined systematically through a graded series of questions such as the following: "Hold up your right hand. Hold up your left foot. Put your right forefinger on your nose. Use your left forefinger to point to your right foot. Point to my right hand. Use your left forefinger to point to my left hand." Tongue twisters such as "Methodist-Episcopal" or "Luke Luck likes lakes" may be used to assess oral-motor coordination, whereas hopping, walking in tandem, and rapid alternating movements are used to evaluate other motor skills. Fine motor skills are evaluated through drawing and writing. After the clinician has assessed many children across a wide range of ages, he or she will gradually develop a sense of what constitutes normal performance on such tests of neurological soft signs for a given child at a given age. Extensive neurological soft signs may serve as an indicator for ordering a more comprehensive laboratory workup including electroencephalography (EEG) or brain scanning.

■ Intellectual Disability (Intellectual Developmental Disorder)

Intellectual disability (intellectual developmental disorder), formerly known as *mental retardation,* is characterized by deficits in general mental abilities and impairment in everyday adaptive functioning with onset in the early developmental period. Typically, intellectual disability is observed and diagnosed in childhood and is usually considered to be present from very early in life. The term *mental retardation* is no longer used because it was considered stigmatizing and was inconsistent with wording adopted into U.S. Federal law that favors the newer terms.

In the past, mental retardation had been defined almost exclusively on the basis of having an IQ less than 70. With intellectual disability, there is no longer an arbitrary reliance on IQ as the main determinant for the diagnosis, and subtypes are now used to classify the person with mild, moderate, severe, or profound levels of severity. Further, the reliance on IQ was limiting because it failed to take into account the individual's adaptive functioning, that is, how well the person functions in important areas of life, including his or her social and behavior interactions, conceptual and intellectual life, and practical day-to-day living skills. Nonetheless, measuring intelligence remains a critical part of the assessment of the person's intellectual functioning.

The diagnosis of an intellectual developmental disorder is based on *both* clinical assessment and standardized testing of intelligence. *Intelligence* has been defined as a general mental ability that involves reasoning, problem solving, planning, thinking abstractly, comprehending complex ideas, judgment, academic learning, and learning from experience, as applied in academic learning and social understanding. See Box 4–1 for the DSM-5 criteria for intellectual developmental disorder.

Box 4–1.   DSM-5 Diagnostic Criteria for Intellectual Disability (Intellectual Developmental Disorder)

Intellectual disability (intellectual developmental disorder) is a disorder with onset during the developmental period that includes both intellectual and adaptive functioning deficits in conceptual, social, and practical domains. The following three criteria must be met:

A. Deficits in intellectual functions, such as reasoning, problem solving, planning, abstract thinking, judgment, academic learning, and learning from experience, confirmed by both clinical assessment and individualized, standardized intelligence testing.

B. Deficits in adaptive functioning that result in failure to meet developmental and sociocultural standards for personal independence and social responsibility. Without ongoing support, the adaptive deficits limit functioning in one or more activities of daily life, such as communication, social participation, and independent living, across multiple environments, such as home, school, work, and community.

C. Onset of intellectual and adaptive deficits during the developmental period.

Note: The diagnostic term *intellectual disability* is the equivalent term for the ICD-11 diagnosis of *intellectual developmental disorders.* Although the term *intellectual disability* is used throughout this manual, both terms are used in the title to clarify relationships with other classification systems. Moreover, a federal statute in the United States (Public Law 111-256, Rosa's Law) replaces the term *mental retardation* with *intellectual disability,* and research journals use the term *intellectual disability.* Thus, *intellectual disability* is the term in common use by medical, educational, and other professions and by the lay public and advocacy groups.

Specify current severity:

Mild
Moderate
Severe
Profound

Standardized intelligence testing usually involves IQ measurement. With such tests, the category of intellectual disorder is considered to be about two standard deviations or more below the population mean, including a margin for error (about ±5 points). On tests with a standard deviation of 15 and a mean of 100, this involves a score in the range of 65–75. Clinical training and judgment are needed to interpret test results, which are generally performed by neuropsychologists. Factors other than intellectual disability may limit performance, such as one's cultural background, native language, or the presence of a communication disorder.

Deficits in *adaptive functioning* are also assessed to determine how well a person meets community standards of personal independence and social responsibility, as compared with others of similar age and sociocultural background, in three crucial domains: conceptual, social, and practical.

- The *conceptual (academic)* domain involves competence in memory, language, reading, writing, math reasoning, and acquisition of practical knowledge; problem solving; and judgment in novel situations, among others.
- The *social* domain involves awareness of others' thoughts, feelings, and experiences; empathy; interpersonal communication skills; friendship abilities; and social judgment, among others.
- The *practical* domain involves learning and self-management across life settings, including personal care, job responsibilities, money management, recreation, self-management of behavior, and school and work task organization, among others.

Intellectual capacity, education, motivation, socialization, personality features, vocational opportunity, cultural experience, and coexisting general medical conditions or mental disorders can influence adaptive functioning.

Children with *mild* disorder represent the majority of cases of intellectual disability, constituting approximately 85% of identified individuals. These children are considered educable, and they usually are able to attend special classes and to work toward the long-term goal of being able to function in the community and to hold some type of job. They usually can learn to read, write, and perform simple arithmetical calculations. Children with *moderate* disorder constitute approximately 10% of the intellectually disabled population. They are considered trainable, in that they can learn to talk, to recognize their name and other simple words, to perform activities of self-care such as bathing or doing their laundry, and to handle small change. They require management and treatment in special education classes. The ideal long-term goal for these individuals is care in a sheltered environment, such as a group home. Children with *severe* and *profound* disorders constitute the smallest groups. Individuals in these categories almost invariably require care in institutionalized settings, usually beginning relatively early in life.

Epidemiology, Clinical Findings, and Course

Intellectual disability is very common, affecting 1%–2% of the general population. It is more common in males, with a male-to-female ratio of approximately 2:1. Mild disorder is more common in the lower social classes, but cases of moderate, severe, and profound intellectual disability are equally common among all social classes.

The long-term outcome is variable. Some severe and profound forms may be characterized by progressive physical deterioration and ultimately premature death, as early as the teens or early 20s (e.g., Tay-Sachs disease). Individuals with mild and moderate disorders have a somewhat reduced life expectancy, but active intervention may enhance their quality of life. Like all children, children with an intellectual developmental disorder may show maturational spurts that could not be predicted at an earlier age. Typically, these children progress through normal milestones, such as sitting, standing, talking, and learning numbers and letters, in a pattern similar to that of nondisabled children but at a slower rate.

Etiology and Pathophysiology

Intellectual developmental disorder is a syndrome that represents a final common pathway produced by a variety of factors that injure the brain and affect its normal development. Individuals with moderate to profound impairment often have an identifiable cause for their mental retardation, whereas those with mild impairment often do not and probably develop their mental retardation through some complex multifactorial and polygenetic combination. Down syndrome is the most common *chromosomal* cause of intellectual disability. Fragile X syndrome is the most common heritable form of intellectual disability and is second only to Down syndrome in frequency. The fragile X gene has been discovered; it contains an unstable segment that expands as it is passed through generations and affects children differently depending on whether it is passed through fathers or mothers (imprinting). Inborn errors of metabolism account for a small percentage of cases; examples include Tay-Sachs disease and untreated phenylketonuria.

In addition to these clearly defined genetic causes, a substantial proportion of cases of intellectual disability probably also reflect polygenic inheritance, possibly interacting with nongenetic factors such as nutrition and psychosocial nurturance. Many prenatal factors also may affect fetal development and lead to neurodevelopmental anomalies. The high rate of Down syndrome (trisomy 21) in children born to older mothers is a prime example. Other prenatal factors that may affect fetal development include maternal malnutrition or substance abuse; exposure to mutagens such as radiation; maternal illnesses such as diabetes, toxemia, or rubella; and maternal abuse and neglect. *Fetal alcohol syndrome* is a common nongenetic cause of intellectual disability. Perinatal and early postnatal factors also may contribute. Examples include traumatic deliveries that cause brain injury, malnutrition, exposure to toxins, infections such as encephalitis, and head injuries occurring during infancy or early childhood. Psychosocial factors obviously contribute to some of these biological factors, and some psychosocial factors also may contribute independently. For example, poor prenatal and perinatal care is more likely to occur in children born in impoverished environments.

Differential Diagnosis

As in other childhood disorders, the differential diagnosis of intellectual developmental disorder (particularly mild impairment) can be complex because of the frequent comorbidity of other childhood disorders. The differential diagnosis includes ADHD, learning disorders, autism spectrum disorder, and childhood psychoses or mood disorders, but all of these conditions can co-occur with intellectual developmental disorder. Seizure disorders also are very common in these children. Children in whom intellectual disability is suspected should be thoroughly evaluated with a careful physical and neurological examination, an electroencephalogram (EEG), an MRI scan, as well as cognitive testing.

Clinical Management

Following a thorough evaluation, a comprehensive program should be developed to determine the best situation in which to place and treat the child, taking the needs and abilities of both the child and the parents into account. Decisions may range from care in the home (supplemented by family support and special education), to placement in a foster or group home, to long-term institutionalization.

Because most children with an intellectual developmental disorder are mildly affected, the majority will remain at home, at least initially. Because the parents of some of these children themselves have intellectual disability, ongoing evaluation through social service agencies may be helpful and even necessary to ensure that the child's needs are being adequately met.

Whatever their own intellectual resources, the parents of intellectually disabled children are confronted with a host of burdens and stresses and can benefit from both supportive counseling and training in behavioral techniques to help manage their child's behavior problems. Comorbid conditions such as seizures require medical management. Cognitive assessment will help to determine the appropriate educational placement for the child, but this should be subjected to periodic review.

■ Communication Disorders

As students might imagine, communication disorders interfere with a child's ability to communicate their needs, desires, and emotions. While not traditionally considered mental disorders, they cause distress and impair the child's ability to function and are important for purposes of differential diagnosis. Autism spectrum disorder needs to be ruled out, as do ADHD, social anxiety disorder, and intellectual disability. The communication disorders are as follows:

Language disorder: a persistent disturbance in the development and use of spoken language, written language, or sign language due to deficits in comprehension or production. Language abilities are substantially below age expectation, significantly interfering with academic achievement, job performance, effective communication, and socialization.

Speech sound disorder: persistent difficulties in speech production that are developmentally inappropriate. They involve articulation, fluency, and voice production in its various aspects. This disorder often coexists with language disorder, intellectual disability, and neurological conditions such as Landau-Kleffner syndrome.

Childhood-onset fluency disorder (stuttering): a disturbance in the normal fluency and time patterning of speech that is inappropriate for the child's age. The disturbance may present as frequent repetitions or prolongations of sounds or syllables or other types of speech dysfluencies, such as broken words (e.g., pauses within a word), audible or silent blocking (e.g., filled or unfilled pauses in speech), or word substitutions to avoid problematic words. Interjections such as "um" or "like" also can occur and may be repeated ("um- um- um") or prolonged ("um-mmm") as the individual struggles to resume speaking. Stuttering can interfere with academic or occupational achievement or social communication; it can also cause humiliation and embarrassment and lead individuals to avoid situations that may be associated with speech, such as using a telephone. The disorder usually begins by age 6 years, although most people recover from the dysfluency as they grow older.

Social (pragmatic) communication disorder: difficulty with the social use of verbal and nonverbal communication. The child may have difficulty with appropriately greeting and sharing information with playmates; changing his or her communication style to match the situation (e.g., speaking differently in a classroom than on a playground); talking differently to a child than to an adult; or avoiding the use of overly formal language. The child may also have trouble taking turns in conversation, using verbal and nonverbal signals to regulate interactions, or understanding what is not explicitly stated (e.g., making inferences) and comprehending nonliteral or ambiguous meanings of language (e.g., idioms, humor, metaphors). The individual comes across to others as socially awkward.

■ Autism Spectrum Disorder

Autism was initially described in 1948 by Leo Kanner as a syndrome of social communication deficits combined with repetitive and stereotyped behaviors in children. Since the early 1990s it has been clear that there are a range of disorders related to autism, including the DSM-IV "pervasive developmental disorders": Rett's disorder, childhood disintegrative disorder, and Asperger's disorder.

DSM-5 has replaced all of these diagnoses with a new diagnosis, *autism spectrum disorder*. Clinicians had found it difficult to distinguish among the various pervasive developmental disorders. Further, investigators realized that these disorders were all defined by a common set of behaviors that lay along a spectrum and were best represented by a single category. Autism spectrum disorder is considered a neurodevelopmental disorder. Present from infancy or early childhood, the disorder may not be detected until later because of minimal social demands and support from parents or caregivers in early years. Essential features include persistent impairment in reciprocal social communication and social interaction and restricted, repetitive patterns of behavior, interests, or activities.

The clinician can specify the child's clinical condition by indicating his or her overall severity of symptoms, intellectual and/or language impairment, and whether there is a known genetic disorder, epilepsy, or comorbid intellectual disability. As an example, rather than receiving a diagnosis of Asperger's disorder, the child is now diagnosed with "autism spectrum disorder, without intellectual impairment and without structural language impairment."

The DSM-5 criteria for autism spectrum disorder appear in Box 4–2. They require that at least 6 of 12 items be present. The items cover the three major domains involved in autism (i.e., social interaction, communication, and behavioral repertoire).

Box 4–2.   DSM-5 Diagnostic Criteria for Autism Spectrum Disorder

A. Persistent deficits in social communication and social interaction across multiple contexts, as manifested by the following, currently or by history (examples are illustrative, not exhaustive; see text):

1. Deficits in social-emotional reciprocity, ranging, for example, from abnormal social approach and failure of normal back-and-forth conversation; to reduced sharing of interests, emotions, or affect; to failure to initiate or respond to social interactions.

2. Deficits in nonverbal communicative behaviors used for social interaction, ranging, for example, from poorly integrated verbal and nonverbal communication; to abnormalities in eye contact and body language or deficits in understanding and use of gestures; to a total lack of facial expressions and nonverbal communication.

3. Deficits in developing, maintaining, and understanding relationships, ranging, for example, from difficulties adjusting behavior to suit various social contexts; to difficulties in sharing imaginative play or in making friends; to absence of interest in peers.

Specify current severity:

Severity is based on social communication impairments and restricted, repetitive patterns of behavior.

B. Restricted, repetitive patterns of behavior, interests, or activities, as manifested by at least two of the following, currently or by history (examples are illustrative, not exhaustive; see text):

1. Stereotyped or repetitive motor movements, use of objects, or speech (e.g., simple motor stereotypies, lining up toys or flipping objects, echolalia, idiosyncratic phrases).

2. Insistence on sameness, inflexible adherence to routines, or ritualized patterns of verbal or nonverbal behavior (e.g., extreme distress at small changes, difficulties with transitions, rigid thinking patterns, greeting rituals, need to take same route or eat same food every day).
3. Highly restricted, fixated interests that are abnormal in intensity or focus (e.g., strong attachment to or preoccupation with unusual objects, excessively circumscribed or perseverative interests).
4. Hyper- or hyporeactivity to sensory input or unusual interest in sensory aspects of the environment (e.g., apparent indifference to pain/temperature, adverse response to specific sounds or textures, excessive smelling or touching of objects, visual fascination with lights or movement).

Specify current severity:

Severity is based on social communication impairments and restricted, repetitive patterns of behavior.

C. Symptoms must be present in the early developmental period (but may not become fully manifest until social demands exceed limited capacities, or may be masked by learned strategies in later life).

D. Symptoms cause clinically significant impairment in social, occupational, or other important areas of current functioning.

E. These disturbances are not better explained by intellectual disability (intellectual developmental disorder) or global developmental delay. Intellectual disability and autism spectrum disorder frequently co-occur; to make comorbid diagnoses of autism spectrum disorder and intellectual disability, social communication should be below that expected for general developmental level.

Note: Individuals with a well-established DSM-IV diagnosis of autistic disorder, Asperger's disorder, or pervasive developmental disorder not otherwise specified should be given the diagnosis of autism spectrum disorder. Individuals who have marked deficits in social communication, but whose symptoms do not otherwise meet criteria for autism spectrum disorder, should be evaluated for social (pragmatic) communication disorder.

Specify if:

With or without accompanying intellectual impairment

With or without accompanying language impairment

Associated with a known medical or genetic condition or environmental factor (**Coding note:** Use additional code to identify the associated medical or genetic condition.)

Associated with another neurodevelopmental, mental, or behavioral disorder (**Coding note:** Use additional code[s] to identify the associated neurodevelopmental, mental, or behavioral disorder[s].)

With catatonia (refer to the criteria for catatonia associated with another mental disorder for definition) (**Coding note:** Use additional code [for] catatonia associated with autism spectrum disorder to indicate the presence of the comorbid catatonia.)

Clinical Findings

Manifestations vary greatly depending on the severity of the syndrome, the child's developmental level, and his or her chronological age. Those with a more severe disorder are usually noted to be developing abnormally relatively soon after birth. Within the child's first 3–6 months of lfie, the parents may note that he or she has not developed a normal pattern of smiling or responding to cuddling. The first clear sign of abnormality is usually in the area of language. As the child grows older, he or he does not progress through developmental milestones such as learning to say words and speak sentences. The failure to develop spoken language typically is what leads parents to seek medical attention. Verbal impairments range from the complete absence of verbal speech to mildly deviant speech and language patterns. Even in patients who develop good facility in verbal expression, the speech lacks spontaneity and has an empty, repetitive quality to it; intonations may be singsong and monotonous.

Severely affected children also may appear to lack the ability to bond with their parents or with others. In milder cases, they have some interaction but lack warmth, sensitivity, and awareness. Interactions, when they occur, tend to have a detached and mechanical quality. Displays of love and affection do not occur or appear stilted and inauthentic. Affected children seem aloof, withdrawn, and detached.

Finally, the behavioral repertoire is impaired. There is an intense and rigid commitment to maintaining specific routines, and severely affected children tend to become quite distressed if routines are interrupted. They may have to sit in a particular chair, dress in a particular way, or eat particular foods. In some cases, the child may engage in self-stimulating behavior, such as rocking or head banging.

Most persons with a severe autism spectrum disorder show some evidence of intellectual disability, but others have normal intelligence, and some have very specific talents or abilities, particularly in the areas of music and mathematics. Those with a milder variant, referred to in DSM-IV as Asperger's disorder, have a similar early onset of impairment in social interaction and abnormal behavior such as stereotypies and rituals, but they have normal language functions and usually have normal intelligence as well.

Epidemiology and Course

Autism spectrum disorder is thought to affect about 1% of the general population, but severe cases are probably much less common. There is some evidence that the prevalence of autism spectrum disorder has increased over the past two decades, a finding thought to be related primarily to better recognition. Other causes for the increase have been suggested, such as environmental toxins or vaccines, but research does not support these claims. Autism is more common in boys than in girls, with a ratio of about 4:1.

The onset of autism spectrum disorder occurs in early childhood, and problems are typically noted during the first or second year of life. For most, the disorder is chronic and lifelong. Some severely affected children show improvement as they mature, although others may worsen. Very few of these individuals are able to progress normally through school or to live independently. Nearly all of the defining features of the disorder, including social aloofness, language abnormalities, and rigid and ritualistic behavior, tend to persist into adulthood. Good prognostic features include higher IQ and better language and social skills.

Mildly affected individuals will perform well in school, providing there is no comorbid intellectual disability, and will have a relatively good long-term outcome. Some will be able to complete college and graduate school and have normal careers.

Etiology and Pathophysiology

Autism spectrum disorder is highly heritable, as shown in family and twin studies. Intellectual disability and both speech and language disorders run in these families as well. Many different chromosomes and candidate genes have been identified. About 15% of cases are associated with a known genetic mechanism. Recent work also suggests that some cases of autism may be a consequence of copy number variants—spontaneous mutations occurring during meiosis that are not inherited.

In brain imaging studies, children with autism spectrum disorder have been found to have large brain size relative to body size, with some evidence for gyral malformation (polymicrogyria). The large cerebral size has been interpreted as reflecting a failure to achieve normal pruning, the process by which neurons are systematically eliminated or "pruned" back. Abnormalities in the cerebellum (particularly the vermis), the temporal lobes, and the hippocampal complex, as well as cerebral asymmetries, also have been reported. Functional imaging studies suggest the presence of an overall impairment in connectivity in brain networks used for attention, consciousness, and self-awareness. Neuropathological studies have reported small, densely packed (and presumably immature) cells in limbic structures in the cerebellum.

Physically, these children have a variety of soft neurological signs and primitive reflexes, an excess of nonright-handedness, and an apparent failure to achieve normal cerebral dominance of language functions in the left hemisphere.

Differential Diagnosis

Children who present with symptoms suggestive of an autism spectrum disorder should receive comprehensive psychiatric and physical examinations, with an emphasis on neurological components. Children should be screened for other disorders that might explain their symptoms, such as phenylketonuria or Down syndrome. Because these children present with profound social withdrawal, hearing and vision should be checked to rule out sensory defects as a cause. Electroencephalography should also be performed when comorbid seizure disorders are suspected. IQ testing will help assess the child's intellectual strengths and weaknesses.

The major differential diagnoses include childhood psychosis, intellectual disability, communication disorders, and selective mutism. The most important distinctions are with intellectual disability and language disorder. These distinctions can be quite difficult, and the differential turns largely on the quality of the social interactions (in the context of the individual's particular intellectual abilities). Intellectually disabled children typically have pervasive intellectual impairments, whereas children with autism spectrum disorder tend to have a much more uneven profile of functional intellectual abilities and may be normal to superior in some areas. Selective mutism also needs to be ruled out; in these cases, the child fails to speak despite an ability to do so, and he or she has none of the cardinal features of autism spectrum disorder. The major distinction between autism spectrum disorder and schizophrenia is the presence or absence of overt psychotic symptoms such as delusions and hallucinations. These symptoms typically do not occur in autism spectrum disorder, although the two disorders are sometimes comorbid.

Clinical Management

Once the diagnosis is made, the disorder should be described and explained to the parents, making it clear that their child has a neurodevelopmental disease and not a psychological disturbance that they caused through poor parenting. Guidelines for behavioral management should be provided so that the parents can help reduce the rigid and stereotyped behaviors and improve language and social skills. Children who are severely affected usually require special education or specialized day care programs that also emphasize improvement in social and language skills. Medications are often used as adjuncts to these supportive and behavioral approaches. Children with seizures require anticonvulsants. Antipsychotics have been found to decrease aggressive and stereotypical patterns of behavior. The second-generation antipsychotics risperidone and aripiprazole have received U.S. Food and Drug Administration (FDA) approval for the treatment of irritability in autistic children and adolescents. Other medications that may be helpful in children with autism spectrum disorder are the selective serotonin reuptake inhibitors for those with depression, anxiety, or obsessive-compulsive symptoms, and stimulants for those with symptoms of inattention or hyperactivity. Management strategies for milder cases (i.e., Asperger's disorder) are similar, but higher expectations can be set.

■ Attention-Deficit/Hyperactivity Disorder

ADHD is one of the most common "bread-and-butter" disorders that are the staple of child psychiatry. Children with ADHD appear to be a caricature of the active child. They are physically overactive, distractible, inattentive, impulsive, and difficult to manage. ADHD is typically evident early in childhood, with signs of increased activity being noted very early (e.g., "As soon as he could crawl, he got into everything"; "He never seemed to sleep and kicked constantly, even before he was born"). Although the disorder improves with maturation, in some individuals it may persist into adulthood.

ADHD is defined by two broad groups of symptoms: 1) inattention and 2) hyperactivity and impulsivity. The DSM-5 criteria for ADHD are shown in Box 4–3. They require that at least 6 of 9 inattention and 6 of 9 hyperactivity/impulsivity symptoms be present for at least 6 months, with onset before age 12. Subtypes can be specified to indicate whether the presentation is predominantly inattentive, predominantly hyperactive/impulsive, or mixed. Because DSM-5 criteria for diagnosis require that impairment occur in at least two settings (e.g., home, school, work), obtaining a schoolteacher's input can be important in preventing the overdiagnosis of ADHD. For those age 17 years and older, only 5 inattention symptoms and 5 hyperactivity/impulsivity symptoms are required.

Box 4–3.   DSM-5 Diagnostic Criteria for Attention-Deficit
           Hyperactivity Disorder

A. A persistent pattern of inattention and/or hyperactivity-impulsivity that inter-
    feres with functioning or development, as characterized by (1) and/or (2):

    1. **Inattention:** Six (or more) of the following symptoms have persisted
        for at least 6 months to a degree that is inconsistent with develop-
        mental level and that negatively impacts directly on social and aca-
        demic/occupational activities:
        Note: The symptoms are not solely a manifestation of oppositional
        behavior, defiance, hostility, or failure to understand tasks or instruc-
        tions. For older adolescents and adults (age 17 and older), at least
        five symptoms are required.

        a. Often fails to give close attention to details or makes careless
            mistakes in schoolwork, at work, or during other activities (e.g.,
            overlooks or misses details, work is inaccurate).
        b. Often has difficulty sustaining attention in tasks or play activities
            (e.g., has difficulty remaining focused during lectures, conversa-
            tions, or lengthy reading).
        c. Often does not seem to listen when spoken to directly (e.g., mind
            seems elsewhere, even in the absence of any obvious distraction).
        d. Often does not follow through on instructions and fails to finish
            schoolwork, chores, or duties in the workplace (e.g., starts tasks
            but quickly loses focus and is easily sidetracked).
        e. Often has difficulty organizing tasks and activities (e.g., difficulty
            managing sequential tasks; difficulty keeping materials and be-
            longings in order; messy, disorganized work; has poor time man-
            agement; fails to meet deadlines).
        f. Often avoids, dislikes, or is reluctant to engage in tasks that re-
            quire sustained mental effort (e.g., schoolwork or homework; for
            older adolescents and adults, preparing reports, completing
            forms, reviewing lengthy papers).
        g. Often loses things necessary for tasks or activities (e.g., school
            materials, pencils, books, tools, wallets, keys, paperwork, eye-
            glasses, mobile telephones).
        h. Is often easily distracted by extraneous stimuli (for older adoles-
            cents and adults, may include unrelated thoughts).
        i. Is often forgetful in daily activities (e.g., doing chores, running er-
            rands; for older adolescents and adults, returning calls, paying
            bills, keeping appointments).

    2. **Hyperactivity and impulsivity:** Six (or more) of the following symp-
        toms have persisted for at least 6 months to a degree that is incon-
        sistent with developmental level and that negatively impacts directly
        on social and academic/occupational activities:

Note: The symptoms are not solely a manifestation of oppositional behavior, defiance, hostility, or a failure to understand tasks or instructions. For older adolescents and adults (age 17 and older), at least five symptoms are required.

   a. Often fidgets with or taps hands or feet or squirms in seat.

   b. Often leaves seat in situations when remaining seated is expected (e.g., leaves his or her place in the classroom, in the office or other workplace, or in other situations that require remaining in place).

   c. Often runs about or climbs in situations where it is inappropriate. (**Note:** In adolescents or adults, may be limited to feeling restless.)

   d. Often unable to play or engage in leisure activities quietly.

   e. Is often "on the go," acting as if "driven by a motor" (e.g., is unable to be or uncomfortable being still for extended time, as in restaurants, meetings; may be experienced by others as being restless or difficult to keep up with).

   f. Often talks excessively.

   g. Often blurts out an answer before a question has been completed (e.g., completes people's sentences; cannot wait for turn in conversation).

   h. Often has difficulty waiting his or her turn (e.g., while waiting in line).

   i. Often interrupts or intrudes on others (e.g., butts into conversations, games, or activities; may start using other people's things without asking or receiving permission; for adolescents and adults, may intrude into or take over what others are doing).

B. Several inattentive or hyperactive-impulsive symptoms were present prior to age 12 years.

C. Several inattentive or hyperactive-impulsive symptoms are present in two or more settings (e.g., at home, school, or work; with friends or relatives; in other activities).

D. There is clear evidence that the symptoms interfere with, or reduce the quality of, social, academic, or occupational functioning.

E. The symptoms do not occur exclusively during the course of schizophrenia or another psychotic disorder and are not better explained by another mental disorder (e.g., mood disorder, anxiety disorder, dissociative disorder, personality disorder, substance intoxication or withdrawal).

Specify whether:

Combined presentation: If both Criterion A1 (inattention) and Criterion A2 (hyperactivity-impulsivity) are met for the past 6 months.

Predominantly inattentive presentation: If Criterion A1 (inattention) is met but Criterion A2 (hyperactivity-impulsivity) is not met for the past 6 months.

Predominantly hyperactive/impulsive presentation: If Criterion A2 (hyperactivity-impulsivity) is met and Criterion A1 (inattention) is not met for the past 6 months.

Specify if:

In partial remission: When full criteria were previously met, fewer than the full criteria have been met for the past 6 months, and the symptoms still result in impairment in social, academic, or occupational functioning.

Specify current severity:

Mild: Few, if any, symptoms in excess of those required to make the diagnosis are present, and symptoms result in no more than minor impairments in social or occupational functioning.

Moderate: Symptoms or functional impairment between "mild" and "severe" are present.

Severe: Many symptoms in excess of those required to make the diagnosis, or several symptoms that are particularly severe, are present, or the symptoms result in marked impairment in social or occupational functioning.

The symptoms of ADHD will vary depending on the age of the child. Younger children (in the 4- to 6-year age range) are "little terrors." They run from one part of the room to another, hop on furniture, knock objects off tables, explore the contents of visitors' handbags, talk incessantly, run outside without telling their parents where they are going, have difficulty learning to look both ways before crossing the street, lose and break toys, stay up late, wake up early, and generally exhaust their parents. When these children enter school and begin the task of learning, the difficulties in focusing attention become more obvious. They may miss things that the teacher says, be unable to finish assignments, forget their pencils or notebooks, and answer the teacher's questions without holding up a hand and often without even waiting to have the question completed. They may annoy their schoolmates by pushing ahead in line, grabbing equipment on the playground, or violating the rules of games without seeming to be aware of them. These children may fall behind their peers in school and develop a poor self-concept. Teachers may complain about their behavior to their parents and request that help be sought.

The following is the case history of a patient with ADHD treated in one of our clinics:

Charlie, a 6-year-old boy, was brought in by his mother after a recent school conference in which it was pointed out that he seemed to be having difficulty in adjusting to first grade.

Charlie's mother described that he had always been a somewhat difficult child. Even as an infant, he was irritable and overactive. He learned to crawl at 7 months and was soon exploring the entire house, leaving a wake of emptied wastepaper baskets and disrupted cupboards behind him. He did not seem to be able to remember or follow through with parental instructions that he should keep his feet off the furniture, not walk on the tops of tables, and not run through the living room carrying melting chocolate popsicles. As he learned to talk, he seemed to talk incessantly and to be continuously in need of attention from his parents.

He began to attend preschool at age 4 years. His teachers complained that he was disruptive and impulsive, seeming to have little consideration for the other children. Charlie's teacher complained that it was difficult to even get through a routine class day because of Charlie's behavior. He would not sit in his seat like the other children and would often get up and run around the room. He could not work on an assignment for more than 5 minutes without being distracted. He would also distract his classmates by talking to them when they were supposed to be working quietly. None of the teacher's efforts seemed to be effective in quieting or calming Charlie.

On initial evaluation, Charlie was noted to be quite active. He entered the doctor's office with a firm, aggressive step. He jumped on his chair rather than sitting down, finally squirming himself into a sitting position, which he maintained for only 2 or 3 minutes. He then jumped up and began pulling books off the bookshelves. When told that they belonged to the doctor and should be placed back on the shelf, he threw one or two on the floor and proceeded to the doctor's desk to examine the pens, pencils, and paperweights. Charlie's mother looked embarrassed and exasperated and tried to get him to sit back down.

The psychiatrist decided to prescribe methylphenidate. Within a week Charlie's mother related that the effects were "amazing." Charlie's behavior had improved, and he showed a distinct increase in his ability to focus attention and a decrease in impulsive, overactive behavior. His teacher also noticed a distinct difference. He was able to complete the first grade with only minimal difficulty and was considered to have appropriate progress for his age in basic skills of learning to read and to do very simple arithmetic.

Increasing numbers of adults also have been given diagnoses of ADHD in recent years, contributing to a rising number of cases and raising concerns about overdiagnosis, as well as the risk for substance abuse because the disorder is treated with stimulants. For that reason, the clinician should exert great care before making the diagnosis. Individuals with adult ADHD may present with difficulties at work caused by inattentiveness as their chief complaint. Alternatively, they may seek treatment because of troublesome impulsive behavior.

Epidemiology, Clinical Findings, and Course

The prevalence of ADHD is about 5% in young and school-age children and 2.5% in adults. It is far more common in boys than in girls, with a male-to-female ratio of approximately 3:1. Approximately one-half of the children with this disorder have a good outcome, completing school on schedule with acceptable grades consistent with their family background and family expectations. Longitudinal studies show that a substantial proportion of children with ADHD remain relatively impaired into adulthood. With adults, the inattentiveness tends to persist as the hyperactivity subsides.

ADHD is most often identified during elementary school years and is relatively stable through early adolescence. Some children have a worsened course with development of antisocial behaviors, some meeting criteria for conduct disorder. Those with antisocial behavior also have higher rates of substance abuse, more arrests, more suicide attempts, and more car accidents; they complete fewer years of school than children without ADHD. Problems with confidence and self-esteem may be prominent because the disorder invites rejection by both parents and peers. Interestingly, treatment with stimulant drugs has been associated with decreased risk for substance abuse. Thus, treating the disorder not only brings symptomatic relief but can lead to a better long-term outcome.

Etiology and Pathophysiology

The etiology and pathophysiology of ADHD are uncertain, but it is well documented that ADHD runs in families and appears to be highly heritable. Genetic studies have begun to identify genes underlying ADHD, but none appear causal. Because dopamine mediates brain reward systems and because the treatments used for ADHD (i.e., stimulants) may work through the dopamine system, genes related to dopamine have received special attention. For example, in one study, a mutation in the dopamine transporter gene was identified in 55% of the patients with ADHD as compared with 8% of controls.

Nongenetic factors also may be important in the development of ADHD. Initial descriptions of ADHD referred to the disorder as *minimal brain dysfunction*. Risk factors include perinatal problems such as maternal smoking, substance abuse, obstetrical complications, malnutrition, exposure to toxins, and viral infections. The possible role of such factors is consistent with the higher prevalence of ADHD in boys because they are more vulnerable than girls to prenatal and perinatal injury. Some children with ADHD have experienced abuse or neglect or have experienced multiple placements in foster care. These same factors predispose to antisocial behavior.

Brain imaging studies using MRI indicate that the prefrontal cortex, basal ganglia, and cerebellum either are reduced in size or have abnormalities in asymmetry in children with ADHD. These findings correlate well with neuropsychological data showing that people with ADHD have difficulties in response inhibition, executive functions mediated through the prefrontal cortex, or timing functions mediated through the cerebellum. Functional imaging studies have shown hypoperfusion in prefrontal and basal ganglia regions that may be reversible with stimulant treatment.

Differential Diagnosis

In making a differential diagnosis, the clinician must be aware that a child with ADHD may have comorbid disorders common in childhood, such as seizure disorders, conduct disorder, oppositional defiant disorder, or learning disorders. When any of these disorders is present, it is often difficult to distinguish which is primary and which is secondary. Childhood bipolar disorder or depression may present with similar or overlapping symptoms. In some cases, ADHD symptoms may appear to be a normal response to an abusive home environment. Neuroendocrine abnormalities such as thyroid disorder also need to be ruled out.

Clinical Management

Most children respond favorably to stimulants. Methylphenidate (10–60 mg/day) is usually the first line of treatment, followed by dextroamphetamine (5–40 mg/day). If neither of these succeeds, atomoxetine (Strattera), an α_2 agonist (e.g., clonidine, guanfacine), imipramine, or bupropion may be used. In general, methylphenidate and dextroamphetamine offer short-term effects, lasting 4–6 hours, whereas the effects of the antidepressants tend to last longer. Stimulant drugs are now available in a number of slow- or extended-release formulations.

Stimulants should be initiated at a low dosage and titrated upward according to response and side effects within the recommended dosage range. They are given after meals to reduce the likelihood of appetite suppression. Starting treatment with a morning dose may be useful in assessing the drug's effect, because morning and afternoon school performance can then be compared. The need for medication on weekends or after school must be determined on an individual basis. Weight should be monitored during the initial titration, and weight and height should be measured several times each year. Feedback from schoolteachers can help to assess the child's response.

Early side effects include appetite suppression, weight loss, irritability, abdominal pain, and insomnia. Mild dysphoria and social withdrawal may occur at higher dosages in some patients. In rare cases, children can develop a depression requiring drug discontinuation. One concern has been the potential for stimulants to cause growth retardation. Research shows that any decrease in expected weight gain is small and probably insignificant. Other side effects include dizziness, nausea, nightmares, dry mouth, constipation, lethargy, anxiety, hyperacusis, and fearfulness.

Parents can benefit from learning basic behavioral management skills, such as the value of positive reinforcement and firm, nonpunitive limit setting, as well as methods for reducing stimulation, thereby diminishing distractibility and inattentiveness. For example, the child with ADHD does better when playing with one friend rather than with groups of children. Noisy or complex toys should be avoided, as should toys that encourage impulsivity and aggression. The parent may want to work closely with the child in completing homework tasks and to teach him or her the value of working on tasks in the single, small increments that are best suited to the child's relatively short attention span, mastering one completely before going on to another.

Clinicians should use caution in treating adolescents and adults who are overly invested in the ADHD diagnosis or its treatment. Clinicians should be wary of patients who seek treatment with stimulants, who request specific drugs by name, or who seem intent on obtaining these drugs. In the last decade the abuse of stimulants has reached epidemic proportions, especially in high schools and colleges, among people who use them for recreation or to enhance their academic performance. In addition to the euphoriant effects that users seek, stimulants—particularly at higher dosages—can induce psychotic symptoms such as hallucinations, delusion, or paranoia. In many cases, the abuse will lead to psychiatric hospitalization because the symptoms can simulate schizophrenia and may require treatment with antipsychotics.

■ Specific Learning Disorder

Specific learning disorder is characterized by an inability to achieve in a designated area of learning at a level consistent with the person's overall intellectual functioning. Typically, a child will have learning problems in one or more areas: reading, mathematics, or written expression. The essential feature is a persistent problem in acquiring or learning academic skills as quickly or as accurately as peers during the years of formal schooling (i.e., the developmental period). Academic skills will be well below the average range for his or her age. Reading disorders are often called *dyslexia*. A commonly used term for mathematic disorders is *dyscalculia*. Specific learning disorder affects about 5%–15% of school-age children; it is from two to three times more common in boys than in girls.

Specific learning disorder is a clinical diagnosis based on a comprehensive evaluation of the child's medical, developmental, family, and educational history, along with school reports and educational testing. The latter is essential and, for example, may indicate that the child is performing markedly below a level expected on the basis of his or her IQ. For example, a 14-year-old with reading disorder may have an IQ of 110 and be reading at a third-grade level.

Specific learning disorder clusters in families. The relative risk for disabilities in reading or mathematics is substantially higher (e.g., 4–8 times and 5–10 times higher, respectively) in first-degree relatives of individuals with these learning difficulties compared with those without them. The disorder is thought to represent a neurodevelopmental defect or the result of a cerebral injury; known risk factors include prematurity, low birth weight, and maternal smoking.

If not diagnosed and treated early and aggressively, specific learning disorder can be extremely handicapping. Although children with this disorder typically have normal intelligence, they often come to view themselves as failures and feel rejected by their peers because of their inability to progress academically in a particular area.

The frustration associated with impairment in academic skills is also associated with a variety of complications, such as truancy, school refusal, conduct disorder, mood disorder, or substance abuse. Rather than being causal, specific learning disorder may be comorbid with these conditions, as well as with ADHD. In this instance, it is important for the clinician to recognize the multiple disorders and to treat both (or all) of them appropriately.

Educational intervention proceeds on two fronts. Children or teenagers usually need remedial instruction to bolster their academic skills, as well as instruction in developing "attack" skills that will assist them in learning strategies to compensate for the neural deficits that underlie their condition. With steady, sympathetic educational support, most children with these deficits are able to develop acceptable skills in reading, writing, and arithmetic.

■ Motor Disorders

Developmental Coordination Disorder

The essential feature of developmental coordination disorder is a marked impairment in the acquisition of skills requiring motor coordination. Manifestations differ by age, but children with the disorder are usually seen by their parents and peers as physically awkward. Younger children may display delays and clumsiness in achieving developmental motor milestones such as crawling, sitting, and walking or in acquiring and using motor skills or mastering tasks such as negotiating stairs, pedaling bicycles, buttoning shirts, and using zippers. Older children may display difficulties with motor aspects of assembling puzzles or building models or with participating in various sports activities. The disorder is diagnosed when the impairment significantly interferes with the performance of or participation in daily activities such as getting dressed, eating meals with appropriate utensils, engaging in games with peers, and participating in sports at school. Children with this disorder can develop low self-esteem and sense of self-worth, and emotional or behavioral problems. For adolescents and adults, impairment in fine motor skills and motor speed may affect performance in the workplace or school setting. Onset is in the early developmental period. Developmental coordination disorder must be distinguished from other medical conditions that may produce coordination problems, such as cerebral palsy, muscular dystrophy, visual impairment, or an intellectual developmental disorder.

Stereotypic Movement Disorder

Stereotypic movement disorder is characterized by repetitive, often seemingly driven, and apparently purposeless motor behaviors that interfere with social, academic, and other activities or result in self-injury. Typical movements can include hand waving, rocking, playing with hands, fiddling with fingers, twirling objects, head banging, self-biting, or hitting various parts of one's own body. These behaviors may cause permanent and disabling tissue damage and may sometimes be life-threatening.

The disorder has an onset in early childhood. The behaviors are not better explained by the physiological effects of a substance, a neurological condition, or another neurodevelopmental or mental disorder (e.g., a compulsion in obsessive-compulsive disorder, a tic in Tourette's disorder, a stereotypy that is part of an autism spectrum disorder, or hair pulling in trichotillomania).

Tic Disorders

The tic disorders are a fascinating group of disorders characterized by the presence of stereotypical but nonrhythmic "jerky" movements and vocalizations called *tics*. DSM-5 lists five tic disorders; the best known is Tourette's disorder, which is described below. The others are persistent (chronic) motor or vocal tic disorder, and provisional tic disorder. There are two residual categories (other specified tic disorder and unspecified tic disorder) that can be used in cases where the tics do not neatly fit within one of the better recognized categories: for example, tic disorders that result from the effect of certain substances (e.g., cocaine) or medical conditions (e.g., Huntington's disease).

Tourette's Disorder

Tourette's disorder is a syndrome involving the production of both motor and vocal tics. The vocal tics can be somewhat socially offensive, such as making loud grunting or barking noises or shouting words. The words are sometimes obscenities such as "shit." The person is aware that he or she is producing the vocal tics and is able to exert a mild degree of control over them, but ultimately has to submit to them. Because people with Tourette's disorder are aware that their tics are socially inappropriate, they find them embarrassing. Motor tics occurring in Tourette's disorder are also often odd or offensive behaviors, such as tongue protrusion, sniffing, hopping, squatting, blinking, or nodding. Because most of the general public is unaware of the nature of Tourette's disorder, the behavior is seen as inappropriate or bizarre. The tics tend to worsen when the individual is anxious, excited, or fatigued. Onset occurs before age 18, and the condition must have lasted at least 1 year. The DSM-5 criteria for Tourette's disorder appear in Box 4–4.

Box 4–4.   DSM-5 Diagnostic Criteria for Tourette's Disorder

A. Both multiple motor and one or more vocal tics have been present at some time during the illness, although not necessarily concurrently.
B. The tics may wax and wane in frequency but have persisted for more than 1 year since first tic onset.
C. Onset is before age 18 years.
D. The disturbance is not attributable to the physiological effects of a substance (e.g., cocaine) or another medical condition (e.g., Huntington's disease, postviral encephalitis).

Epidemiology, clinical findings, and course.   Once considered relatively rare, the disorder affects about 3 to 8 schoolchildren per 1,000. Tics themselves are very common in childhood but tend to be transient. Up to 20% of children, however, experience transient simple tics. Tourette's disorder is more common in boys than girls, with a ratio of approximately 3:1. As with ADHD, a gender threshold effect has been observed with Tourette's disorder; that is, girls appear to have higher genetic loading than boys, suggesting that there is a lower penetrance for the disorder in females.

Tourette's disorder begins in childhood or early adolescence. Tics often begin between the ages of 4 and 6 years, with motor tics generally preceding the appearance of vocal tics. Tic severity tends to peak between ages 10 and 12. People tend to have fewer symptoms as they age, although a small percentage will have persistently severe or worsening symptoms in adulthood. Patients with Tourette's disorder typically experience shame and embarrassment about their disorder, which may lead them to avoid public or social situations or even close interpersonal relationships.

Etiology and pathophysiology.   Tourette's disorder is highly familial and comorbid with obsessive-compulsive disorder (OCD). Clinically, tics and compulsions have a superficial resemblance, suggesting that these symptoms may lie along a continuum. Two-thirds of the first-degree relatives of patients with Tourette's disorder have tics, and a substantial number also have OCD.

The search for candidate genes is ongoing, particularly genes related to dopamine neurotransmission, prompted by the observation that the symptoms of Tourette's disorder can be markedly improved through treatment with antipsychotic medications, which work primarily by blocking dopaminergic pathways. Because of its prominent motor component, investigators suspect that the primary abnormalities in Tourette's disorder may lie within nigrostriatal projections, but (given the complex feedback loops of the dopamine system, as described in Chapter 3, "The Neurobiology and Genetics of Mental Illness") many other localizations are also possible.

Some children with Tourette's disorder have their onset of symptoms after infection with group A β-hemolytic *Streptococcus*. Streptococcal infections are a well-known cause of Sydenham's chorea, and it now appears that Tourette's disorder is a related condition. This group of syndromes is now referred to as a pediatric autoimmune neuropsychiatric disorder associated with streptococcal infections (PANDAS).

Differential diagnosis. The evaluation of a patient presenting with Tourette's disorder should include a comprehensive neurological evaluation to rule out other possible causes of the tics. The patient should be examined for the stigmata of Wilson's disease, and a family history should be obtained to evaluate the possibility of Huntington's disease. The patient also should be evaluated for other psychiatric conditions. Comorbidity with ADHD and learning disorders may occur, as may symptoms of mood and anxiety disorders, or OCD.

Tourette's disorder also must be differentiated from persistent (chronic) motor or vocal tic disorder, which is characterized by the presence of either motor tics or vocal tics but not both. Other clinical features are the same for both conditions, including onset before age 18 years. The diagnosis of a persistent tic disorder cannot be made if the individual has ever met the criteria for Tourette's disorder.

Clinical management. The clinical management of Tourette's disorder has emphasized the use of antipsychotics, although treatment is often started with low dosages of α-adrenergic drugs (e.g., clonidine, 0.2–0.3 mg/day; guanfacine, 1.5–4 mg/day). Haloperidol and pimozide are the best-studied antipsychotics, but due to their many side effects, second-generation antipsychotics (e.g., risperidone, 1–3 mg/day; ziprasidone, 20–40 mg/day) are generally prescribed if adrenergic medications are ineffective. In addition to prescribing medication, it is important to educate the family about the disorder and to assist them in providing psychological support to the patient. Because of the social embarrassment that it produces, Tourette's disorder has a potential for serious long-term social complications, and supportive psychotherapy for the patient or family may help minimize these problems.

■ Other "Adult" Disorders Frequently Seen in Children

Several common "adult" disorders may have their first onset during childhood or adolescence. Because these are syndromally similar across all ages, they are classified with the adult disorders. Common examples are schizophrenia, major depression, and bipolar disorder. In general, children with these disorders meet the criteria that have been defined for adults. There may be subtle differences in presentation and management, however.

Schizophrenia often presents initially during adolescence, but in rare instances the onset is during childhood. Schizophrenia in adolescents typically begins insidiously, with apathy, a change in personal hygiene, and withdrawal. Schizophrenia may be particularly difficult to distinguish from depression, and it is usually preferable to make an initial diagnosis of depression if there is any doubt; after an unsuccessful trial of several different antidepressants, the diagnosis of schizophrenia is more certain, particularly when the clinical picture is consistent with the adult presentation. The major challenge in assessing childhood schizophrenia involves determining the difference between normal childhood fantasies and frank delusions and hallucinations. In addition, the symptoms of disorganization of speech and behavior must be distinguished from abnormalities of speech and behavior that are simply due to developmental slowness or intellectual disability. Children with a definite diagnosis of schizophrenia usually are treated with antipsychotic medications, but the dosage is typically lower than that used in adults.

Mood disorders in adolescents are extremely common and are also more common in children than was thought several decades ago. Up to 5% of children and 8% of adolescents meet diagnostic criteria for major depression. The patient with major depression may present initially with physical complaints rather than the psychological complaint of depression. In young children, the complaints may be abdominal pain, nightmares, or trouble sleeping. In teenagers, complaints of fatigue, insomnia or hypersomnia, headache, or tension are common. Depression also may present initially with disruptive behavior such as that seen in oppositional defiant disorder or conduct disorder. A combination of medication and psychotherapy might provide the best chance for recovery. Fluoxetine and escitalopram are approved by the FDA for the treatment of pediatric depression and should be used as first-line medications.

In 2003, the FDA issued a black box warning about the risk of increased suicidal behavior in children, adolescents, and young adults (<25 years) taking antidepressants and advised "close supervision" of such patients. This warning was based on an analysis of pooled results of treatment studies that showed there might be an increased risk for broadly defined suicidal behavior with short-term antidepressant use in these patients, although no actual suicides were reported. Unfortunately, this warning had the unintended result of reducing prescriptions for antidepressants, without any increase in doctor visits. There is some evidence that the warning may have led to an increase in suicidal behaviors because many cases of depression have gone untreated.

Bipolar disorder presenting with mania is also becoming increasingly recognized in children and adolescents. This has led to some controversy, because many of its symptoms overlap with ADHD and other disruptive behavior disorders. The essential element that distinguishes the syndromes is the distinct quality of the mood. In mania, the child will be overly happy, giddy, or euphoric. Sometimes the child will just be irritable. Bipolar disorder in children is generally treated with the same medications used in adults.

In response to concerns that bipolar disorder has been overdiagnosed in children, DSM-5 has included the new diagnosis *disruptive mood dysregulation disorder,* characterized by severe and repeated temper outbursts (described in Chapter 6, "Mood Disorders"). Many children formerly diagnosed with bipolar disorder will fit this new category. Research has shown that children diagnosed with bipolar disorder differ in fundamental ways from adolescents and adults with bipolar disorder, including clinical symptoms, family history, and outcome, leading to the conclusion that many if not most of the children were probably not bipolar after all.

■ Self-Assessment Questions

1. Describe some techniques that are useful in assessing children and establishing rapport with them.
2. List and describe the various types of nonphysician clinicians who may be helpful in assessing and managing children and adolescents.
3. Describe the various levels used to define intellectual developmental disorder. How are they assigned?
4. Discuss the distinction between autism spectrum disorder, intellectual disability, and specific learning disorder.

Clinical points for the neurodevelopmental (child) disorders

1. In assessing children and adolescents, the clinician should be imaginative and meet each patient on his or her own terms.
    -   Problem-solving and motor skills can be evaluated by playing games.
    -   Dolls and toys should be used with young children to create pretend situations that will provide insight about personal and social interactions.
2. Normal maturational levels are highly variable in children and adolescents.
3. Children and adolescents often do not have a level of cognitive development suitable for the insight-oriented and introspective approaches used with adults.
4. Establishing rapport with adolescents is difficult but may be crucial to creating a therapeutic alliance.
    -   The therapist should find out what the patient is interested in and relate to him or her through these interests.
5. The clinician must not preach or judge.
6. The basic maturational task of adolescents is to disengage themselves from their parents, become independent, and define their own identities; reliance on peers is an important crutch for adolescents in this transitional period.
7. The therapist should remain neutral and try not to criticize either parents or peers.
8. The adolescent's first reaction may be to see the therapist as a parent. The therapist should try to use this to therapeutic advantage, or at least try to prevent it from being a therapeutic handicap.
9. It is best to strike a balance between being perceived as a good parent and being perceived as a good peer, but this balance cannot and should not (usually) be achieved by attacking the real parent or real peer.
10. Because the parents and peers of adolescents may vary in quality, the therapist needs to be flexible, insightful, and creative in dealing with the patient's perceptions of him or her.
11. The clinician must be aware of the pervasiveness of comorbidity in childhood and adolescent disorders.

5. List three well-recognized causes of intellectual disability.
6. Describe the three major domains that are abnormal in autism spectrum disorder and give examples of signs and symptoms within these domains. How common is autism spectrum disorder?

What are its long-term course and outcome? What methods are used to treat it?

7. List the two broad categories of symptoms used to define ADHD and give several examples of each. Describe the long-term course and outcome of ADHD. Identify the medications commonly used to treat ADHD.

8. Define *specific learning disorder* and list the three skills that are commonly affected.

9. Describe the clinical features of Tourette's disorder. Describe two pharmacological strategies for treating Tourette's disorder.

Chapter 5

Schizophrenia Spectrum and Other Psychotic Disorders

I felt a Cleaving in my Mind—
As if my Brain had split—
I tried to match it—Seam by Seam—
But could not make them fit.

Emily Dickinson

Schizophrenia is not a "split personality,"** as many people assume, based on its name. The illness is called "schizo" (fragmented or split apart) "phrenia" (mind) because it causes its victims to experience profound disabilities in their capacity to think clearly and to feel normal emotions. It is probably the most devastating illness that psychiatrists treat. Schizophrenia strikes people just when they are preparing to enter the phase of their lives in which they can achieve their highest growth and productivity—typically in the teens or early 20s—leaving most of them unable to return to normal young adult lives: to go to school, to find a job, or to marry and have children. According to *The Global Burden of Disease*, a World Health Organization–sponsored study of the cost of medical illnesses worldwide, schizophrenia is among the 10 leading causes of disability in the world among people in the 15–44 age range.

In addition to schizophrenia, DSM-5 recognizes an entire spectrum of psychotic disorders that also includes delusional disorder, brief psychotic disorder, schizophreniform disorder, schizoaffective disorder, substance and medication-related psychotic disorders, and catatonic disorder due to another medical condition (Table 5–1). Although *schizotypal personality disorder* is considered to fall within the schizophrenia

TABLE 5–1.   **DSM-5 schizophrenia spectrum and other psychotic disorders**

Schizotypal personality disorder (see Chapter 17)

Delusional disorder

Brief psychotic disorder

Schizophreniform disorder

Schizophrenia

Schizoaffective disorder

Substance/medication-induced psychotic disorder

Psychotic disorder due to another medical condition

Catatonia associated with another mental disorder (catatonia specifier)

Catatonic disorder due to another medical condition

Unspecified catatonia

Other specified schizophrenia spectrum and other psychotic disorder

Unspecified schizophrenia spectrum and other psychotic disorder

spectrum, its criteria and description are to be found in Chapter 17 ("Personality Disorders"). For individuals who do not fit into any of the better-defined categories, the residual categories *other specified schizophrenia spectrum and other psychotic disorder* and *unspecified schizophrenia spectrum and other psychotic disorder* are available. Catatonia is defined with specific criteria and can be used to subtype other disorders.

■ Delusional Disorder

Delusional disorder is characterized by the presence of well-systematized delusions accompanied by affect appropriate to the delusion occurring in the presence of a relatively well-preserved personality. The delusions will have lasted at least 1 month; behavior is generally not odd or bizarre apart from the delusion or its ramifications; active-phase symptoms that may occur in schizophrenia (e.g., disorganized speech. negative symptoms) are absent; and the disorder is not due to a mood disorder, is not substance induced, and is not due to a medical condition (see Box 5–1).

Box 5–1.   DSM-5 Diagnostic Criteria for Delusional Disorder

A. The presence of one (or more) delusions with a duration of 1 month or longer.
B. Criterion A for schizophrenia has never been met.
   Note: Hallucinations, if present, are not prominent and are related to the delusional theme (e.g., the sensation of being infested with insects associated with delusions of infestation).
C. Apart from the impact of the delusion(s) or its ramifications, functioning is not markedly impaired, and behavior is not obviously bizarre or odd.
D. If manic or major depressive episodes have occurred, these have been brief relative to the duration of the delusional periods.
E. The disturbance is not attributable to the physiological effects of a substance or another medical condition and is not better explained by another mental disorder, such as body dysmorphic disorder or obsessive-compulsive disorder.

Specify whether:
   Erotomanic type: This subtype applies when the central theme of the delusion is that another person is in love with the individual.
   Grandiose type: This subtype applies when the central theme of the delusion is the conviction of having some great (but unrecognized) talent or insight or having made some important discovery.
   Jealous type: This subtype applies when the central theme of the individual's delusion is that his or her spouse or lover is unfaithful.
   Persecutory type: This subtype applies when the central theme of the delusion involves the individual's belief that he or she is being conspired against, cheated, spied on, followed, poisoned or drugged, maliciously maligned, harassed, or obstructed in the pursuit of long-term goals.
   Somatic type: This subtype applies when the central theme of the delusion involves bodily functions or sensations.
   Mixed type: This subtype applies when no one delusional theme predominates.
   Unspecified type: This subtype applies when the dominant delusional belief cannot be clearly determined or is not described in the specific types (e.g., referential delusions without a prominent persecutory or grandiose component).

Specify if:
   With bizarre content: Delusions are deemed bizarre if they are clearly implausible, not understandable, and not derived from ordinary life experiences (e.g., an individual's belief that a stranger has removed his or her internal organs and replaced them with someone else's organs without leaving any wounds or scars).

Specify if:
The following course specifiers are only to be used after a 1-year duration of the disorder:

First episode, currently in acute episode: First manifestation of the disorder meeting the defining diagnostic symptom and time criteria. An *acute episode* is a time period in which the symptom criteria are fulfilled.

First episode, currently in partial remission: *Partial remission* is a time period during which an improvement after a previous episode is maintained and in which the defining criteria of the disorder are only partially fulfilled.

First episode, currently in full remission: *Full remission* is a period of time after a previous episode during which no disorder-specific symptoms are present.

Multiple episodes, currently in acute episode

Multiple episodes, currently in partial remission

Multiple episodes, currently in full remission

Continuous: Symptoms fulfilling the diagnostic symptom criteria of the disorder are remaining for the majority of the illness course, with subthreshold symptom periods being very brief relative to the overall course.

Unspecified

Specify current severity:

Severity is rated by a quantitative assessment of the primary symptoms of psychosis, including delusions, hallucinations, disorganized speech, abnormal psychomotor behavior, and negative symptoms. Each of these symptoms may be rated for its current severity (most severe in the last 7 days) on a 5-point scale ranging from 0 (not present) to 4 (present and severe). (See Clinician-Rated Dimensions of Psychosis Symptom Severity in the chapter "Assessment Measures.")

Note: Diagnosis of delusional disorder can be made without using this severity specifier.

The core feature of delusional disorder is the presence of a delusion in the absence of obviously odd or bizarre behavior. The person may be unimpaired, other than for the immediate impact of the delusion. If hallucinations are present, they are not prominent and are related to the theme of the delusion.

Epidemiology, Etiology, and Course

Delusional disorder is relatively rare, having a prevalence of about 0.2% in the general population; the persecutory type is the most common. There are no major gender differences in frequency. It is considered a disorder of middle to late adult life. Delusional disorder has a significant familial relationship with schizophrenia and schizotypal personality disorder. Although the disorder is thought to be chronic for most, people with delusional disorder are generally employed and self-supporting.

Clinical Findings

People with delusional disorder tend to be socially isolated and chronically suspicious. Those with persecutory or jealous delusions sometimes become angry and hostile, emotions that can lead to violent outbursts. They can be overtalkative and circumstantial, particularly when discussing their delusions. One observation is that many people with delusional disorder will become litigious and end up as lawyers' clients rather than as psychiatrists' patients.

The following DSM-5 subtypes are based on the predominant delusional theme:

- *Persecutory type*: The belief that one is being treated in some way or conspired against
- *Erotomanic type* (de Clerambault's syndrome): The belief that a person, usually of higher status, is in love with the patient
- *Grandiose type*: The belief that one is of inflated worth, power, knowledge, or identity or that one has a special relationship to a deity or famous person
- *Jealous type*: The belief that one's sexual partner is unfaithful
- *Somatic type*: The belief that one has some physical defect, disorder, or disease, such as AIDS

The residual category *unspecified type* is for patients who do not fit the previous categories (e.g., those who have been ill less than 1 month). The category *mixed type* is used for those with delusions characteristic of more than one subtype but without any single theme predominating.

The following patient seen in our hospital illustrates the erotomanic subtype:

> Doug, a 33-year-old restaurant manager, was brought to the hospital under court order. He allegedly had harassed and threatened a young woman. The following story gradually unfolded.
>
> Doug was convinced that an attractive young woman who worked in a local bookstore was in love with him, even though they had never met. He took as evidence of her affection glances and smiles they had exchanged when crossing paths in their small town. After learning her name and address, he sent her a "sexual business letter." Doug continued to send additional love letters over the next few years and carefully tracked her whereabouts. There were no other communications, but the letters indicated his belief that she was infatuated with him.
>
> The young woman reported her concerns to the police; they warned Doug not to call or write her, but this had little effect. Eventually a court order was sought when Doug's letters took a more threatening tone and

a "no contact" order failed to keep him away from the bookshop where she worked.

Doug was indignant about his hospitalization. Although he was circumstantial in describing his fantasy relationship, there was no evidence of a mood disorder, hallucinations, or bizarre delusions. He reported a history of a similar relationship 10 years earlier, consisting mostly of letters, which ended only when the girl moved out of town. Doug was a loner with few friends but functioned well in his position at work and was active in several community organizations.

At his mental health hearing, Doug denied that his behavior was inappropriate, but he agreed to undergo outpatient psychiatric treatment. The young woman eventually moved out of town.

Differential Diagnosis

The major differential diagnosis involves distinguishing delusional disorder from the mood disorders, schizophrenia, paranoid personality disorder, and body dysmorphic disorder. The chief distinction from psychotic mood disorders is that with delusional disorder, a depressive or manic syndrome is absent, develops after the psychotic symptoms, or is brief in relation to the psychotic symptoms. Unlike patients with schizophrenia, delusional disorder patients are free of disorganized speech, negative symptoms, and catatonic behavior. If hallucinations are present, they are not prominent. For example, tactile and olfactory hallucinations may be present when they are related to the delusional theme. Furthermore, the delusional disorder patient's personality is generally preserved. Persons with paranoid personality disorder may be suspicious and hypervigilant, but they are not delusional. With body dysmorphic disorder, patients may have delusional beliefs about their appearance (i.e., that a body part is misshapen or disfigured), but this does not meet criteria for delusional disorder because their somatic belief does not involve bodily functions or sensations.

Clinical Management

Because delusional disorder is uncommon, treatment recommendations are based on clinical observation and not careful research. Clinical experience suggests that response to antipsychotics is often poor; they may help relieve agitation and anxiety, but the core delusion remains intact. Any of the antipsychotics can be used, including one of the high-potency conventional antipsychotics (e.g., haloperidol 5–10 mg/day) or a second-generation antipsychotic (e.g., risperidone 2–6 mg/day). Monohypochondriacal paranoia (i.e., delusional disorder, somatic subtype) has been specifically reported to respond to the antipsychotic pimozide (4–8 mg/day). Selective serotonin reuptake inhibitors (e.g., fluoxetine, paroxetine) also have been reported to be helpful in reducing delusional beliefs in some patients.

The physician should make an effort to develop a trusting relationship with the patient, after which he or she may gently challenge the patient's beliefs by showing how they interfere with the patient's life. The patient should be assured of the confidential nature of the doctor-patient relationship. Tact and skill are necessary to persuade a patient to accept treatment, and the physician must neither condemn nor collude in the delusional beliefs. Group therapy is not recommended because patients with delusional disorder are often suspicious and tend to misinterpret situations that can arise in the course of the therapy.

Clinical points for delusional disorder

1. Because the patient with delusional disorder is suspicious, it may be very difficult to establish a therapeutic relationship.

   - Building a relationship will take time and patience.

   - The therapist must neither condemn nor collude in the delusional beliefs of the patient.

   - The patient must be assured of complete confidentiality.

2. Once rapport is established, the patient's delusional beliefs can be gently challenged by pointing out how they interfere with his or her functioning.

   - Tact and skill are needed to convince the patient to accept treatment.

3. A patient with delusional disorder may be more accepting of medication if it is explained as a treatment for the anxiety, dysphoria, and stress that may result from or accompany his or her delusions.

   - Antipsychotic medication should be tried, although results are unpredictable.

   - Patients with the somatic subtype may preferentially respond to pimozide.

■ Brief Psychotic Disorder

Patients with a *brief psychotic disorder* have psychotic symptoms that last at least 1 day but no more than 1 month, with gradual recovery. Psychotic mood disorders, schizophrenia, and the effects of drugs or medical conditions have been ruled out as causing the symptoms. Signs and symptoms are similar to those seen in schizophrenia, including hallucinations, delusions, and disorganized speech or grossly disorganized behavior. The four subtypes are: 1) with marked stressor(s), 2) without marked stressor(s), 3) with postpartum onset, and 4) with catatonia.

Patients with postpartum onset generally develop symptoms during pregnancy or within 4 weeks after delivery. *Postpartum psychosis,* as it is often called, tends to arise in otherwise normal individuals and resolves within 2–3 months. The disorder should be distinguished from *postpartum blues,* which occurs in up to 80% of new mothers, lasts for a few days after delivery, and is considered normal.

The prevalence of brief psychotic disorder may be as high as 9% of new-onset psychoses, and it is twice as common in women. The disorder is thought to occur more commonly in lower-income groups and among individuals with personality disorders, especially of the borderline and schizotypal types.

Hospitalization may be necessary for the safety of the patient or others. Because a brief psychotic disorder is probably self-limiting, no specific treatment is indicated, and the hospital milieu itself may be sufficient to help the patient recover. Antipsychotics may be helpful early on, especially when the patient is highly agitated or experiencing great emotional turmoil. After the patient has sufficiently recovered, the clinician can help him or her explore the meaning of the psychotic reaction and of the triggering stressor. Supportive psychotherapy may help restore morale and self-esteem.

■ Schizophreniform Disorder

Schizophreniform disorder is a diagnosis used for patients who present with symptoms typical of schizophrenia but have been ill for less than 6 months. In DSM-5, the definition requires that the following features be present: 1) the patient has psychotic symptoms characteristic of schizophrenia, such as hallucinations, delusions, or disorganized speech; 2) the symptoms are not due to a substance of abuse, a medication, or a medical condition; 3) schizoaffective disorder and mood disorder with psychotic features have been ruled out; and 4) the duration is at least 1 month but less than 6 months.

The diagnosis changes to schizophrenia if the condition persists past 6 months, even if only residual symptoms such as blunted affect remain. The diagnosis appears to identify a widely varying group of patients, most of whom eventually develop schizophrenia, a mood disorder, or schizoaffective disorder.

Clearly, the proper boundaries of this diagnosis remain in question; its main use is to guard against premature diagnosis of schizophrenia. Treatment of schizophreniform disorder has not been systematically evaluated. The principles for its management are similar to those for an acute exacerbation of schizophrenia, described below.

■ Schizophrenia

Definition

One of the greatest challenges to the student of schizophrenia is to understand the broad range of signs and symptoms that arise from its underlying cognitive and emotional impairments. Its symptoms include dysfunctions in nearly every capacity of which the human brain is capable—perception, inferential thinking, language, memory, and executive functions.

In DSM-5, *schizophrenia* is defined by a group of characteristic symptoms, such as hallucinations, delusions, or negative symptoms (i.e., affective flattening, alogia, avolition); deterioration in social, occupational, or interpersonal relationships; and continuous signs of the disturbance for at least 6 months. (See Box 5–2 for the DSM-5 diagnostic criteria for schizophrenia.)

Box 5–2.   DSM-5 Diagnostic Criteria for Schizophrenia

A. Two (or more) of the following, each present for a significant portion of time during a 1-month period (or less if successfully treated). At least one of these must be (1), (2), or (3):

1. Delusions.
2. Hallucinations.
3. Disorganized speech (e.g., frequent derailment or incoherence).
4. Grossly disorganized or catatonic behavior.
5. Negative symptoms (i.e., diminished emotional expression or avolition).

B. For a significant portion of the time since the onset of the disturbance, level of functioning in one or more major areas, such as work, interpersonal relations, or self-care, is markedly below the level achieved prior to the onset (or when the onset is in childhood or adolescence, there is failure to achieve expected level of interpersonal, academic, or occupational functioning).

C. Continuous signs of the disturbance persist for at least 6 months. This 6-month period must include at least 1 month of symptoms (or less if successfully treated) that meet Criterion A (i.e., active-phase symptoms) and may include periods of prodromal or residual symptoms. During these prodromal or residual periods, the signs of the disturbance may be manifested by only negative symptoms or by two or more symptoms listed in Criterion A present in an attenuated form (e.g., odd beliefs, unusual perceptual experiences).

D. Schizoaffective disorder and depressive or bipolar disorder with psychotic features have been ruled out because either 1) no major depressive or manic episodes have occurred concurrently with the active-phase symptoms, or 2) if mood episodes have occurred during active-phase symptoms, they have been present for a minority of the total duration of the active and residual periods of the illness.

E. The disturbance is not attributable to the physiological effects of a substance (e.g., a drug of abuse, a medication) or another medical condition.

F. If there is a history of autism spectrum disorder or a communication disorder of childhood onset, the additional diagnosis of schizophrenia is made only if prominent delusions or hallucinations, in addition to the other required symptoms of schizophrenia, are also present for at least 1 month (or less if successfully treated).

Specify if:

The following course specifiers are only to be used after a 1-year duration of the disorder and if they are not in contradiction to the diagnostic course criteria.

First episode, currently in acute episode: First manifestation of the disorder meeting the defining diagnostic symptom and time criteria. An *acute episode* is a time period in which the symptom criteria are fulfilled.

First episode, currently in partial remission: *Partial remission* is a period of time during which an improvement after a previous episode is maintained and in which the defining criteria of the disorder are only partially fulfilled.

First episode, currently in full remission: *Full remission* is a period of time after a previous episode during which no disorder-specific symptoms are present.

Multiple episodes, currently in acute episode: Multiple episodes may be determined after a minimum of two episodes (i.e., after a first episode, a remission and a minimum of one relapse).

Multiple episodes, currently in partial remission

Multiple episodes, currently in full remission

Continuous: Symptoms fulfilling the diagnostic symptom criteria of the disorder are remaining for the majority of the illness course, with subthreshold symptom periods being very brief relative to the overall course.

Unspecified

Specify if:

With catatonia (refer to the criteria for catatonia associated with another mental disorder for definition).

Coding note: Use additional code [for] catatonia associated with schizophrenia to indicate the presence of the comorbid catatonia.

Specify current severity:

Severity is rated by a quantitative assessment of the primary symptoms of psychosis, including delusions, hallucinations, disorganized speech, abnormal psychomotor behavior, and negative symptoms. Each of these symptoms may be rated for its current severity (most severe in the last 7 days) on a 5-point scale ranging from 0 (not present) to 4 (present and severe). (See Clinician-Rated Dimensions of Psychosis Symptom Severity in the chapter "Assessment Measures.")

Note: Diagnosis of schizophrenia can be made without using this severity specifier.

Epidemiology

The worldwide prevalence of schizophrenia is about 0.5%–1%. Schizophrenia can develop at any age, but the age at first psychotic episode is typically 18–25 years for men and 21–30 years for women. Patients with schizophrenia tend not to marry and are less likely to have children than people without schizophrenia.

People with schizophrenia are at high risk for suicidal behavior. About one-third attempt suicide, and 1 in 10 eventually kill themselves. Risk factors for suicide include male gender, age less than 30 years, unemployment, chronic course, prior depression, past treatment for depression, history of substance abuse, and recent hospital discharge.

Clinical Findings

Using factor analysis, researchers have repeatedly identified three dimensions (or groups of related symptoms) in schizophrenia: psychoticism, negative symptoms, and disorganization. The psychotic dimension includes *positive symptoms* (i.e., symptoms characterized by the presence of something that should be absent, such as hearing voices). The negative dimension includes *negative symptoms* (i.e., symptoms characterized by the absence of something that should be present, such as avolition [lack of motivation]). The disorganized dimension includes disorganized speech and behavior and inappropriate affect.

The Psychotic Dimension

The *psychotic dimension* refers to hallucinations and delusions, two classic "psychotic" symptoms that reflect a patient's confusion about the loss of boundaries between himself or herself and the external world. *Hallucinations* are perceptions experienced without an external stimulus to the sense organs and have a quality similar to a true perception. Patients with schizophrenia commonly report auditory, visual, tactile, gustatory, or olfactory hallucinations or a combination of these. Auditory hallucinations are the most frequent; they are typically experienced as speech ("voices"). The voices may be mumbled or heard clearly, and they may speak words, phrases, or sentences. Visual hallucinations may be simple or complex and include flashes of light, persons, animals, or objects. Olfactory and gustatory hallucinations are often experienced together, especially as unpleasant tastes or odors. Tactile hallucinations may be experienced as sensations of being touched or pricked, electrical sensations, or *formication*, which is the sensation of insects crawling under the skin.

Delusions involve disturbance in thought rather than perception; they are firmly held beliefs that are untrue as well as contrary to a person's educational and cultural background. Delusions typically have somatic, grandiose, religious, nihilistic, sexual, or persecutory themes (Table 5–2) and often differ according to the patient's cultural background.

While very common in schizophrenia, delusions and hallucinations also occur in other conditions, such as the neurocognitive disorders and the mood disorders. Kurt Schneider, a German psychiatrist working in the early twentieth century, argued that certain types of hallucinations and delusions were of the "first rank," meaning that they are especially characteristic of schizophrenia. Examples include delusions of being forced to do things against one's will or that thoughts are being withdrawn from or inserted into one's mind. These symptoms tend to reflect a patient's confusion about the loss of boundaries between himself or herself and the external world.

The following case is of a patient evaluated in our hospital and illustrates symptoms characteristic of schizophrenia:

Jane, a 55-year-old woman, was admitted to the hospital for evaluation of agitation and paranoia. A former schoolteacher, she had lived in a series of rooming houses and had held only temporary jobs in the past 10 years.

Shy and socially awkward during her youth, Jane was an avid reader and a model student. She briefly joined a convent before attending college. She eventually obtained a teaching certificate but continued to live with her mother.

TABLE 5–2.   Varied content in delusions

Delusions	Foci of preoccupation
Grandiose	Possessing wealth or great beauty or having a special ability (e.g., extrasensory perception); having influential friends; being an important figure (e.g., Napoleon, Hitler)
Nihilistic	Believing that one is dead or dying; believing that one does not exist or that the world does not exist
Persecutory	Being persecuted by friends, neighbors, or spouse; being followed, monitored, or spied on by the government (e.g., FBI, CIA) or other important organizations (e.g., the Catholic church)
Somatic	Believing that one's organs have stopped functioning (e.g., that the heart is no longer beating) or are rotting away; believing that the nose or another body part is terribly misshapen or disfigured
Sexual	Believing that one's sexual behavior is commonly known; that one is a prostitute, pedophile, or rapist; that masturbation has led to illness or insanity
Religious	Believing that one has sinned against God, that one has a special relationship to God or some other deity, that one has a special religious mission, or that one is the Devil or is condemned to burn in Hell

She was first hospitalized at age 25 after becoming convinced that her neighbors were harassing her. For the next 20 years, Jane believed she was at the center of a government cabal to change her identity. The FBI, the judicial system, the Roman Catholic Church, hospital personnel, and, it seems, most of her neighbors were involved in the plot. At age 49, Jane was hospitalized after her landlord discovered her pounding on the ceiling and walls of her apartment with a broom in an effort to stop the perceived harassment.

At admission, Jane reported that she was simply responding to the discomfort the landlord and neighbors had caused by "zapping" her with electronic beams. She believed that electromagnetic waves were being used to control her actions and thoughts, and she described a bizarre sensation of electricity moving around her body when the landlord was nearby.

Jane cooperated fully but was upset about her hospitalization, which she believed to be unnecessary. Jane was circumstantial but spoke in a clear, strong voice that one might expect after years of teaching. After 1 month of antipsychotic therapy, Jane remained delusional but was less concerned about her perceived harassment. Because of her poor insight and history of medication noncompliance, Jane was given an intramuscular antipsychotic before discharge.

The Negative Dimension

DSM-5 lists two negative symptoms as characteristic of schizophrenia: diminished emotional expression and avolition. Other negative symptoms common in schizophrenia are alogia and anhedonia. These symptoms are described below:

- *Diminished emotional expression (affective flattening or blunting)* is a reduced intensity of emotional expression and response. It is manifested by unchanging facial expression, decreased spontaneous movements, poverty of expressive gestures, poor eye contact, lack of voice inflections, and slowed speech.
- *Avolition* is a loss of the ability to initiate goal-directed behavior and to carry it through to completion. Patients seem inert and unmotivated.
- *Alogia* is characterized by a diminution in the amount of spontaneous speech or a tendency to produce speech that is empty or impoverished in content when the amount is adequate.
- *Anhedonia* is the inability to experience pleasure. Patients may describe themselves as feeling emotionally empty and unable to enjoy activities that previously gave them pleasure, such as playing sports or visiting with family or friends.

The Disorganization Dimension

The *disorganization dimension* refers to disorganized speech, disorganized or bizarre behavior, and inappropriate affect.

Disorganized speech, or *thought disorder,* was regarded as the most important symptom by Eugen Bleuler, who was responsible for coining the term *schizophrenia* to highlight the importance of fragmenting of thought. Standard definitions for various types of thought disorders have been developed that stress objective aspects of language and communication (which are empirical indicators of "thought"), such as derailment (loose associations), poverty of speech, poverty of content of speech, and tangential replies, and all have been found to occur frequently in both schizophrenia and mood disorders. Manic patients often have a thought disorder characterized by tangentiality, derailment, and illogicality. Depressed patients manifest thought disorder less frequently than do manic patients but often have poverty of speech, tangentiality, or circumstantiality. Other types of formal thought disorder include perseveration, distractibility, clanging, neologisms, echolalia, and blocking. With the possible exception of clanging in mania, none appears to be disorder specific.

Many patients with schizophrenia have various types of disorganized motor and social behavior, another aspect of this dimension. Abnormal motor behaviors include

- *Catatonic stupor:* The patient is immobile, mute, and unresponsive, yet fully conscious.
- *Catatonic excitement:* The patient has uncontrolled and aimless motor activity. Patients sometimes assume bizarre or uncomfortable postures (e.g., squatting) and maintain them for long periods.
- *Stereotypy:* The patient has a repeated but non-goal-directed movement, such as back-and-forth rocking.
- *Mannerisms:* The patient has goal-directed activities that are either odd in appearance or out of context, such as grimacing.
- *Echopraxia:* The patient imitates movements and gestures of another person.
- *Automatic obedience:* The patient carries out simple commands in a robot-like fashion.
- *Negativism:* The patient refuses to cooperate with simple requests for no apparent reason.

Disorganized behavior is common in schizophrenia patients, particularly as the illness advances. Patients neglect themselves, become messy or unkempt, and wear dirty or inappropriate clothing. They ignore their surroundings so that they become cluttered and untidy. Patients sometimes develop other odd behaviors that break social conventions, such as foraging through garbage bins or shouting obscenities. Many of today's street people have schizophrenia.

Inappropriate affect is another component of the disorganized dimension. Patients may smile inappropriately when speaking of neutral or sad topics or giggle for no apparent reason.

Other Symptoms

Many patients *lack insight;* they do not believe they are ill and reject the idea that they need treatment. Orientation and memory usually are normal, unless they are impaired by the patient's psychotic symptoms, inattention, or distractibility.

Nonlocalizing *neurological soft signs* occur in some patients and include abnormalities in stereognosis, graphesthesia, balance, and proprioception. Some patients have disturbances of sleep, sexual interest, and other bodily functions. Many schizophrenic patients have inactive sex drives and avoid sexual intimacy.

Substance abuse is common and includes alcohol and other drugs. Patients who abuse substances tend to be young, male, and poorly adherent with treatment; they also have more frequent hospitalizations than those who do not abuse substances. It is thought that many schizophrenic patients abuse substances in an attempt to lift their mood, boost their level of motivation, or reduce their medication side effects (e.g., akinesia).

Common symptoms of schizophrenia are shown in Table 5–3.

Course of Illness

Schizophrenia typically begins with a prodromal phase in the mid to late teens that is characterized by subtle changes in emotional, cognitive, and social functioning. This is followed by an active phase, during which psychotic symptoms develop. Many patients go for as long as 2 years before symptoms become so troubling that a psychiatrist is consulted. The psychotic symptoms usually respond relatively well to antipsychotic treatment, but ongoing problems such as blunted emotions or odd behavior tend to persist as the person passes into a residual phase. Acute exacerbations tend to occur from time to time, even when the patient continues to take medication. Typical stages of schizophrenia are outlined in Table 5–4.

Breaking the news about the diagnosis to the patient and his or her family can be very difficult. The first question that they will ask is "What does the future hold?" While it is always difficult to know for sure in any particular case, many clinicians were taught the "rule of thirds": about one-third of patients first diagnosed with schizophrenia will have a relatively good outcome, with minimal symptoms and mild impairments in cognition and social functioning; one-third will have a poor outcome, with persistence of psychotic symptoms, prominent negative symptoms, and significant psychosocial impairment; and one-third will have an outcome somewhere in the middle. As originally formulated, the rule of thirds was based on relatively limited clinical observation rather than rigorous scientific studies. Nonetheless, these studies stressed an important fact: schizophrenia has a variable outcome. In fact, follow-up studies show that a variety of features are associated with outcome (summarized in Table 5–5). Among these, IQ is one of the strongest predictors of outcome, with age at onset, gender, severity and type of initial symptoms, and structural brain abnormalities also having predictive value.

Cross-cultural studies show that patients in less developed countries tend to have better outcomes than those in more developed ones.

TABLE 5–3. Frequency of symptoms in 111 patients with schizophrenia

Negative symptoms	%	Positive symptoms	%
Affective flattening		**Hallucinations**	
Unchanging facial expression	96	Auditory	75
Decreased spontaneous movements	66	Voices commenting	58
Paucity of expressive gestures	81	Voices conversing	57
Poor eye contact	71	Somatic-tactile	20
Affective nonresponsivity	64	Olfactory	6
Inappropriate affect	63	Visual	49
Lack of vocal inflections	73	**Delusions**	
Alogia		Persecutory	81
Poverty of speech	53	Jealous	4
Poverty of content of speech	51	Guilt, sin	26
Blocking	23	Grandiose	39
Increased response latency	31	Religious	31
Avolition-apathy		Somatic	28
Impaired grooming and hygiene	87	Delusions of reference	49
Lack of persistence at work		Delusions of	
or school	95	being controlled	46
Physical anergia	82	Delusions of	
Anhedonia-asociality		mind reading	48
Few recreational interests/activities	95	Thought broadcasting	23
Little sexual interest/activity	69	Thought insertion	31
Impaired intimacy/closeness	84	Thought withdrawal	27
Few relationships with friends/		**Bizarre behavior**	
peers	96	Clothing, appearance	20
Attention		Social, sexual behavior	33
Social inattentiveness	78	Aggressive-agitated	27
Inattentiveness during testing	64	Repetitive-stereotyped	28
		Positive formal thought	
		disorder	
		Derailment	45
		Tangentiality	50
		Incoherence	23
		Illogicality	23
		Circumstantiality	35
		Pressure of speech	24
		Distractible speech	23
		Clanging	3

Source. Adapted from Andreasen 1987.

Individuals with schizophrenia may be better accepted in less developed societies, have fewer external demands (e.g., work, school), and be more likely to be taken care of by family members.

TABLE 5–4.   Typical stages of schizophrenia

Stage	Typical features
Prodromal phase	Insidious onset occurs over months or years; subtle behavior changes include social withdrawal, work impairment, blunting of emotion, avolition, and odd ideas and behavior.
Active phase	Psychotic symptoms develop, including hallucinations, delusions, or disorganized speech and behavior. These symptoms eventually lead to medical intervention.
Residual phase	Active-phase symptoms are absent or no longer prominent. There is often role impairment, negative symptoms, or attenuated positive symptoms. Acute-phase symptoms may reemerge during the residual phase ("acute exacerbation").

TABLE 5–5.   Features associated with good and poor outcome in schizophrenia

Feature	Good outcome	Poor outcome
Onset	Acute	Insidious
Duration of prodrome	Short	Since childhood
Age at onset	Late 20s to 30s	Early teens
Mood symptoms	Present	Absent
Psychotic or negative symptoms	Mild to moderate	Severe
Obsessions/compulsions	Absent	Present
Gender	Female	Male
Premorbid functioning	Good	Poor
Marital status	Married	Never married
Psychosexual functioning	Good	Poor
Neurological functioning	Normal	+ Soft signs
Structural brain abnormalities	None	Present
Intelligence level	High	Low
Family history of schizophrenia	Negative	Positive

Differential Diagnosis

Schizophrenia should be diagnosed only after a thorough evaluation in which alternative explanations for the patient's symptoms have been ruled out. A physical examination and history should be performed to help rule out medical causes of schizophrenic symptoms. Psychotic symptoms are found in many other illnesses, including substance use disorder (e.g., stimulants, hallucinogens, phencyclidine), intoxication due to commonly prescribed medications (e.g., corticosteroids, anticholinergics, levodopa), infections, metabolic and endocrine disorders, tumors and mass lesions, and temporal lobe epilepsy. Routine laboratory tests can help to rule out medical etiologies: a complete blood count, urinalysis, liver enzymes, serum creatinine, blood urea nitrogen, thyroid function tests, and serologic tests for evidence of an infection with syphilis or HIV. MRI scans can be helpful in selected patients to rule out focal brain disorder (e.g., tumors, strokes) during the initial workup for new-onset cases.

The major differential diagnosis involves separating schizophrenia from schizoaffective disorder, the mood disorders, delusional disorder, and personality disorders. (See Table 5–6 for the differential diagnosis of schizophrenia.) The chief distinction from schizoaffective disorder and a psychotic mood disorder is that in schizophrenia, a full depressive or manic syndrome either is absent, develops after the psychotic symptoms, or is brief relative to the duration of psychotic symptoms. With delusional disorder, the person's behavior is not obviously bizarre or odd. Patients with personality disorders, particularly those disorders within the "eccentric cluster" (e.g., schizoid, schizotypal, and paranoid), may be indifferent to social relationships and have a restricted affect, bizarre ideation, or odd speech, but they are not psychotic.

Other psychiatric disorders also must be ruled out, including schizophreniform disorder, brief psychotic disorder, factitious disorder with psychological symptoms, and malingering.

Etiology and Pathophysiology

Schizophrenia is best considered a "multiple-hit" illness similar to cancer, diabetes, and cardiovascular disease. Individuals may carry a genetic predisposition, but this vulnerability is not "released" unless other factors also intervene. Although most of these factors are considered environmental, in the sense that they are not encoded in DNA and could potentially produce mutations or influence gene expression, most are also biological rather than psychological and include factors such as

---

TABLE 5–6. Differential diagnosis of schizophrenia

Psychiatric illness	Other medical illness
Bipolar disorder	Temporal lobe epilepsy
Major depression	Tumor, stroke, brain trauma
Schizoaffective disorder	Endocrine/metabolic disorders
Brief psychotic disorder	(e.g., porphyria)
Schizophreniform disorder	Vitamin deficiency (e.g., B_{12})
Delusional disorder	Infectious disease (e.g.,
Panic disorder	neurosyphilis)
Depersonalization disorder	Autoimmune disorder (e.g.,
Obsessive-compulsive disorder	systemic lupus erythematosus)
Personality disorders	Toxic illness (e.g., heavy metal
	poisoning)

Drugs

Stimulants (e.g., amphetamine, cocaine)
Hallucinogens
Anticholinergics (e.g., belladonna alkaloids)
Alcohol withdrawal
Barbiturate withdrawal

---

birth injuries, poor maternal nutrition, or maternal substance abuse. Current studies of the neurobiology of schizophrenia examine a multiplicity of factors, including genetics, anatomy (primarily through structural neuroimaging), functional circuitry (through functional neuroimaging), neuropathology, electrophysiology, neurochemistry and neuropharmacology, and neurodevelopment.

Genetics

There is substantial evidence that schizophrenia has a strong genetic component. Family studies have shown that siblings of schizophrenic patients have about a 10% chance of developing schizophrenia, whereas children who have one parent with schizophrenia have a 5%–6% chance. The risk of family members developing schizophrenia increases markedly when two or more family members have the illness. The risk of developing schizophrenia is 17% for persons with one sibling and one parent with schizophrenia and 46% for the children of two schizophrenic parents. Twin studies have been remarkably consistent in demonstrating high concordance rates for monozygotic twins—an average of 46%, compared with 14% concordance in dizygotic twins. Adoption studies show that the risk for schizophrenia is greater in the biological relatives of index adoptees with schizophrenia than in the biological relatives of mentally healthy control adoptees.

Numerous attempts have been made to identify genes using linkage and candidate gene methods and, more recently, genome-wide association studies. However, obtaining robust and consistent results has been difficult. For instance, positive mapping studies have been reported on chromosomes 1, 6, 8, 10, 11, 13, and 22, but often to very broad chromosomal regions and with different groups often mapping to nonoverlapping regions of the same chromosome arm. A possible exception to this pessimistic outcome are a few vulnerability genes that have recently been identified for schizophrenia. These genes include neuregulin 1 (*NRG1*); dystrobrevin binding protein, or dysbindin (*DTNBP1*); catechol-O-methyltransferase (*COMT*); Disrupted-in-Schizophrenia 1 (*DISC1*); D-amino acid oxidase activator (*DAOA*); metabotropic glutamate receptor 3 (*GRM3*); and brain-derived neurotrophic factor (*BDNF*). Most of these genes were identified through follow-up on linkage and candidate gene studies using fine mapping and guided by hypotheses about their role in neurodevelopment or neurotransmission, and they now have had several replications. An intriguing feature of these candidate susceptibility genes is that they may explain selected features of the pathophysiology of the disease. For example, *COMT* affects the production of dopamine, a neurotransmitter considered to be functionally overactive in schizophrenia and that is blocked or down-regulated by antipsychotic medications. Similarly, *NRG1, DAOA,* and *GRM3* have effects on GABAergic and glutamatergic neurotransmission, which are also thought to be dysfunctional in schizophrenia.

Structural Neuroimaging and Neuropathology

Cerebral ventricular enlargement in schizophrenia has been confirmed in numerous studies. Sulcal enlargement and cerebellar atrophy also are found. Examination of ventricular size in persons with and without schizophrenia over a broad age range suggests that enlargement progresses over time at a greater rate in schizophrenic patients than normally and that structural brain abnormalities are present from the outset. Ventricular enlargement is associated with poor premorbid functioning, negative symptoms, poor response to treatment, and cognitive impairment.

MRI also has been used to explore possible abnormalities in other specific brain subregions. Studies comparing both first-episode and chronic schizophrenia patients with healthy control subjects indicate that on average, frontal lobe size is decreased in both groups of patients.

Longitudinal studies show that progressive tissue loss occurs over time in some patients; the mechanism is as yet unknown, but genes that regulate synaptic plasticity (e.g., *BDNF*) may play a role. Several studies also indicate that the size of temporal regions is decreased in schizophrenia and that there may even be a relatively specific abnormality in the superior temporal gyrus or planum temporale that is correlated with the presence of hallucinations or formal thought disorder.

Several studies have found decreased thalamus size in patients with schizophrenia. The thalamus is a major relay station that could serve functions such as gating or filtering or even generating input and output because it receives afferent input from and sends efferent output to widely distributed areas in the association cortices and primary sensory and motor regions.

Most studies have consistently shown a decrease in total brain tissue volume in schizophrenia and an increase in cerebrospinal fluid in the ventricles and on the brain surface. There appears to be a selective decrease in cortical gray matter, although some investigators have found white matter decreases as well.

Functional Circuitry and Functional Neuroimaging

Studies of regional cerebral blood flow have been used to explore the possibility of functional or metabolic abnormalities in schizophrenia. Early work suggested that patients with schizophrenia have a relative "hypofrontality," which is associated with prominent negative symptoms. Functional imaging studies have become more sophisticated, and it is now clear that functional MRI and positron emission tomography (PET) can be used to explore the functional circuitry used by healthy individuals while they perform a variety of mental tasks and to identify circuits that are dysfunctional in schizophrenia. Although no single group of regions has definitely emerged as the "schizophrenia circuit," a consensus is developing about some of the nodes that may be involved, including a variety of subregions within the frontal cortex (orbital, dorsolateral, medial), the anterior cingulate gyrus, the thalamus, several temporal lobe subregions, and the cerebellum.

Current thinking on the mechanics of schizophrenia postulates that it is a disease of multiple distributed circuits in the brain. Some experts have suggested that the disease is characterized by a *cognitive dysmetria* caused by a disruption in the pontine-cerebellar-thalamic-frontal feedback loop. The thalamus is a crucial way station in the brain that has complex interconnections to many other regions. Various parts of the prefrontal cortex (i.e., dorsolateral, orbital, and medial) are connected to it, as are other regions such as the basal ganglia and anterior cingulate. Furthermore, various thalamic nuclei have relay connections to virtually all other parts of the cerebral cortex, including sensory, motor, and association regions. Finally, the cerebellum also projects to multiple cortical regions via thalamic relay nuclei. This distributed circuitry is disrupted, leading to the multiple kinds of symptoms and cognitive impairment seen in schizophrenia.

Neurodevelopmental Influences

Several lines of evidence suggest schizophrenia is a neurodevelopmental disorder that results from brain injury occurring early in life or during later stages of brain development in adolescence. For example, patients with schizophrenia are more likely than controls to have a history of birth injury and perinatal complications that could result in a subtle brain injury, thus setting the stage for the development of schizophrenia. Minor physical anomalies (slight anatomical defects of the head, hands, feet, and face) are sometimes observed in schizophrenic patients and are themselves thought to reflect abnormal neurodevelopment.

Neurochemistry and Neuropharmacology

For many years, the most popular pathophysiological explanation for schizophrenia has been the *dopamine hypothesis*. This hypothesis suggests that the symptoms of schizophrenia arise from a functional hyperactivity in the dopamine system in limbic regions and a functional hypoactivity in frontal regions. Drugs that enhance dopamine transmission in limbic regions, such as the amphetamines, tend to worsen the symptoms of schizophrenia and can sometimes precipitate psychotic symptoms in normal individuals. The efficacy of many of the antipsychotic drugs used to treat schizophrenia is highly correlated with their ability to block dopamine (D_2) receptors. Therefore, the dopamine hypothesis suggests that the abnormality in this illness might lie specifically in the D_2 receptors.

The newer second-generation antipsychotics were developed to have a broader pharmacological profile. In addition to dopamine receptor blockade, they also block serotonin type 2 ($5\text{-}HT_2$) receptors, suggesting a role for serotonin in the pathophysiology of schizophrenia. Another neurotransmitter, glutamate, is also being studied as a possible contributor to the development of schizophrenia. The *glutamate hypothesis* suggests that there is a hypofunction in the NMDA receptors within the glutamate system; the normal balance between the excitatory glutamate and inhibitory GABA systems is thereby destabilized, potentially leading to a combination of excitotoxicity and impaired neuroplasticity. Thus, it is unlikely that schizophrenia can be conceptualized as a single-neurotransmitter disease.

Clinical Management

Antipsychotic medication is the treatment mainstay. The probable mechanism of action is their ability to block postsynaptic dopamine D_2 receptors in the limbic forebrain. This blockade is thought to initiate a cascade of events responsible for both acute and chronic therapeutic actions. These drugs also block serotonergic, noradrenergic, cholinergic, and histaminic receptors to differing degrees, accounting for the unique side effect profile of each agent.

Treatment of Acute Psychosis

High-potency conventional antipsychotics (e.g., haloperidol) and second-generation antipsychotics (e.g., risperidone, olanzapine) are considered first-line treatments. Second-generation antipsychotics are generally better tolerated because they have less potential to cause extrapyramidal side effects, but they can cause weight gain, glucose intolerance, and lipid dysregulation. Clozapine is a second-line choice because it can—in rare cases—cause agranulocytosis. Nonetheless, it is associated with a reduction in suicidal behavior and may be particularly useful in patients with schizophrenia at high risk for suicide. The rational use of these drugs is further described in Chapter 21, "Psychopharmacology and Electroconvulsive Therapy."

Maintenance Therapy

Sustained control of psychotic symptoms is the goal of maintenance treatment. At least 1–2 years of treatment with antipsychotic medication are recommended after the initial psychotic episode because of the high risk of relapse and the possibility of social deterioration from further relapses. At least 5 years of treatment for multiple episodes is recommended because a high risk of relapse remains. Beyond this, data are incomplete, but indefinite—perhaps lifelong—treatment is likely to be needed by most patients. Long-acting injectable antipsychotics are available and are particularly useful in patients who lack insight or have been shown to be noncompliant with medication. Some patients may prefer injections to oral medication.

Adjunctive Treatments

Adjunctive psychotropic medications are sometimes useful in the schizophrenic patient, but their role has not been clearly defined. Many patients benefit from anxiolytics (e.g., benzodiazepines) when anxiety is prominent. Lithium carbonate, valproate, and carbamazepine can be used to reduce impulsive and aggressive behaviors, hyperactivity, or mood swings, although their effectiveness in patients with schizophrenia has not been fully determined. Antidepressants are sometimes used to treat depression in schizophrenic patients and appear effective. Electroconvulsive therapy is sometimes used, particularly to treat concurrent depression or catatonic symptoms.

Psychosocial Interventions

Most treatment occurs in the community and not in the hospital. Hospitalization should be reserved for patients who pose a danger to themselves or others; are unable to properly care for themselves (e.g., refuse food or fluids); or require special medical observation, tests, or treatments. (See Table 5–7 for the reasons to hospitalize patients with schizophrenia.)

The outpatient clinic will be the best setting in which to coordinate care for most schizophrenic patients. A well-equipped clinic should be able to provide medication management, adjunctive behavioral and cognitive treatments, and case management.

Partial hospital or day treatment programs can be helpful for patients with symptoms that have not responded well to medication (e.g., psychosis, depression) and who need more structure. These programs generally operate on weekdays, and patients return home in the evenings and on weekends. Medication management and various psychosocial services are provided.

Assertive community treatment (ACT) programs are available in some areas. They employ careful monitoring of patients through mobile mental health teams and individually tailored programming. ACT programs have staff available 24 hours a day and have been shown to reduce hospital admission rates and to improve the quality of life for many patients.

Other Approaches

Family therapy, combined with antipsychotic medication, has been shown to reduce relapse rates in schizophrenia. Families need realistic and accurate information about the symptoms, course of illness, and

TABLE 5–7. Reasons to hospitalize patients with schizophrenia

1. When the illness is new, to rule out alternative diagnoses and to stabilize the dosage of antipsychotic medication

2. For special medical procedures such as electroconvulsive therapy

3. When aggressive or assaultive behavior presents a danger to the patient or others

4. When the patient becomes suicidal

5. When the patient is unable to properly care for himself or herself (e.g., refuses to eat or take fluids)

6. When medication side effects become disabling or potentially life threatening (e.g., severe pseudoparkinsonism, neuroleptic malignant syndrome)

available treatments. They also will benefit from learning how to improve communications with their schizophrenic relative and how to provide constructive support.

Cognitive rehabilitation involves the remediation of abnormal thought processes known to occur in schizophrenia, using methods pioneered in the treatment of brain-injured persons.

Social skills training (SST) aims to help patients develop more appropriate behavior.

Psychosocial rehabilitation serves to integrate the patient back into his or her community rather than segregating the patient in separate facilities as has occurred in the past. This may involve patient clubhouses available in some areas to encourage socialization.

Vocational rehabilitation may help a patient obtain supported employment, competitive work in integrated settings, and more formal job training programs.

Appropriate and affordable housing is a major concern for many patients. Depending on the community, options may range from supervised shelters and group homes ("halfway houses") to boarding homes to supervised apartments. Group homes provide peer support and companionship, along with on-site staff supervision. Supervised apartments provide greater independence and offer the availability and backup of trained staff.

Clinical points for schizophrenia

1. Psychotic symptoms should be treated aggressively with medication.

   - High-potency conventional antipsychotics and second-generation antipsychotics are considered first-line therapy because they are effective and well tolerated.

   - Intramuscular medication is useful in noncompliant patients or those who prefer the convenience of bimonthly or monthly injections.

2. The clinician should engage the patient in an empathic relationship.

   - This task may at times be challenging because some patients are unemotional, aloof, and withdrawn.

   - The clinician should be practical and help the patient with problems that matter to him or her, such as finding adequate housing.

3. The clinician should help the patient find a daily routine that he or she can manage, to help improve socialization and reduce boredom.

   - Partial hospitalization or day treatment programs are available in many areas.

   - Sheltered workshops that provide simple, repetitive chores may be helpful.

4. The clinician should develop a close working relationship with local social services.

   - Patients tend to be poor and disabled; finding adequate housing and food takes the skills of a social worker.

   - The clinician should help the patient obtain disability benefits.

5. Family therapy is important for the patient who lives at home or who still has close family ties.

   - As a result of the illness, many patients will have broken their family ties.

   - Families desperately need education about schizophrenia.

   - The clinician should help family members find a support group through referral to a local chapter of the National Alliance on Mental Illness (NAMI).

Schizoaffective Disorder

The term *schizoaffective* was first used in 1933 by Jacob Kasanin to describe a small group of severely ill patients who had a mixture of psychotic and mood symptoms. In DSM-5, its hallmark is the presence of either a depressive or a manic episode concurrent with symptoms characteristic of schizophrenia, such as delusions, hallucinations, or disorganized speech (see Box 5–3). During the illness, hallucinations or delusions must be present for 2 weeks or more in the absence of prominent mood symptoms, but mood symptoms must be present for a majority of the total duration of the illness. Finally, medical conditions and drugs of abuse must be excluded as having caused the symptoms. There are two subtypes: the bipolar type, marked by a current or previous manic syndrome, and the depressive type, marked by the absence of any manic syndromes.

Box 5–3.   DSM-5 Diagnostic Criteria for Schizoaffective Disorder

---

A. An uninterrupted period of illness during which there is a major mood episode (major depressive or manic) concurrent with Criterion A of schizophrenia.

   Note: The major depressive episode must include Criterion A1: Depressed mood.

B. Delusions or hallucinations for 2 or more weeks in the absence of a major mood episode (depressive or manic) during the lifetime duration of the illness.

C. Symptoms that meet criteria for a major mood episode are present for the majority of the total duration of the active and residual portions of the illness.

D. The disturbance is not attributable to the effects of a substance (e.g., a drug of abuse, a medication) or another medical condition.

Specify whether:

   Bipolar type: This subtype applies if a manic episode is part of the presentation. Major depressive episodes may also occur.

   Depressive type: This subtype applies if only major depressive episodes are part of the presentation.

Specify if:

   With catatonia (refer to the criteria for catatonia associated with another mental disorder, [DSM-5] pp. 119–120, for definition).

Specify if:

The following course specifiers are only to be used after a 1-year duration of the disorder and if they are not in contradiction to the diagnostic course criteria.

First episode, currently in acute episode: First manifestation of the disorder meeting the defining diagnostic symptom and time criteria. An *acute episode* is a time period in which the symptom criteria are fulfilled.

First episode, currently in partial remission: *Partial remission* is a time period during which an improvement after a previous episode is maintained and in which the defining criteria of the disorder are only partially fulfilled.

First episode, currently in full remission: *Full remission* is a period of time after a previous episode during which no disorder-specific symptoms are present.

Multiple episodes, currently in acute episode: Multiple episodes may be determined after a minimum of two episodes (i.e., after a first episode, a remission and a minimum of one relapse).

Multiple episodes, currently in partial remission

Multiple episodes, currently in full remission

Continuous: Symptoms fulfilling the diagnostic symptom criteria of the disorder are remaining for the majority of the illness course, with subthreshold symptom periods being very brief relative to the overall course.

Unspecified

Specify current severity:

Severity is rated by a quantitative assessment of the primary symptoms of psychosis, including delusions, hallucinations, disorganized speech, abnormal psychomotor behavior, and negative symptoms. Each of these symptoms may be rated for its current severity (most severe in the last 7 days) on a 5-point scale ranging from 0 (not present) to 4 (present and severe). (See Clinician-Rated Dimensions of Psychosis Symptom Severity in the chapter "Assessment Measures.")

Note: Diagnosis of schizoaffective disorder can be made without using this severity specifier.

Schizoaffective disorder has an estimated prevalence of less than 1% and occurs more often in women. The diagnosis is common in psychiatric hospitals and clinics but is primarily a diagnosis of exclusion. The differential diagnosis for schizoaffective disorder consists primarily of schizophrenia, the mood disorders, and disorders induced by medical conditions or drugs of abuse. In schizophrenia, mood episodes have been present for a minority of the total duration of the illness. Although psychotic symptoms may occur in persons with mood disorders, they are generally not present in the absence of depression or mania, helping to set the boundary between schizoaffective disorder and psychotic mania or depression. It is usually clear from the history, physical examination, or laboratory tests when a drug or a medical condition has initiated and maintained the disorder.

The signs and symptoms of schizoaffective disorder include those seen in schizophrenia and the mood disorders. The symptoms may present together or in an alternating fashion, and psychotic symptoms may be mood congruent or mood incongruent. The course of schizoaffective disorder is variable but represents a middle ground between that of schizophrenia and the mood disorders. A worse outcome is associated with poor premorbid adjustment, insidious onset, lack of a precipitating stressor, predominance of psychotic symptoms, early onset, unremitting course, and a family history of schizophrenia.

The treatment of schizoaffective disorder should target both mood and psychotic symptoms. With second-generation antipsychotics, a single drug may adequately target both; these drugs may represent an ideal first-line treatment. Paliperidone has been approved as monotherapy by the U.S. Food and Drug Administration for the treatment of schizoaffective disorder. Some patients may benefit from the addition of a mood stabilizer (e.g., lithium, valproate) or an antidepressant. Patients not responding to medication may respond to electroconvulsive therapy, although medication is typically reinstituted for long-term maintenance. Schizoaffective patients who are a danger to themselves or others or who are unable to properly care for themselves should be hospitalized.

■ Self-Assessment Questions

1. How does delusional disorder differ from schizophrenia?
2. What are the subtypes of delusional disorder?
3. Describe brief psychotic disorder.
4. How is schizophrenia diagnosed? What is its differential diagnosis?
5. What are typical signs and symptoms of schizophrenia?
6. What are the subtypes of schizophrenia?
7. What evidence supports a neurobiological basis for schizophrenia?
8. What is the natural history of schizophrenia?
9. How is schizophrenia managed pharmacologically and psychosocially?
10. How does schizoaffective disorder differ diagnostically from both schizophrenia and psychotic mood disorders?

Chapter 6

Mood Disorders

I see the lost are like this, and their curse
To be, as I am mine, their sweating selves. But worse.

Gerard Manley Hopkins

ood disorders have a high prevalence, a high morbidity, and a high mortality rate. Masked as complaints about insomnia, fatigue, or unexplained pain, mood disorders often lead people to seek medical care in primary care settings. For people ages 15–45 years, depression accounts for an astonishing 10.3% of all costs of biomedical illnesses worldwide. Bipolar disorder, characterized by extreme mood swings, ranks sixth among the world's most disabling illnesses. Yet these substantial costs to society from disability due to mood disorders may be unnecessary. When correctly diagnosed and treated, mood disorders usually respond well. Therefore, all physicians who have direct personal contact with patients should learn the fundamentals about diagnosing and treating mood disorders.

In DSM-5, there are separate chapters for bipolar and related disorders and for depressive disorders. For convenience, they are all described in this single chapter, starting with the bipolar disorders.

■ Bipolar Disorders

This diagnostic class recognizes disorders characterized by marked swings in mood, activity, and behavior. The classic form of bipolar disorder was described by the German psychiatrist Emil Kraepelin as an episodic and nondeteriorating illness in contrast to schizophrenia. A milder form of the disorder, bipolar II disorder, was given its own category in DSM-IV. In DSM-5, bipolar and related disorders are placed be-

---

TABLE 6–1.   DSM-5 bipolar and related disorders

Bipolar I disorder

Bipolar II disorder

Cyclothymic disorder

Substance/medication-induced bipolar and related disorder

Bipolar and related disorder due to another medical condition

Other specified bipolar and related disorder

Unspecified bipolar and related disorder

---

tween the chapters on schizophrenia spectrum and other psychotic disorders and the depressive disorders, in recognition of their place in bridging these diagnostic classes.

The class includes bipolar I and bipolar II disorders, cyclothymic disorder, substance/medication-induced bipolar and related disorder, and bipolar and related disorder due to another medical condition. Two residual categories are available for those who do not fit one of the more specific diagnoses (Table 6–1).

Manic Episode

The DSM-5 criteria for a manic episode require the presence of an abnormally elevated, expansive, or irritable mood lasting at least 1 week plus three of seven characteristic symptoms (Box 6–1). The criteria are similar to those used to define depression in that the mood disturbance must be sufficiently severe to cause marked impairment or to require hospitalization. As in the case of depression, the symptoms cannot be due to the physiological effects of drugs of abuse, medications, or another medical condition.

Box 6–1.   DSM-5 Criteria for Manic Episode

A. A distinct period of abnormally and persistently elevated, expansive, or irritable mood and abnormally and persistently increased goal-directed activity or energy, lasting at least 1 week and present most of the day, nearly every day (or any duration if hospitalization is necessary).

B. During the period of mood disturbance and increased energy or activity, three (or more) of the following symptoms (four if the mood is only irritable) are present to a significant degree and represent a noticeable change from usual behavior:

1. Inflated self-esteem or grandiosity.
2. Decreased need for sleep (e.g., feels rested after only 3 hours of sleep).
3. More talkative than usual or pressure to keep talking.
4. Flight of ideas or subjective experience that thoughts are racing.
5. Distractibility (i.e., attention too easily drawn to unimportant or irrelevant external stimuli), as reported or observed.
6. Increase in goal-directed activity (either socially, at work or school, or sexually) or psychomotor agitation (i.e., purposeless non-goal-directed activity).
7. Excessive involvement in activities that have a high potential for painful consequences (e.g., engaging in unrestrained buying sprees, sexual indiscretions, or foolish business investments).

C. The mood disturbance is sufficiently severe to cause marked impairment in social or occupational functioning or to necessitate hospitalization to prevent harm to self or others, or there are psychotic features.

D. The episode is not attributable to the physiological effects of a substance (e.g., a drug of abuse, a medication, other treatment) or to another medical condition.

Note: A full manic episode that emerges during antidepressant treatment (e.g., medication, electroconvulsive therapy) but persists at a fully syndromal level beyond the physiological effect of that treatment is sufficient evidence for a manic episode and, therefore, a bipolar I diagnosis.

Note: Criteria A–D constitute a manic episode. At least one lifetime manic episode is required for the diagnosis of bipolar I disorder.

Bipolar I disorder is defined by the occurrence of at least one manic or mixed episode. Typically, bipolar I disorder is characterized by recurrent episodes of both mania and depression, which can be separated by intervals of months to years. Although the episodes may lead to psychosocial morbidity because of the effect of a severe recurrent illness on interpersonal relationships or work functioning, interepisode functioning may be good or even excellent.

Clinical Findings

The patient's mood is typically cheerful, enthusiastic, and expansive. The cheerfulness often has an infectious quality, making interviewing an enjoyable and sometimes amusing experience. Sometimes, however, the patient's mood is simply irritable, particularly if the person feels thwarted, and such irritable manic patients can be quite difficult to manage. Because of their euphoria, manic patients usually have very little insight into their problems. In fact, they may deny that anything is wrong with them and instead blame friends or family for attributing an abnormality to them that is not actually present.

Manic patients may believe that they have special abilities or powers that clearly are outside the normal range for their educational background or intellectual achievement. Inflated self-esteem and grandiosity, if present, may reach delusional proportions. Patients may develop plans to write books, record compact discs, lead religious movements, or undertake expansive business ventures. When the grandiosity reaches delusional proportions, patients may report that they are rock stars, famous athletes or politicians, or even religious figures such as Christ.

Patients typically experience increased goal-directed energy or activity. This is often a noteworthy change from their usual behavior. They may be physically restless and unable to sit still. The increased level of activity is often accompanied by poor judgment. Patients with mania tend to overextend themselves in ways that lead them into serious trouble after the manic episode is over. They spend money excessively, commit themselves to projects that they are unable to complete, become involved in extramarital affairs, or engage in quarrels with business associates or family members who disagree with them or try to slow them down.

Patients may also experience an increase in their cognitive speed, feeling smarter and more creative than usual. Patients with mania usually require less sleep than usual, often getting by on only 2 or 3 hours per night. Patients may become more social and gregarious, going to bars, planning parties, or calling friends at all hours of the night. Interest in sex is often increased, leading the manic patient to exhaust his or her partner or to make inappropriate overtures to casual acquaintances or strangers.

Manic patients tend to talk excessively and to manifest pressured speech. Thus, they answer questions at great length, continue to talk even when interrupted, and sometimes talk when no one is listening. Their speech usually is rapid, loud, and emphatic. Underlying the pressured speech is probably a rapid flow of thought, sometimes referred to as *flight of ideas*. This increased speed in cognitive functioning is inferred by listening to the patient's speech, which manifests derailment, incoherence, and distractibility. Manic patients tend to skip from one topic to another as they describe their experiences, ideas, or symptoms. Distractibility is observed in both their speech and their social behavior. While speaking, they may shift their topic in response to some stimulus in the environment, and they manifest the same pattern of distractibility when trying to perform tasks or complete activities.

Many manic patients—perhaps 50% of hospitalized patients—have psychotic symptoms, which may include either delusions or hallucinations that express themes consistent with the mood, such as delusions about special abilities or powers. Less commonly, the delusions will be mood incongruent and express themes not related to the patient's euphoric and grandiose mood.

The following case illustrates a manic episode:

Charles, a 43-year-old man, was brought to the emergency room by the local police after he had jumped from his seat in the middle of a performance of *Les Misérables*, run onto the stage, and begun yelling that the injustices of the Bush administration were as extensive and profound as those portrayed in the performance. He had begun conversing with Jean Valjean, urging him to leave the performance, to join the Democratic Party, and to assist in the effort to place a Democrat in the White House. This speech was accompanied by an extensive speech on the injustice of packing the Supreme Court with a group of extreme conservatives.

In the emergency room, Charles indicated that he did not live in Iowa City but had come from Des Moines (100 miles away) to attend the performance and to consult with friends and colleagues at the law school. He described himself as a prominent lawyer, a graduate of Harvard Law School who had edited the *Law Review,* a close friend of the Clinton family and other prominent Democrats, and a dedicated crusader against social injustice. He described the Bush administration as a rerun of the industrial-totalitarian axis that had been created in Nazi Germany, complained about a conspiracy that he believed was under way to destroy the Democratic Party by either persecution or assassination of key figures, and indicated that one of the purposes of his trip to Iowa City was to warn his colleagues at the law school about these dangerous circumstances.

His appearance was unkempt and disheveled, inconsistent with his description of his prominent status. Although he was attired in an expensive-appearing pinstripe suit, his hair was uncombed, his eyes were red, and he was unshaven. Charles spoke excitedly in a rapid manner, and his voice rose to a shout at times. His speech was disjointed and difficult to follow as his topic changed from his own special importance and abilities to the various conspiracies that he thought were under way in the Bush administration.

When admission to the hospital was proposed, he became physically agitated and tried to run away. He became physically combative at attempts to restrain him. A decision was made to obtain an emergency hospitalization order. His claims of special importance and abilities were discounted and attributed to his manic state. Later, as more history was obtained, it became evident that Charles was indeed a prominent attorney with many important national connections. The conspiracy against the Democratic Party, although potentially bearing some credence, contained enough implausible elaborations to qualify as delusional thinking. Interviews with his family members revealed that he had had one prior hospitalization for mania and had been treated for depression as an outpatient. He had been taking maintenance lithium but had decided to discontinue it abruptly about 3 days earlier.

Charles was given a therapeutic dose of lithium, and his symptoms cleared over the course of 5–7 days. He was able to leave the hospital and to return to work within 1 week.

Course and Outcome

The onset of mania is frequently abrupt, although it may begin gradually over the course of a few weeks. The episodes usually last from a few days to months. They tend to be briefer and to have a more abrupt termination than depressive episodes. Although the prognosis for any particular episode is reasonably good, especially with the availability of effective treatments such as lithium and antipsychotics, the risk for recurrence is significant. Not uncommonly, an episode of mania is followed by an episode of depression. Some patients with bipolar disorder recover relatively fully, but a substantial subset continues to have chronic instability of mood, particularly recurrent episodes of mild depression.

The complications of mania are primarily social: marital discord, divorce, business difficulties, financial extravagance, and sexual indiscretions. Drug or alcohol abuse may occur during a manic episode. When mania is relatively severe, the patient may be almost completely incapacitated and require protection from the consequences of poor judgment or hyperactivity. The excessive activity level continues to be a significant risk in patients with cardiac problems. A manic syndrome can switch rapidly to depression, and the risk for suicide is heightened when the patient becomes remorsefully aware of inappropriate behavior that occurred during the manic episode.

Some patients present with a mixture of manic and depressive symptoms within a single episode of illness. When this occurs, the clinician designates this by adding a "with mixed features" specifier to the diagnosis. Typically, the patient with this presentation will have a full manic syndrome that is accompanied by some depressive symptoms, such as feelings of sadness, or guilty ruminations. The clinical presentation can be quite confusing because the patient's mood and symptom picture tend to alternate rapidly. The patient at one moment will be talkative, energetic, and expansive, yet minutes later may burst into tears and complain of feeling hopeless and suicidal.

The presence of mixed features has been associated with course (earlier onset), greater number of episodes, higher likelihood of alcohol abuse and suicide attempts, greater likelihood of rapid cycling, and greater likelihood of a lifetime diagnosis of bipolar disorder. Therefore, it is important that mixed states be recognized when present.

Hypomanic Episode

Hypomania is another important form of mood disorder. The syndrome is similar to mania, but it is milder and briefer. During a hypomanic episode, the patient experiences the elevated mood and other classic symptoms that define mania, but they are not accompanied by delusional beliefs or hallucinations, and they are not severe enough to require hospitalization or to markedly impair social and occupational functioning. Many patients with hypomania also have chronic mild depression, so it can sometimes be difficult to determine whether they are "back to their usual selves" or "just feeling good for a change." Obtaining information from family and friends usually is helpful in determining whether the presence of a good mood is indeed pathological rather than a patch of normal happiness in the midst of feeling chronically blue.

Bipolar II disorder is characterized by periods of hypomania that typically occur either before or after periods of depression but also may occur independently. These mild manic episodes are not sufficiently severe to require hospitalization, although they can lead to personal, social, or work difficulties. During the mild bipolar phase, the patient is upbeat, shows signs of poor judgment, and has other indices of mania such as increased energy or insomnia, but the symptoms do not meet full criteria for a manic episode. Bipolar II disorder appears to breed true within families, in that relatives of bipolar II patients themselves have higher rates of bipolar II disorder than either bipolar I (i.e., criteria are met for a full manic episode) or unipolar major depression. Bipolar II disorder also tends to have a high rate of comorbidity with other disorders, such as substance abuse. Patients with bipolar II tend to experience a greater burden of depressive symptoms than their bipolar I counterparts.

Course of illness may also be informative, because like manic episodes, hypomanic episodes are often followed by a crash into a depressive episode.

Cyclothymic Disorder

Cyclothymic disorder is the mildest form of bipolar disorder and is a condition in which the patient has mild swings between the two poles of depression and hypomania. While in the hypomanic phase the person appears to be high, but not so high as to be socially or professionally incapacitated. During the depressed phase the individual has some symptoms of depression, but these are not severe enough to meet criteria for a full major depressive episode (i.e., five symptoms persisting for

2 weeks). Thus, the individual with cyclothymic disorder tends to swing from high to low with a chronic mild instability of mood.

■ Depressive Disorders

The DSM-5 depressive disorders are listed in Table 6–2. They include disruptive mood dysregulation disorder, major depressive disorder (single episode and recurrent), persistent depressive disorder (dysthymia), premenstrual dysphoric disorder, substance/medication-induced depressive disorder, and depressive disorder due to another medical condition. Two residual categories are available for those who do not fit one of the more specific diagnoses: other specified and unspecified depressive disorder.

Disruptive Mood Dysregulation Disorder

Disruptive mood dysregulation disorder (DMDD) is new to DSM-5 and is characterized by chronic, severe, and persistent irritability. The diagnosis helps fill an important gap for children with mood disorders. In the past few decades, there has been a near 40-fold increase in the number of youth diagnosed with bipolar disorder, based on their frequent "mood swings"—usually from sad to angry. Research has shown, however, that these children have a different outcome, gender ratio, and family history from those with bipolar disorder. Furthermore, they do not go on to develop manic or hypomanic episodes, but they primarily appear to be depressed, which is expressed as anger and irritability. The children may also meet DSM-5 criteria for one of the anxiety disorders and attention-deficit/hyperactivity disorder. Many will also meet criteria for oppositional defiant disorder (due to overlapping symptoms); in these cases, the child should be assigned only the diagnosis of DMDD.

Diagnostic criteria for DMDD are shown in Box 6–2. The symptoms must have been present for at least 12 months and have begun before age 10. The symptoms occur in at least two settings, such as at home and school. This diagnosis is not made before the child is age 6 nor after the child turns age 18. Neurodevelopmental syndromes likely to have earlier onset (e.g., autism spectrum disorder) should be ruled out as a cause of the symptoms, and symptoms are not due to adult misbehavior arising from an antisocial personality disorder (which is not diagnosed in persons under age 18 years).

TABLE 6–2.   DSM-5 depressive and related disorders

Disruptive mood dysregulation disorder

Major depressive disorder, single episode

Major depressive disorder, recurrent

Persistent depressive disorder (dysthymia)

Substance/medication-induced depressive disorder

Premenstrual dysphoric disorder

Depressive disorder due to another medical condition

Other specified depressive disorder

Unspecified depressive disorder

Box 6–2.   DSM-5 Diagnostic Criteria for Disruptive Mood
Dysregulation Disorder

A. Severe recurrent temper outbursts manifested verbally (e.g., verbal rages) and/or behaviorally (e.g., physical aggression toward people or property) that are grossly out of proportion in intensity or duration to the situation or provocation.

B. The temper outbursts are inconsistent with developmental level.

C. The temper outbursts occur, on average, three or more times per week.

D. The mood between temper outbursts is persistently irritable or angry most of the day, nearly every day, and is observable by others (e.g., parents, teachers, peers).

E. Criteria A–D have been present for 12 or more months. Throughout that time, the individual has not had a period lasting 3 or more consecutive months without all of the symptoms in Criteria A–D.

F. Criteria A and D are present in at least two of three settings (i.e., at home, at school, with peers) and are severe in at least one of these.

G. The diagnosis should not be made for the first time before age 6 years or after age 18 years.

H. By history or observation, the age at onset of Criteria A–E is before 10 years.

I. There has never been a distinct period lasting more than 1 day during which the full symptom criteria, except duration, for a manic or hypomanic episode have been met.
Note: Developmentally appropriate mood elevation, such as occurs in the context of a highly positive event or its anticipation, should not be considered as a symptom of mania or hypomania.

J. The behaviors do not occur exclusively during an episode of major depressive disorder and are not better explained by another mental disorder (e.g., autism spectrum disorder, posttraumatic stress disorder, separation anxiety disorder, persistent depressive disorder [dysthymia]).

Note: This diagnosis cannot coexist with oppositional defiant disorder, intermittent explosive disorder, or bipolar disorder, though it can coexist with others, including major depressive disorder, attention-deficit/hyperactivity disorder, conduct disorder, and substance use disorders. Individuals whose symptoms meet criteria for both disruptive mood dysregulation disorder and oppositional defiant disorder should only be given the diagnosis of disruptive mood dysregulation disorder. If an individual has ever experienced a manic or hypomanic episode, the diagnosis of disruptive mood dysregulation disorder should not be assigned.

K. The symptoms are not attributable to the physiological effects of a substance or to another medical or neurological condition.

Children with DMDD stand apart from other boys and girls because of the severity and regularity of their temper outbursts, which tend to be inconsistent with the situation. Most parents would see these as indicating the child is out of control; they are also not consistent with the child's developmental level (i.e., the child is outside the range of the "terrible twos"). Between outbursts the child's mood is persistently irritable or angry, and the symptoms are not just a passing phase. As any parent knows, children may experience "developmentally appropriate" episodes of mood elevation in the context of highly positive events (e.g., a birthday party, a visit to an amusement park); in the context of DMDD, these are not a reason to confuse the disorder with bipolar disorder.

DMDD is common among children presenting to pediatric mental health clinics. It occurs mostly in boys. Based on rates of chronic and persistent irritability—the core feature of the disorder—the overall 6-month to 1-year period-prevalence of DMDD may fall in the 2%–5% range. Approximately half of children with severe, chronic irritability will have a presentation that continues to meet criteria for the condition 1 year later. Rates of conversion from severe, nonepisodic irritability to bipolar disorder are very low. These children appear to be at high risk for depressive and anxiety disorders in adulthood.

Major Depressive Episode

In DSM-5, patients with an episode of major depression must have at least five of nine symptoms of depression (and one of them must be depressed mood or loss of interest or pleasure). These characteristic symptoms define major depression, and they must be present for at least 2 weeks to rule out transient mood fluctuations. Also, the symptoms must cause distress or impairment in order to differentiate a disorder from normal fluctuations in mood. Other conditions must be ruled out, such as a bipolar disorder, abnormalities in mood due to the effects of a substance (e.g., amphetamines) or to a general medical condition (e.g., hypothyroidism) (Box 6–3).

Box 6–3. DSM-5 Criteria for Major Depressive Episode

A. Five (or more) of the following symptoms have been present during the same 2-week period and represent a change from previous functioning; at least one of the symptoms is either (1) depressed mood or (2) loss of interest or pleasure.

Note: Do not include symptoms that are clearly attributable to another medical condition.

1. Depressed mood most of the day, nearly every day, as indicated by either subjective report (e.g., feels sad, empty, or hopeless) or observation made by others (e.g., appears tearful). (**Note:** In children and adolescents, can be irritable mood.)
2. Markedly diminished interest or pleasure in all, or almost all, activities most of the day, nearly every day (as indicated by either subjective account or observation).
3. Significant weight loss when not dieting or weight gain (e.g., a change of more than 5% of body weight in a month), or decrease or increase in appetite nearly every day. (**Note:** In children, consider failure to make expected weight gain.)
4. Insomnia or hypersomnia nearly every day.
5. Psychomotor agitation or retardation nearly every day (observable by others; not merely subjective feelings of restlessness or being slowed down).
6. Fatigue or loss of energy nearly every day.
7. Feelings of worthlessness or excessive or inappropriate guilt (which may be delusional) nearly every day (not merely self-reproach or guilt about being sick).
8. Diminished ability to think or concentrate, or indecisiveness, nearly every day (either by subjective account or as observed by others).
9. Recurrent thoughts of death (not just fear of dying), recurrent suicidal ideation without a specific plan, or a suicide attempt or a specific plan for committing suicide.

B. The symptoms cause clinically significant distress or impairment in social, occupational, or other important areas of functioning.
C. The episode is not attributable to the physiological effects of a substance or another medical condition.

Note: Criteria A–C constitute a major depressive episode. Major depressive episodes are common in bipolar I disorder but are not required for the diagnosis of bipolar I disorder.

Note: Responses to a significant loss (e.g., bereavement, financial ruin, losses from a natural disaster, a serious medical illness or disability) may include the feelings of intense sadness, rumination about the loss, insomnia, poor appetite, and weight loss noted in Criterion A, which may resemble a depressive episode. Although such symptoms may be understandable or considered appropriate to the loss, the presence of a major depressive episode in addition to the normal response to a significant loss should also be carefully considered. This decision inevitably requires the exercise of clinical judgment based on the individual's history and the cultural norms for the expression of distress in the context of loss.[1]

Because major depression is the most common psychiatric illness that clinicians in any branch of medicine are likely to encounter, it is worthwhile to commit the nine characteristic symptoms to memory. When interviewing patients to determine whether they are depressed, the clinician must mentally run through this list of symptoms. Consequently, it is convenient to have it stored in an accessible memory bank so that the evaluation can be done fluently and smoothly. This can be facilitated through the use of a simple mnemonic: "**D**epression **I**s **W**orth **S**tudiously **M**emorizing **E**xtremely **G**rueling **C**riteria. **S**orry." (DIWSMEGCS). The initials stand for **D**epressed mood, **I**nterest, **W**eight, **S**leep, **M**otor activity, **E**nergy, **G**uilt, **C**oncentration, **S**uicide.

---

[1]In distinguishing grief from a major depressive episode (MDE), it is useful to consider that in grief the predominant affect is feelings of emptiness and loss, while in MDE it is persistent depressed mood and the inability to anticipate happiness or pleasure. The dysphoria in grief is likely to decrease in intensity over days to weeks and occurs in waves, the so-called pangs of grief. These waves tend to be associated with thoughts or reminders of the deceased. The depressed mood of MDE is more persistent and not tied to specific thoughts or preoccupations. The pain of grief may be accompanied by positive emotions and humor that are uncharacteristic of the pervasive unhappiness and misery characteristic of MDE. The thought content associated with grief generally features a preoccupation with thoughts and memories of the deceased, rather than the self-critical or pessimistic ruminations seen in MDE. In grief, self-esteem is generally preserved, whereas in MDE, feelings of worthlessness and self-loathing are common. If self-derogatory ideation is present in grief, it typically involves perceived failings vis-à-vis the deceased (e.g., not visiting frequently enough, not telling the deceased how much he or she was loved). If a bereaved individual thinks about death and dying, such thoughts are generally focused on the deceased and possibly about "joining" the deceased, whereas in MDE such thoughts are focused on ending one's own life because of feeling worthless, undeserving of life, or unable to cope with the pain of depression.

Clinical Findings

The basic abnormality in depression is an alteration in mood: a person who is depressed feels sad, despondent, down in the dumps, or full of despair. Occasional patients will complain of feeling tense or irritable, with only a small component of sadness, or of having lost their ability to feel pleasure or to experience interest in things they normally enjoy.

The depressive syndrome is frequently accompanied by a group of *vegetative* (or *somatic*) symptoms, such as decreased appetite or insomnia. Decreased appetite often leads to some weight loss, although some depressed persons will force themselves to eat despite decreased appetite, or they may be urged to eat by a parent or spouse. Less frequently, depression expresses itself as a desire to eat excessively and is accompanied by weight gain.

Insomnia may be initial, middle, or terminal. *Initial insomnia* means that the patient has difficulty falling asleep, often tossing or turning for several hours before dozing off. *Middle insomnia* refers to awakening in the middle of the night, remaining awake for an hour or two, and finally falling asleep again. *Terminal insomnia* refers to awakening early in the morning and being unable to return to sleep. Patients with insomnia will often worry and ruminate while they are lying awake. Patients who have terminal insomnia may have more severe depressive syndromes. Occasionally, the sleep difficulty may involve a need to sleep excessively: the patient may complain of feeling chronically tired and needing to spend 10–14 hours in bed each day.

Motor activity is often altered in depression. Patients with *psychomotor retardation* may sit quietly in a chair for hours without speaking to anyone, simply staring into space. When these patients get up and move about, they walk at a snail's pace; their speech is slow, and their replies are brief. If asked about their thinking, they may complain that it is markedly slowed. Conversely, patients with *psychomotor agitation* are restless and seem extremely nervous. Agitated patients may complain more of irritability or tenseness than of depression. They are unable to sit in a chair and frequently pace about. They may wring their hands or perform repetitive gestures such as drumming their fingers on a table or pulling on their hair or clothing.

Depressed patients also complain of fatiguing too easily or lacking energy. In a primary care setting, this may be one of the most common presenting complaints of depression.

Feelings of worthlessness and guilt are very common. Depressed persons may lose confidence in themselves so that they are fearful of going to work, taking examinations, or assuming responsibility for household tasks. They may not answer the telephone or return telephone calls to avoid responsibilities or social relationships that they feel unable to handle. They may become completely hopeless and full of despair, believing that their situation can never be improved or even that they do not deserve to feel better. Depressed patients may feel guilty over actual or fantasized misdeeds they have committed in the past. Usually the misdeed is seen as more terrible than it actually was, so that depressed persons believe that they should be social pariahs because of a lie told as a child or sent to prison for a long term because of a questionable deduction taken on an income tax return.

Complaints of difficulty in concentrating or thinking clearly are also common in depression. Depressed patients feel that they function less well at work, are unable to study, or in severe cases are even unable to perform simple cognitive tasks such as watching a football game on television or reading.

Depressed patients may think a great deal about death or dying. Suicide may be seen either as an escape from their suffering or as a deserved punishment for their various misdeeds. The suicidal patient often expresses the notion that "everyone would be better off without me." Suicide risk is high in depressed patients and should always be assessed carefully. (See Chapter 18, "Psychiatric Emergencies," for a description of the evaluation and management of the suicidal patient.)

In addition to the nine core symptoms summarized in the diagnostic criteria, other symptoms may occur in patients with depression. *Diurnal variation* is a fluctuation in mood during the course of a 24-hour day. Most typically, patients state that their mood is worse in the morning but that it improves as the day progresses, so that they feel best in the evening.

Sex drive may decrease markedly, so that the patient has no interest in sex or even begins to experience impotence or anorgasmia. The depressed patient also may complain of other physical symptoms such as constipation or dry mouth.

Occasionally, patients experience *masked depression*. This term means that the full depressive syndrome is not immediately obvious because the patient does not report a depressed mood. Masked depression may be especially important in primary care settings. For example, an older person may come in complaining primarily of somatic symptoms (e.g., insomnia, loss of energy and appetite) so troubling that he or she is unable to concentrate, work, and sleep. Although a careful medical workup reveals no physical abnormalities, the patient continues to insist on the troubling nature of the various somatic and depressive symptoms. When the masked depression is diagnosed and remits with appropriate treatment, physical complaints tend to disappear, making it clear that they were related to a depression.

About one-fifth of severely depressed patients experience *psychotic symptoms* such as delusions or hallucinations. These are usually congruent with the depressed mood ("mood-congruent"). For example, people who are depressed may hear the voice of the Devil telling them that they have fallen from God's ways and that they will be tormented in Hell. They may think that a fatal disease is consuming their bodies and rotting away their internal organs. Less frequently, the delusions will be inconsistent with depressed mood ("mood-incongruent"). For example, patients may report that they are being spied on because they are on the verge of developing some great invention that others are attempting to steal—a persecutory delusion that is not directly related to depressed mood.

The following case is that of a patient with major depressive episode:

> Wilma, a 41-year-old woman, was brought to the hospital by her family. She described herself as being despondent and demoralized because her husband, Bill, was having an affair with Lydia, a woman who had been his office assistant. Her husband adamantly denied having an affair.
>
> Wilma admitted to having a depressed mood plus feelings of worthlessness, suicidal thoughts, hypersomnia, increased appetite and weight gain, and decreased interest in and enjoyment of activities she normally found pleasurable. Wilma had had one prior episode of depression that had been successfully treated with antidepressants approximately 5 years earlier.
>
> Wilma attributed most of her depressive symptoms to this situation, which she believed had been going on for at least 6 months. She had no conclusive evidence to support the occurrence of the affair, but she said that her husband had been away more in the evenings, had a marked decrease in sexual interest, and had talked frequently about Lydia's administrative skills until Wilma became jealous and angry. Because of pressure from Wilma, her husband eventually urged Lydia to seek another position, but Wilma believed that her husband was continuing to see Lydia secretly.
>
> Major depression was diagnosed, and Wilma was given imipramine, with the dosage gradually increased to 150 mg/day. She showed some improvement on this medication, and both Bill and Wilma also were seen for marital counseling. Their relationship improved somewhat, but Wilma continued to be suspicious.
>
> After 3 months of psychotherapy, she came in one day with a new firmness of step and her eyes flashing with anger. While cleaning out the pockets of one of her husband's suits in preparation for sending it to the cleaners, she had found a love letter from Lydia. She did not confront Bill immediately but instead followed him the next night when he indicated that he was going back to the office to get caught up on some

work. Ten minutes after his departure, Wilma left, drove past Lydia's house and found Bill's car parked in her garage. She confronted him, and he finally confessed to an affair that had been going on for nearly 2 years.

The direction of marital counseling changed sharply, and Bill was urged to seek individual psychotherapy himself. Wilma continued to take antidepressant medication for another 6 months, and she gradually came to terms with the fact of her husband's infidelity. Eventually, however, the couple was able to work through this situation, to remain married, and eventually to establish a reasonably good relationship with each other.

Course and Outcome

A depressive episode may begin either suddenly or gradually. The duration of an untreated episode may range from a few weeks to months or even years, although most depressive episodes clear spontaneously within approximately 6 months. The prognosis for any single depressive episode is quite good, particularly in view of the efficacy of the available treatment. Unfortunately, a substantial number of patients will have a recurrence of depression at some time in their lives, and about 20% will develop a chronic form of depression.

Suicide is the most serious complication of depression. Approximately 10%–15% of all patients hospitalized for major depression will eventually take their own lives. Several factors suggest an increase in suicidal risk: being divorced or living alone, having a history of alcohol or drug abuse, being older than 40, having a history of a prior suicide attempt, and expressing suicidal ideation (particularly when detailed plans have been formulated). Suicidal risks always should be carefully evaluated in any patient with depression (or a depressed affect), beginning with a direct inquiry as to whether the patient has considered taking his or her life. A patient considered at risk for suicide usually should be treated as an inpatient to minimize the risk. Suicide and suicidal behavior are discussed in more detail in Chapter 18 ("Psychiatric Emergencies").

A broad range of other social and personal complications also may occur. Decreased energy, poor concentration, and lack of interest may cause poor performance at school or work. Apathy and decreased sexual interest may lead to marital discord. Patients may attempt to treat depressive symptoms themselves with sedatives, alcohol, or stimulants, thereby initiating problems with drug and alcohol abuse.

Persistent Depressive Disorder (Dysthymia)

Persistent depressive disorder (dysthymia) is a chronic and persistent disturbance in mood that has been present for at least 2 years and is characterized by relatively typical depressive symptoms such as anorexia, insomnia, decreased energy, low self-esteem, difficulty concentrating, and feelings of hopelessness. Because this is a chronic, mild disorder, only two of six symptoms are necessary, but they must have persisted more or less continuously for at least a 2-year period (Box 6–4). Major depression may precede persistent depressive disorder, and major depressive episodes may occur during persistent depressive disorder. Individuals whose symptoms meet major depressive disorder criteria for 2 years should be given a diagnosis of persistent depressive disorder as well as major depressive disorder.

Persistent depressive disorder often has an early onset, typically in childhood, adolescence, or early adult life, and by definition is chronic. Early onset (i.e., before age 21) is associated with a higher likelihood of comorbid personality disorders and substance use disorders.

Patients with persistent depressive disorder are chronically unhappy and miserable. Some of them also develop the relatively more severe major depressive syndrome. When the major depressive episode clears, these patients usually return to their chronic low mood. The coexistence of these mild and severe forms of depression is sometimes referred to as *double depression*.

Box 6–4.   DSM-5 Diagnostic Criteria for Persistent Depressive Disorder (Dysthymia)

This disorder represents a consolidation of DSM-IV-defined chronic major depressive disorder and dysthymic disorder.

A. Depressed mood for most of the day, for more days than not, as indicated by either subjective account or observation by others, for at least 2 years.

   Note: In children and adolescents, mood can be irritable and duration must be at least 1 year.

B. Presence, while depressed, of two (or more) of the following:

   1. Poor appetite or overeating.
   2. Insomnia or hypersomnia.
   3. Low energy or fatigue.
   4. Low self-esteem.
   5. Poor concentration or difficulty making decisions.
   6. Feelings of hopelessness.

C. During the 2-year period (1 year for children or adolescents) of the disturbance, the individual has never been without the symptoms in Criteria A and B for more than 2 months at a time.

D. Criteria for a major depressive disorder may be continuously present for 2 years.

E. There has never been a manic episode or a hypomanic episode, and criteria have never been met for cyclothymic disorder.

F. The disturbance is not better explained by a persistent schizoaffective disorder, schizophrenia, delusional disorder, or other specified or unspecified schizophrenia spectrum and other psychotic disorder.

G. The symptoms are not attributable to the physiological effects of a substance (e.g., a drug of abuse, a medication) or another medical condition (e.g. hypothyroidism).

H. The symptoms cause clinically significant distress or impairment in social, occupational, or other important areas of functioning.

Note: Because the criteria for a major depressive episode include four symptoms that are absent from the symptom list for persistent depressive disorder (dysthymia), a very limited number of individuals will have depressive symptoms that have persisted longer than 2 years but will not meet criteria for persistent depressive disorder. If full criteria for a major depressive episode have been met at some point during the current episode of illness, they should be given a diagnosis of major depressive disorder. Otherwise, a diagnosis of other specified depressive disorder or unspecified depressive disorder is warranted.

Specify if:
With anxious distress
With mixed features
With melancholic features
With atypical features
With mood-congruent psychotic features
With mood-incongruent psychotic features
With peripartum onset

Specify if:
In partial remission
In full remission

Specify if:
Early onset: If onset is before age 21 years.
Late onset: If onset is at age 21 years or older.

Specify if (for most recent 2 years of persistent depressive disorder):
With pure dysthymic syndrome: Full criteria for a major depressive episode have not been met in at least the preceding 2 years.
With persistent major depressive episode: Full criteria for a major depressive episode have been met throughout the preceding 2-year period.

With intermittent major depressive episodes, with current episode: Full criteria for a major depressive episode are currently met, but there have been periods of at least 8 weeks in at least the preceding 2 years with symptoms below the threshold for a full major depressive episode.

With intermittent major depressive episodes, without current episode: Full criteria for a major depressive episode are not currently met, but there has been one or more major depressive episodes in at least the preceding 2 years.

Specify current severity:

Mild

Moderate

Severe

Premenstrual Dysphoric Disorder

Premenstrual dysphoric disorder is a new diagnosis in DSM-5 (Box 6–5). Since the disorder was initially proposed in the 1980s as "late luteal phase dysphoric disorder," research evidence has accumulated to show that the disorder is common and causes significant distress and impairment. Clinical research and epidemiological studies have shown that many women experience depressive symptoms that begin during the luteal phase of the menstrual cycle and terminate around the onset of menses. Additionally, these studies identify a subset of women (about 2% in the community) who suffer intermittently from severe symptoms associated with the luteal phase of the menstrual cycle.

Box 6–5.   DSM-5 Diagnostic Criteria for Premenstrual
              Dysphoric Disorder

A. In the majority of menstrual cycles, at least five symptoms must be present in the final week before the onset of menses, start to *improve* within a few days after the onset of menses, and become *minimal* or absent in the week postmenses.

B. One (or more) of the following symptoms must be present:

1. Marked affective lability (e.g., mood swings; feeling suddenly sad or tearful, or increased sensitivity to rejection).

2. Marked irritability or anger or increased interpersonal conflicts.

3. Marked depressed mood, feelings of hopelessness, or self-deprecating thoughts.

4. Marked anxiety, tension, and/or feelings of being keyed up or on edge.

C. One (or more) of the following symptoms must additionally be present, to reach a total of *five* symptoms when combined with symptoms from Criterion B above.

1. Decreased interest in usual activities (e.g., work, school, friends, hobbies).
2. Subjective difficulty in concentration.
3. Lethargy, easy fatigability, or marked lack of energy.
4. Marked change in appetite; overeating; or specific food cravings.
5. Hypersomnia or insomnia.
6. A sense of being overwhelmed or out of control.
7. Physical symptoms such as breast tenderness or swelling, joint or muscle pain, a sensation of "bloating," or weight gain.

Note: The symptoms in Criteria A–C must have been met for most menstrual cycles that occurred in the preceding year.

D. The symptoms are associated with clinically significant distress or interference with work, school, usual social activities, or relationships with others (e.g., avoidance of social activities; decreased productivity and efficiency at work, school, or home).
E. The disturbance is not merely an exacerbation of the symptoms of another disorder, such as major depressive disorder, panic disorder, persistent depressive disorder (dysthymia), or a personality disorder (although it may co-occur with any of these disorders).
F. Criterion A should be confirmed by prospective daily ratings during at least two symptomatic cycles. (**Note:** The diagnosis may be made provisionally prior to this confirmation.)
G. The symptoms are not attributable to the physiological effects of a substance (e.g., a drug of abuse, a medication, other treatment) or another medical condition (e.g., hyperthyroidism).

■ Mood Disorder Specifiers

The mood disorders may be further specified based on patterns of symptoms detected during a careful evaluation. The importance of these specifiers is that they may indicate a specific treatment or may describe a particular course and outcome. Specifiers listed in DSM-5 include with anxious distress, with mixed features, with rapid cycling, with melancholic features, with atypical features, with psychotic features, with catatonia, with peripartum onset, and with seasonal pattern. Each may be used with either the bipolar and related disorders or the depressive disorders, with the exception of "with rapid cycling," which is only used in the case of the former.

Melancholic, Anxious Distress, and Mixed Features

The *melancholic features* specifier describes a relatively severe form of depression that is more likely to respond to somatic therapy. The concept is based on an older historic distinction between endogenous and reactive depression, a distinction that was based on both presumed etiology and a characteristic clustering of symptoms. In the original definition of *endogenous depression,* it had no precipitating factors (*endogenous* means "grows from within"), whereas a *reactive depression* occurred in reaction to some stressful life event such as a divorce or loss of a job.

Melancholia requires the presence of one of two specific characteristic features: loss of pleasure and inability to respond to pleasurable stimuli. Three from a list of six additional features also are required: distinct quality of depressed mood, regularly worse in the morning (diurnal variation), early morning awakening (terminal insomnia), marked psychomotor agitation or retardation, significant anorexia or weight loss, and excessive or inappropriate guilt.

Melancholic features are more common in inpatients, as opposed to outpatients, and are more likely to occur in severe major depressive episodes, particularly ones marked by psychosis. A substantial body of research has suggested that this clustering of symptoms predicts a good response to antidepressant medication or to electroconvulsive therapy (ECT).

Anxious distress has been noted as a prominent feature of both bipolar and major depressive disorders in primary care and mental health settings. High levels of anxiety have been associated with higher suicide risk, longer duration of illness, and greater likelihood of treatment nonresponse. As a result, it is clinically useful to specify accurately the presence and severity levels of anxious distress for treatment planning and monitoring of response to treatment.

Mixed features that occur with a major depressive episode have been found to be a significant risk factor for the development of bipolar I or bipolar II disorder. As a result, it is clinically useful to note the presence of this specifier for treatment planning and monitoring of response to treatment.

Atypical Features

Atypical features have an important historical context. Patients with these features do not present with the classic vegetative symptoms such as insomnia, weight loss, or anorexia but instead have weight gain and hypersomnia. The hypersomnia may include extended nighttime sleep or excessive daytime napping. In addition, instead of having a nonreactive mood, they are quite responsive to their life situation. The individual's *mood reactivity* is the capacity to be easily cheered by positive events (e.g., an unexpected compliment, a visit from one's children) but potentially to feel devastated by perceived slights or rejections. This rejection sensitivity often leads to difficulties in interpersonal relationships, with a stormy personal life characterized by being easily hurt, having many partners, and experiencing frequent breakups. Subjectively, these patients often express their somatic state by complaining of "leaden paralysis," the feeling that their arms and legs weigh them down and make activities difficult for them. Monoamine oxidase inhibitors (MAOIs) have proved particularly useful with this group of patients. Selective serotonin reuptake inhibitors (SSRIs) also may be effective.

Peripartum, Catatonia, Seasonal, and Rapid-Cycling Specifiers

DSM-5 also recognizes other aspects of a recent episode that may be clinically important.

The *peripartum onset* specifier identifies those patients who experience a depressive, manic, or hypomanic episode during pregnancy or within the first 4 weeks postpartum. Although feeling a bit depressed before or after delivery is common, some women develop a full mood syndrome that requires treatment. Although the estimates differ, 3%–6% of women will experience the onset of a major depressive episode during pregnancy or in the weeks or months following delivery. About 50% of "postpartum" depressive episodes actually begin prior to delivery. These episodes may be accompanied by severe anxiety and even panic attacks. Mood and anxiety symptoms during pregnancy, as well as the "baby blues," increase the risk for a postpartum major depressive episode. At its most severe, the mood episode may become psychotic and/or life threatening to the mother or child.

The *catatonic features* specifier identifies a subgroup of patients who have catatonic features similar to those that historically have been observed primarily in schizophrenia (e.g., posturing, waxy flexibility, catalepsy, negativism, and mutism). The presence of this specifier serves to remind clinicians that such symptoms also may occur in the mood disorders.

Another useful descriptor in DSM-5 recognizes that some depressed patients have a *seasonal pattern.* Clinicians have long recognized that some individuals have a characteristic onset of mood symptoms in relation to changes of season, with depression typically occurring more frequently during the winter months and remissions or changes from depression to mania occurring during the spring. Light therapy is reported to be an effective treatment for seasonal affective disorder (i.e., depressive illness that recurs in winter months and tends to remit in the spring). Exposure to bright light (minimum of 2,500 lux for 2 hours each morning) alleviates depressive symptoms. Most patients who respond to light therapy tend to use it daily during the winter months. Patients can also be treated with standard antidepressant therapy. The U.S. Food and Drug Administration (FDA) has approved an extended-release form of bupropion as a preventive treatment for seasonal affective disorder.

A *rapid-cycling* specifier identifies those patients who have had at least four major depressive, manic, hypomanic, or mixed episodes during the past 12 months. Rapid-cycling bipolar disorder is a particularly severe form of the disorder and is associated with a younger age at onset, more frequent depressive episodes, and greater risk for suicide attempts than other forms of the disorder.

■ Differential Diagnosis of Mood Disorders

When evaluating a patient with a mood disorder, the physician should always consider that the illness might result from some specific extrinsic factor that can induce a manic or depressive syndrome, such as drugs of abuse, sedatives, tranquilizers, antihypertensives, oral contraceptives, or glucocorticoids. General medical conditions such as hypothyroidism and systemic lupus erythematosus also may present with prominent depressive symptoms. If the episode of mood disorder is judged to be the result of a specific drug or medical illness, the disorder is diagnosed as secondary to it. Treatment usually involves withdrawing or reducing the drug or treating the underlying general medical illness.

Dysphoric mood may also occur in schizophrenia. In schizophrenia the dysphoric mood is more typically apathetic or empty, whereas in depression the dysphoric mood usually is experienced as intensely painful. The onset of schizophrenia usually is more gradual, and patients with schizophrenia also typically have a more severe deterioration in function than do patients with depression. Patients with schizophrenia and patients with major depression may both have psychotic symptoms; thus severe psychotic depression is sometimes difficult to distinguish from schizophrenia with acute onset. In this relatively difficult case, it is often best to treat the depression and to observe the course of illness over time. When psychotic symptoms persist after mood symptoms remit, then the diagnosis of schizophrenia or schizoaffective disorder is more likely.

The differential diagnosis between mania and schizophrenia is also quite important. Several features are useful in making this distinction. Personality and general functioning are usually satisfactory before and after a manic episode, even though mild disturbances in mood may occur. Although manic episodes may present with disorganized speech that is indistinguishable from the speech sometimes observed in schizophrenia, speech abnormalities in mania are always accompanied by a disturbance in mood and usually by overactivity and physical agitation. Manic patients may experience delusions or hallucinations, but these typically reflect the underlying disturbance in mood. (Mood-incongruent psychotic symptoms occur occasionally, making the differential diagnosis more difficult.) Additional guidelines that make the diagnosis of manic episode more likely include a family history of a mood disorder, good premorbid adjustment, and a previous episode of a mood disorder from which the patient completely or substantially recovered. When psychotic symptoms persist in the absence of an abnormality in mood, the diagnosis of schizophrenia or schizoaffective disorder is more likely.

People with *bereavement* may have many depressive symptoms and experience them for a sufficient duration to meet criteria for a depressive episode. In DSM-5, these individuals are now diagnosed with major depression. In the past, bereavement excluded a person from receiving the diagnosis unless the depressive symptoms were particularly severe or were accompanied by suicidal wishes or psychotic features. The change was made because researchers have shown that the loss of a loved one is about as likely as other stressors to trigger a major depressive episode. Although bereavement may be painful, most persons do not develop a major depressive episode. Those who do, however, typically experience more suffering, feel worthless, and may have suicidal ideation. Further, bereavement-induced depression has most of the characteristics of a major depressive episode; that is, it is most likely to occur in individuals with past personal and family history of a major depressive episode, is genetically influenced, and is associated with similar personality characteristics, patterns of comorbidity, and outcome. Finally, the symptoms associated with a bereavement-related major depressive disorder respond to antidepressant medication.

■ Epidemiology of Mood Disorders

The National Comorbidity Study reported a lifetime prevalence of nearly 17% for major depression and about 2% for bipolar I and II disorders combined. Persistent depressive disorder has a prevalence of around 2%–3%. Combined, these disorders affect just over one in five persons. Depression is more common in women than in men. The current ratio in the United States is approximately 2:1. Bipolar disorder also is more common in women than in men, with a ratio of approximately 3:2. This study also showed the median age at onset for major depression to be 32 years, for bipolar disorder 25 years, and for dysthymia 31 years. Men tend to have an earlier onset of bipolar disorder than women.

■ Etiology and Pathophysiology of Mood Disorders

The etiology of mood disorders is not well understood; however, genetic, social and environmental, and neurobiological factors may all play a role.

Genetics

Mood disorders tend to run in families, an observation confirmed by many investigators. However, familiality does not necessarily indicate genetic transmission, because role modeling, learned behavior, social environmental factors such as economic deprivation, and physical environmental factors such as prenatal and perinatal birth complications all may provide nongenetic contributions to the development of a disorder, and these contributions could themselves be familial. (For example, before the advent of antibiotics, tuberculosis tended to run in families for environmental rather than genetic reasons.)

Nearly all family studies show significantly increased rates of mood disorder, especially bipolar disorder, in the first-degree relatives of bipolar patients compared with control subjects. Unipolar depressed patients tend to have much less bipolar illness among their first-degree relatives but a high rate of unipolar illness. Thus these disorders not only are familial but also tend to breed true. However, the fact that they do not breed perfectly true (i.e., bipolar illness *only* in the relatives of bipolar patients and unipolar illness *only* in the relatives of unipolar patients) also suggests that these two forms of mood disorder may not be totally distinct from each other. Twin and adoption studies have complemented these family studies and have provided evidence that mood disorders are genetic in addition to being familial. If one averages together all the twin studies of mood disorder (slightly fewer than 500 twin pairs), the overall monozygotic-to-dizygotic ratio is approximately 4:1 (65% vs. 14%).

Efforts to identify genes implicated in mood disorders face several challenges. There has been debate about the definition of the phenotype. One view treats bipolar and unipolar mood disorders as distinct phenotypes. Within bipolar disorder, it is not clear whether a narrow definition limited to bipolar I is preferable or whether a broader model that includes bipolar II should be used. Alternatively, some argue that all mood disorders, ranging from bipolar to unipolar, should be grouped together. Because depression is so common, including it undoubtedly introduces phenocopies. Genome-wide studies have implicated several chromosomal regions, including 9p, 10q, 14q, 18p-q, and 8q. Candidate genes showing replicated associations with bipolar disorder include the D-amino-acid oxidase gene *(G72)*, brain-derived neurotrophic factor gene *(BDNF)*, neuregulin 1 gene *(NRG1)*, and dysbindin *(DTNBP1)*. Genes associated with the regulation of circadian rhythm *(CLOCK, TIMELESS, PERIOD3)* have also been implicated. Additionally, a polymorphism in the serotonin transporter gene has been associated with a vulnerability to developing depression when experiencing stresses such as job loss or divorce. Clearly, the task of identifying genes for the mood disorders is difficult, and the search will continue for many years to come.

Social and Environmental Factors

One of the fundamental questions about the nature of depression is how to draw the line between a normal response to a painful personal life experience and a clinically significant depression. Everyone experiences transient episodes of sadness after breaking up with a girlfriend or boyfriend, getting a divorce, performing badly on an examination, or losing a loved one. Diagnostic criteria were developed to assist in drawing this line by setting a relatively high bar to receiving a diagnosis of major depressive disorder. However, the criteria do not help with disentangling the effects of less serious life experiences.

People who experience a loss or disappointment often develop symptoms similar to those of major depression: feelings of sadness, difficulties with sleep or appetite, indecisiveness, poor concentration, or guilt or self-criticism. We all know people who continue to have these symptoms for more than a few weeks after a personal loss or other psychosocial stressor. When the symptoms persist long enough, then the person who experienced the stressor does in fact meet criteria for major depression, and this person may respond well to treatment with an antidepressant. Therefore, it is intuitively obvious that psychosocial stressors may play a role in the etiology of depression. The crucial question is not "Do psychosocial and environmental factors play a role in precipitating depression?" but rather "What is the nature of the role that psychosocial and environmental factors play? Do they tip a predisposed person over the edge, or are they sufficient in and of themselves?"

A plausible model for the role of stressful life events is that they do induce a biological reaction (e.g., an outpouring of cortisol). Once this biological reaction is initiated, it is difficult to stop and may trigger or exacerbate a depressive syndrome, particularly in individuals who have been previously primed because of either a genetic diathesis or experiences that made them particularly vulnerable to stress. In fact, a tendency to be neurobiologically oversensitive to the effects of psychosocial stress may be one of the genetic factors that are transmitted within families, as suggested by the polymorphism that has been identified in the serotonin transporter gene. These individuals may be unable to increase serotonergic tone in their brains to help them cope with stress and therefore develop a depressive response. Early life events, such as harsh or abusive parenting during childhood, could create a diathesis by making a person more psychologically sensitive to rejection and more biologically sensitive to stress.

Neurobiology

The *catecholamine hypothesis*, perhaps the earliest formulation concerning the role of neurotransmitters in depression, suggested that depression is caused by a deficit of norepinephrine at crucial nerve terminals throughout the brain. This hypothesis received support from studies of the mechanism of action of antidepressant medications used during the 1970s and 1980s. Classic work by Julius Axelrod, which led to his Nobel

Prize, demonstrated that antidepressants such as imipramine increase the amount of norepinephrine functionally available at nerve terminals by inhibiting reuptake. The MAOIs also increase the amount of norepinephrine available by inhibiting breakdown of norepinephrine through monoamine oxidase. Reserpine, which depletes monoamines, worsens depression.

The development of other types of antidepressant medications has indicated, however, that other neurotransmitters also may play a role in depression. The selective serotonin reuptake inhibitors (SSRIs) also are very effective treatments for depression, yet they do not act on the norepinephrine system. Instead, they appear to exert their therapeutic effect by increasing the amount of serotonin functionally available at nerve terminals. Furthermore, patients with severe depression have been found to have a decrease in a major serotonin metabolite, 5-hydroxyindoleacetic acid (5-HIAA), in their cerebrospinal fluid. In addition, numbers of serotonin type 2 (5-HT$_2$) receptors are decreased in postmortem brains of persons who have committed suicide.

Either a catecholamine hypothesis or a serotonin hypothesis is an oversimplification, although these hypotheses have been helpful. They have turned attention to examining the biological mechanisms of emotional and cognitive states and the role that these mental systems play in disease processes.

Neuroimaging Studies

Both structural and functional brain imaging techniques have been applied to study the mechanisms of mood disorders. A convergence of findings indicates that the subgenual prefrontal cortex (SGPFC) has particular importance among the various brain structures thought to play a role in depression. Positron emission tomography studies have demonstrated increased blood flow in this area when sadness is induced in non-ill subjects, and such changes are particularly marked in depressed patients. Lesions of this area block the extinction of fear conditioning in animal studies, and in humans the area is thought to be important in the evaluation of the consequences of social behavior. It may thus play a role in the heightened self-criticism and pessimistic ruminations that characterize depressive episodes. Several anatomic magnetic resonance studies have also found volumetric reductions in the SGPFC. Efforts to characterize the projections of the SGPFC in primates have shown direct connections to a number of areas important to the pathophysiology of depressive disorders. Particularly plentiful are projections to the hypothalamus, a structure central to the regulation of the hypothalamic-pituitary-adrenal axis. Another magnetic resonance abnormality observed in some patients is an increased number of focal signal hyperintensities in white matter; the functional significance of this abnormality is unclear, but it has been noted in both bipolar and unipolar mood disorders.

Abnormalities in Neurophysiological Function

Neurophysiological abnormalities also have been extensively studied in mood disorders. The largest and most consistent body of data involves the use of sleep electroencephalography (EEG). (Sleep EEG, or polysomnography, is further discussed in Chapter 12, "Sleep-Wake Disorders.") Studies have consistently found that patients with depression have a variety of abnormal electroencephalographic findings during sleep, including decreased slow-wave sleep (i.e., deep sleep), a shortened time before the onset of rapid eye movement (REM) sleep (the period when dreams and nightmares occur), and longer periods of REM sleep, compared with subjects without depression. These three types of abnormality are referred to as decreased delta sleep, decreased REM latency, and increased REM density, respectively. All of these abnormalities in sleep EEG correspond with the subjective sleep complaints of depressed patients. A recent positron emission tomography study suggests that depressed patients, in contrast with control subjects, have a relative hypermetabolism in frontoparietal regions and thalamus during the transition from wakefulness to non-REM sleep, which may help to explain their sleep anomalies.

Abnormalities in Neuroendocrine Function

Neuroendocrine abnormalities also have been extensively explored in patients with depression. Early research in this area suggested that depressed patients have abnormal diurnal variation in cortisol production. The dexamethasone suppression test (DST) has been used extensively to explore the possibility of neuroendocrine dysregulation in depression and to attempt to determine the place on the hypothalamic-pituitary-adrenal axis where this abnormality might occur. Up to 70% of patients with severe depression have abnormal suppression of cortisol secretion after the administration of dexamethasone. Rates of dexamethasone nonsuppression in other psychiatric conditions, such as anorexia nervosa, dementia, and substance abuse, are also relatively high.

In addition to the hypothalamic-pituitary-adrenal axis, other aspects of the neuroendocrine system have been explored. Depressed patients have been shown to have a blunting of growth hormone output in response to insulin challenge as well as a blunted production of thyroid-stimulating hormone in response to thyrotropin-releasing hormone. The abnormalities across a variety of neuroendocrine target organs (e.g., adrenals, pancreas, thyroid) indicate that the problem is not in these organs, and the patterns of abnormal response to challenge suggest that it is also not in the pituitary. More likely, the abnormality is at the level of the hypothalamus, a brain region regulated largely through monoamine neurotransmitters.

■ Clinical Management of Mood Disorders

Treatment of Mania

Lithium, valproate, and carbamazepine are all approved by the FDA for the acute treatment of mania. Lamotrigine is approved for maintenance treatment of bipolar disorder. Several additional anticonvulsant drugs (including gabapentin and topiramate) have been used to treat bipolar patients but have had mixed results. In addition, nearly all second-generation antipsychotics (SGAs) are approved to treat acute mania except clozapine, and several have received indications for maintenance treatment of bipolar disorder or as adjuncts to lithium or valproate. The rational use of these drugs, and their dosing, is described in Chapter 21 ("Psychopharmacology and Electroconvulsive Therapy").

Electroconvulsive therapy is highly effective in treatment of manic patients when medication is ineffective.

Treatment of Depression

Various medications are available to treat depression: tricyclics and other related compounds, MAOIs, SSRIs, and other antidepressants that are not easily categorized, such as bupropion and mirtazapine. These drugs are all thought to work by altering levels of various neurotransmitters at crucial nerve terminals in the central nervous system. They are largely similar in their overall effectiveness, and from 65% to 70% of persons who receive antidepressants will markedly improve. Unfortunately, and despite adequate treatment, some patients develop a tendency to become treatment refractory, a phenomenon called *tachyphylaxis* or "poop out."

Clinical points for mania

1. Somatic therapies should be used aggressively to treat manic symptoms as rapidly as possible.

2. The patient should be followed up closely as the mania "breaks" to determine whether a subsequent depression is emerging.

3. After an episode of mania, patients should receive maintenance medication; typically they will continue to take mood stabilizers for several years, and perhaps for the remainder of their lives, to prevent subsequent relapses.

4. Patients should be advised about the importance of getting sufficient sleep and of following sensible sleep hygiene measures (described in Chapter 12, "Sleep-Wake Disorders").

5. Even when they are stable, patients should be followed up regularly to ensure continued compliance with medication and to monitor blood levels (if applicable).

6. Manic episodes can have devastating personal, social, and economic consequences; patients will usually require (at a minimum) supportive psychotherapy to help them cope with these consequences and maintain their self-esteem.

7. Family members should be provided with both psychological support, as needed, and educational materials to help them understand the disorder, its symptoms, and the need for continued treatment.

8. Patients with bipolar illness are often appreciative of being told about the "good side" of their illness: its association with creativity and high achievement.

Treatment should begin with one of the SSRIs because they are well tolerated and safe in overdose. Low dosages are generally effective, and frequent dosage adjustments are usually unnecessary. In particular, patients with cardiac conduction defects should receive an SSRI (or one of the other new agents). Likewise, impulsive or suicidal patients should receive an SSRI or one of the newer medications that are unlikely to be dangerous in overdose. Most patients will actually start to improve relatively quickly, even within the first 1 or 2 weeks after starting medication. Although the SSRIs are relatively safe in overdose as compared with the older tricyclic antidepressants and MAOIs, they have also been reported to increase the risk for impulsive behavior and even suicidality. Therefore, patients treated with SSRIs should be carefully monitored, and these medications should be used with caution in teenagers and young adults.

Drug trials should generally last from 4 to 8 weeks. If the patient fails to respond within 4 weeks of treatment, the dosage should be increased or the patient switched to another drug, preferably from another class (e.g., providing a different balance of norepinephrine, serotonin, and acetylcholine).

One useful strategy to boost the effectiveness of antidepressants is to augment treatment with another drug. Augmentation with lithium carbonate is the best-researched option. Other agents have been used for augmentation and include triiodothyronine, a thyroid preparation; psychostimulants such as methylphenidate; pindolol, a beta-blocker; and benzodiazepines. Antipsychotics have also been used, and in fact aripiprazole, a second-generation antipsychotic, is approved by the FDA for this purpose. The combination of the SGA olanzapine and the SSRI fluoxetine is FDA approved for use in cases of treatment-resistant depression.

When the depressed patient is psychotic, we generally recommend co-administering an antipsychotic, such as one of the SGAs. Benzodiazepines co-administered with the antidepressant may help calm the anxious or agitated depressed patient relatively quickly.

For patients who are experiencing their first episode of depression, the drug should be continued for another 16–36 weeks after the patient is considered to have recovered. Thereafter, the clinician may decide to discontinue the medication while monitoring the patient closely. Because some antidepressants produce undesirable side effects such as weight gain, and because conservative prescription of medications is always a good clinical practice, discontinuation should almost always be attempted in patients who do not have a history of recurrent depression. The medication should be discontinued gradually because many patients experience mild withdrawal symptoms, particularly if tricyclics or SSRIs (except fluoxetine) are discontinued abruptly. Patients sometimes subjectively experience these withdrawal symptoms as a recurrence or relapse. Symptoms that can occur on withdrawal of antidepressants include insomnia and nervousness, nightmares, and gastrointestinal symptoms such as nausea or vomiting. Patients with recurrent depressions often will need long-term maintenance, typically at the full treatment dosage. Research shows that long-term maintenance can significantly reduce the risk of relapse and increase the patient's quality of life.

MAOIs may be used to treat those patients whose symptoms do not respond to the first-line antidepressants or who are unable to tolerate their side effects. MAOIs should be used with caution because they have potentially more dangerous side effects and interactions than do the other antidepressants. MAOIs may be particularly useful in patients characterized by *atypical depression,* with symptoms such as hypersomnia, increased appetite, and rejection sensitivity.

Clinical points for depression

1. A hopeful, optimistic tone should be established at the initial interview.

    • The severity of the depressive syndrome should be assessed, remembering that there may be individual and cultural differences in the way depression is experienced and expressed.

    • Extensive psychological probing should not be attempted when the patient is deeply depressed.

    • Suicidal risk should be determined initially and reassessed frequently.

2. Moderate to severe depression should be treated aggressively with somatic therapy.

    • Severely depressed or suicidal patients may require hospitalization.

    • Severely depressed outpatients may need frequent (e.g., twice-weekly) brief (e.g., 10- to 15-minute) contacts for support and medication management until their depression lifts.

    • Most patients will require at least 16–20 weeks of maintenance medication following an initial episode and thereafter should be given a trial of decreasing or discontinuing the medication. If symptoms reemerge, medication should be reinstituted, and consideration should be given to long-term drug administration.

3. The clinician should determine whether psychosocial stressors are present that are contributing to the depressed mood and should counsel the patient on ways to cope with them.

4. Depressed patients tend to "get down" on themselves because they have been depressed; the clinician should help the patient learn to abandon negative or self-deprecating attitudes through cognitive-behavioral therapy or other psychotherapeutic techniques.

ECT is another option for the treatment of depression. Methods for administering and monitoring ECT, as well as its side effects, are described in more detail in Chapter 21, "Psychopharmacology and Electroconvulsive Therapy." In general, indications for ECT include severe depression, high potential for suicide, cardiovascular disease (which may preclude use of some antidepressants), and pregnancy. ECT often produces a rapid remission of depressive symptoms. Patients will need maintenance antidepressant treatment after the course of ECT is completed.

Both repetitive transcranial magnetic stimulation (rTMS) and vagal nerve stimulation (VNS) are FDA approved to treat adults with treatment-refractory depression. Neither treatment is widely available, and their respective roles in treating depression are not yet clear. With rTMS, magnetic pulses are applied to the scalp using a handheld coil. The magnetic field passes through the scalp and induces a current in underlying tissue, depolarizing neurons. Patients can experience headache, nausea, and dizziness. With VNS, a device is implanted under the skin of the chest wall and an electrode is connected to the vagus nerve. The device sends small electrical pulses to the vagus nerve on the left side of the neck, which in turn delivers these pulses to the brain. Problems include the discomfort of surgical implantation and adverse effects related to vagus nerve function, including hoarseness, cough, and dysphagia. Both treatments are thought to alter levels of neurotransmitters and functional activity of the central nervous system dysregulated in depression.

Other Treatments

Experiencing an episode of mood disorder is often a major blow to the patient's confidence and self-esteem. Consequently, most patients will require supportive psychotherapy in addition to whatever medications are prescribed. During the acute episode, the clinician will typically let the depressive wound begin to heal. As the patient recovers, the clinician may begin to review with him or her the various social and psychological factors that may be causing distress or that may have worsened as a consequence of depression. Work, school performance, and interpersonal relationships all may be impaired because of a mood disorder. It is important to help patients assess these problems and recognize that the illness is responsible—rather than feeling that they themselves are responsible—and to instill confidence that they can now begin to restore and repair whatever injuries have occurred as a consequence of their episode of mood disorder.

Some depressed patients will respond well to brief psychotherapy alone. Both cognitive-behavioral therapy and interpersonal therapy are as effective as medication in the treatment of mild to moderately severe depression, and their combination with psychotherapy is even more powerful. Psychotherapy is described in greater detail in Chapter 20, "Behavioral, Cognitive, and Psychodynamic Treatments."

■ Self-Assessment Questions

1. What are the nine symptoms used to define a major depressive episode in DSM-5?

2. What is the difference between delusions that are mood congruent and those that are mood incongruent?
3. What is the lifetime prevalence for bipolar disorder and for major depression?
4. Review the evidence that suggests that mood disorders are familial and may be genetic.
5. Which neurotransmitter systems have been proposed to be dysfunctional in mood disorders?
6. Identify at least four genes that have been implicated as playing a role in mood disorders.
7. What is the difference between bereavement and major depression?
8. Describe the first-line treatment for a manic episode. What alternative treatments are available?
9. Describe the first-line treatments for depression as well as the various alternative treatments and their indications.

Chapter 7

Anxiety Disorders

I stood stunned, my hair rose, the voice stuck in my throat.

Virgil

Anxiety disorders are among the most prevalent psychiatric conditions worldwide, and are a leading cause of distress and impairment. The word *anxiety* has been used to describe diverse phenomena, but in the clinical literature refers to the presence of fear or apprehension that is out of proportion to the situation. Anxiety was considered to play an important role in several conditions identified in the nineteenth century. Da Costa described the "irritable heart syndrome," characterized by chest pain, palpitations, and dizziness, a disorder thought due to a functional cardiac disturbance. He described the syndrome in a Civil War veteran, and later it was variously referred to as *soldier's heart, effort syndrome,* or *neurocirculatory asthenia.*

While internists were emphasizing cardiovascular aspects of the anxiety syndrome, psychiatrists and neurologists focused on its psychological aspects. Freud was among the first to recognize that feelings related to earlier trauma could express themselves in anxious symptoms and behaviors. He introduced the term *anxiety neurosis* to describe a disorder characterized by feelings of fearfulness, panic, and doom. Today we call this syndrome *panic disorder.*

DSM-III gave shape to the anxiety disorders class by grouping panic disorder with phobic disorders, obsessive-compulsive disorder, and posttraumatic stress disorder (PTSD), a new diagnosis created to better describe the symptoms that war veterans and trauma victims had experienced. Acute stress disorder was added to the class in DSM-IV.

In DSM-5, the anxiety disorders have been reconceptualized. Obsessive-compulsive disorder now has its own chapter (see Chapter 8, "Obsessive-Compulsive and Related Disorders"). Posttraumatic stress disorder and acute stress disorder have been moved to "Trauma- and Stressor-

Related Disorders" (see Chapter 9). The changes were made in response to scientific data showing that these disorders stand apart from the other anxiety disorders. Last, separation anxiety disorder and selective mutism are new to the chapter, having been formerly included with DSM-IV's "Disorders Usually First Diagnosed in Infancy, Childhood, or Adolescence." They were moved because of research linking them to the anxiety disorders and the growing recognition that both conditions can also occur in adults. Categories are included for those whose anxiety syndrome is due to the effects of a substance, medication, or another medical condition. For those who do not fit into any of the better defined categories, the residual categories *other specified anxiety disorder* and *unspecified anxiety disorder* are available. The DSM-5 anxiety disorders are listed in Table 7–1.

■ Separation Anxiety Disorder

With separation anxiety disorder, a person has excessive anxiety regarding separation from places or people to whom he or she has a strong emotional attachment. The 12-month prevalence estimate of separation anxiety disorder in childhood is about 4%; in adults the figure is about 1%–2%. In fact, the majority of adults with separation anxiety disorder had a first onset in adulthood. In children, the strong emotional attachment is likely to a parent, but with adults the attachment might be to a spouse or friend. Disorders that start in childhood generally do not persist into adulthood.

Separation anxiety disorder should not be confused with separation anxiety that occurs as a normal stage of development for healthy, secure babies. Most infants and children experience fear at the possibility (or reality) of being separated from their parents. Once infants learn to recognize maternal and paternal faces and shapes, they also learn to cry when the parent leaves the room or hands them to a stranger. (Stranger anxiety first develops at about age 9 months.) No doubt this pattern of behavior reflects some type of primal fear of loss or fear of the unknown. As the child grows older, he or she also experiences natural fears of being left with a babysitter, being sent to preschool, or entering kindergarten. Crying, tenseness, or physical complaints may appear and last for minutes, hours, or days in such situations.

As specified in DSM-5, separation anxiety disorder is defined largely by the persistence of such symptoms for a long enough duration to be considered pathological (see Box 7–1). At least three of eight char-

---

TABLE 7–1. DSM-5 anxiety disorders

Separation anxiety disorder

Selective mutism

Specific phobia

Social anxiety disorder (social phobia)

Panic disorder

Agoraphobia

Generalized anxiety disorder

Substance/medication-induced anxiety disorder

Anxiety disorder due to another medical condition

Other specified anxiety disorder

Unspecified anxiety disorder

---

acteristic symptoms must be present for at least 4 weeks (6 months or more in adults) and include three types of distress or worry (distress at being separated from home, worry that some harm will come to major attachment figures [i.e., parents], and worry that an untoward event will cause the separation [e.g., kidnapping]), three types of behaviors (school or work refusal, sleep refusal, and clinging), and two physiological symptoms (nightmares and physical complaints such as headache or nausea).

Box 7–1. DSM-5 Diagnostic Criteria for Separation Anxiety Disorder

---

A. Developmentally inappropriate and excessive fear or anxiety concerning separation from those to whom the individual is attached, as evidenced by at least three of the following:

1. Recurrent excessive distress when anticipating or experiencing separation from home or from major attachment figures.
2. Persistent and excessive worry about losing major attachment figures or about possible harm to them, such as illness, injury, disasters, or death.
3. Persistent and excessive worry about experiencing an untoward event (e.g., getting lost, being kidnapped, having an accident, becoming ill) that causes separation from a major attachment figure.
4. Persistent reluctance or refusal to go out, away from home, to school, to work, or elsewhere because of fear of separation.

5. Persistent and excessive fear of or reluctance about being alone or without major attachment figures at home or in other settings.
6. Persistent reluctance or refusal to sleep away from home or to go to sleep without being near a major attachment figure.
7. Repeated nightmares involving the theme of separation.
8. Repeated complaints of physical symptoms (e.g., headaches, stomachaches, nausea, vomiting) when separation from major attachment figures occurs or is anticipated.

B. The fear, anxiety, or avoidance is persistent, lasting at least 4 weeks in children and adolescents and typically 6 months or more in adults.
C. The disturbance causes clinically significant distress or impairment in social, academic, occupational, or other important areas of functioning.
D. The disturbance is not better explained by another mental disorder, such as refusing to leave home because of excessive resistance to change in autism spectrum disorder; delusions or hallucinations concerning separation in psychotic disorders; refusal to go outside without a trusted companion in agoraphobia; worries about ill health or other harm befalling significant others in generalized anxiety disorder; or concerns about having an illness in illness anxiety disorder.

In children, this disorder may present as school phobia, school refusal, or school absenteeism. Children with this problem develop a fear of going to school, typically during grade school or junior high school. A child who has previously been attending school (albeit with some anxiety) begins to develop methods for staying home. He or she may have repeated episodes of "illness" such as headache or nausea. Such children may be truant, leaving home with the appearance of going to school and then returning home without their parents' knowledge or going to some other environment that they experience as safe. They may simply refuse to go to school and give only some vague explanation such as "I don't like it." Not all children who refuse to attend school have a separation anxiety disorder, and for that reason clinicians need to rule out other diagnostic possibilities (e.g., truancy secondary to conduct disorder, avoidance of school as a complication of mood disorder, school avoidance secondary to a psychosis), or even stressors such as bullying.

Treatment of separation anxiety disorder involves a combination of medication and individual psychotherapy (often combined with family therapy or parental guidance). Medication can help control the feelings of anxiety and fear. Selective serotonin reuptake inhibitors (SSRIs) have been used with some success, as have benzodiazepines. Cognitive-behavioral methods can help the child (or adult) to correct dysfunctional beliefs (e.g., "No one likes me"), promote a positive self-image, and learn problem-solving skills. This can be combined with social skills training, graded exposure and desensitization, and anxiety reduction techniques (e.g., relaxation training). Parental involvement can help reinforce the child's successes and promote the child's social participation, and model appropriate behavior. If school refusal is the main problem, it is important to emphasize to both the child and the family that the child must attend school regularly and that absenteeism or refusal cannot be tolerated.

■ Selective Mutism

Selective mutism is the persistent failure to speak in specific social situations where speaking is expected despite being able to speak in other situations (e.g., at home). The disorder is uncommon and most likely to manifest in young children. Selective mutism should be distinguished from normal shyness and other reasons for reluctance to speak such as unfamiliarity with the language.

In specific social interactions, children and adults with selective mutism do not initiate speech (or reciprocally respond) when spoken to by others. These same individuals, however, can interact normally at home. Because children are frequently quiet when entering an unfamiliar classroom, this diagnosis should not be given when the lack of speech occurs only during the first month of school, as the diagnosis requires a consistent failure to speak in a social situation.

Selective mutism is associated with significant impairment. As these children mature they may face increasing social isolation, and in school settings suffer academic impairment because often they do not communicate appropriately with teachers regarding academic or personal needs. Brief periods of selective silence lasting less than a month do not qualify an individual for this diagnosis.

Children in families that have immigrated to a country where a different language is spoken may refuse to speak the new language because of lack of knowledge of the language. If comprehension of the new language is adequate but refusal to speak persists, a diagnosis of selective mutism is warranted.

Although children with selective mutism generally have normal language skills, there may occasionally be an associated communication disorder. Selective mutism should be distinguished from speech disturbances that are better explained by a communication disorder, such as language disorder, speech sound disorder (previously phonological disorder), childhood-onset fluency disorder (stuttering), or pragmatic (social) communication disorder. Unlike selective mutism, the speech disturbance in these conditions is not restricted to a specific social situation. Individuals with an autism spectrum disorder, schizophrenia or another psychotic disorder, or severe intellectual disability may have problems in social communication and be unable to speak appropriately in social situations. In contrast, selective mutism should be diagnosed only when a child has an established capacity to speak in some social situations (typically at home).

Treatment of selective mutism is difficult and usually involves the use of SSRIs and behavior therapy techniques such as contingency management, positive reinforcement, desensitization, and assertiveness training. Parental counseling is also important. Parents (and teachers) often make accommodations to the child's muteness, but it is generally useful to maintain the expectation that the child will talk and communicate, at least for a certain amount of time at home and at school.

DSM-5 criteria for selective mutism are shown in Box 7–2.

Box 7–2.   DSM-5 Diagnostic Criteria for Selective Mutism

A. Consistent failure to speak in specific social situations in which there is an expectation for speaking (e.g., at school) despite speaking in other situations.
B. The disturbance interferes with educational or occupational achievement or with social communication.
C. The duration of the disturbance is at least 1 month (not limited to the first month of school).
D. The failure to speak is not attributable to a lack of knowledge of, or comfort with, the spoken language required in the social situation.
E. The disturbance is not better explained by a communication disorder (e.g., childhood-onset fluency disorder) and does not occur exclusively during the course of autism spectrum disorder, schizophrenia, or another psychotic disorder.

■ Specific Phobia and Social Anxiety Disorder (Social Phobia)

Phobias are irrational fears of specific objects, places or situations, or activities. Although fear can be adaptive to some extent, the fear in phobias is irrational, excessive, and disproportionate to any actual danger. *Social anxiety disorder (social phobia)* is the fear of humiliation or embarrassment in social settings, while *specific phobia* is a category that includes isolated phobias such as the irrational and intense fear of snakes.

Persons with social anxiety disorder fear situations in which they might be observed by other people. These persons also commonly fear performance situations such as speaking in public, eating in restaurants, writing in front of other persons, or using public restrooms. Sometimes the fear becomes generalized, so that phobic persons avoid most social situations. Specific phobias are usually well circumscribed and involve objects that could conceivably cause harm, such as snakes, heights, flying, or blood, but the person's reaction to them is excessive and inappropriate.

The DSM-5 criteria for specific phobia and social anxiety disorder are presented in Boxes 7–3 and 7–4, respectively. For these diagnoses, the phobia must have lasted at least 6 months (a requirement meant to exclude those with transient fears). The phobia causes clinically significant distress or impairment, and other causes for the disorder have been ruled out including another mental disorder or medical condition. Patients with social phobia are ill at ease in the interview situation. They often appear anxious or fearful, and their verbal responses may be restricted.

Box 7–3.   DSM-5 Diagnostic Criteria for Specific Phobia

A. Marked fear or anxiety about a specific object or situation (e.g., flying, heights, animals, receiving an injection, seeing blood).

   Note: In children, the fear or anxiety may be expressed by crying, tantrums, freezing, or clinging.

B. The phobic object or situation almost always provokes immediate fear or anxiety.

C. The phobic object or situation is actively avoided or endured with intense fear or anxiety.

D. The fear or anxiety is out of proportion to the actual danger posed by the specific object or situation and to the sociocultural context.

E. The fear, anxiety, or avoidance is persistent, typically lasting for 6 months or more.

F. The fear, anxiety, or avoidance causes clinically significant distress or impairment in social, occupational, or other important areas of functioning.

G. The disturbance is not better explained by the symptoms of another mental disorder, including fear, anxiety, and avoidance of situations associated with panic-like symptoms or other incapacitating symptoms (as in agoraphobia); objects or situations related to obsessions (as in obsessive-compulsive disorder); reminders of traumatic events (as in posttraumatic stress disorder); separation from home or attachment figures (as in separation anxiety disorder); or social situations (as in social anxiety disorder).

Specify if:
Animal (e.g., spiders, insects, dogs).
Natural environment (e.g., heights, storms, water).
Blood-injection-injury (e.g., needles, invasive medical procedures).
Situational (e.g., airplanes, elevators, enclosed places).
Other (e.g., situations that may lead to choking or vomiting; in children, e.g., loud sounds or costumed characters).

Box 7–4. DSM-5 Diagnostic Criteria for Social Anxiety Disorder (Social Phobia)

A. Marked fear or anxiety about one or more social situations in which the individual is exposed to possible scrutiny by others. Examples include social interactions (e.g., having a conversation, meeting unfamiliar people), being observed (e.g., eating or drinking), and performing in front of others (e.g., giving a speech).

   Note: In children, the anxiety must occur in peer settings and not just during interactions with adults.

B. The individual fears that he or she will act in a way or show anxiety symptoms that will be negatively evaluated (i.e., will be humiliating or embarrassing; will lead to rejection or offend others).

C. The social situations almost always provoke fear or anxiety.

   Note: In children, the fear or anxiety may be expressed by crying, tantrums, freezing, clinging, shrinking, or failing to speak in social situations.

D. The social situations are avoided or endured with intense fear or anxiety.

E. The fear or anxiety is out of proportion to the actual threat posed by the social situation and to the sociocultural context.

F. The fear, anxiety, or avoidance is persistent, typically lasting for 6 months or more.

G. The fear, anxiety, or avoidance causes clinically significant distress or impairment in social, occupational, or other important areas of functioning.

H. The fear, anxiety, or avoidance is not attributable to the physiological effects of a substance (e.g., a drug of abuse, a medication) or another medical condition.

I. The fear, anxiety, or avoidance is not better explained by the symptoms of another mental disorder, such as panic disorder, body dysmorphic disorder, or autism spectrum disorder.

J. If another medical condition (e.g., Parkinson's disease, obesity, disfigurement from burns or injury) is present, the fear, anxiety, or avoidance is clearly unrelated or is excessive.

Specify if:
   Performance only: If the fear is restricted to speaking or performing in public.

Epidemiology, Clinical Findings, and Course

Specific phobias and social anxiety disorder are surprisingly common, with prevalence rates in the National Comorbidity Survey of 11% for specific phobias and 13% for social anxiety disorder. Specific phobias are more common in women, whereas social anxiety disorder affects men and women about equally. Specific phobias begin in childhood, most starting before age 12. Social anxiety disorder begins during adolescence, and almost always before age 25. Among specific phobias, the most commonly feared objects or situations are animals, storms, heights, illness, injury, and death.

Despite the frequency of phobias in the general population, few phobic persons seek treatment, because they are generally symptom free apart from contact with feared objects or situations. Most individuals simply avoid the object of their fears and in doing so find that it does not interfere with their work or social life. Fear of snakes, for instance, is not likely to keep a person from succeeding socially or occupationally, but fear of flying may do so (for example, a salesperson who is expected to travel around the country). This may help to explain why phobia patients constitute only 2%–3% of psychiatric outpatients.

Persons with social anxiety disorder or specific phobias experience anxiety when exposed to feared objects or situations and manifest autonomic arousal and avoidance behavior. Initially, exposure leads to an unpleasant subjective state of anxiety. This state is accompanied by physical symptoms such as rapid heartbeat, shortness of breath, and jitteriness. Individuals with social anxiety disorder may fear doing or saying something that might cause humiliation or embarrassment in social situations. Others are afraid that people will recognize their anxiety through some outward sign (e.g., blushing, sweating, trembling). In severe cases, the socially anxious person may avoid almost all social encounters and become isolated. For the person with a specific phobia, distress varies with exposure to the feared object or situation. For example, a hospital employee who fears blood might experience considerable distress in a surgical suite.

The following case is of a boy with a specific phobia and the problems the disorder caused for him:

> John, a 13-year-old boy, was brought to the clinic by his mother. She reported that John would not wear shirts that had buttons on them and was worried that this peculiarity would cause problems for John when he was older. Already, his mother pointed out, not being able to wear regular collared shirts had kept John out of scouting troops and the school orchestra because of the uniforms he would have had to wear. Doctors had told John's mother in the past that he would outgrow this fear. John clearly was uncomfortable and appeared embarrassed by his mother's recitation of the story but admitted that it was true. John said that at about age 4, he had developed a fear of buttons but was not sure why. Since then, he had worn only T-shirts or sweaters and had refused to wear collared shirts. In fact, John said, just thinking about such shirts bothered him, and he even avoided touching his brother's shirts that hung in the closet they shared.
>
> Ten years later, John had finished college and had enrolled in graduate school. He had overcome the phobia by himself at age 16 and was able to wear regular collared shirts, but he still reported that he avoided wearing these shirts whenever possible.

Social anxiety disorder tends to develop slowly, is chronic, and has no obvious precipitating events. Whether the disorder is perceived as disabling depends on the nature and extent of the fear as well as one's occupation and social position. A business executive whose job requires meeting with the public, for instance, would face much greater disability from social anxiety disorder than would a software designer or computer programmer who works in isolation.

About one in eight persons with social anxiety disorder develops a substance use disorder, and about one-half meet criteria for another psychiatric disorder, such as major depression.

Unlike social anxiety disorder, specific phobias tend to subside (or remit) as a person ages, as illustrated in the case of John. When they persist into adulthood, specific phobias often become chronic, though rarely causing disability.

Etiology and Pathophysiology

Phobic disorders tend to run in families. Studies show that relatives of phobic persons were significantly more likely to have phobias than those of nonphobic control subjects. Further, the disorders breed true—that is, people with social anxiety disorder are likely to have relatives with social anxiety disorder, and not a specific phobia.

The biological underpinnings of the phobias are not well understood. Research suggests that dopaminergic pathways play a role in social anxiety disorder. These patients show a preferential response to monoamine oxidase inhibitors (MAOIs), which have dopaminergic activity. Lower levels of dopamine metabolites in cerebrospinal fluid have been linked to introversion, a facet of social anxiety disorder. Additionally, functional brain imaging studies have found decreased striatal dopamine D_2 receptor and dopamine transporter binding in patients with social anxiety disorder.

Learning also may play an important role in the etiology of phobias. Behaviorists have pointed out that many phobias tend to arise in association with traumatic events, for example developing a fear of heights after a fall. Psychoanalysts have long held that phobias result from unresolved conflicts in childhood and attribute phobias to the use of displacement and avoidance as defense mechanisms.

Differential Diagnosis

The differential diagnosis of phobic disorders includes other anxiety disorders (e.g., panic disorder), obsessive-compulsive disorder, mood disorders, schizophrenia, and both schizoid and avoidant personality disorders. The irrational fear that characterizes phobias needs to be distinguished from a delusion, which involves a fixed false belief (e.g., "The people I'm avoiding are plotting to kill me"). The person with obsessive-compulsive disorder has multiple fears and phobias, not isolated, circumscribed fears. The distinction between schizoid and avoidant personality disorders and social anxiety disorder can be difficult. Generally, the person with avoidant personality disorder does not fear specific social situations but feels insecure about social relationships and fears being hurt by others. In contrast, the person with schizoid personality disorder has little interest in social situations, but does not fear embarrassment or humiliation.

Clinical Management

Fluoxetine (10–30 mg/day), paroxetine (20–50 mg/day), sertraline (50–200 mg/day), and a long-acting form of venlafaxine (75–225 mg/day) are all approved by the U.S. Food and Drug Administration for the treatment of social anxiety disorder. Other SSRIs are probably also effective, as are the MAOIs and benzodiazepines. Tricyclic antidepressants (TCAs) are probably less effective, and socially anxious patients may be overly sensitive to their activating side effects (e.g., jitteriness). Other drugs, including gabapentin and pregabalin, have been investigated and may be effective; buspirone is ineffective. β-Blocking drugs are effective for the short-term treatment of performance-related anxiety but are ineffective for social anxiety disorder. Patients tend to relapse when the drugs are discontinued.

Medication is generally ineffective in the treatment of specific phobias. Benzodiazepines may provide temporary relief from a specific phobia. Because these disorders tend to be chronic and benzodiazepines have the potential for abuse and habituation, their long-term use is not recommended.

Behavior therapy can be very effective in the treatment of social anxiety disorder and specific phobias and involves exposure through the techniques of systematic desensitization and flooding. In the former, patients are gradually exposed to feared situations, beginning with the one they fear the least. With flooding, patients are instructed to enter situations that are associated with anxiety until the anxiety associated with the exposure (e.g., eating in restaurants) subsides. Patients tend not to improve unless they are willing to confront feared situations. (Commonly used behavioral techniques are discussed further in Chapter 20, "Behavioral, Cognitive, and Psychodynamic Treatments.")

Cognitive-behavioral therapy can be used to correct dysfunctional thoughts about fear of failure, humiliation, or embarrassment. For example, it may help to point out to the socially anxious person that he or she is receiving no more scrutiny than any other people receive. A therapist also can help to restore the patient's generally low self-confidence and poor morale.

■ Panic Disorder

Panic disorder consists of recurrent, unexpected panic (or anxiety) attacks accompanied by at least 1 month of persistent concern about having another attack, worry about the implications of having an attack (e.g., dying, going crazy), or significant maladaptive change in behavior related to the attacks (e.g., avoiding places where attacks had occurred). For an episode of anxiety to be defined as a panic attack, at least 4 of 13 characteristic symptoms, such as shortness of breath, dizziness, palpitations, and trembling or shaking, must occur (see Box 7–5 for panic attack criteria). The clinician should determine that the attacks are not induced by a substance (e.g., caffeine) or a medical condition (e.g., hyperthyroidism) and that the anxiety is not better accounted for by another mental disorder. The DSM-5 diagnostic criteria for panic disorder are shown in Box 7–6.

Box 7–5.   DSM-5 Criteria for Panic Attack Specifier

Note: Symptoms are presented for the purpose of identifying a panic attack; however, panic attack is not a mental disorder and cannot be coded. Panic attacks can occur in the context of any anxiety disorder as well as other mental disorders (e.g., depressive disorders, posttraumatic stress disorder, substance use disorders) and some medical conditions (e.g., cardiac, respiratory, vestibular, gastrointestinal). When the presence of a panic attack is identified, it should be noted as a specifier (e.g., "posttraumatic stress disorder with panic attacks"). For panic disorder, the presence of panic attack is contained within the criteria for the disorder and panic attack is not used as a specifier.

An abrupt surge of intense fear or intense discomfort that reaches a peak within minutes, and during which time four (or more) of the following symptoms occur:

Note: The abrupt surge can occur from a calm state or an anxious state.

1. Palpitations, pounding heart, or accelerated heart rate.
2. Sweating.
3. Trembling or shaking.
4. Sensations of shortness of breath or smothering.
5. Feelings of choking.
6. Chest pain or discomfort.
7. Nausea or abdominal distress.
8. Feeling dizzy, unsteady, light-headed, or faint.
9. Chills or heat sensations.
10. Paresthesias (numbness or tingling sensations).
11. Derealization (feelings of unreality) or depersonalization (being detached from oneself).
12. Fear of losing control or "going crazy."
13. Fear of dying.

Note: Culture-specific symptoms (e.g., tinnitus, neck soreness, headache, uncontrollable screaming or crying) may be seen. Such symptoms should not count as one of the four required symptoms.

Box 7–6.   DSM-5 Diagnostic Criteria for Panic Disorder

A. Recurrent unexpected panic attacks. A panic attack is an abrupt surge of intense fear or intense discomfort that reaches a peak within minutes, and during which time four (or more) of the following symptoms occur:

Note: The abrupt surge can occur from a calm state or an anxious state.

1. Palpitations, pounding heart, or accelerated heart rate.
2. Sweating.
3. Trembling or shaking.

4. Sensations of shortness of breath or smothering.
5. Feelings of choking.
6. Chest pain or discomfort.
7. Nausea or abdominal distress.
8. Feeling dizzy, unsteady, light-headed, or faint.
9. Chills or heat sensations.
10. Paresthesias (numbness or tingling sensations).
11. Derealization (feelings of unreality) or depersonalization (being detached from oneself).
12. Fear of losing control or "going crazy."
13. Fear of dying.

Note: Culture-specific symptoms (e.g., tinnitus, neck soreness, headache, uncontrollable screaming or crying) may be seen. Such symptoms should not count as one of the four required symptoms.

B. At least one of the attacks has been followed by 1 month (or more) of one or both of the following:

1. Persistent concern or worry about additional panic attacks or their consequences (e.g., losing control, having a heart attack, "going crazy").
2. A significant maladaptive change in behavior related to the attacks (e.g., behaviors designed to avoid having panic attacks, such as avoidance of exercise or unfamiliar situations).

C. The disturbance is not attributable to the physiological effects of a substance (e.g., a drug of abuse, a medication) or another medical condition (e.g., hyperthyroidism, cardiopulmonary disorders).

D. The disturbance is not better explained by another mental disorder (e.g., the panic attacks do not occur only in response to feared social situations, as in social anxiety disorder; in response to circumscribed phobic objects or situations, as in specific phobia; in response to obsessions, as in obsessive-compulsive disorder; in response to reminders of traumatic events, as in posttraumatic stress disorder; or in response to separation from attachment figures, as in separation anxiety disorder).

The following case illustrates how panic disorder and agoraphobia (which is described later in the chapter) affected one of our patients:

Susan, a 32-year-old homemaker, came to the clinic for evaluation of anxiety. She reported the onset of panic attacks at age 13, which she remembered as terrifying. She vividly recalled her first attack, which occurred during history class. "I was just sitting in class when my heart began to beat wildly, my skin began to tingle, and I began to feel like I was dying. There was no need for me to feel nervous," she observed. Over the following 19 years, attacks became frequent and unrelenting, occurring up to 10 times daily. To Susan, the panic was devastating: "I grew up all those years feeling that I wasn't quite normal." The attacks made her feel different from others and kept her from having a normal social life.

Along with her fear of attacks, Susan began to avoid crowded places, particularly shopping centers, grocery stores, movie theaters, and restaurants. She was a regular churchgoer but would sit in a pew near an exit. Her phobic avoidance tended to wax and wane, and although she never became housebound, Susan would insist on having her husband or a friend accompany her when she went shopping.

Susan had not previously sought treatment and thought that no one could help her. On occasion, she had gone to the emergency department for evaluation, but she had never received a diagnosis of panic disorder. Because she believed that admitting her symptoms was a sign of weakness, she had not even told her husband of 15 years about her panic attacks.

Susan was given fluvoxamine and within 1 month was free of attacks; within 3 months, she was no longer avoiding crowded places. At a 6-month follow-up, she remained free of all anxiety-related symptoms. Susan reported feeling like a new person.

Nine years later, Susan continued to be well, although she was now taking fluoxetine (20 mg/day). In the interim, she had divorced her husband, who had been unable to cope with a more confident and independent spouse. She eventually remarried, enrolled at a community college, and moved away from her small town.

Epidemiology, Clinical Findings, and Course

According to the National Comorbidity Survey, 5% of women and 2% of men have met criteria for panic disorder at some point in their life. Rates for panic disorder are elevated threefold in primary care patients and are even higher among patients seen in specialty clinics. For example, in patients seeking cardiology evaluations for chest pain, the rate may exceed 50% in those found to have normal coronary arteries.

Panic disorder typically has an onset in the mid-20s, although age at onset may vary; nearly 8 in 10 patients develop the disorder before age 30. There are usually no precipitating stressors before the onset of either panic disorder. Some patients, however, report that the attacks began after an illness, an accident, or the breakup of a relationship; developed postpartum; or occurred after using mind-altering drugs such as lysergic acid diethylamide (LSD) or marijuana.

The initial panic attack is alarming and may prompt a visit to an emergency department, where routine laboratory tests and electrocardiograms generally produce normal results. Many patients undergo extensive, often unnecessary medical workups that focus on the target symptoms (see Table 7–2). Psychiatrists may be consulted when no obvious physical cause for the patient's symptoms is found.

TABLE 7–2.   Specialists consulted depending on target symptoms of panic disorder

Specialist	Target symptoms
Pulmonologist	Shortness of breath, hyperventilation, smothering sensations
Cardiologist	Palpitations, chest pain or discomfort
Neurologist	Tingling and numbness, trembling, imbalance
Otolaryngologist	Dizziness, choking sensation, dry mouth
Gynecologist	Hot flashes, sweating
Gastroenterologist	Nausea, diarrhea, abdominal pain or discomfort
Urologist	Frequent urination

Panic attacks typically develop suddenly, peak within 10 minutes, and last 5–20 minutes. During attacks, patients hyperventilate; they appear fearful, pale, diaphoretic, and restless. Many patients report that their attacks last hours to days, but it is more likely that their continuing symptoms represent anxiety that persists after an attack. Common symptoms are presented in Table 7–3.

Panic disorder is chronic, although symptoms fluctuate in frequency and severity. Total remission is uncommon, yet up to 70% of patients with panic disorder will have some degree of improvement. Panic disorder patients are at increased risk for peptic ulcer disease and cardiovascular disease, including hypertension, and have higher death rates than expected. An increased risk of suicide is largely due to co-occurring depression and substance misuse.

A number of other physical conditions have been found in patients with panic disorder including joint hypermobility syndrome, mitral valve prolapse, migraine, fibromyalgia, chronic fatigue syndrome, irritable bowel syndrome, asthma, allergic rhinitis, and sinusitis. The disorder appears to share connective tissue, pain perception, and autoimmune abnormalities with these conditions. Mitral valve prolapse in patients with panic disorder may result from an interaction between lax connective tissue and noradrenergic activation of the circulation.

The most common comorbid psychiatric disorders are major depression and alcohol use disorder. Major depression occurs in up to half of the patients with panic disorder and may be severe. Misuse of alcohol or other drugs complicates panic disorder in about 20% of the cases and

TABLE 7–3. Common symptoms of panic disorder

Symptoms	%	Symptoms	%
Fearfulness or worry	96	Restlessness	80
Nervousness	95	Trouble breathing	80
Palpitations	93	Easy fatigability	76
Muscle aching or tension	89	Trouble concentrating	76
Trembling or shaking	89	Irritability	74
Apprehension	83	Trouble sleeping	74
Dizziness or imbalance	82	Chest pain or discomfort	69
Fear of dying or going crazy	81	Numbness or tingling	65
Faintness/light-headedness	80	Tendency to startle	57
Hot or cold sensations	80	Choking or smothering sensations	54

Source. Adapted from Noyes et al. 1987b.

may start in an attempt at self-medication. This complication is important to keep in mind when evaluating patients who abuse substances, because they may also have an underlying, treatable anxiety disorder. A person with panic disorder may also have another anxiety disorder requiring evaluation and treatment, such as social anxiety disorder or generalized anxiety disorder.

Etiology and Pathophysiology

Family and twin studies strongly suggest that panic disorder is hereditary. When the results of family studies are pooled, the morbidity risk for the disorder is nearly 20% among the first-degree relatives of patients with panic disorder compared with only 2% among the relatives of controls. Twin studies show higher concordance rates for panic disorder among identical twins than among nonidentical twins, a finding that genetic influences predominate over environmental influences. Molecular genetic studies just getting under way are targeting genes thought to be associated with fear and anxiety (e.g., norepinephrine and serotonin), but they have produced inconsistent results.

Among the biological mechanisms possibly underlying panic disorder are increased catecholamine levels in the central nervous system, an abnormality in the locus coeruleus (an area of the brain stem regulating alertness), carbon dioxide (CO_2) hypersensitivity, a disturbance in lactate metabolism, and abnormalities of the γ-aminobutyric acid (GABA) neurotransmitter system. There are data to support each of these possibilities, although none explains all of the symptoms of panic disorder.

Many of the competing theories are based on the ability of different substances to induce panic attacks, such as isoproterenol (a β antagonist), yohimbine (an α_2-receptor blocker), CO_2, and sodium lactate. For example, the observation that exposure to 5% CO_2 induces panic attacks has led to the "false suffocation alarm" theory. The theory posits that patients with panic disorder are hypersensitive to CO_2 because they have an overly sensitive brainstem suffocation alarm system that produces respiratory distress, hyperventilation, and anxiety.

Psychoanalysts postulate that *repression,* a common defense mechanism, may be involved in the development of panic. Freud theorized that repression holds unacceptable thoughts, impulses, or desires out of conscious reach. When the psychic energy attached to these unacceptable thoughts, impulses, or desires becomes too strong to hold back, they find their way into conscious awareness in disguised form, leading to anxiety and panic.

Meanwhile, behaviorists argue that anxiety attacks are a *conditioned response* to a fearful situation; a car accident might be paired with the experience of heart palpitations and anxiety. Long after the accident, palpitations alone, whether from vigorous exercise or emotional upset, might provoke the conditioned response of panic.

Differential Diagnosis

The clinician should rule out other medical and psychiatric disorders as a cause of anxiety when evaluating patients with panic disorder (see Table 7–4). The symptoms of panic attacks are sometimes caused by medical conditions, including hyperthyroidism, pheochromocytoma, diseases of the vestibular nerve, hypoglycemia, and supraventricular tachycardia; these diagnostic possibilities must be ruled out.

Other mental disorders also must be ruled out. Patients with major depression often develop anxiety and panic attacks, which resolve when the depression is treated. Panic attacks also may occur in patients with GAD, schizophrenia, depersonalization disorder, somatization disorder, or borderline personality disorder. When anxiety symptoms occur in response to a recognizable stressor but are out of proportion to the stressor and cause impairment, the diagnosis of adjustment disorder with anxiety may be appropriate (see Chapter 9, "Trauma- and Stressor-Related Disorders").

In many cases, panic attacks are isolated, and while the person may not meet diagnostic criteria for panic disorder, the panic attacks can

---

TABLE 7–4. **Differential diagnosis of panic disorder and other anxiety disorders**

Medical illnesses	Drugs
Angina	Caffeine
Cardiac arrhythmias	Aminophylline and related
Congestive heart failure	compounds
Hypoglycemia	Sympathomimetic agents (e.g.,
Hypoxia	decongestants and diet pills)
Pulmonary embolism	Monosodium glutamate
Severe pain	Psychostimulants and
Thyrotoxicosis	hallucinogens withdrawal
Carcinoid	Withdrawal from benzodiazepines
Pheochromocytoma	and other sedative-hypnotics
Menière's disease	Thyroid hormones
Psychiatric illnesses	Antipsychotic medication
Schizophrenia	
Mood disorders	
Avoidant personality disorder	
Adjustment disorder with	
anxious mood	

---

cause distress and impairment. In DSM-5, the presence of such panic attacks can be specified by indicating their presence ("with panic attacks"). The panic attack specifier can be used with any DSM-5 disorder.

Clinical Management

Panic disorder is usually treated with a combination of medication and individual psychotherapy. SSRIs are the medications of choice and are effective in blocking panic attacks in 70%–80% of patients. The U.S. Food and Drug Administration (FDA) has approved fluoxetine, paroxetine, and sertraline for the treatment of panic disorder. The serotonin–norepinephrine reuptake inhibitor (SNRI) venlafaxine is also effective, and a long-acting formulation is also FDA approved. Although these medications are called antidepressants, they also treat anxiety.

In the past, TCAs and MAOIs were used, but SSRIs are safer and better tolerated. Benzodiazepines can be effective in blocking panic attacks, but they are potentially habit-forming. β-blocking drugs, such as propranolol, are sometimes prescribed to patients with panic disorder but are much less effective than SSRIs or benzodiazepines. The pharmacological treatment of panic disorder is discussed in more detail in Chapter 21 ("Psychopharmacology and Electroconvulsive Therapy").

In general, patients who respond well to medication tend to have milder anxiety symptoms, later age at onset, fewer panic attacks, and a relatively normal personality.

The antidepressant dosage depends on the specific medication but is usually similar to that used to treat major depression. Typical dosages for the SSRIs are fluoxetine, 20 mg/day; sertraline, 50 mg/day; paroxetine, 20 mg/day; and citalopram, 20 mg/day. Once panic attacks have remitted, the patient should continue taking medication for at least 1 year to prevent relapse. After this period, the medication may be gradually tapered and discontinued. Panic symptoms may recur, but some patients will not relapse after cessation of medication. When a patient relapses or panic attacks recur, the medication can be restarted. Some patients will benefit from taking medication chronically.

Patients should avoid caffeine because it can induce anxiety. Patients often fail to realize how much caffeine they are ingesting with coffee (50–150 mg), tea (20–50 mg), cola drinks (30–60 mg), and even milk chocolate (1–15 mg).

Cognitive-behavioral therapy also is effective in the treatment of panic disorder and is frequently combined with medication. Cognitive-behavioral therapy usually involves distraction and breathing exercises, along with education to help the patient make more appropriate attributions for distressing somatic symptoms. For example, patients learn that panic-induced chest pain will not cause a heart attack. Psychodynamic psychotherapy has also been shown to be beneficial in the treatment of panic disorder.

A therapist can help to boost the patient's low morale and poor self-esteem. Books and other reading materials about panic disorder can be recommended, and the patient can be referred to the Web site of the Anxiety Disorders Association of America.

■ Agoraphobia

Agoraphobia is a condition in which an individual fears being unable to get out of a place or situation quickly in the event of a panic attack. As a consequence of this fear, he or she avoids places or situations where this might occur (see Box 7–7). Agoraphobia often occurs as a complication of panic disorder. Agoraphobia is nearly as common as panic disorder; women are more likely than men to develop agoraphobia. When panic disorder and agoraphobia are both present, each disorder should be diagnosed.

Box 7–7. DSM-5 Diagnostic Criteria for Agoraphobia

A. Marked fear or anxiety about two (or more) of the following five situations:

1. Using public transportation (e.g., automobiles, buses, trains, ships, planes).
2. Being in open spaces (e.g., parking lots, marketplaces, bridges).
3. Being in enclosed places (e.g., shops, theaters, cinemas).
4. Standing in line or being in a crowd.
5. Being outside of the home alone.

B. The individual fears or avoids these situations because of thoughts that escape might be difficult or help might not be available in the event of developing panic-like symptoms or other incapacitating or embarrassing symptoms (e.g., fear of falling in the elderly; fear of incontinence).
C. The agoraphobic situations almost always provoke fear or anxiety.
D. The agoraphobic situations are actively avoided, require the presence of a companion, or are endured with intense fear or anxiety.
E. The fear or anxiety is out of proportion to the actual danger posed by the agoraphobic situations and to the sociocultural context.
F. The fear, anxiety, or avoidance is persistent, typically lasting for 6 months or more.
G. The fear, anxiety, or avoidance causes clinically significant distress or impairment in social, occupational, or other important areas of functioning.
H. If another medical condition (e.g., inflammatory bowel disease, Parkinson's disease) is present, the fear, anxiety, or avoidance is clearly excessive.
I. The fear, anxiety, or avoidance is not better explained by the symptoms of another mental disorder—for example, the symptoms are not confined to specific phobia, situational type; do not involve only social situations (as in social anxiety disorder); and are not related exclusively to obsessions (as in obsessive-compulsive disorder), perceived defects or flaws in physical appearance (as in body dysmorphic disorder), reminders of traumatic events (as in posttraumatic stress disorder), or fear of separation (as in separation anxiety disorder).

Note: Agoraphobia is diagnosed irrespective of the presence of panic disorder. If an individual's presentation meets criteria for panic disorder and agoraphobia, both diagnoses should be assigned.

The term *agoraphobia* translates literally from Greek as "fear of the marketplace," and although many patients with agoraphobia are uncomfortable in shops and markets, their true fear is being separated from a source of security. Agoraphobic patients often fear having a panic attack in a public place, thereby embarrassing themselves, or having an attack and not being near a physician or medical clinic. They tend to avoid crowded places, such as malls, restaurants, theaters, and churches, because they feel trapped. Many have difficulty driving (because they fear being away from help should an attack occur), crossing bridges, and driving through tunnels. Many agoraphobic patients are able to go places they might otherwise avoid if accompanied by a trusted person or even a pet. People with severe agoraphobia may be unable to leave their home. Common situations that either provoke or relieve anxiety in people with agoraphobia are shown in Table 7–5.

Agoraphobia can be challenging to treat. Because many people with agoraphobia will have panic disorder, medication is usually recommended, with the agents and doses described earlier for that condition. Exposure therapy is the most effective behavioral intervention and in its most basic form consists of encouraging patients to gradually enter feared situations, such as a grocery store. Some patients may require direct supervision by a therapist during the process of exposure to the various feared situations.

■ Generalized Anxiety Disorder

Patients with generalized anxiety disorder worry excessively about life circumstances, such as their health, finances, social acceptance, job performance, and marital adjustment. This worry is central to the diagnosis.

Generalized anxiety disorder is not diagnosed when the symptoms occur exclusively during the course of another mental disorder such as major depression or schizophrenia or when the generalized anxiety occurs in the context of panic disorder, social phobia, or OCD. The anxiety or worry in generalized anxiety disorder should not relate solely to anxiety about having a panic attack, being embarrassed in social situations, being contaminated, or gaining weight (as in anorexia nervosa). The criteria also require that the individual have at least three of six symptoms, which include feeling restless or keyed up, being easily fatigued, having difficulty concentrating, being irritable, having muscle tension, or experiencing poor sleep. The symptoms must be present more days than not and cause significant distress or impairment in social, occupational, or other important areas of functioning. Finally, the effects of a substance or a general medical condition should be ruled out as a cause of the symptoms. The condition must persist for 6 months or longer (see Box 7–8 for the DSM-5 diagnostic criteria for generalized anxiety disorder).

TABLE 7–5. Common situations that either provoked or relieved anxiety in 100 agoraphobic patients

Situations that provoke anxiety	%	Situations that relieve anxiety	%
Standing in line at a store	96	Being accompanied by spouse	85
Having an appointment	91	Sitting near the door in church	76
Feeling trapped at hairdresser, etc.	89	Focusing thoughts on something else	63
Increasing distance from home	87	Taking the dog, baby carriage, etc., along	62
Being at particular places in neighborhood	66	Being accompanied by a friend	60
Being in cloudy, depressing weather	56	Reassuring self	52
		Wearing sunglasses	36

Source. Adapted from Burns and Thorpe 1977.

Box 7–8. DSM-5 Diagnostic Criteria for Generalized Anxiety Disorder

A. Excessive anxiety and worry (apprehensive expectation), occurring more days than not for at least 6 months, about a number of events or activities (such as work or school performance).

B. The individual finds it difficult to control the worry.

C. The anxiety and worry are associated with three (or more) of the following six symptoms (with at least some symptoms having been present for more days than not for the past 6 months):

Note: Only one item is required in children.

1. Restlessness or feeling keyed up or on edge.
2. Being easily fatigued.
3. Difficulty concentrating or mind going blank.
4. Irritability.
5. Muscle tension.
6. Sleep disturbance (difficulty falling or staying asleep, or restless, unsatisfying sleep).

D. The anxiety, worry, or physical symptoms cause clinically significant distress or impairment in social, occupational, or other important areas of functioning.

E. The disturbance is not attributable to the physiological effects of a substance (e.g., a drug of abuse, a medication) or another medical condition (e.g., hyperthyroidism).

F. The disturbance is not better explained by another mental disorder (e.g., anxiety or worry about having panic attacks in panic disorder, negative evaluation in social anxiety disorder [social phobia], contamination or other obsessions in obsessive-compulsive disorder, separation from attachment figures in separation anxiety disorder, reminders of traumatic events in posttraumatic stress disorder, gaining weight in anorexia nervosa, physical complaints in somatic symptom disorder, perceived appearance flaws in body dysmorphic disorder, having a serious illness in illness anxiety disorder, or the content of delusional beliefs in schizophrenia or delusional disorder).

Epidemiology, Clinical Findings, and Course

Generalized anxiety disorder is relatively common, with a lifetime prevalence between 4% and 7% in the general population. Rates are higher in women, African-Americans, and persons younger than 30 years. The disorder often has an onset in the early 20s, yet persons at any age can develop the disorder. Few persons with generalized anxiety disorder seek psychiatric treatment, although many seek evaluations from medical specialists for specific symptoms, such as muscle tension or sleep disturbance. The disorder is usually chronic, with symptoms that fluctuate in severity. Some patients who initially have generalized anxiety later develop panic disorder.

Patients with generalized anxiety disorder appear worried. They are often restless, tremulous, and distractible, and they may appear tired from lack of sleep.

The most frequent complications of generalized anxiety disorder are major depression and substance use disorder. Many patients experience one or more episodes of major depression over the course of their illness, and some meet criteria for social anxiety disorder or specific phobia. Some patients use alcohol or drugs to control their symptoms, which can lead to a substance use disorder.

Etiology and Pathophysiology

Research shows that generalized anxiety disorder runs in families. Twin studies imply that it is genetic as well, although nongenetic factors are important. Several different neurotransmitter systems—including the norepinephrine, GABAergic, and serotonergic systems in the frontal lobe and limbic system—are believed to play a role in mediating the disorder.

Differential Diagnosis

The differential diagnosis of generalized anxiety disorder is similar to that for panic disorder. It is particularly important to rule out drug-induced conditions such as caffeine intoxication, stimulant abuse, and alcohol, benzodiazepine, and sedative-hypnotic withdrawal. The mental status examination and patient history should cover the diagnostic possibilities of panic disorder, specific phobias, social anxiety disorder, obsessive-compulsive disorder, schizophrenia, and major depression.

Clinical Management

The treatment of generalized anxiety disorder usually involves individual psychotherapy and medication. The patient should be educated about the chronic nature of the disorder and the tendency of symptoms to wax and wane, often along with external stressors that the patient may be experiencing. Behavior therapy may help the patient to recognize and control anxiety symptoms. Relaxation training, re-breathing exercises, and meditation can be easily taught and may be effective, especially if the condition is mild.

The following case is of a patient seen in our outpatient clinic who benefited from behavior therapy:

> Kelly, a 19-year-old college student, presented for evaluation of "nerves." He had been anxious for as long as he could remember but denied being sad or blue. The problem had been worse since he finished high school and moved away from home to attend college.
>
> Kelly worried about everything—his physical appearance, his grades in school, whether he had the right kind of friends, the health of his parents, and even his sexual inexperience.
>
> Kelly was mildly tremulous and swallowed frequently; sweat was beaded on his brow. He acknowledged being tense and unable to relax and had recently been evaluated for stress headaches. He chewed gum to counter his chronically dry mouth. He often had clammy hands and a feeling of a lump in his throat.
>
> There was no apparent explanation for his chronic anxiety, but stress made his condition worse. He requested tranquilizers but agreed to try re-breathing exercises and progressive muscle relaxation as an initial treatment. After learning to use these techniques, he remained anxious but no longer felt that he needed tranquilizers.

Several medications have been approved by the FDA to treat generalized anxiety disorder. These include the SSRIs paroxetine (20–50 mg/ day) and escitalopram (10–20 mg/day); the SNRIs venlafaxine (75–225 mg/day) and duloxetine (60–120 mg/day); and the nonbenzodiazepine anxiolytic buspirone (10–40 mg/day). These drugs are generally well tolerated but take several weeks to take full effect. Benzodiazepines are rapidly effective but have the potential to lead to tolerance and dependence. Their use should be reserved for short periods (e.g., weeks or months) when the anxiety is severe. Sedating TCAs, such as doxepin or amitriptyline, also may be useful when given in low dosages (e.g., 25–100 mg/day), but they are used infrequently because of their side effects and danger in overdose. The antihistamine hydroxyzine (25–50 mg/day) may be helpful to some patients and has the advantage of being relatively safe.

■ Other Anxiety Disorders

For individuals with a *substance/medication-induced anxiety disorder*, clinically significant symptoms of panic, worry, phobia, or obsessions result from prescribed or illicit substance use. For example, stimulants (e.g., methamphetamine, cocaine) can produce relatively marked degrees of anxiety. Clinicians should be particularly attuned to substance misuse when encountering an anxious individual. If misuse is present, the clinician should determine whether it has any relationship to the ongoing anxiety symptoms. Although no definitive test exists to establish such a causal relationship, several factors can help confirm the diagnosis. These include the timing of the symptoms, the existing literature pertaining to the strength of the association between anxiety and the potential complicating factor, and signs or symptoms that are atypical for an anxiety disorder.

With *anxiety disorder due to another medical condition*, anxiety symptoms develop in the context of an identifiable medical syndrome (e.g., hyperthyroidism). The clinician needs to rule out medical conditions as possible etiologies.

■ Self-Assessment Questions

1. When is anxiety normal and when is it abnormal? What is the irritable heart syndrome?
2. Describe separation anxiety disorder and discuss its relationship to school refusal. In children, what other disorders can be a cause of school refusal?
3. What are the various treatments for selective mutism?
4. What are the specific and social phobias? How do they differ?
5. What is the differential diagnosis of panic disorder?

Clinical points for anxiety disorders

1. Separation anxiety disorder and selective mutism are disorders of children in most cases. Treatment necessarily involves the parents, along with medication.

2. Mild cases of panic may respond to cognitive-behavioral therapy, but many patients will need medication.

    -   SSRIs are the drugs of first choice because of their effectiveness and tolerability. TCAs and MAOIs work well but are second-line treatments due to their many adverse effects and dangerousness in overdose.

3. The agoraphobic patient should be gently encouraged to get out and explore the world.

    -   Progress will not occur unless the phobic patient confronts the feared places or situations. Some patients will need formal behavior therapy.

4. Patients with anxiety disorders should minimize intake of caffeine, a known anxiogenic.

5. Behavioral techniques (e.g., exposure, flooding, desensitization) will help most persons with social anxiety disorder and specific phobias.

    -   Some people with a social phobia respond well to medication. SSRIs and venlafaxine are the drugs of choice because of their effectiveness and tolerability.

6. Generalized anxiety disorder may respond to simple behavioral techniques (e.g., relaxation training), but many patients will need medication.

    -   Buspirone, venlafaxine, and the SSRIs paroxetine and escitalopram are effective FDA-approved treatments.

    -   Benzodiazepines, when used, should be prescribed for a limited time (e.g., weeks or months). Hydroxyzine is a relatively benign alternative.

6. What is the pharmacological treatment of social anxiety disorder? Panic disorder? Generalized anxiety disorder?
7. What is the relation between panic disorder and agoraphobia?
8. What is the natural history of the different anxiety disorders?
9. What behavioral treatments are useful in the various anxiety disorders?

Chapter 8

Obsessive-Compulsive and Related Disorders

> He had another peculiarity — This was his anxious care to go out or in at a door
> or passage by a certain number of steps from a certain point.
>
> *James Boswell,* Life of Johnson

Johnson, whose behavior was so carefully observed by Boswell, probably had obsessive-compulsive disorder. Shakespeare, in describing the guilt-laden handwashing rituals of Lady Macbeth, appears also to have had some familiarity with the symptoms of the disorder. More recently, industrialist Howard Hughes had crippling obsessions in late adulthood that led to a fanatical preoccupation with germs and contamination.

Like most mental illnesses, obsessive-compulsive disorder has been recognized for centuries, and by the late nineteenth century Freud and his contemporaries had described the syndrome, known as *obsessional neurosis,* which was widely thought to result from intrapsychic conflicts. Renamed *obsessive-compulsive disorder* in DSM-III, the disorder has been the focus of intense study and, with the development of effective treatments, its once poor prognosis has been transformed.

In the past two decades, researchers became interested in a spectrum of disorders thought related to obsessive-compulsive disorder based on new data regarding its phenomenology, genetics, and pathophysiology. In response to the emerging evidence, the authors of DSM-5 created a new chapter that brings together disorders considered to fall within the obsessive-compulsive spectrum. They include, along with obsessive-compulsive disorder, body dysmorphic disorder, hoarding disorder, trichotillomania (hair-pulling disorder), and excoriation (skin-picking) disorder. Clinicians are now encouraged to screen for these conditions and consider their overlap. Residual categories are also available for persons with an obsessive-compulsive-related disorder thought to result from effects of a substance, a medication, or a medical condition, and for those whose symptoms do not fit the criteria for a more specific disorder. The DSM-5 obsessive-compulsive and related disorders are listed in Table 8–1.

TABLE 8–1.   DSM-5 obsessive-compulsive and related disorders

Obsessive-compulsive disorder

Body dysmorphic disorder

Hoarding disorder

Trichotillomania (hair-pulling disorder)

Excoriation (skin-picking) disorder

Substance/medication-induced obsessive-compulsive and related disorder

Obsessive-compulsive and related disorder due to another medical condition

Other specified obsessive-compulsive and related disorder

Unspecified obsessive-compulsive and related disorder

■ Obsessive-Compulsive Disorder

Obsessions and compulsions are the hallmarks of obsessive-compulsive disorder. According to DSM-5 (see Box 8–1), *obsessions* are recurrent and persistent ideas, thoughts, impulses, or images that are experienced as intrusive and inappropriate and that cause marked anxiety or distress. Common obsessions include fears of germs and contamination. The content of typical obsessions is shown in Table 8–2.

Box 8–1.   DSM-5 Diagnostic Criteria for Obsessive-Compulsive
           Disorder

A. Presence of obsessions, compulsions, or both:

   Obsessions are defined by (1) and (2):

   1. Recurrent and persistent thoughts, urges, or images that are experienced, at some time during the disturbance, as intrusive and unwanted, and that in most individuals cause marked anxiety or distress.
   2. The individual attempts to ignore or suppress such thoughts, urges, or images, or to neutralize them with some other thought or action (i.e., by performing a compulsion).

Compulsions are defined by (1) and (2):

1. Repetitive behaviors (e.g., hand washing, ordering, checking) or mental acts (e.g., praying, counting, repeating words silently) that the individual feels driven to perform in response to an obsession or according to rules that must be applied rigidly.
2. The behaviors or mental acts are aimed at preventing or reducing anxiety or distress, or preventing some dreaded event or situation; however, these behaviors or mental acts are not connected in a realistic way with what they are designed to neutralize or prevent, or are clearly excessive.

   Note: Young children may not be able to articulate the aims of these behaviors or mental acts.

B. The obsessions or compulsions are time-consuming (e.g., take more than 1 hour per day) or cause clinically significant distress or impairment in social, occupational, or other important areas of functioning.

C. The obsessive-compulsive symptoms are not attributable to the physiological effects of a substance (e.g., a drug of abuse, a medication) or another medical condition.

D. The disturbance is not better explained by the symptoms of another mental disorder (e.g., excessive worries, as in generalized anxiety disorder; preoccupation with appearance, as in body dysmorphic disorder; difficulty discarding or parting with possessions, as in hoarding disorder; hair pulling, as in trichotillomania [hair-pulling disorder]; skin picking, as in excoriation [skin-picking] disorder; stereotypies, as in stereotypic movement disorder; ritualized eating behavior, as in eating disorders; preoccupation with substances or gambling, as in substance-related and addictive disorders; preoccupation with having an illness, as in illness anxiety disorder; sexual urges or fantasies, as in paraphilic disorders; impulses, as in disruptive, impulse-control, and conduct disorders; guilty ruminations, as in major depressive disorder; thought insertion or delusional preoccupations, as in schizophrenia spectrum and other psychotic disorders; or repetitive patterns of behavior, as in autism spectrum disorder).

Specify if:

With good or fair insight: The individual recognizes that obsessive-compulsive disorder beliefs are definitely or probably not true or that they may or may not be true.

With poor insight: The individual thinks obsessive-compulsive disorder beliefs are probably true.

With absent insight/delusional beliefs: The individual is completely convinced that obsessive-compulsive disorder beliefs are true.

Specify if:

Tic-related: The individual has a current or past history of a tic disorder.

TABLE 8–2.   **Varied content in obsessions**

Obsession	Foci of preoccupation
Aggression	Physical or verbal assault on self or others (includes suicidal and homicidal thoughts); accidents; mishaps; wars and natural disasters; death
Contamination	Excreta, human or otherwise; dirt, dust; semen; menstrual blood; other bodily excretions; germs; illness, especially venereal diseases; AIDS
Symmetry	Orderliness in arrangements of any kind (e.g., books on the shelf, shirts in the dresser)
Sexual	Sexual advances toward self or others; incestuous impulses; genitalia of either gender; homosexuality; masturbation; competence in sexual performance
Hoarding	Collecting items of any kind, typically items with little or no intrinsic value (e.g., string, shopping bags); inability to throw things out
Religious	Existence of God; validity of religious stories, practices, or holidays; committing sinful acts
Somatic	Preoccupation with body parts (e.g., nose); concern with appearance; belief in having disease or illness (e.g., cancer)

Source.   Adapted from Akhtar et al. 1975.

Compulsions are repetitive and intentional behaviors (or mental acts) performed in response to obsessions or according to certain rules that must be applied rigidly. Examples include repetitive hand washing and ritualistic checking. Compulsions are meant to neutralize or reduce discomfort or to prevent a dreaded event or situation. The rituals are not connected in a realistic way to the event or situation or are clearly excessive. For example, a person may believe that failing to reread the directions on a box of detergent may cause harm to her child. In short, obsessions create anxiety, which is relieved by compulsive rituals. The frequency of common obsessions and compulsions in a series of 560 patients is presented in Table 8–3.

To receive a diagnosis of obsessive-compulsive disorder, a person must have either obsessions or compulsions that cause marked anxiety or distress, are time-consuming (more than 1 hour daily), or significantly interfere with the person's normal routine, occupational functioning, or usual social activities and relationships. In addition, the person recognizes that the obsessions and compulsions are intrusive and unwanted, and the clinician will have determined that the symp-

TABLE 8–3. Frequency of common obsessions and compulsions in 560 patients with obsessive-compulsive disorder

Obsessions	%	Compulsions	%
Contamination	50	Checking	61
Pathological doubt	42	Washing	50
Somatic	33	Counting	36
Need for symmetry	32	Need to ask or confess	34
Aggressive impulse	31	Symmetry and precision	28
Sexual impulse	24	Hoarding	18
Multiple obsessions	72	Multiple compulsions	58

Source. Adapted from Rasmussen and Eisen 1998.

toms are not due to another mental disorder, such as major depression, nor are they caused by the effects of a substance or medical condition.

Many people—especially children—will have occasional obsessional thoughts or repetitive behaviors, but these tend not to cause distress or interfere with living. In fact, in many ways rituals add needed structure to our lives (e.g., daily routines that have probably changed little in years). These rituals are viewed as desirable and are easily adapted to changing circumstances. To the obsessive-compulsive person, rituals are a distressing and unavoidable way of life.

The following case describes a patient treated in our clinic who endured the crippling effects of obsessive-compulsive disorder:

> Todd, a 24-year-old man, was accompanied to the clinic by his mother for evaluation of obsessions and compulsive rituals. The rituals had begun in childhood and included touching objects a certain number of times and rereading prayers in church, but these symptoms were not disabling. After graduating from college, he moved to a large Midwestern city to work as an accountant for a major firm. He began to check the locks on his doors frequently and to check his automobile for signs of intruders. In time, the checking also included appliances, water faucets, and electrical switches in his apartment, fearing that they might be unsafe. Fearing contamination, he also developed extensive grooming and bathing rituals. Because of his time-consuming rituals, he was often late for work, and in fact his workload became too much for him. He would find himself adding columns of numbers over and over to make sure that he had "done it right." He eventually quit his accounting job.
>
> Todd moved back into his parents' home. His rituals became even more extensive and eventually took up nearly his entire day. The rituals mostly involved bathing (he showered for a half hour and had to wash

his body in a specific order), dressing in a certain way, and repeating activities, such as walking in and out of doorways a certain number of times.

Todd was a slender, unkempt young man with a scraggly beard, long hair, and unclipped fingernails. His shoelaces were untied, and he wore several layers of clothing. His rituals had become so time-consuming that he had found it easier not to shave or wash at all. He wore the same clothes every day for the same reason.

Todd began treatment with fluoxetine (20 mg/day), and his daily dosage was gradually increased to 80 mg. Within 2 months, his rituals were reduced to less than 1 hour per day and his grooming improved. After 6 months, Todd still had minor rituals but reported that he felt like his old self. He had obtained a job and was coaching track at a nearby high school.

Ten years later, Todd remained well. Attempts to stop the medication had always led to an increase in symptoms. In the interim, Todd had received a law degree, had married, and had developed a growing law practice.

In DSM-5, obsessive-compulsive disorder is subtyped according to the patient's degree of current insight (good or fair, poor, absent), as well as whether the disorder is tic related. This subtyping allows clinicians to designate a broad range of insight that can characterize obsessive-compulsive beliefs, including delusional beliefs. Poor insight tends to be associated with poor outcome.

Research evidence provides support for the inclusion of a *tic-related* subtype. This subtype is highly familial with specific clinical characteristics (early onset, male predominance) and high rates of symmetry and exactness obsessions and of ordering and arranging compulsions. Individuals with this subtype may respond better with an antipsychotic added to the selective serotonin reuptake inhibitor (SSRI).

Epidemiology, Clinical Findings, and Course

Obsessive-compulsive disorder typically begins in the late teens or early 20s, and most persons with the disorder will have developed it by age 30 years. Onset is generally gradual but may occur relatively suddenly and in the absence of any obvious stressor.

The disorder has a lifetime prevalence of 2%–3% in the general population. Men and women are equally likely to develop obsessive-compulsive disorder, but men tend to have an earlier onset.

In a study of 250 patients, 85% had a chronic course, 10% a progressive or deteriorating course, and 2% an episodic course with periods of remission. Because effective treatment is available, it is likely that future outcome studies will show a more favorable course. A study of youth with obsessive-compulsive disorder seems to bear this out. At a 5-year follow-up, most of the subjects still had obsessive-compulsive symptoms, but they were much less severe, and 6% of the youth had achieved full remission.

Mild symptoms and good premorbid adjustment have been associated with a better outcome. Early onset and the presence of a personality disorder have been associated with poor outcome. Patients typically report that their obsessive-compulsive symptoms are worse when they are depressed or are experiencing stressful situations. Recurrent episodes of major depression occur in 70%–80% of obsessive-compulsive disorder patients.

Etiology and Pathophysiology

The cause of obsessive-compulsive disorder is unknown, but many experts favor a neurobiological model. Evidence supporting this model includes the fact that obsessive-compulsive disorder occurs more often in persons who have various neurological disorders, such as epilepsy, Sydenham's chorea, and Huntington's chorea, as well as in cases of brain trauma. Obsessive-compulsive disorder has been linked to birth injury, abnormal electroencephalographic findings, abnormal auditory evoked potentials, growth delays, and abnormal neuropsychological test results. One particular type of obsessive-compulsive disorder, PANDAS (pediatric autoimmune neuropsychiatric disorders associated with streptococcal infections), has been identified in children following a group A β-streptococcal infection. These children not only develop obsessions and compulsions but also have emotional lability, separation anxiety, and tics.

The neurotransmitter serotonin has been the focus of great interest, perhaps because antidepressant drugs that block its reuptake—the SSRIs—are effective in treating obsessive-compulsive disorder, whereas other antidepressants are ineffective. Other evidence supporting the "serotonin hypothesis" is indirect but is consistent with the view that either levels of the neurotransmitter or variations in the number or function of serotonin receptors are disturbed in patients with obsessive-compulsive disorder.

Brain imaging studies have shown basal ganglia involvement in some persons with obsessive-compulsive disorder. Studies using positron emission tomography (PET) or single photon emission computed tomography (SPECT) scanning in obsessive-compulsive disorder patients have found increased glucose metabolism in the caudate nuclei and the orbital cortex of the frontal lobes, abnormalities that partially reverse with treatment. One hypothesis is that basal ganglia dysfunction leads to the complex motor programs involved in obsessive-compulsive disorder, whereas the prefrontal hyperactivity may be related to the tendency to worry and plan excessively. As discussed in Chapter 3 ("The Neurobiology and Genetics of Mental Illness"), the prefrontal cortex has important connections with the basal ganglia.

Finally, obsessive-compulsive disorder appears to have a considerable genetic component based on family and twin studies. It appears linked with Tourette's disorder.

Behaviorists have explained the development of obsessive-compulsive disorder in terms of learning theory. They believe that anxiety, at least initially, becomes paired with specific environmental events (i.e., classical conditioning), for example, becoming dirty or contaminated. The person then engages in compulsive rituals, such as compulsive hand washing, to decrease the anxiety. When the rituals successfully reduce the anxiety, the compulsive behavior is reinforced and is more likely to be repeated in the future (i.e., operant conditioning).

Differential Diagnosis

Obsessive-compulsive disorder overlaps with many other psychiatric syndromes that must be ruled out, including schizophrenia, major depression, posttraumatic stress disorder, hypochondriasis, anorexia nervosa, Tourette's disorder, and obsessive-compulsive personality disorder. Schizophrenia is the most important disorder to exclude, because obsessional thoughts can resemble delusional thinking. In most patients the distinction between obsessions and delusions is clear-cut. Obsessions are unwanted, resisted, and recognized by the patient as having an internal origin, whereas delusions are typically not resisted and are looked on as having an external origin. Nonetheless, rare patients appear to have both conditions.

The obsessions reported by patients must be distinguished from the morbid preoccupations and guilty ruminations of some patients with major depression (e.g., "I have sinned!"). In such patients, the ruminations are viewed as reasonable, although perhaps exaggerated, and are seldom resisted. Whereas the depressed patient tends to focus on past events, the obsessional patient focuses on the prevention of future events.

Other disorders need to be ruled out as well. Tourette's disorder, characterized by vocal and motor tics, may coexist with obsessive-compulsive disorder. Posttraumatic stress disorder is characterized by recurrent, intrusive thoughts that may suggest obsessional thinking. Anorexia nervosa also resembles obsessive-compulsive disorder because both disorders involve ritualistic behavior; however, the patient with anorexia views the behavior as desirable and rarely resists it. Some patients with anorexia nervosa appear to meet criteria for obsessive-compulsive disorder and, in addition to their food-related rituals, will have symptoms typical of obsessive-compulsive disorder, such as frequent hand washing and checking.

Obsessive-compulsive personality disorder and obsessive-compulsive disorder should not be confused. Obsessive-compulsive personality is characterized by perfectionism, orderliness, and obstinacy, traits that most persons with obsessive-compulsive disorder do not have. Obsessive-compulsive disorder patients are more likely to have dependent, avoidant, or passive-aggressive personality traits. Admittedly, distinguishing between the two disorders can sometimes be difficult. For example, we saw a 45-year-old man whose wife was "sick and tired" of his book collecting, which had "taken over" their house. He saw nothing wrong with his hobby, which he enjoyed. He pointed out that many of the books were quite valuable. In this case, the patient viewed his obsessive-compulsive personality traits as desirable and had not resisted them. Based on his history of a rigid and aloof demeanor, miserliness, and perfectionism, in addition to the collecting, he received a diagnosis of obsessive-compulsive personality disorder. (A further discussion of obsessive-compulsive personality disorder is found in Chapter 17, "Personality Disorders.")

Clinical Management

The treatment for obsessive-compulsive disorder usually involves medication and behavior therapy, mainly exposure paired with response prevention. For example, a patient might be exposed to a dreaded situation, event, or stimulus by various techniques (e.g., imaginal exposure, systematic desensitization, flooding) and then prevented from carrying out the compulsive behavior that usually results. A compulsive washer may be asked to handle "contaminated" objects (e.g., a dirty tissue) and then be prevented from washing his or her hands.

The SSRIs are particularly effective, and several are approved by the U.S. Food and Drug Administration for the treatment of obsessive-compulsive disorder, including fluoxetine, fluvoxamine, paroxetine, and sertraline. Clomipramine, a tricyclic antidepressant that is a relatively specific serotonin reuptake blocker, is also approved to treat obsessive-compulsive disorder. Because of its many side effects, it is used less frequently than are the SSRIs. Venlafaxine may also be effective, as one randomized clinical trial suggests. The addition of an antipsychotic may boost the likelihood of response of patients whose disorder appears refractory to SSRIs. Typically, higher dosages of the SSRIs are needed to treat obsessive-compulsive disorder than to treat major depression, and response is often delayed. For that reason, patients should have relatively lengthy trials (i.e., 12–16 weeks).

Research shows that nearly half of patients with treatment-refractory illness who undergo specific psychosurgical procedures (e.g., cingulotomy, deep brain stimulation) can benefit from them. None of these options is widely available.

Apart from behavior therapy, individual psychotherapy is beneficial in helping to restore a patient's low morale and self-esteem, in helping the patient solve day-to-day problems, and in encouraging treatment compliance.

Family therapy also has a role in managing obsessive-compulsive disorder. Family members are often ignorant about obsessive-compulsive disorder and get drawn into their relative's rituals in a misguided effort to be helpful. A mother, for example, may be asked to assist in her daughter's cleaning and checking rituals ("Is the stove turned off? Can you check it for me, please?"). In family therapy, the relatives can learn to accept the illness, learn to cope with its symptoms, and learn how not to encourage obsessive-compulsive behavior.

■ Body Dysmorphic Disorder

A patient with *body dysmorphic disorder,* formerly called *dysmorphophobia,* is preoccupied with an imagined defect or flaws in physical appearance that are not observable or appear slight to others (Box 8–2). For this reason, body dysmorphic disorder is sometimes referred to as the disease of imagined ugliness.

Box 8–2.   DSM-5 Diagnostic Criteria for Body Dysmorphic
            Disorder

A. Preoccupation with one or more perceived defects or flaws in physical appearance that are not observable or appear slight to others.
B. At some point during the course of the disorder, the individual has performed repetitive behaviors (e.g., mirror checking, excessive grooming,

skin picking, reassurance seeking) or mental acts (e.g., comparing his or her appearance with that of others) in response to the appearance concerns.

C. The preoccupation causes clinically significant distress or impairment in social, occupational, or other important areas of functioning.

D. The appearance preoccupation is not better explained by concerns with body fat or weight in an individual whose symptoms meet diagnostic criteria for an eating disorder.

Specify if:

With muscle dysmorphia: The individual is preoccupied with the idea that his or her body build is too small or insufficiently muscular. This specifier is used even if the individual is preoccupied with other body areas, which is often the case.

Specify if:

Indicate degree of insight regarding body dysmorphic disorder beliefs (e.g., "I look ugly" or "I look deformed").

With good or fair insight: The individual recognizes that the body dysmorphic disorder beliefs are definitely or probably not true or that they may or may not be true.

With poor insight: The individual thinks that the body dysmorphic disorder beliefs are probably true.

With absent insight/delusional beliefs: The individual is completely convinced that the body dysmorphic disorder beliefs are true.

Body dysmorphic disorder has an estimated prevalence of 1%–3% in the general population and is equally common in men and women. Onset occurs in adolescence or early adulthood. Body dysmorphic disorder tends to be chronic but fluctuates in intensity and severity; patients rarely experience full remission. The disorder can be highly incapacitating and impair the person's social and occupational functioning. About three-quarters of body dysmorphic disorder patients choose not to marry, and divorce is common among those who do. Some will become housebound. Nearly all attribute their disability to the embarrassment associated with their imagined defect. Patients who are particularly concerned with their facial appearance sometimes undergo repeated plastic surgery procedures in their quest for a defect-free appearance but are rarely satisfied with the results.

Patients with body dysmorphic disorder tend to focus on imagined defects involving their face and head, but any body part may become a focus of concern. Mirror checking, comparing oneself with others, camouflaging the affected body part, ritualized grooming, and requests for reassurance are common symptoms and behaviors. Body dysmorphic disorder is associated with high rates of major depression and social phobia. Suicidal ideation and attempts are unfortunately common in these patients.

Some individuals with body dysmorphic disorder are delusional (i.e., cannot be persuaded that their appearance beliefs are false). In these cases, the patient receives the diagnosis of body dysmorphic disorder with absent insight/delusional beliefs, and not a diagnosis of delusional disorder.

The following case is of a patient with body dysmorphic disorder seen in our clinic:

> Arthur, a 20-year-old man, first began to think of his face as a problem when he was a senior in high school. He noticed that when his face was in repose, his brows would droop over his eyes and give him a "devious look." He also noticed that his jawline seemed weak and receding. He tried to camouflage these "defects" by keeping his lower jaw jutted forward and his eyebrows raised. His attempts at camouflage became almost habitual; eventually he consulted a surgeon about obtaining a jaw augmentation and having his eyebrows raised, because he felt the camouflaging made him self-conscious and decreased his spontaneity.
>
> Arthur was a good student in high school but participated in relatively few activities. Although he had occasionally dated, he had not had a close relationship with a girl. He experienced a brief rebellious period during high school in which he stopped studying and smoked marijuana. After several months of this behavior, he began to feel depressed, apathetic, guilt-ridden, and paranoid. He did not meet criteria for major depression and did not have delusions or hallucinations. The episode passed when he stopped rebelling and using marijuana. He later completed 1 year of college but then dropped out to work and thus obtain money for cosmetic surgery. After the surgery, he planned to return to college. One day he hoped to attend medical school.
>
> Arthur was a handsome young man with heavy, dark eyebrows but a perfectly normal jawline. He related his motivation for seeking surgery to his general pattern of pursuing perfection in all aspects of life. He considered himself well adjusted and normal and, in fact, superior to most people. He saw no need for psychiatric treatment and refused a medication trial.

Body dysmorphic disorder is often treated with medication and cognitive-behavioral therapy. SSRIs are the medications of choice and are effective in treating body dysmorphic disorder. A positive response to medication means that the patient is less distressed and preoccupied by his or her thoughts about the "defect" and reports improved social and occupational functioning. In delusional forms of body dysmorphic disorder, a second-generation antipsychotic (e.g., olanzapine, risperidone) added to the SSRI may boost response. With cognitive-behavioral therapy, patients are encouraged to reassess their distorted beliefs about the "defect" and to modify behaviors that appear to encourage their preoccupation, such as mirror gazing. Supportive counseling can help to boost morale, provide hope, and offer insight into the disorder. Cosmetic surgery can lead to surgical complications, provides few benefits, and does not change the patient's preoccupation. For these reasons, surgery should be avoided.

■ Hoarding Disorder

Hoarding disorder is new to DSM-5 and involves the collection of objects that are of limited value or are worthless and the inability to discard them (Box 8–3). Many people refer to this as the "pack rat" syndrome, though patients are more likely to think of themselves as collectors. Hoarding is surprisingly common and potentially disabling. Significant hoarding has been shown to occur in up to 5% of the general population. The high prevalence and serious consequences of hoarding disorder, together with research on its distinctiveness from obsessive-compulsive disorder and obsessive-compulsive personality disorder, led the authors of DSM-5 to classify it as an independent disorder.

Box 8–3.   DSM-5 Diagnostic Criteria for Hoarding Disorder

A. Persistent difficulty discarding or parting with possessions, regardless of their actual value.
B. This difficulty is due to a perceived need to save the items and to distress associated with discarding them.
C. The difficulty discarding possessions results in the accumulation of possessions that congest and clutter active living areas and substantially compromises their intended use. If living areas are uncluttered, it is only because of the interventions of third parties (e.g., family members, cleaners, authorities).
D. The hoarding causes clinically significant distress or impairment in social, occupational, or other important areas of functioning (including maintaining a safe environment for self and others).
E. The hoarding is not attributable to another medical condition (e.g., brain injury, cerebrovascular disease, Prader-Willi syndrome).
F. The hoarding is not better explained by the symptoms of another mental disorder (e.g., obsessions in obsessive-compulsive disorder, decreased energy in major depressive disorder, delusions in schizophrenia or another psychotic disorder, cognitive deficits in major neurocognitive disorder, restricted interests in autism spectrum disorder).

Specify if:
   With excessive acquisition: If difficulty discarding possessions is accompanied by excessive acquisition of items that are not needed or for which there is no available space.

Specify if:
   With good or fair insight: The individual recognizes that hoarding-related beliefs and behaviors (pertaining to difficulty discarding items, clutter, or excessive acquisition) are problematic.
   With poor insight: The individual is mostly convinced that hoarding-related beliefs and behaviors (pertaining to difficulty discarding items, clutter, or excessive acquisition) are not problematic despite evidence to the contrary.
   With absent insight/delusional beliefs: The individual is completely convinced that hoarding-related beliefs and behaviors (pertaining to difficulty discarding items, clutter, or excessive acquisition) are not problematic despite evidence to the contrary.

The central feature of hoarding disorder is the intention to save possessions. Clutter that results is due to purposeful saving and reluctance to discard items because they have sentimental significance, are potentially useful, or have intrinsic aesthetic value. Frequently hoarded items include clothes, newspapers, and magazines. Many items, especially clothes, are new and never worn or used.

The nature of emotional attachment is reflected in the person's reaction to getting rid of a possession; the emotion experienced is either anxiety or a feeling of grief at the loss. Associated with this is the tendency to assign humanlike qualities to possessions. Patients may say something like, "Getting rid of things is like getting rid of part of myself." Another form of emotional attachment concerns a sense of comfort and security provided by possessions. The thought of getting rid of a possession appears to violate feelings of safety.

Hoarding disorder causes substantial distress (often more to family members than to the patient) and impairment, particularly in the ability to use living areas of the home for their intended purposes. Disorganized clutter, typical for the disorder, elicits great concern by family and friends because it makes space unusable or unsanitary; finding important items may be nearly impossible. In some cases, family members will keep the living area from being cluttered, often antagonizing the hoarder in the process.

People are often unable to use living spaces in the home, and in severe cases appliances are not functional and utilities such as water and electricity are shut off. The hoarder may find it too embarrassing to have a repair person in the home, or may worry that he or she will be reported to the authorities because of concerns with fire hazards or infestations.

Several other conditions can lead to clutter and difficulty discarding possessions and need to be ruled out. For example, hoarding behaviors can occur in people with lesions in the anterior ventromedial prefrontal and cingulate cortices. Also, people with Prader-Willi syndrome (a rare genetic disorder associated with short stature, hyperphagia, insatiability, and food-seeking behavior) display hoarding behavior, mostly associated with food but with nonfood items as well.

In some people, hoarding may be related to obsessive-compulsive disorder, generalized anxiety disorder, or major depressive disorder rather than being an independent disorder. Hoarding can also occur in individuals with severe dementia; when it occurs in association with dementia, hoarding appears to stem from significant cognitive deterioration and not an attachment to objects. Hoarding has been described in patients with schizophrenia, but also does not appear motivated by an attachment to objects. Obsessive-compulsive disorder is the condition most closely associated with hoarding, and up to 30% of individuals with the disorder will have some degree of hoarding behavior. If the hoarding appears to be secondary to typical obsessive-compulsive disorder symptoms, such as contamination fears, the diagnosis of hoarding disorder is not appropriate.

DSM-5 includes the specifier "with excessive acquisition." Research shows that many hoarders tend to buy and spend excessively (and may qualify for the term "compulsive shopper"). Stealing is another form of excessive acquisition associated with hoarding. When the hoarding is particularly severe, it may appear to take on delusional proportions. Many individuals with hoarding recognize the problem with their behavior, but their unreasonable ideas about the value of their possessions make it impossible for them to discard anything. This may appear to others—family members, for instance—as lack of insight, but in reality these beliefs about the value and usefulness of possessions may represent part of the disorder.

The treatment of hoarding disorder is challenging. Some patients, particularly those with milder syndromes, may benefit from SSRIs. Cognitive-behavioral therapy treatment models have been developed for hoarding but have not provided consistent benefit. The clinician may need to think "outside the box" and, for example, recommend that the patient hire a personal organizer (or a trusted friend or relative) who can both help with cleaning up the person's home and property and provide consistent monitoring afterwards, since reaccumulation begins almost immediately.

■ Trichotillomania (Hair-Pulling Disorder)

Trichotillomania (hair-pulling disorder) is characterized by recurrent pulling out of one's hair that results in noticeable hair loss. This is usually associated with an increasing sense of tension before pulling out the hair and pleasure, gratification, or relief when pulling out the hair. Persons with trichotillomania usually report substantial subjective distress or develop other evidence of impairment (see Box 8–4).

Box 8–4.   DSM-5 Diagnostic Criteria for Trichotillomania
           (Hair-Pulling Disorder)

A. Recurrent pulling out of one's hair, resulting in hair loss.
B. Repeated attempts to decrease or stop hair pulling.
C. The hair pulling causes clinically significant distress or impairment in social, occupational, or other important areas of functioning.
D. The hair pulling or hair loss is not attributable to another medical condition (e.g., a dermatological condition).
E. The hair pulling is not better explained by the symptoms of another mental disorder (e.g., attempts to improve a perceived defect or flaw in appearance in body dysmorphic disorder).

The disorder is generally chronic, although it tends to wax and wane in symptom severity. It can affect any site where hair grows, including the scalp, eyelids, eyebrows, body, and axillary and pubic regions. Most hair pullers are female, and they typically report a childhood onset. Surveys show that it affects 1%–4% of adolescents and college students. Compulsive hair pullers frequently have comorbid mood and anxiety disorders.

The diagnosis is easily made once alternative diagnoses and medical conditions have been ruled out. Most patients have no obvious balding, but they may have small, easily disguised bald spots or patches or missing eyebrows and eyelashes. The following case example describes a patient seen in our clinic:

> Shirley, a 42-year-old married homemaker, presented for evaluation of compulsive hair pulling. She had grown up in a small Midwestern farming community and described her childhood as happy and her family life as harmonious. As a young girl, she began to twist and twirl her hair and later, before age 10, began to pull out scalp, eyebrow, and eyelash hair.

The amount of hair pulling had fluctuated, but she had never been free of it. The pulling was sometimes automatic, such as when she was reading or watching television, but at other times, it was more deliberate. Shirley reported that she was unable to stop pulling her hair.

At the interview, Shirley removed her wig, revealing an essentially bald scalp. She had no eyebrows or eyelashes, which she disguised with makeup and eyeglasses. She was embarrassed by her hair pulling and tearfully recalled how classmates had made fun of her as a child. Over the years Shirley had received many medical and dermatological evaluations. Ointments and solutions had been prescribed but did not alter the hair pulling.

A trial of clomipramine (up to 150 mg/day) boosted her mood but had little effect on the hair pulling. Supportive psychotherapy helped to boost her low self-esteem. On follow-up 13 years later, Shirley's hair pulling behavior was unchanged, but she reported being happy and feeling fulfilled. She continued to disguise the disorder with a wig and make-up.

Treatment consists of medication and behavioral therapy, often in combination. With behavior therapy, patients learn to identify when their hair pulling occurs (it is often automatic) and to substitute a benign behavior such as squeezing a ball. Some patients benefit from learning to apply barriers to prevent hair pulling, such as wearing gloves or a hat. These techniques are often collectively referred to as *habit reversal,* and research studies show they can be effective.

SSRIs or clomipramine are probably the most frequently prescribed medications for trichotillomania and may help to reduce urges to pull. A recent study suggested that the glutamate modulator N-acetylcysteine might be effective in reducing hair pulling.

Some patients also will benefit from cognitive-behavioral psychotherapy to help boost their often low self-esteem, addressing relationship and family issues, and helping to correct faulty cognitions (e.g., "No one likes me because my eyebrows are missing"). Topical steroids may be helpful to patients who describe localized itching that prompts hair pulling. Hypnosis also has been used and is reported to benefit some persons.

■ Excoriation (Skin-Picking) Disorder

Excoriation (skin-picking) disorder is new to DSM-5. People with this disorder repetitively and compulsively pick at their skin, leading to tissue damage. There are significant clinical similarities between excoriation disorder and trichotillomania, and the criteria for the two disorders are very similar (see Box 8–5). Skin picking is relatively common, occurring in about 1%–5% of the general population. Often considered chronic, the disorder fluctuates in intensity and severity. Few people with this disorder seek treatment.

Box 8–5.   DSM-5 Diagnostic Criteria for Excoriation (Skin-Picking) Disorder

A. Recurrent skin picking resulting in skin lesions.
B. Repeated attempts to decrease or stop skin picking.
C. The skin picking causes clinically significant distress or impairment in social, occupational, or other important areas of functioning.
D. The skin picking is not attributable to the physiological effects of a substance (e.g., cocaine) or another medical condition (e.g., scabies).
E. The skin picking is not better explained by symptoms of another mental disorder (e.g., delusions or tactile hallucinations in a psychotic disorder, attempts to improve a perceived defect or flaw in appearance in body dysmorphic disorder, stereotypies in stereotypic movement disorder, or intention to harm oneself in nonsuicidal self-injury).

All people pick at their skin at some time, either to smooth out irregularities or to improve blemishes or acne, but with excoriation disorder the picking is recurrent and result in lesions. The face is the most common site of picking; other areas such as the hands, fingers, torso, arms, and legs are also common targets. People with this disorder use their fingernails, knives, and even tweezers and pins for picking. Picking may result in significant tissue damage and may lead to medical complications such as localized infections or septicemia. The person may try to decrease or stop the picking, but usually without success. The picking can also lead people to be late for work, school, or social activities, lowers self-esteem, and interferes with personal relationships. In rare cases, stimulants can cause skin picking behaviors, and so these need to be ruled out. Dermatological conditions such as scabies, atopic dermatitis, psoriasis, and blistering skin disorders also need to be ruled out.

Treatment is not well established, but often consists of the same elements as treating trichotillomania: SSRIs to lessen urges, and habit reversal techniques to address the skin picking.

Clinical points for obsessive-compulsive and related disorders

1.   Educate the patient about his or her obsessive-compulsive disorder:

   •   To reduce feelings of isolation, fear, and confusion.

Clinical points for obsessive-compulsive and related disorders *(continued)*

- To reassure worried patients that people with obsessive-compulsive disorder rarely act on their frightening or violent obsessions.
- To point out the "up" side of obsessive-compulsive disorder: that people with the disorder tend to be conscientious, dependable, and likeable.

2. Establish an empathic relationship.

- Do not tell patients to stop their rituals; they can't. That's why they are seeking help.
- Explain that talking about their obsessions and compulsions will not make them worse.

3. Patients generally do best with both medication and behavior therapy.

- Clomipramine and the SSRIs are usually effective. With SSRIs, higher doses will be needed than for the treatment of depression.
- The lag time to improvement on medication is months, not weeks as in the treatment of depression.

4. Body dysmorphic disorder often responds well to SSRIs.

- Even delusional forms of the disorder tend not to require the addition of an antipsychotic medication.

5. With hoarding disorder, the clinician needs to think "outside the box."

- Medication and psychotherapy do not appear especially helpful, but some patients with more typical obsessive-compulsive symptoms may benefit from SSRIs.
- Some patients benefit from hiring a personal organizer to help clear out the house, if feasible.
- Personal organizers will need to periodically monitor the hoarder's home because clutter begins to reaccumulate almost immediately.

6. Trichotillomania probably responds best to behavior therapy.

- Habit reversal methods have been shown to be beneficial.
- SSRIs or clomipramine may reduce the urge to pull, but response to these drugs is inconsistent.
- For patients with extensive hair loss, wigs and other forms of hair replacement may be the most sensible solution to restore self-esteem and boost morale.

7. Because excoriation disorder strongly resembles trichotillomania, habit reversal techniques may be beneficial.

■ Self-Assessment Questions

1. How is obsessive-compulsive disorder diagnosed? What are its characteristic features?
2. What evidence supports the neurobiological model of obsessive-compulsive disorder?
3. What is the differential diagnosis of obsessive-compulsive disorder?
4. How are obsessions distinguished from delusions?
5. What are some of the behavioral techniques used to treat obsessive-compulsive disorder?
6. What are the common features of body dysmorphic disorder?
7. In what way does hoarding disorder overlap with obsessive-compulsive disorder? Why is it so difficult to treat?
8. What is trichotillomania and how is it treated? Describe habit reversal therapy.
9. How is excoriation (skin-picking) disorder similar to trichotillomania?

Chapter 9

Trauma- and Stressor-Related Disorders

Whether 'tis nobler in the mind to suffer
The slings and arrows of outrageous fortune...

William Shakespeare, Hamlet

Trauma- and stressor-related disorders is a new diagnostic class in DSM-5 that brings together acute stress disorder, posttraumatic stress disorder (PTSD), reactive attachment disorder, disinhibited social engagement disorder, and adjustment disorders. Disorders in this class each result from exposure to traumatic or stressful situations or events explicitly recognized in the diagnostic criteria. These are among the few diagnoses in DSM-5 in which there is a direct cause-and-effect relationship.

These diagnoses link the all-too-common experiences of wartime combat, terrorist attacks, and gross parental neglect, all of which are direct causes of mental disorders. Included in this class are the adjustment disorders, which affect the many "walking wounded"; that is, individuals who experience everyday stressors that contribute directly to the onset of depression, anxiety, or behavioral problems. Included are two residual categories that can be used for those with trauma- or stressor-related disorders that do not meet the criteria for a more specific disorder. The DSM-5 trauma- and stressor-related disorders are listed in Table 9–1.

TABLE 9–1.   DSM-5 trauma- and stressor-related disorders

Reactive attachment disorder

Disinhibited social engagement disorder

Posttraumatic stress disorder

Acute stress disorder

Adjustment disorders

Other specific trauma- and stressor-related disorder

Unspecified trauma- and stressor-related disorder

■ Reactive Attachment Disorder and Disinhibited Social Engagement Disorder

Reactive attachment disorder and disinhibited social engagement disorder are characterized by disturbances in attachment behaviors that normally occur between a child and caregiver (most often a parent). These disorders result from parental neglect or abuse.

With *reactive attachment disorder,* attachment is either absent or underdeveloped (see Box 9–1). Because the disorder results from grossly inadequate parenting, it may be associated with signs of severe neglect (e.g., malnutrition, poor hygiene) and may be accompanied by delays in speaking and in cognitive development. Children with this condition show little responsiveness to others and make scant effort to obtain comfort, support, nurturance, or protection from caregivers. In addition, they have episodes of negative emotions (e.g., fear, sadness, irritability) that are not easily explained. The diagnosis is not appropriate for children developmentally unable to form selective attachments. (See Box 9–1 for the DSM-5 criteria.)

Box 9–1.   DSM-5 Diagnostic Criteria for Reactive Attachment Disorder

---

A. A consistent pattern of inhibited, emotionally withdrawn behavior toward adult caregivers, manifested by both of the following:

1. The child rarely or minimally seeks comfort when distressed.
2. The child rarely or minimally responds to comfort when distressed.

B. A persistent social and emotional disturbance characterized by at least two of the following:

1. Minimal social and emotional responsiveness to others.
2. Limited positive affect.
3. Episodes of unexplained irritability, sadness, or fearfulness that are evident even during nonthreatening interactions with adult caregivers.

C. The child has experienced a pattern of extremes of insufficient care as evidenced by at least one of the following:

1. Social neglect or deprivation in the form of persistent lack of having basic emotional needs for comfort, stimulation, and affection met by caregiving adults.
2. Repeated changes of primary caregivers that limit opportunities to form stable attachments (e.g., frequent changes in foster care).
3. Rearing in unusual settings that severely limit opportunities to form selective attachments (e.g., institutions with high child-to-caregiver ratios).

D. The care in Criterion C is presumed to be responsible for the disturbed behavior in Criterion A (e.g., the disturbances in Criterion A began following the lack of adequate care in Criterion C).

E. The criteria are not met for autism spectrum disorder.

F. The disturbance is evident before age 5 years.

G. The child has a developmental age of at least 9 months.

Specify if:

Persistent: The disorder has been present for more than 12 months.

Specify current severity:

Reactive attachment disorder is specified as **severe** when a child exhibits all symptoms of the disorder, with each symptom manifesting at relatively high levels.

A requirement in DSM-5 is that the child must have reached a developmental age of 9 months; the purpose of this requirement is to ensure that reactive attachment disorder is not diagnosed in children who are developmentally incapable of having a focused attachment. Children typically begin to develop stranger wariness and separation protest at around ages 7 to 9 months, in addition to selective comfort seeking or behavioral indicators of selective attachment.

Reactive attachment disorder is rare in clinical settings, and even among severely neglected children the disorder is uncommon, occurring in fewer than 10% of such children.

The evaluation of children is especially difficult and involves assessing the child, the parents (or caregivers), and often other family members as well. Please refer to Chapter 4, "Neurodevelopmental (Child) Disorders," for a "how-to" description of assessing infants, children, and adolescents.

According to DSM-5, there is a pattern of extremes of insufficient care; this can include disregard of a child's need for comfort, stimulation, and affection; repeated changes of caregivers; and rearing in unusual settings such as institutions with a high child to caregiver ratio. The diagnosis is complicated by the unwillingness of many (if not most) caregivers to admit their inadequate parenting and the inability of young children to describe their own experiences. For that reason, the diagnosis is not made when the clinician is unaware of the child's maltreatment. On the other hand, there are no case reports of young children exhibiting reactive attachment disorder without at least a reasonable inference of seriously inadequate caregiving.

As part of a differential diagnosis, autism spectrum disorder needs to be ruled out. The disorders can be distinguished on the basis of developmental histories of neglect, the presence of restricted interests or ritualized behaviors, specific deficits in social communication, and the presence of selective attachment behaviors.

In terms of treatment, it is crucial that children with reactive attachment disorder be removed from the home in which there is abuse or neglect and be placed in foster care. Typically, clinicians are legally obligated to report evidence of a child's abuse or neglect to the authorities. Other elements include assuring the child a secure and stable living situation, providing access to medical care and treatment of medical illnesses, and having an appropriately nurturing caregiver reversing the pervasive neglect and/or abuse. As the child becomes older, he or she should be educated about the condition. Psychotherapy, including varying types of family therapies, should be directed at the disturbed emotions and relationships.

Disinhibited social engagement disorder is new to DSM-5, having been split off from the DSM-IV "reactive attachment disorder of infancy or early childhood." Unlike reactive attachment disorder, its essential feature is a pattern of behavior that involves inappropriate and overly familiar behavior with relative strangers, thus violating the social boundaries of the culture (Box 9–2).

Box 9–2.   DSM-5 Diagnostic Criteria for Disinhibited Social
            Engagement Disorder

A. A pattern of behavior in which a child actively approaches and interacts with unfamiliar adults and exhibits at least two of the following:

   1. Reduced or absent reticence in approaching and interacting with unfamiliar adults.

2. Overly familiar verbal or physical behavior (that is not consistent with culturally sanctioned and with age-appropriate social boundaries).
3. Diminished or absent checking back with adult caregiver after venturing away, even in unfamiliar settings.
4. Willingness to go off with an unfamiliar adult with minimal or no hesitation.

B. The behaviors in Criterion A are not limited to impulsivity (as in attention-deficit/hyperactivity disorder) but include socially disinhibited behavior.

C. The child has experienced a pattern of extremes of insufficient care as evidenced by at least one of the following:

1. Social neglect or deprivation in the form of persistent lack of having basic emotional needs for comfort, stimulation, and affection met by caregiving adults.
2. Repeated changes of primary caregivers that limit opportunities to form stable attachments (e.g., frequent changes in foster care).
3. Rearing in unusual settings that severely limit opportunities to form selective attachments (e.g., institutions with high child-to-caregiver ratios).

D. The care in Criterion C is presumed to be responsible for the disturbed behavior in Criterion A (e.g., the disturbances in Criterion A began following the pathogenic care in Criterion C).

E. The child has a developmental age of at least 9 months.

Specify if:

Persistent: The disorder has been present for more than 12 months.

Specify current severity:

Disinhibited social engagement disorder is specified as **severe** when the child exhibits all symptoms of the disorder, with each symptom manifesting at relatively high levels.

The prevalence of disinhibited social engagement disorder is unknown, but its occurrence in foster care or shared residential facilities may be as high as 20%. The disorder has been described from the second year of life through adolescence. At very young ages, children are typically shy around strangers. Children with this disorder not only lack such reticence, but willingly engage with strangers and will even go off with unfamiliar adults.

In preschool children, verbal and social intrusiveness are common, often accompanied by attention-seeking behaviors. Verbal and physical overfamiliarity continues through middle childhood, and by adolescence indiscriminate behavior extends to peers.

Disinhibited social engagement disorder is associated with cognitive and language delays, stereotypies, and other signs of severe neglect, including malnutrition and poor hygiene. Signs of the disorder may persist even when the neglect is no longer present. Thus, disinhibited social engagement disorder may be seen in children with a history of neglect who lack attachments, or whose attachment to their caregivers ranges from disturbed to secure.

The diagnosis requires the presence of two or more of four examples of disinhibited behavior. These include reduced (or absent) reticence with unfamiliar adults, overly familiar behavior, diminished or absent checking back, and little hesitation about going off with an unfamiliar adult. These behaviors are unusual in many cultures, where most children typically become upset in these situations.

Insufficient care is described exactly as it is for reactive attachment disorder because there is no evidence to suggest that certain types of pathogenic care are more or less likely to lead to reactive attachment disorder than to disinhibited social engagement disorder. Interestingly, children with adequate caregiving but a chromosome 7 deletion demonstrate phenotypically similar behavior to those with disinhibited social engagement disorder.

Treatment tends to be directed at improving relatedness and interpersonal functioning.

■ Posttraumatic Stress Disorder

PTSD occurs in individuals who have been exposed to actual or threatened death, serious physical injury, or sexual violence. The event is typically outside the range of normal human experience. Examples of such events include combat, physical assault, rape, and disasters (e.g., home fires). A person's age, history of psychiatric illness, level of social support, and proximity to the stressor are all factors that affect the likelihood of developing PTSD.

The major elements of PTSD are 1) reexperiencing of the trauma through dreams or recurrent and intrusive thoughts, 2) persistent avoidance of stimuli associated with the event; 3) negative alterations in mood (e.g., emotional numbing such as feeling detached from others, and 4) alterations in arousal and reactivity such as irritability/angry outbursts and exaggerated startle response. Two subtypes are specified in DSM-5: *with dissociative symptoms,* when derealization or depersonalization is present, and *with delayed expression,* if onset is delayed more than 6 months after the traumatic event. The DSM-5 criteria for PTSD are included in Box 9–3.

Box 9–3. DSM-5 Diagnostic Criteria for Posttraumatic Stress
Disorder

Posttraumatic Stress Disorder

Note: The following criteria apply to adults, adolescents, and children older
than 6 years. For children 6 years and younger, see corresponding criteria
below.

A. Exposure to actual or threatened death, serious injury, or sexual violence in one (or more) of the following ways:

1. Directly experiencing the traumatic event(s).
2. Witnessing, in person, the event(s) as it occurred to others.
3. Learning that the traumatic event(s) occurred to a close family member or close friend. In cases of actual or threatened death of a family
member or friend, the event(s) must have been violent or accidental.
4. Experiencing repeated or extreme exposure to aversive details of
the traumatic event(s) (e.g., first responders collecting human remains; police officers repeatedly exposed to details of child abuse).

Note: Criterion A4 does not apply to exposure through electronic
media, television, movies, or pictures, unless this exposure is work
related.

B. Presence of one (or more) of the following intrusion symptoms associated with the traumatic event(s), beginning after the traumatic event(s)
occurred:

1. Recurrent, involuntary, and intrusive distressing memories of the
traumatic event(s).

Note: In children older than 6 years, repetitive play may occur in
which themes or aspects of the traumatic event(s) are expressed.

2. Recurrent distressing dreams in which the content and/or affect of
the dream are related to the traumatic event(s).

Note: In children, there may be frightening dreams without recognizable content.

3. Dissociative reactions (e.g., flashbacks) in which the individual feels
or acts as if the traumatic event(s) were recurring. (Such reactions
may occur on a continuum, with the most extreme expression being
a complete loss of awareness of present surroundings.)

Note: In children, trauma-specific reenactment may occur in play.

4. Intense or prolonged psychological distress at exposure to internal
or external cues that symbolize or resemble an aspect of the traumatic event(s).

5. Marked physiological reactions to internal or external cues that symbolize or resemble an aspect of the traumatic event(s).

C. Persistent avoidance of stimuli associated with the traumatic event(s),
beginning after the traumatic event(s) occurred, as evidenced by one or
both of the following:

1. Avoidance of or efforts to avoid distressing memories, thoughts, or feelings about or closely associated with the traumatic event(s).
2. Avoidance of or efforts to avoid external reminders (people, places, conversations, activities, objects, situations) that arouse distressing memories, thoughts, or feelings about or closely associated with the traumatic event(s).

D. Negative alterations in cognitions and mood associated with the traumatic event(s), beginning or worsening after the traumatic event(s) occurred, as evidenced by two (or more) of the following:

1. Inability to remember an important aspect of the traumatic event(s) (typically due to dissociative amnesia and not to other factors such as head injury, alcohol, or drugs).
2. Persistent and exaggerated negative beliefs or expectations about oneself, others, or the world (e.g., "I am bad," "No one can be trusted," "The world is completely dangerous," "My whole nervous system is permanently ruined").
3. Persistent, distorted cognitions about the cause or consequences of the traumatic event(s) that lead the individual to blame himself/herself or others.
4. Persistent negative emotional state (e.g., fear, horror, anger, guilt, or shame).
5. Markedly diminished interest or participation in significant activities.
6. Feelings of detachment or estrangement from others.
7. Persistent inability to experience positive emotions (e.g., inability to experience happiness, satisfaction, or loving feelings).

E. Marked alterations in arousal and reactivity associated with the traumatic event(s), beginning or worsening after the traumatic event(s) occurred, as evidenced by two (or more) of the following:

1. Irritable behavior and angry outbursts (with little or no provocation) typically expressed as verbal or physical aggression toward people or objects.
2. Reckless or self-destructive behavior.
3. Hypervigilance.
4. Exaggerated startle response.
5. Problems with concentration.
6. Sleep disturbance (e.g., difficulty falling or staying asleep or restless sleep).

F. Duration of the disturbance (Criteria B, C, D, and E) is more than 1 month.
G. The disturbance causes clinically significant distress or impairment in social, occupational, or other important areas of functioning.
H. The disturbance is not attributable to the physiological effects of a substance (e.g., medication, alcohol) or another medical condition.

Specify whether:

With dissociative symptoms: The individual's symptoms meet the criteria for posttraumatic stress disorder, and in addition, in response to the stressor, the individual experiences persistent or recurrent symptoms of either of the following:

1. **Depersonalization:** Persistent or recurrent experiences of feeling detached from, and as if one were an outside observer of, one's mental processes or body (e.g., feeling as though one were in a dream; feeling a sense of unreality of self or body or of time moving slowly).
2. **Derealization:** Persistent or recurrent experiences of unreality of surroundings (e.g., the world around the individual is experienced as unreal, dreamlike, distant, or distorted).

Note: To use this subtype, the dissociative symptoms must not be attributable to the physiological effects of a substance (e.g., blackouts, behavior during alcohol intoxication) or another medical condition (e.g., complex partial seizures).

Specify if:

With delayed expression: If the full diagnostic criteria are not met until at least 6 months after the event (although the onset and expression of some symptoms may be immediate).

Posttraumatic Stress Disorder for Children 6 Years and Younger

A. In children 6 years and younger, exposure to actual or threatened death, serious injury, or sexual violence in one (or more) of the following ways:

1. Directly experiencing the traumatic event(s).
2. Witnessing, in person, the event(s) as it occurred to others, especially primary caregivers.

    Note: Witnessing does not include events that are witnessed only in electronic media, television, movies, or pictures.

3. Learning that the traumatic event(s) occurred to a parent or caregiving figure.

B. Presence of one (or more) of the following intrusion symptoms associated with the traumatic event(s), beginning after the traumatic event(s) occurred:

1. Recurrent, involuntary, and intrusive distressing memories of the traumatic event(s).

    Note: Spontaneous and intrusive memories may not necessarily appear distressing and may be expressed as play reenactment.

2. Recurrent distressing dreams in which the content and/or affect of the dream are related to the traumatic event(s).

    Note: It may not be possible to ascertain that the frightening content is related to the traumatic event.

3. Dissociative reactions (e.g., flashbacks) in which the child feels or acts as if the traumatic event(s) were recurring. (Such reactions may

occur on a continuum, with the most extreme expression being a complete loss of awareness of present surroundings.) Such trauma-specific reenactment may occur in play.

4. Intense or prolonged psychological distress at exposure to internal or external cues that symbolize or resemble an aspect of the traumatic event(s).
5. Marked physiological reactions to reminders of the traumatic event(s).

C. One (or more) of the following symptoms, representing either persistent avoidance of stimuli associated with the traumatic event(s) or negative alterations in cognitions and mood associated with the traumatic event(s), must be present, beginning after the event(s) or worsening after the event(s):

Persistent Avoidance of Stimuli

1. Avoidance of or efforts to avoid activities, places, or physical reminders that arouse recollections of the traumatic event(s).
2. Avoidance of or efforts to avoid people, conversations, or interpersonal situations that arouse recollections of the traumatic event(s).

Negative Alterations in Cognitions

3. Substantially increased frequency of negative emotional states (e.g., fear, guilt, sadness, shame, confusion).
4. Markedly diminished interest or participation in significant activities, including constriction of play.
5. Socially withdrawn behavior.
6. Persistent reduction in expression of positive emotions.

D. Alterations in arousal and reactivity associated with the traumatic event(s), beginning or worsening after the traumatic event(s) occurred, as evidenced by two (or more) of the following:

1. Irritable behavior and angry outbursts (with little or no provocation) typically expressed as verbal or physical aggression toward people or objects (including extreme temper tantrums).
2. Hypervigilance.
3. Exaggerated startle response.
4. Problems with concentration.
5. Sleep disturbance (e.g., difficulty falling or staying asleep or restless sleep).

E. The duration of the disturbance is more than 1 month.

F. The disturbance causes clinically significant distress or impairment in relationships with parents, siblings, peers, or other caregivers or with school behavior.

G. The disturbance is not attributable to the physiological effects of a substance (e.g., medication or alcohol) or another medical condition.

Specify whether:

> **With dissociative symptoms:** The individual's symptoms meet the criteria for posttraumatic stress disorder, and the individual experiences persistent or recurrent symptoms of either of the following:

1. **Depersonalization:** Persistent or recurrent experiences of feeling detached from, and as if one were an outside observer of, one's mental processes or body (e.g., feeling as though one were in a dream; feeling a sense of unreality of self or body or of time moving slowly).
2. **Derealization:** Persistent or recurrent experiences of unreality of surroundings (e.g., the world around the individual is experienced as unreal, dreamlike, distant, or distorted).

Note: To use this subtype, the dissociative symptoms must not be attributable to the physiological effects of a substance (e.g., blackouts) or another medical condition (e.g., complex partial seizures).

Specify if:

> **With delayed expression:** If the full diagnostic criteria are not met until at least 6 months after the event (although the onset and expression of some symptoms may be immediate).

Epidemiology, Clinical Findings, and Course

PTSD has a prevalence of nearly 7% in the general population. Most men with the disorder have experienced combat. Fifteen percent of veterans of the Vietnam War suffered from PTSD. For women, the most frequent precipitating event is a physical assault or rape. The disorder can occur at any age, and even young children may develop the disorder, as occurred after the terrorist attacks of September 11, 2001, or several of the more recent school shooting incidents. The frequency of PTSD among survivors of catastrophes varies, but in one well-studied tragedy, the Cocoanut Grove nightclub fire that occurred in Boston in 1942, 57% of the patients still had a posttraumatic syndrome 1 year later.

The following case is of a woman seen in our clinic who had developed PTSD after a sexual assault:

> Megan, a 21-year-old college student, presented for evaluation of depression and flashbacks. At a fraternity party 3 months earlier, she had become interested in one of the men. The man suggested they go elsewhere to have sexual relations. Although intoxicated, Megan objected, but the man persisted. He forced her into another room, tore off her clothing, and raped her. Later, feeling embarrassed and humiliated, Megan chose not to tell her friends, nor did she seek a medical evaluation. She thought that the police would ignore what they might consider consensual sex.

Although she never missed a class or her part-time clerical job, Megan became depressed and anxious and began to experience episodes of anger and irritability. She ruminated about the rape, would recall its unpleasant details, and withdrew from her friends. Several concerned friends convinced her to seek help.

Based on the history and symptoms, PTSD was diagnosed and explained to Megan. She was referred for group therapy at a local rape crisis advocacy center. Fluoxetine (20 mg/day) was prescribed to treat symptoms of depression and anxiety. With treatment, Megan gradually improved and was able to overcome her symptoms of PTSD.

PTSD generally begins soon after experiencing the stressor, but its onset may be delayed for months or years. The disorder is chronic for many, but symptoms fluctuate and typically worsen during stressful periods. Rapid onset of symptoms, good premorbid functioning, strong social support, and the absence of psychiatric or medical comorbidity are factors associated with a good outcome. Many patients with PTSD develop comorbid psychiatric disorders such as major depression, other anxiety disorders, or alcohol and drug abuse.

Children and adolescents are also at risk for PTSD. Preschool children are dependent on parents and guardians for their well-being and therefore especially vulnerable. Common traumas affecting young children and adolescents include emotional and physical abuse, accidents, and effects of war and disasters. As in adults, the prevalence in children and adolescents may be underreported, and research suggests that up to 60% of child disaster survivors may develop PTSD and that about 40% of high school students have witnessed or experienced trauma or violence, with about 3%–6% of those meeting PTSD criteria.

Etiology and Pathophysiology

The major etiological factor leading to PTSD is a traumatic event, which by definition must be severe enough to be outside the range of normal human experience. Business losses, marital conflicts, and the death of a loved one are *not* considered stressors that cause PTSD. Research shows that the more severe the trauma, the greater the risk of developing PTSD. During wartime, for example, certain experiences are linked to the development of the disorder: witnessing a friend being killed, witnessing atrocities, or participating in atrocities.

A person's age, history of emotional disturbance, level of social support, and proximity to the stressor are all factors that affect the likelihood of developing PTSD. Eighty percent of young children who sustain burn injuries show symptoms of posttraumatic stress 1–2 years after the injury, but only 30% of adults who sustain similar injuries do so. Those who have received prior psychiatric treatment are more likely to develop PTSD, presumably because the previous illness reflects the person's greater vulnerability to stress. Persons with adequate social support are less likely to develop PTSD than are persons with poor support.

Certain biological abnormalities have been found in persons with PTSD, and these abnormalities may play a role in its development. Research suggests that the sustained levels of high emotional arousal can lead to dysregulation of the hypothalamic-pituitary-adrenal axis. The noradrenergic and serotonergic pathways in the central nervous system also have been implicated in the genesis of PTSD.

Brain imaging is also helping researchers to understand the underlying neurobiology of PTSD. Reduced hippocampal volume and increased metabolic activity in limbic regions, particularly the amygdala, are the most replicated findings. These findings may help to explain the role of disturbed emotional memory in PTSD.

Differential Diagnosis

The differential diagnosis of PTSD includes major depression, adjustment disorder, panic disorder, generalized anxiety disorder, acute stress disorder, obsessive-compulsive disorder, depersonalization/derealization disorder, factitious disorder, or malingering. In some cases, a physical injury may have occurred during the traumatic event, necessitating a physical and neurological examination.

Clinical Management

Both paroxetine (20–50 mg/day) and sertraline (50–200 mg/day) have been approved by the U.S. Food and Drug Administration for the treatment of PTSD, but the other selective serotonin reuptake inhibitors (SSRIs) are probably effective as well. These drugs help to decrease depressive symptoms, to reduce intrusive symptoms such as nightmares and flashbacks, and to normalize sleep. A long-acting form of the serotonin-norepinephrine reuptake inhibitor venlafaxine also appears effective based on large clinical trials. Benzodiazepines (e.g., diazepam, 5–10 mg twice daily; clonazepam, 1–2 mg twice daily) may help reduce anxiety but should be used for short-term treatment (e.g., days to weeks) because of their potential for abuse. The α_1-adrenergic antagonist prazosin (up to 10 mg/day) appears to be effective in alleviating the intractable nightmares that some PTSD patients report.

Establishing a sense of safety and separation from the trauma is an important first step in the treatment of PTSD. Cultivating a therapeutic working relationship requires time for the patient to develop trust. Research has shown that cognitive-behavioral therapy is effective in reducing PTSD symptoms. With cognitive-behavioral therapy, patients are provided the skills to control anxiety and to counter dysfunctional thoughts (e.g., "I deserved to be raped"). Controlled exposure to cues associated with the trauma may be helpful in decreasing avoidance. Group therapy and family therapy are also useful and have been widely recommended for veterans of war. The Department of Veterans Affairs has organized groups for distressed veterans across the country.

■ Acute Stress Disorder

Acute stress disorder occurs in some individuals after a traumatic experience and is considered a precursor to PTSD. By definition, the individual must have 9 or more of 14 symptoms from five categories: intrusion symptoms, negative mood, dissociative symptoms, avoidance symptoms, and arousal symptoms. The symptoms must cause clinically significant difficulties in functioning and last from 3 days to 1 month after trauma exposure (see Box 9–4).

Box 9–4.   DSM-5 Diagnostic Criteria for Acute Stress Disorder

A. Exposure to actual or threatened death, serious injury, or sexual violation in one (or more) of the following ways:
 1. Directly experiencing the traumatic event(s).
 2. Witnessing, in person, the event(s) as it occurred to others.
 3. Learning that the event(s) occurred to a close family member or close friend. **Note:** In cases of actual or threatened death of a family member or friend, the event(s) must have been violent or accidental.
 4. Experiencing repeated or extreme exposure to aversive details of the traumatic event(s) (e.g., first responders collecting human remains, police officers repeatedly exposed to details of child abuse).

 Note: This does not apply to exposure through electronic media, television, movies, or pictures, unless this exposure is work related.

B. Presence of nine (or more) of the following symptoms from any of the five categories of intrusion, negative mood, dissociation, avoidance, and arousal, beginning or worsening after the traumatic event(s) occurred:

Intrusion Symptoms

1. Recurrent, involuntary, and intrusive distressing memories of the traumatic event(s). **Note:** In children, repetitive play may occur in which themes or aspects of the traumatic event(s) are expressed.
2. Recurrent distressing dreams in which the content and/or affect of the dream are related to the event(s). **Note:** In children, there may be frightening dreams without recognizable content.
3. Dissociative reactions (e.g., flashbacks) in which the individual feels or acts as if the traumatic event(s) were recurring. (Such reactions may occur on a continuum, with the most extreme expression being a complete loss of awareness of present surroundings.) **Note:** In children, trauma-specific reenactment may occur in play.
4. Intense or prolonged psychological distress or marked physiological reactions in response to internal or external cues that symbolize or resemble an aspect of the traumatic event(s).

Negative Mood

5. Persistent inability to experience positive emotions (e.g., inability to experience happiness, satisfaction, or loving feelings).

Dissociative Symptoms

6. An altered sense of the reality of one's surroundings or oneself (e.g., seeing oneself from another's perspective, being in a daze, time slowing).
7. Inability to remember an important aspect of the traumatic event(s) (typically due to dissociative amnesia and not to other factors such as head injury, alcohol, or drugs).

Avoidance Symptoms

8. Efforts to avoid distressing memories, thoughts, or feelings about or closely associated with the traumatic event(s).
9. Efforts to avoid external reminders (people, places, conversations, activities, objects, situations) that arouse distressing memories, thoughts, or feelings about or closely associated with the traumatic event(s).

Arousal Symptoms

10. Sleep disturbance (e.g., difficulty falling or staying asleep, restless sleep).
11. Irritable behavior and angry outbursts (with little or no provocation), typically expressed as verbal or physical aggression toward people or objects.
12. Hypervigilance.
13. Problems with concentration.
14. Exaggerated startle response.

C. Duration of the disturbance (symptoms in Criterion B) is 3 days to 1 month after trauma exposure.

Note: Symptoms typically begin immediately after the trauma, but persistence for at least 3 days and up to a month is needed to meet disorder criteria.

D. The disturbance causes clinically significant distress or impairment in social, occupational, or other important areas of functioning.

E. The disturbance is not attributable to the physiological effects of a substance (e.g., medication or alcohol) or another medical condition (e.g., mild traumatic brain injury) and is not better explained by brief psychotic disorder.

The diagnosis was first included in DSM-IV after research had shown that dissociative symptoms occurring immediately following a traumatic event predicted the development of PTSD. In introducing the diagnosis, the goal was to enable clinicians to more accurately identify persons less likely to recover from their traumatic experience and to develop PTSD. Later research showed that other symptoms are also likely to predict the development of PTSD including emotional numbing.

Acute stress disorder occurs in less than 20% of cases following a traumatic event. Higher rates have been reported after interpersonal traumatic events such as assaults, rape, or witnessing a mass shooting. Women appear to be at greater risk for developing an acute stress disorder.

The differential diagnosis of acute stress disorder is between PTSD, brief psychotic disorder, a dissociative disorder, or an adjustment disorder. PTSD lasts more than 1 month, and although dissociative symptoms may be present, they are usually not prominent. Brief psychotic disorder lasts less than 1 month but is characterized by hallucinations, delusions, or disorganized speech/behavior. Dissociative disorders do not necessarily occur in response to traumatic situations or involve emotional numbing, reexperiencing of the trauma, or signs of autonomic hyperarousal. An adjustment disorder occurs in response to stressful situations (e.g., personal bankruptcy) but not necessarily a traumatic event involving serious personal threats; adjustment disorders may last up to 6 months, and the diagnosis is mainly used when criteria for other mental disorders are not met. The diagnosis of acute stress disorder preempts a diagnosis of adjustment disorder.

Cognitive-behavioral therapy involving exposure and anxiety management (e.g., relaxation training, re-breathing) has been shown to help prevent the progression to full-blown PTSD. When anxiety is severe, a brief course of a benzodiazepine tranquilizer may be helpful (e.g., clonazepam, 1–2 mg twice daily). There is some evidence that the administration of β-blockers immediately after a trauma may reduce the later development of symptoms of PTSD.

■ Adjustment Disorders

A student learns he has failed an important exam and may lose a scholarship; a physician discovers her husband has been unfaithful; a CEO must deal with an impending bankruptcy and staff layoffs. These are examples of everyday stressful events that most persons adjust to and cope with. Some people, however, feel overwhelmed by these situations and develop symptoms of emotional distress, such as depression, anxiety, or impaired work ability. These symptoms may be sufficiently severe to require brief periods of psychiatric care, usually on an outpatient basis. The term *adjustment disorder* acknowledges the fact that some people develop symptoms that are a direct consequence of a stressful though non–life-threatening situation.

Definition

DSM-5 specifies that the emotional or behavioral symptoms causing an adjustment disorder must arise within 3 months of a stressor and must be clinically significant. The symptoms cannot merely represent an exacerbation of a preexisting disorder, and they cannot be accounted for by normal bereavement. Furthermore, the maladaptive reaction cannot persist for more than 6 months after the termination of the stressor or its consequences (see Box 9–5).

Box 9–5.   DSM-5 Diagnostic Criteria for Adjustment Disorders

A. The development of emotional or behavioral symptoms in response to an identifiable stressor(s) occurring within 3 months of the onset of the stressor(s).

B. These symptoms or behaviors are clinically significant, as evidenced by one or both of the following:

　1. Marked distress that is out of proportion to the severity or intensity of the stressor, taking into account the external context and the cultural factors that might influence symptom severity and presentation.

　2. Significant impairment in social, occupational, or other important areas of functioning.

C. The stress-related disturbance does not meet the criteria for another mental disorder and is not merely an exacerbation of a preexisting mental disorder.

D. The symptoms do not represent normal bereavement.

E. Once the stressor or its consequences have terminated, the symptoms do not persist for more than an additional 6 months.

Specify whether:
   With depressed mood: Low mood, tearfulness, or feelings of hope-
   lessness are predominant.
   With anxiety: Nervousness, worry, jitteriness, or separation anxiety is
   predominant.
   With mixed anxiety and depressed mood: A combination of depression and anxiety is predominant.
   With disturbance of conduct: Disturbance of conduct is predominant.
   With mixed disturbance of emotions and conduct: Both emotional
   symptoms (e.g., depression, anxiety) and a disturbance of conduct are
   predominant.
   Unspecified: For maladaptive reactions that are not classifiable as one
   of the specific subtypes of adjustment disorder.

Five subtypes of adjustment disorder are listed. For that reason, the specific diagnosis depends on the predominant symptoms that develop in response to the stressor, such as depressed mood, anxiety, mixed anxiety and depressed mood, disturbance of conduct, or mixed disturbance of emotions and conduct. An unspecified subtype also exists for reactions that do not fit into any specific categories (e.g., a patient who responds to a new diagnosis of AIDS with denial and noncompliance with his or her treatment regimen).

Epidemiology

Adjustment disorders are common, but there are no good prevalence estimates. The frequency of these disorders in psychiatric clinics and hospitals is estimated to range from 5% to 20%. Adjustment disorders are even more common on psychiatric consultation-liaison services at general hospitals. For example, in one study, 51% of cardiac surgery patients received a diagnosis of an adjustment disorder. In another study, medical illness was the most common stressor for patients with adjustment disorders seen by a consultation service. These patients were largely free of preexisting psychiatric illness and had endured prolonged hospitalizations for serious physical illnesses such as cancer or diabetes. Those in whom medical illness was not the stressor were more likely to have established psychiatric histories and recurrent problems with relationships or finances.

The diagnosis is more common in women, unmarried persons, and young people. Common symptoms in adolescents include behavioral changes or acting out. Adults typically develop mood or anxiety symptoms. Adjustment disorders can occur at any age from childhood through senescence, but the mean age at diagnosis tends to be in the mid-20s to early 30s.

Clinical Findings

Different subtypes of adjustment disorder reflect the varied symptoms that can occur in response to a stressor:

- *Depressed mood:* dysphoria, tearfulness, hopelessness
- *Anxiety:* psychic anxiety, palpitations, jitteriness, hyperventilation
- *Conduct disturbance:* violating the rights of others or disregarding age-appropriate societal norms and rules (e.g., vandalism, reckless driving, fighting)
- *Mixed disturbance of emotions and conduct:* emotional symptoms, such as depression or anxiety, in addition to a behavioral disturbance
- *Unspecified:* for example, a person who has developed difficulty functioning at work

Table 9–2 presents the frequency of psychosocial stressors thought to have contributed to an adjustment disorder in a study of adults and adolescents. Many of these people had multiple, recurrent, or continuous stressors. School problems were the most frequently cited stressor in adolescents. Parental rejection, alcohol and/or drug problems, and parental separation or divorce also were common. In adults, the most common stressors were marital problems, separation or divorce, moving, and financial problems. Stressors were sometimes chronic. For example, among adolescents, nearly 60% of the stressors had been present for a year or more, and only 9% had been present for 3 months or less. Among adults, stressors showed more variation, but 36% had been present for a year or more, and nearly 40% had been present for 3 months or less. Another study suggests that stressors are gender specific in adolescents. School and legal problems were common stressors for boys as was parental illness for girls.

The following case is of a patient who developed an adjustment disorder with depressed mood:

Joanne, a 34-year-old homemaker, was admitted to the hospital following a tricyclic antidepressant overdose. She had felt well until earlier that day when she learned she had lost custody of her 13-year-old daughter to her ex-husband; she became upset, anxious, and tearful. That evening, feeling desperate, Joanne took a handful of nortriptyline tablets she had in her medicine chest (prescribed months earlier for migraine) because she felt life was no longer worth living. When her current husband returned home from work, Joanne told him what she had done. An ambulance was called, and Joanne was taken to the hospital emergency department, where she underwent charcoal lavage. There was no prior psychiatric history.

TABLE 9–2. Stressors occurring in adolescents and adults with adjustment disorders

Adolescents		Adults	
Stressor	**%**	**Stressor**	**%**
School problems	60	Marital problems	25
Parental rejection	27	Separation or divorce	23
Alcohol and/or drug problems	26	Move	17
Parental separation or divorce	25	Financial problems	14
Girlfriend or boyfriend problems	20	School problems	14
Marital problems in parents	18	Work problems	9
Move	16	Alcohol and/or drug problems	8
Legal problems	12	Illness	6
Work problems	8	Legal problems	6
Other	60	Other	81

Source. Adapted from Andreasen and Wasek 1980.

After calming down, Joanne explained that her current husband had been accused of sexually molesting her daughter, an allegation reported to local social service agencies. This led to her daughter's placement in foster care. Although she denied her husband had ever touched the girl inappropriately, she conceded that such an allegation was serious and would be taken into account by a judge in determining custody. After considering her situation, Joanne reported she was no longer depressed or suicidal and was now in an appropriate frame of mind to work with her lawyer to regain custody of her child.

Course and Outcome

Data are somewhat mixed for adolescents who receive the diagnosis. In a 5-year follow-up of 52 adolescents with adjustment disorders, 57% were well at follow-up, but 43% had a current mental disorder, including schizophrenia, major depression, alcohol or drug abuse, and antisocial personality disorder. Adolescents were also more likely to be suicidal at admission and had readmission rates similar to those of comparison subjects. These findings suggest that the diagnosis may be less useful in adolescents because they tend to have more varied outcomes. However, some clinicians consider the diagnosis of adjustment disorder appealing for younger patients because it is relatively nonpejorative. They believe the diagnosis avoids stereotyping patients with a harsher, more severe diagnosis that may lead to self-fulfilling prophecies.

Etiology

Most people are remarkably resilient and do not develop psychiatric symptoms in response to stressful situations, which suggests that individuals who develop an adjustment disorder may have an underlying psychological vulnerability.

One way to conceptualize this is to recognize that each person has his or her own "breaking point," depending on the amount of stress applied, underlying constitution, personality structure, and temperament. To draw an analogy, if enough pressure is applied to a bone, it will fracture; however, the amount of pressure required will differ from person to person, depending on age, gender, and physical well-being. To carry the analogy a bit further, adjustment disorders can occur in psychiatrically "normal" people, just as healthy bones will break if subjected to sufficient stress. At the other end of the continuum, people with fragile personalities, like bones with osteoporosis, will "break" more readily.

Differential Diagnosis

In making a diagnosis of adjustment disorder, the crucial question is: "What is the patient having trouble adjusting to?" Without a stressor, there is no adjustment disorder. Yet even when a stressor exists, other mental disorders need to be ruled out as causing the symptoms, and the stressor cannot represent normal bereavement. Another more specific mental disorder takes precedence over—or preempts—a diagnosis of adjustment disorder. A person who experiences an important stressor (e.g., recent marital separation) and develops depressed mood receives a diagnosis of adjustment disorder *only* when his or her symptoms fail to meet criteria for major depression.

The differential diagnosis reflects the broad range of symptoms seen in adjustment disorders. The differential diagnosis includes mood disorders (such as major depression), anxiety disorders (such as panic disorder or generalized anxiety disorder), and conduct disorder in the child or adolescent. Personality disorders should be considered because they are frequently associated with mood instability and behavior problems. For example, patients with borderline personality disorder often react to stressful situations in maladaptive ways (e.g., verbal outbursts, suicide threats), so an additional diagnosis of adjustment disorder usually is unnecessary, unless the new reaction differs from their usual maladaptive pattern. Psychotic disorders are often preceded by the development of social withdrawal, work or academic inhibition, or dysphoria and need to be differentiated from adjustment disorders. Other mental disorders that are believed to occur in reaction to a stressor also must be considered, including brief psychotic disorder, in which a person develops psychotic symptoms, and acute stress disorder or posttraumatic stress disorder, which develops after a traumatic event that involves actual or threatened death or serious injury (e.g., wartime experiences).

As with the assessment of any mental disorder, the patient being evaluated for an adjustment disorder should undergo a thorough physical examination and mental status examination to rule out alternative diagnoses.

Clinical Management

Supportive psychotherapy is probably the most widely used treatment for adjustment disorders. The therapist can help the patient to adapt to the stressor when it is ongoing or to better understand the stressor once it has passed. The patient may also have an opportunity to review the meaning and significance of the stressor. Group psychotherapy can provide a supportive atmosphere for persons who have experienced similar stressors, such as people who have received a diagnosis of breast cancer.

Medications can also be beneficial and should be prescribed based on the patient's predominant symptoms. For example, a patient with initial insomnia may benefit from a hypnotic (e.g., zolpidem, 5–10 mg at bedtime) for a few days. A patient experiencing anxiety may benefit from a brief course (e.g., days to weeks) of a benzodiazepine (e.g., lorazepam, 0.5–2.0 mg twice daily). If the disorder persists, the clinician should reconsider the diagnosis. At some point, an adjustment disorder with depressed mood, for example, may develop into major depression, which would respond best to antidepressant medication.

**Clinical points
for trauma- and stressor-related disorders**

1. Reactive attachment disorder and disinhibited social engagement disorder result from pathogenic care. In many cases the best response is to remove the child from the home and place him or her in a more nurturing environment.

2. PTSD tends to be chronic, but many patients will benefit from a combination of medication and cognitive-behavioral therapy.

   - Paroxetine and sertraline are approved for the treatment of PTSD. The other SSRIs are probably effective as well.

   - Prazosin may be effective in treating disturbing dreams and nightmares.

> **Clinical points**
> **for trauma- and stressor-related disorders** *(continued)*
>
> - Many PTSD patients will benefit from the mutual support found in group therapy.
>
> - Group therapy has become especially popular with veterans. Most veterans' organizations can offer help in finding a local group.
>
> 3. Adjustment disorders can evolve into other, better defined disorders, such as major depression, so be alert to changes in mental status and the evolution of symptoms.
>
>   - Most adjustment disorders are transient. Tincture of time and supportive therapy are usually all that is needed.
>
>   - Psychotropic medication taken short-term (i.e., days to weeks) should be targeted to the predominant symptoms.
>
>   - Hypnotics (e.g., zolpidem, 5–10 mg at bedtime) for those with insomnia.
>
>   - Benzodiazepines (e.g., lorazepam, 0.5–2.0 mg twice daily) for those with anxiety.
>
>   - If long-term treatment is needed, the patient may have another disorder (e.g., major depression), that will need to be diagnosed and treated.

■ Self-Assessment Questions

1. How do reactive attachment disorder and disinhibited social engagement disorder develop? Why are they included in the class of trauma- and stressor-related disorders? What steps are essential to their treatment?
2. When does PTSD develop? What factors predispose to its development? What medications are used to treat PTSD?
3. What behavioral treatments are useful in PTSD?
4. How common are adjustment disorders, and what are their typical precipitants and manifestations? What is the differential diagnosis of the adjustment disorders?
5. What is the "cause" of adjustment disorders? Why do some persons develop adjustment disorders and others do not? How do the stressors differ between adolescents and adults?
6. Describe the clinical management of the adjustment disorders.

Chapter 10

Somatic Symptom Disorders and Dissociative Disorders

So it is that a patient can confront his doctor with his symptoms, and put on him the whole onus of their cure.

Mayer-Gross, Slater, and Roth, Clinical Psychiatry

Somatic symptom disorders are characterized by physical symptoms that defy medical investigation. They cause significant distress to individuals and can cause serious functional impairment. People with these disorders report troublesome medical symptoms, visit doctors, take unnecessary medications, and even undergo needless medical procedures. Some become disabled socially and occupationally or seek disability payments. The disorders tend to baffle and frustrate clinicians, who must balance their concern to investigate the patient's complaints against the real concern of inadvertently encouraging help-seeking behavior.

These disorders are surprisingly common. For example, up to 30% of primary care patients present with medically unexplained symptoms, and a large proportion of them will have a somatic symptom disorder. Many of these individuals see primary care physicians rather than psychiatrists, motivated by the belief that their symptoms are medically based. Transient health-related complaints are even more common, affecting 60%–80% of healthy persons in any given week, with intermittent worry about illness occurring in 10%–20%. Unlike those with a somatic symptom disorder, most other people can be readily reassured that their symptoms are benign.

In DSM-5, the somatic symptom disorders have been reconceptualized. Rather than a focus on somatic symptoms, the focus has been redirected to the patient's excessive thoughts, feelings, and behaviors that arise in response to his or her somatic symptoms. A new diagnosis—*somatic symptom disorder*—consolidates DSM-IV's somatization disorder, hypochondriasis, pain disorder, and undifferentiated somatoform disorder. These four diagnoses were rarely used and created confusion for clinicians and patients. The new diagnosis will be more user friendly to clinicians and will be perceived as less stigmatizing by patients.

Seven somatic symptom disorders are listed in DSM-5 (see Table 10–1). They include somatic symptom disorder, illness anxiety disorder, conversion disorder, psychological factors affecting other medical conditions, and factitious disorder. Two residual categories (*other specified somatic symptom and related disorder* and *unspecified somatic symptom and related disorder*) can be used to diagnose patients whose somatic symptoms do not meet criteria for one of the more specific disorders.

Dissociative disorders and malingering are discussed later in this chapter.

■ Somatic Symptom Disorder

Somatic symptom disorder is characterized by the presence of one or more somatic symptoms that are distressing and/or result in significant disruption in daily life. To qualify for the diagnosis, the concerns have to have been present for at least 6 months, but not necessarily with any one symptom continuously (see Box 10–1). Symptom migration, in which an individual previously preoccupied with a particular symptom will focus on a new symptom, is not uncommon. If the symptom predominantly involves pain, that can be specified by the clinician ("with predominant pain").

TABLE 10–1. DSM-5 somatic symptom and related disorders

Somatic symptom disorder

Illness anxiety disorder

Conversion disorder

Psychological factors affecting other medical conditions

Factitious disorder imposed on self and imposed on another

Other specified somatic symptom and related disorder

Unspecified somatic symptom and related disorder

Box 10–1. DSM-5 Diagnostic Criteria for Somatic Symptom Disorder

---

A. One or more somatic symptoms that are distressing or result in significant disruption of daily life.

B. Excessive thoughts, feelings, or behaviors related to the somatic symptoms or associated health concerns as manifested by at least one of the following:

1. Disproportionate and persistent thoughts about the seriousness of one's symptoms.
2. Persistently high level of anxiety about health or symptoms.
3. Excessive time and energy devoted to these symptoms or health concerns.

C. Although any one somatic symptom may not be continuously present, the state of being symptomatic is persistent (typically more than 6 months).

Specify if:

With predominant pain (previously pain disorder): This specifier is for individuals whose somatic symptoms predominantly involve pain.

Specify if:

Persistent: A persistent course is characterized by severe symptoms, marked impairment, and long duration (more than 6 months).

Specify current severity:

Mild: Only one of the symptoms specified in Criterion B is fulfilled.

Moderate: Two or more of the symptoms specified in Criterion B are fulfilled.

Severe: Two or more of the symptoms specified in Criterion B are fulfilled, plus there are multiple somatic complaints (or one very severe somatic symptom).

In contrast to the four disorders that this diagnosis replaces, somatic symptom disorder deemphasizes medically unexplained symptoms, which played a central role for many of DSM-IV's somatoform disorders. The class is now defined on the basis of an individual's response to the distressing symptoms, and not specific medical symptoms or a required symptom count that many clinicians believed was arbitrary.

For these individuals, health concerns typically trump all others, including work and family life obligations. They may see their medical complaints as unduly threatening and fear the potential seriousness of them (i.e.: Could this mole be a melanoma? Is this swelling a tumor?). The complaints can involve multiple organ systems at once—or over time—and often present in a dramatic fashion. By way of illustration, the many symptoms reported by one of our somatic symptom disorder patients are shown in Table 10–2.

People with somatic symptom disorder tend to invest substantial time and energy in their symptoms and health concerns. Quality of life is often significantly impaired, particularly when the disorder leads to a high level of medical care utilization. For some patients, this means frequent clinic visits, "doctor shopping" (while searching for a particular medical diagnosis or treatment), emergency department visits, hospital stays, and unnecessary medical procedures. Their preoccupation with medical symptoms typically begins early in life and can last many years or even decades.

The following case shows the variety and stability of symptoms that can be found in persons with a somatic symptom disorder. The case also illustrates how these patients can receive inappropriate diagnoses and unnecessary evaluations from physicians unfamiliar with the syndrome:

> Carol, a 26-year-old homemaker, presented for evaluation of weakness and malaise of 1 year's duration. She also reported a burning pain in her eyes, muscular aches and pains in her lower back, headaches, a stiff neck, abdominal pain "on both sides and below the navel," and vomiting "glassy white stuff—as if I were poisoned."
>
> Six months earlier, Carol had developed blurry vision, complained of a sharp shooting pain in her rectum with walking, and reported passing blood and mucus in her stools. A sigmoidoscopic examination was unremarkable, but she was nevertheless given a diagnosis of mild ulcerative colitis and started on sulfasalazine therapy. Another barium enema examination produced negative results. Five months before her clinic visit, she noted "wasting" of her hands and reported needing a larger glove size for the right hand. She also was concerned with a pulsating vessel and whitish nodules on her hand.
>
> Carol identified additional symptoms during her clinic visit: a burning pain in her pelvis, hands, and feet; heavy vaginal bleeding, passing "clots as large as a fist"; abdominal bloating; malodorous stools with "bits of sudsy mucus"; urinary urgency; cough incontinence; tingling in hands and feet; and a belief that her bowel movements "just don't look right."
>
> Carol was next seen at the same clinic 21 years later, at age 47, for evaluation of multiple somatic complaints. Her symptoms were remarkably similar to those reported earlier, and it was clear that she had never been free of them. Her complaints included a right-sided tremor that caused her to spill food, migratory aches and pains, a feeling of coldness in her extremities, and a heavy menstrual flow ("I used 48 sanitary pads in a single day"). In addition, she reported feeling sick; having abdominal bloating, flatulence, and frequent nausea and vomiting; and being constipated. She was concerned that her skin was becoming darker and that her scalp hair was falling out. An extended medical workup was negative.
>
> Six years later, she was admitted to the psychiatric service. During the intervening years, she had received a total hysterectomy and oopho-

---

TABLE 10–2. **Medical symptoms reported by a patient with a somatic symptom disorder**

Organ system	Complaint
Neuropsychiatric	"The two hemispheres of my brain aren't working properly." "I couldn't name familiar objects around the house when asked." "I was hospitalized with tingling and numbness all over, and the doctors didn't know why."
Cardiopulmonary	"I had extreme dizziness after climbing stairs." "It hurts to breathe." "My heart was racing and pounding and thumping. . . . I thought I was going to die."
Gastrointestinal	"For 10 years I was treated for nervous stomach, spastic colon, and gallbladder, and nothing the doctor did seemed to help." "I got a violent cramp after eating an apple and felt terrible the next day." "The gas was awful—I thought I was going to explode."
Genitourinary	"I'm not interested in sex, but I pretend to be to satisfy my husband's needs." "I've had red patches on my labia, and I was told to use boric acid." "I had difficulty with bladder control and was examined for a tipped bladder, but nothing was found." "I had nerves cut going into my uterus because of severe cramps."
Musculoskeletal	"I have learned to live with weakness and tiredness all the time." "I thought I pulled a back muscle, but my chiropractor says it's a disc problem."
Sensory	"My vision is blurry. It's like seeing through a fog, but the doctor said that glasses wouldn't help." "I suddenly lost my hearing. It came back, but now I have whistling noises, like an echo."
Metabolic/endocrine	"I began teaching half days because I couldn't tolerate the cold." "I was losing hair faster than my husband."

rectomy, but apart from menstruation-related symptoms, she continued to have the same unrelenting physical complaints. Again, a protracted medical workup was negative.

This patient's remarkable history that spans 27 years leaves little doubt that she had an unrecognized somatic symptom disorder. Her complaints were consistent over the years and had led to many unnecessary evaluations and procedures. The distress she conveyed to her physicians, and the intensity of her preoccupation, belied the benign nature of the symptoms. Despite the complaints—many alarming—Carol remained fit and physically healthy.

The prevalence of somatic symptom disorder is around 5%–7% in the general population but higher in primary care. Women tend to report more somatic symptoms, so it follows that the prevalence among women is higher than in men. The disorder typically has an onset in the 20s, although excessive health worries can begin even in elderly persons. Low levels of education and income are risk factors for the disorder. While the cause is unknown, the more restricted DSM-IV concept of *somatization disorder* runs in families and likely has a genetic component. Many women with somatic symptom disorder report histories of childhood sexual abuse.

The differential diagnosis of somatic symptom disorder includes panic disorder, major depression, and schizophrenia. Patients with panic disorder typically report multiple autonomic symptoms (e.g., palpitations, shortness of breath), but they occur almost exclusively during panic attacks. Patients with major depression often report multiple physical complaints, but these are overshadowed by the dysphoria and vegetative symptoms of depression (e.g., appetite loss, lack of energy, insomnia). Schizophrenic patients sometimes have physical complaints, but they are often bizarre or delusional (e.g., "My spine is a set of twirling plates").

■ Illness Anxiety Disorder

Illness anxiety disorder is a new diagnosis in DSM-5 and is used in patients who are preoccupied with the possibility of having or acquiring a serious illness (Box 10–2). The person may amplify normal physiological sensations and misinterpret them as signs of disease, yet the distress comes mainly from his or her anxiety regarding the meaning, significance, or cause of the symptoms—and not the symptoms themselves. Under DSM-IV, some of these individuals would have been diagnosed with *hypochondriasis*, which involved the belief that one had a serious disease despite reassurance that one did not.

Box 10–2. DSM-5 Diagnostic Criteria for Illness Anxiety Disorder

A. Preoccupation with having or acquiring a serious illness.
B. Somatic symptoms are not present or, if present, are only mild in intensity. If another medical condition is present or there is a high risk for developing a medical condition (e.g., strong family history is present), the preoccupation is clearly excessive or disproportionate.

C. There is a high level of anxiety about health, and the individual is easily alarmed about personal health status.

D. The individual performs excessive health-related behaviors (e.g., repeatedly checks his or her body for signs of illness) or exhibits maladaptive avoidance (e.g., avoids doctor appointments and hospitals).

E. Illness preoccupation has been present for at least 6 months, but the specific illness that is feared may change over that period of time.

F. The illness-related preoccupation is not better explained by another mental disorder, such as somatic symptom disorder, panic disorder, generalized anxiety disorder, body dysmorphic disorder, obsessive-compulsive disorder, or delusional disorder, somatic type.

Specify whether:

Care-seeking type: Medical care, including physician visits or undergoing tests and procedures, is frequently used.

Care-avoidant type: Medical care is rarely used.

If a physical sign or symptom is present, it is often a normal physiological sensation, a benign and self-limited dysfunction, or a bodily discomfort not generally considered indicative of disease. If a diagnosable medical condition is present, the person's anxiety and preoccupation is disproportionate to its severity. Individuals with this condition are easily alarmed about ill health and tend not to be reassured by negative medical tests or a benign course. Incessant worry becomes frustrating to family members and may lead to considerable strain within marriages and families.

Their preoccupation with the idea of having a serious illness directs attention away from other activities and undermines relationships. The following vignette concerns Mabel, a patient seen in our hospital, who clearly had an illness anxiety disorder:

> Mabel, an 80-year-old retired schoolteacher, was admitted for evaluation of an 8-month preoccupation with having colon cancer. The patient had a history of single vessel coronary artery disease and diabetes mellitus (controlled by oral hypoglycemic agents) but was otherwise well. She had no history of mental illness. On admission, Mabel reported her concern about having colon cancer, which her two brothers had developed. As evidence of a possible tumor, she reported having diffuse abdominal pain and cited an abnormal barium enema examination 1 year earlier. (The examination had revealed diverticulosis.) Because of her concern about having cancer, Mabel had seen 11 physicians, but each in turn had been unable to reassure her that she did not have cancer.
>
> Mabel was pleasant and cooperated well with the ward team. Her physical examination and routine admission laboratory tests were unremarkable. Despite her complaint, Mabel denied depressed mood and displayed a full affect. She reported sleeping less than usual but attrib-

uted this to her abdominal discomfort. She chose not to socialize with
other patients, whom she characterized as "crazy." She remained preoccupied with the possibility that she had cancer, despite our reassurance.
A benzodiazepine was prescribed for her sleep disturbance, but she refused any other type of psychiatric treatment.

People with illness anxiety disorder are typically hypervigilant about
their health. They monitor their bodies seeking evidence of disease,
while exaggerating the importance of every ache, pain, discoloration,
bowel change, or noise. Like the person with obsessive-compulsive
disorder, they engage in significant checking behaviors (e.g., to ensure
there are no lumps or swellings). By definition, the preoccupation must
last 6 months or longer, but with many patients the preoccupation will
have lasted for many years.

Physicians find these patients frustrating and difficult. Patients, on
the other hand, feel ignored or rejected by physicians or are made to feel
ashamed by those who tell them that their complaints are not legitimate
(e.g., "It's all in your head"). Like patients with somatic symptom disorder, people with this condition sometimes "doctor-shop" and receive
unnecessary evaluations, tests, or surgeries. They also are at risk for alcohol or drug addiction.

The prevalence of illness anxiety disorder is estimated to range from
1% to 10% of the general population, based on estimates of the earlier
diagnosis hypochondriasis. The prevalence is similar in men and
women.

The development and course of illness anxiety disorder are unclear.
Illness anxiety disorder is generally thought to be chronic or relapsing,
and to have age at onset in early and middle adulthood. In older adults,
health-related anxiety tends to center on memory loss. Although the
disorder can be found in children, it is thought to be rare.

Because some mental disorders can be associated with excessive
health concerns, other causes of health preoccupations need to be
ruled out, as well as medical conditions. Health complaints tend to be
common in persons with mood or anxiety disorders. Individuals with
obsessive-compulsive disorder will have other symptoms (e.g., hand
washing rituals). Although individuals with panic disorder may have
concerns about having a heart attack, this concern occurs in the context
of a panic attack. When illness anxiety symptoms occur in the course
of another illness (e.g., panic disorder), treatment of the primary disorder may lead to a reduction in or resolution of the symptoms.

■ Conversion Disorder (Functional Neurological Symptom Disorder)

Conversion disorders have a long history in psychiatry. In DSM-5, *conversion disorder (functional neurological symptom disorder)* is defined by the presence of one or more symptoms of altered voluntary motor or sensory function that suggest a neurological or medical condition (see Box 10–3). Notably, patients whose major complaint is limited to pain receive a diagnosis of *somatic symptom disorder.* Importantly, the symptoms are not consistent with known neurological or medical conditions. In DSM-III and DSM-IV, psychological factors were linked with the development and expression of the symptoms; the authors of DSM-5 concluded that this requirement was too difficult to prove, and set too high a bar to the diagnosis, so it was dropped.

Box 10–3.   DSM-5 Diagnostic Criteria for Conversion Disorder (Functional Neurological Symptom Disorder)

A. One or more symptoms of altered voluntary motor or sensory function.
B. Clinical findings provide evidence of incompatibility between the symptom and recognized neurological or medical conditions.
C. The symptom or deficit is not better explained by another medical or mental disorder.
D. The symptom or deficit causes clinically significant distress or impairment in social, occupational, or other important areas of functioning or warrants medical evaluation.

Specify symptom type:
   With weakness or paralysis
   With abnormal movement (e.g., tremor, dystonic movement, myoclonus, gait disorder)
   With swallowing symptoms
   With speech symptom (e.g., dysphonia, slurred speech)
   With attacks or seizures
   With anesthesia or sensory loss
   With special sensory symptom (e.g., visual, olfactory, or hearing disturbance)
   With mixed symptoms

Specify if:
   Acute episode: Symptoms present for less than 6 months.
   Persistent: Symptoms occurring for 6 months or more.

Specify if:
   With psychological stressor (specify stressor)
   Without psychological stressor

Conversion symptoms are surprisingly common in hospital and clinic settings. For example, an estimated 20%–25% of the patients admitted to neurology wards have conversion symptoms. Conversion symptoms are more frequent in women, in patients from rural areas, and in persons with lower levels of education and income. Onset tends to be in late childhood or early adulthood. Onset in middle or late age suggests a medical condition.

Typical symptoms include paralysis, abnormal movements, inability to speak (aphonia), blindness, and deafness. *Pseudoseizures* are also common and may occur in patients with genuine epileptic seizures. (Pseudoseizures are spells that resemble true seizures but are unaccompanied by abnormal brain waves.) Conversion symptoms often conform to the patient's concept of disease rather than to recognized physiological patterns. For example, symptoms of anesthesia may follow a stocking-and-glove pattern, not a dermatomal distribution. Patients sometimes mimic symptoms based on prior experience with an illness or base them on illness symptoms modeled by an important person in their life (e.g., parent, grandparent).

Clinicians should be alert to the possibility that the symptoms are medically based, because some patients who receive a diagnosis of conversion disorder are later discovered to have a medical or neurological illness that, in retrospect, accounted for their symptoms. For that reason, clinicians need to remain tentative in their diagnosis of conversion disorder. The phenomenon of *la belle indifférence* (i.e., lack of concern about the nature or implications of the symptom) has been associated with the disorder, but it is not diagnostic.

The cause of conversion disorder is not well understood, but most people who receive the diagnosis have a history of mental illness, such as a mood disorder, a somatic symptom disorder, or a psychotic disorder. Conversion disorder is often associated with dissociative symptoms, such as depersonalization, derealization, and dissociative amnesia, particularly at symptom onset or during attacks. Of interest is the high rate of conversion symptoms in individuals with brain injuries. A study of conversion disorder patients in Australia and Great Britain found that nearly two-thirds had coexisting or antecedent brain disorders, such as epilepsy, tumor, or stroke, compared with 6% of control subjects.

Onset may occur at any point throughout life. While most conversion symptoms tend to be transient, for persons receiving a diagnosis of conversion disorder a favorable outcome is generally associated with acute onset, a precipitating stressor, good premorbid adjustment, and the absence of medical or neurological comorbidity. In one study, 83%

of the patients had improved or were well at a 4- to 6-year follow-up. When conversion symptoms occur in the context of another psychiatric disorder, their outcome reflects the natural history of the primary disorder, such as major depression or schizophrenia.

■ Clinical Management of Somatic Symptom Disorder, Illness Anxiety Disorder, and Conversion Disorder

There are several important principles that guide the treatment of the somatic symptom disorders. First, the physician should follow the Hippocratic Oath and "do no harm." Because symptoms are often embellished or misidentified (e.g., minor spotting during the menses may be reported as "gushing"), physicians tend to overreact and pursue the diagnostic equivalent of a wild goose chase. It comes as no surprise that the symptoms of the various somatic symptom disorders can prompt unnecessary diagnostic evaluations, surgical procedures, or medication prescriptions that have little relevance to the underlying condition. For that reason, it is essential that physicians who evaluate patients preoccupied with somatic symptoms learn about—and learn to diagnose—somatic symptom disorders. Physicians should understand that the patient's suffering is real and should be legitimized.

Regular scheduled clinic visits may reduce unnecessary utilization of health resources by these patients. Implicit in this approach is the message that new symptoms are *not* necessary in order to see a physician. The physician should listen attentively and convey genuine concern but refrain from focusing on the symptoms, thereby communicating the message that somatic complaints are not the most important or interesting feature about the patient. Ideally, the doctor should become the patient's primary and only physician.

The physician's goal becomes one of helping the patient cope with the symptoms and, in doing so, enable him or her to function at as high a level as possible. To this end, patients will benefit from receiving an explanation for their symptoms, appropriate advice regarding diet and exercise, and encouragement to return to meaningful activity and work. Perhaps the most important therapeutic element is an empathic doctor-patient relationship.

Psychotropic medications and analgesics should be prescribed with caution. They are rarely indicated unless prescribed for a co-occurring mental disorder known to respond to the medication. For example, antidepressants may help relieve major depression or block panic attacks, yet they have little effect on an underlying somatic symptom disorder. As a general rule, benzodiazepines should be avoided because of their abuse potential.

These simple measures have been shown to lower health care costs in patients with DSM-IV's somatization disorder and appear to reduce the likelihood of the patient's doctor-shopping and undergoing costly and unnecessary tests and procedures. In one study, patients receiving a psychiatric consultation with recommendations for conservative care (i.e., essentially the above measures) had a 53% decline in health care costs, mostly as a result of fewer hospitalizations, and improved physical functioning. The patients' general health status and satisfaction with their health care were unchanged. Health care costs of control subjects did not change.

The patient with illness anxiety disorder may further benefit from individual psychotherapy that involves education about illness attitudes and selective perception of symptoms. Controlled trials have shown that cognitive-behavioral therapy (CBT) can help to correct faulty beliefs about illness and counter the patient's tendency to seek inappropriate care. Selective serotonin reuptake inhibitors (SSRIs) are reported to be effective in treating DSM-IV hypochondriasis and may well help in treating illness anxiety disorder.

The treatment of conversion disorder is not well established, but symptom removal is the goal. Reassurance and gentle suggestion (for example, the idea that gradual improvement is expected) are appropriate, along with efforts to resolve stressful situations that may have accompanied the symptoms. The spontaneous remission rate for acute conversion symptoms is high, so that even without any specific intervention, most patients will improve and probably not suffer any serious complications.

A treatment approach for persistent conversion symptoms using behavioral modification for psychiatric inpatients has been described. The patient is placed at complete bed rest and informed that use of ward facilities will parallel his or her improvement. As the patient improves, the time out of bed is gradually increased until full privileges are restored. Nearly all patients (84%) who had conversion symptoms (ranging from blindness to bilateral wrist drop) treated in this manner remitted. By allowing the patient to save face, this method has the advantage of keeping secondary gain (e.g., escaping from noxious activities, obtaining desired attention from family, friends, and others) to a minimum.

In treating conversion disorder, hospital staff should remain supportive and show concern while encouraging self-help. It is rarely helpful to confront patients about their symptoms or make them feel ashamed or embarrassed. The pain, weakness, or disability is quite real to the patient. The physician should explain that treatment will be conservative and will emphasize rehabilitation rather than medication.

Clinical points for somatic symptom disorders

1. The physician should validate the patient's suffering and acknowledge his or her symptoms.

2. An empathic relationship should be established to reduce the patient's tendency to doctor-shop.

   - The primary physician should preferably become the patient's only physician.

3. Patients benefit from brief, scheduled visits.

   - As the patient improves, the time between visits can be extended.

4. The physician's goal is not to remove symptoms but to improve function and quality of life.

5. The use of psychotropic drugs should be minimized.

   - No medication has proven value in somatic symptom disorder.

   - Illness anxiety disorder may respond to selective serotonin reuptake inhibitors.

   - Psychotropic drugs with abuse potential (e.g., benzodiazepines, opioids) should be avoided.

6. Medical evaluations should be minimized to reduce expense and iatrogenic complications.

   - Conservative management has been shown to reduce health care costs.

■ Psychological Factors Affecting Other Medical Conditions

The essential feature of *psychological factors affecting other medical conditions* is the presence of one or more clinically significant psychological or behavioral factors that adversely affect a medical condition by increasing the risk for suffering, death, or disability (see Box 10–4). These factors can adversely affect the medical condition by influencing its course or treatment, by constituting an additional health risk factor, or by exacerbating the physiology related to the medical condition. Psychological or behavioral factors include psychological distress, patterns of interpersonal interaction, coping styles, and maladaptive help behaviors such as denial of symptoms or poor adherence to medical recommendations. Common examples are the person with anxiety exacerbating his or her asthma, denial of the need for treatment of acute chest pain, or manipulation of insulin by a person with diabetes wishing to lose weight.

Box 10–4.   DSM-5 Diagnostic Criteria for Psychological Factors Affecting Other Medical Conditions

---

A. A medical symptom or condition (other than a mental disorder) is present.
B. Psychological or behavioral factors adversely affect the medical condition in one of the following ways:

1. The factors have influenced the course of the medical condition as shown by a close temporal association between the psychological factors and the development or exacerbation of, or delayed recovery from, the medical condition.
2. The factors interfere with the treatment of the medical condition (e.g., poor adherence).
3. The factors constitute additional well-established health risks for the individual.
4. The factors influence the underlying pathophysiology, precipitating or exacerbating symptoms or necessitating medical attention.

C. The psychological and behavioral factors in Criterion B are not better explained by another mental disorder (e.g., panic disorder, major depressive disorder, posttraumatic stress disorder).

Specify current severity:
Mild: Increases medical risk (e.g., inconsistent adherence with antihypertension treatment).
Moderate: Aggravates underlying medical condition (e.g., anxiety aggravating asthma).
Severe: Results in medical hospitalization or emergency room visit.
Extreme: Results in severe, life-threatening risk (e.g., ignoring heart attack symptoms).

With this disorder, a medical condition—involving any of the organ systems—must be present. Also required is that the "psychological or behavioral factors" adversely affect the medical condition. There must be a clear-cut temporal relationship between these factors and the development of, exacerbation of, or recovery from the medical condition.

Other mental disorders need to be ruled out as a cause of the disturbance.

■ Factitious Disorder

Factitious disorder is characterized by the intentional production or feigning of physical or psychological signs or symptoms (see Box 10–5). Patients with factitious disorder have no obvious external incentive for the behavior, such as economic gain. Instead, these individuals are thought to be motivated by an unconscious desire to occupy the sick role.

Box 10–5.   DSM-5 Diagnostic Criteria for Factitious Disorder

---

Factitious Disorder Imposed on Self

A. Falsification of physical or psychological signs or symptoms, or induction of injury or disease, associated with identified deception.
B. The individual presents himself or herself to others as ill, impaired, or injured.
C. The deceptive behavior is evident even in the absence of obvious external rewards.
D. The behavior is not better explained by another mental disorder, such as delusional disorder or another psychotic disorder.

Specify:

Single episode

Recurrent episodes (two or more events of falsification of illness and/ or induction of injury)

Factitious Disorder Imposed on Another
(Previously Factitious Disorder by Proxy)

A. Falsification of physical or psychological signs or symptoms, or induction of injury or disease, in another, associated with identified deception.
B. The individual presents another individual (victim) to others as ill, impaired, or injured.
C. The deceptive behavior is evident even in the absence of obvious external rewards.
D. The behavior is not better explained by another mental disorder, such as delusional disorder or another psychotic disorder.

Note: The perpetrator, not the victim, receives this diagnosis.

Specify:

Single episode

Recurrent episodes (two or more events of falsification of illness and/ or induction of injury)

Some factitious disorder patients appear to make hospitalization a way of life and have been called "hospital hobos" or "peregrinating problem patients." The term *Munchausen syndrome* also has been used to describe patients who move from hospital to hospital simulating various illnesses. The name comes from the fictitious wanderings of the nineteenth-century Baron von Munchausen, known for his tall tales and fanciful exaggeration.

The prevalence of factitious disorder is unknown because most cases are probably never recognized or go undetected. In one study involving persons with a fever of unknown origin, up to 10% of the fevers were diagnosed as factitious. In rare cases, factitious disorder may be imposed on another person. For example, a parent induces (or simulates) illness in his or her child so that the child is repeatedly hospitalized.

Most cases of factitious disorder involve the simulation of physical illness. Patients typically use one of three strategies to feign illness: 1) they report symptoms suggesting an illness, without having them; 2) they produce false evidence of an illness (e.g., a factitious fever produced by applying friction to a thermometer to raise the temperature); or 3) they intentionally produce symptoms of illness (e.g., by injecting feces to produce infection or taking warfarin orally to induce a bleeding disorder). Some of the more common methods for producing symptoms are presented in Table 10–3.

Factitious disorders begin in early adulthood and can become chronic. They tend to develop in people who have had experience with hospitalization or severe illness involving either themselves or someone close to them (e.g., a parent). The disorder can severely impair social and occupational functioning and is typically associated with the presence of a personality disorder (e.g., borderline personality disorder). In one study, most of the factitious disorder patients had worked in health care occupations. Most had maladaptive personality traits, but none had a diagnosis of a major mental disorder, such as major depression or schizophrenia. Nearly all were women.

The diagnosis of a factitious disorder requires almost as much inventiveness as is shown by the patient in producing symptoms. Clues to the diagnosis include a lengthy and involved medical history that does not correspond to the patient's apparent health and vigor, a clinical presentation that too closely resembles textbook descriptions, a sophisticated medical vocabulary, demands for specific medications or treatments, and a history of excessive surgeries. Previous hospital charts should be gathered and prior clinicians contacted when a factitious disorder is suspected.

TABLE 10–3.   Methods used to produce symptoms in patients with a factitious disorder

Method	%
Injection or insertion of contaminated substance	29
Surreptitious use of medications	24
Exacerbation of wounds	17
Thermometer manipulation	10
Urinary tract manipulation	7
Falsification of medical history	7
Self-induced bruises or deformities	2
Phlebotomy	2

Source.   Adapted from Reich and Gottfried 1983.

In one intriguing case reported in the literature, the authors were able to document at least 15 different hospitalizations in a 2-year period and found that medical evaluations had included repeated cardiac catheterizations and angiograms. Complications from the procedures had eventually resulted in the loss of a limb. In this particular patient, clues to the diagnosis included the manner in which the patient presented his story, the absence of family or friends at the hospital, the presence of multiple surgical scars, and an absence of distress despite complaints of crushing retrosternal pain.

The treatment of factitious disorder is difficult and frustrating. The first task is to make the diagnosis so that additional and potentially harmful procedures can be avoided. Because many of these patients are hospitalized on medical and surgical wards, a psychiatric consultation should be obtained. The psychiatrist can help make the diagnosis and educate the treatment team about the nature of factitious disorders. Once sufficient evidence has been assembled to support the diagnosis, the patient should be confronted in a nonthreatening manner by the attending physician and the consulting psychiatrist. In a follow-up of 42 patients with factitious disorder, 33 were confronted. None signed out of the hospital or became suicidal, but only 13 acknowledged causing their disorders. Nevertheless, most improved after the confrontation, and 4 became asymptomatic. The authors reported that their lawyers had advised that room searches could be justified legally and ethically in the pursuit of a diagnosis. Like the suicidal patient whose belongings may be searched for dangerous objects, the factitious disorder patient also has a potentially life-threatening condition that justifies such measures.

■ Malingering

Malingering is not considered one of DSM-5's somatic symptom disorders but is included here because it is important to the differential diagnosis of these conditions. In DSM-5, it is included in the category "Other Conditions That May Be a Focus of Clinical Attention" that are not considered attributable to a mental disorder (i.e., the V/Z code diagnoses). Malingering is the intentional production of false or grossly exaggerated physical or psychological symptoms motivated by external incentives, such as avoiding military conscription or duty, avoiding work, obtaining financial compensation, evading criminal prosecution, obtaining drugs, or securing better living conditions.

Malingering is differentiated from factitious disorder by the intentional reporting of symptoms for personal gain (e.g., money, time off work). In contrast, the diagnosis of factitious disorder requires the absence of obvious rewards.

Most malingerers are male, and most have obvious reasons to feign illness. Many are prisoners, factory workers, or persons living in unpleasant situations (e.g., homeless persons). An illness may provide an escape from a harsh reality, while the hospital may offer a temporary sanctuary.

Malingering should be suspected when any of the following clues are present: medicolegal context of presentation (e.g., the person is being referred by his or her attorney for examination); marked discrepancy between the person's claimed disability and objective findings; lack of cooperation during the diagnostic evaluation and noncompliance with the treatment regimen; and the presence of an antisocial personality disorder. Symptoms reported by malingering patients are often vague, subjective, and unverifiable.

There is little consensus on the correct approach to take with malingerers. Some experts believe that malingering patients should be confronted once sufficient evidence has been collected to confirm the diagnosis. Others feel that confrontations simply disrupt the doctor-patient relationship and make the patient even more alert to possible future detection. Clinicians who take the second position feel that the best approach is to treat the patient as though the symptoms were real. The symptoms can then be given up in response to treatment without the patient losing face.

■ Dissociative Disorders

The hallmark of dissociative disorders is a disturbance of or alteration in the normally well-integrated functions of identity, memory, and consciousness. Dissociative disorders include dissociative identity disorder (formerly known as *multiple personality disorder*), dissociative amnesia, and depersonalization/derealization disorder. Two residual categories exist for people with dissociative symptoms who do not meet criteria for a more specific disorder: *other specified dissociative disorder* and *unspecified dissociative disorder.* (See Table 10–4 for a list of the DSM-5 dissociative disorders.)

TABLE 10–4. DSM-5 dissociative disorders
Dissociative identity disorder
Dissociative amnesia
Depersonalization/derealization disorder
Other specified dissociative disorder
Unspecified dissociative disorder

Dissociation occurs along a spectrum, but at the milder end is a common and normal part of human consciousness. For example, most people have had the experience of driving somewhere and not remembering the trip ("highway hypnosis"). An even more common example is the daydreaming that nearly all of us engage in at one time or another. These are both examples of normative dissociation, while hypnosis and meditation are examples of induced forms of dissociation. In these situations, it has been suggested that dissociation serves an adaptive function by allowing the mind to process the events of daily life. In some people, however, the dissociative process becomes distorted and actively interferes with one's functioning, causing distress and disability. Symptoms can be experienced as unwanted intrusions into awareness and behavior with accompanying loss of continuity in subjective experience, or as an inability to access information or control mental functions that are normally amenable to access or control.

Dissociative Identity Disorder

Dissociative identity disorder is characterized by the presence of two or more distinct personality states, which in some cultures may be likened to possession (see Box 10–6). According to DSM-5, this involves a marked discontinuity in sense of self and sense of agency, accompanied by related alterations in affect, behavior, consciousness, memory, perception, cognition, and/or sensory-motor functioning, as observed by others or reported by oneself. For example, people with dissociative identity disorder may feel they have suddenly become outside observers of their own speech and actions, which they may feel powerless to stop.

Most lay conceptions of dissociative identity disorder, which has been described for centuries, are based on media portrayals, the most famous of which are found in the film adaptations of the books *The Three Faces of Eve* and *Sybil*. Both provide detailed accounts of women with many strikingly different personalities.

Box 10–6.   DSM-5 Diagnostic Criteria for Dissociative Identity Disorder

---

A. Disruption of identity characterized by two or more distinct personality states, which may be described in some cultures as an experience of possession. The disruption in identity involves marked discontinuity in sense of self and sense of agency, accompanied by related alterations in affect, behavior, consciousness, memory, perception, cognition, and/ or sensory-motor functioning. These signs and symptoms may be observed by others or reported by the individual.
B. Recurrent gaps in the recall of everyday events, important personal information, and/or traumatic events that are inconsistent with ordinary forgetting.
C. The symptoms cause clinically significant distress or impairment in social, occupational, or other important areas of functioning.
D. The disturbance is not a normal part of a broadly accepted cultural or religious practice.
   Note: In children, the symptoms are not better explained by imaginary playmates or other fantasy play.
E. The symptoms are not attributable to the physiological effects of a substance (e.g., blackouts or chaotic behavior during alcohol intoxication) or another medical condition (e.g., complex partial seizures).

Surveys show that dissociative identity disorder has a prevalence of around 1.5% in the general population. It has also been reported to be fairly common (5%–15%) in inpatient and outpatient psychiatric settings. Because it was once thought rare, the apparent increase in frequency has led some to question whether well-meaning therapists have unknowingly induced the disorder through suggestion and the process of hypnosis. These methods are thought by some to lead to the creation of additional personalities in suggestible patients.

The case of a patient with dissociative identity disorder follows:

Cindy, a 24-year-old woman, was transferred to the psychiatry service to facilitate community placement. Over the years, she had received many different diagnoses, including schizophrenia, borderline personality disorder, schizoaffective disorder, and bipolar disorder. Dissociative identity disorder was her current diagnosis.

Cindy had been well until 3 years before admission, when she developed depression, "voices," multiple somatic complaints, periods of amnesia, and wrist cutting. Her family and friends considered her a pathological liar because she would do or say things that she would later deny. Chronic depression and recurrent suicidal behavior led to frequent hospitalizations. Cindy had trials of antipsychotics, antidepressants, mood stabilizers, and anxiolytics, all without benefit. Her condition continued to worsen.

Cindy was a petite, neatly groomed woman who cooperated well with the treatment team. She reported having nine distinct alters that ranged in age from 2 to 48 years; two were masculine. Cindy's main concern was her inability to control the switches among her alters, which made her feel out of control. She reported having been sexually abused by her father as a child and described visual hallucinations of him threatening her with a knife. We were unable to confirm the history of sexual abuse but thought it likely, based on what we knew of her chaotic early home life.

Nursing staff observed several episodes in which Cindy switched to a troublesome alter. Her voice would change in inflection and tone, becoming childlike as Joy, an 8-year-old alter, took control. Arrangements were made for individual psychotherapy and Cindy was discharged.

At a follow-up 3 years later, Cindy still had many alters but was functioning better, had fewer switches, and lived independently. She continued to see a therapist weekly and hoped to one day integrate her many alters.

Most persons diagnosed with dissociative identity disorder are women. The disorder is thought to have a childhood onset, usually before age 9 years, and is often chronic. The disorder is reported to run in families and as occurring in multiple generations.

Some researchers believe that dissociative identity disorder results from severe physical and sexual abuse in childhood. They hypothesize that the disorder results from self-induced hypnosis, used by the individual to cope with abuse, emotional maltreatment, or neglect. Some compare dissociative identity disorder to posttraumatic stress disorder (PTSD), a condition that develops in response to life-threatening situations.

Like persons with PTSD, dissociative identity disorder patients are reported to have smaller hippocampal and amygdalar volumes, suggesting that early traumatic experiences may affect neural circuitry alterations in brain areas associated with memory.

In one case series, the mean number of personalities (or "alters") in dissociative identity disorder patients was 7, and approximately one-half had more than 10. Different alters are reported to control an individual's behavior for varying lengths of time. The transition from one alter to another may be sudden or gradual, often prompted by stressful situations.

Some of the more common symptoms reported by patients with dissociative identity disorder, as well as characteristics of their alters, are shown in Table 10–5.

Patients with dissociative identity disorder often meet criteria for other mental disorders. Like Cindy, many have unexplained physical complaints and fulfill criteria for somatic symptom disorder. Headaches and amnesia ("losing time") are particularly common symptoms. Borderline personality disorder, found in up to 70% of dissociative identity disorder patients, is diagnosed on the basis of mood instability, identity disturbance, deliberate self-harm, and other symptoms characteristic of the disorder. Many dissociative identity disorder patients report psychotic symptoms such as auditory hallucinations ("voices"), and many will have a past diagnosis of schizophrenia, schizoaffective disorder, or psychotic mood disorder. These diagnoses need to be ruled out.

Patients with dissociative identity disorder tend to report that the voices originate within their heads, are not experienced with the ears, and are not associated with mood changes; insight generally is preserved. By contrast, patients with psychotic disorders usually report that auditory hallucinations "come from the outside," have the quality of a percept (as opposed to one's own thoughts), and are accompanied by changes in mood; insight is minimal. Hallucinations that accompany dissociative identity disorder are probably best considered *pseudohallucinations*—that is, hallucinations that are a product of one's own mind and are accompanied by the realization that the experience is due to illness and is not real.

There is no standard treatment for dissociative identity disorder, but many clinicians recommend long-term individual psychotherapy to help patients integrate their many alters. At least one study has shown that motivated patients treated by experienced therapists can achieve integration and remission of symptoms. Other aspects of treatment remain controversial. Some experts use hypnosis to help access the different alters in the context of psychotherapy. Cognitive-behavioral therapy has also been used to help patients achieve reintegration. All agree that therapy is lengthy and challenging.

TABLE 10–5. Common symptoms in 50 patients with dissociative identity disorder and characteristics of alternate personalities ("alters")

Symptoms	%	Alternate-personality characteristics	%
Markedly different moods	94	Amnestic personalities	100
Exhibiting an alter	84	Personalities with proper names	
Different accents	68	(e.g., Nick, Sally)	98
Inability to remember angry		Angry alternate personality	80
outbursts	58	Depressed alternate personality	74
Inner conversations	58	Personalities of different ages	66
Different handwriting	34	Suicidal alternate personality	62
Different dress or makeup	32	Protector alternate personality	30
Unfamiliar people know them		Self-abusive alternate	
well	18	personality	30
Amnesia for a previously		Opposite-sexed alternate	
learned subject	14	personality	26
Discovery of unfamiliar		Personality with nonproper	
possessions	14	names (e.g., "observer,"	
Different handedness	14	"teacher")	24
		Unnamed alternate personality	18

Source. Adapted from Coons et al. 1988.

Although the core features of dissociative identity disorder do not respond to medication, these patients often have co-occurring mood and anxiety disorders that can benefit from medication. For example, antidepressants may relieve coexisting major depression and block panic attacks.

Dissociative Amnesia

Dissociative amnesia is defined as the inability to recall important autobiographical information considered too extensive to be explained by ordinary forgetfulness (see Box 10–7). With dissociative amnesia, the person is typically confused and perplexed. He or she may not recall significant personal information or even his or her own name. The amnesia can develop suddenly and last minutes to days or longer. In one case series, 79% of amnestic episodes lasted less than a week.

Box 10–7.   DSM-5 Diagnostic Criteria for Dissociative Amnesia

A. An inability to recall important autobiographical information, usually of a traumatic or stressful nature, that is inconsistent with ordinary forgetting. **Note:** Dissociative amnesia most often consists of localized or selective amnesia for a specific event or events; or generalized amnesia for identity and life history.
B. The symptoms cause clinically significant distress or impairment in social, occupational, or other important areas of functioning.
C. The disturbance is not attributable to the physiological effects of a substance (e.g., alcohol or other drug of abuse, a medication) or a neurological or other medical condition (e.g., partial complex seizures, transient global amnesia, sequelae of a closed head injury/traumatic brain injury, other neurological condition).
D. The disturbance is not better explained by dissociative identity disorder, posttraumatic stress disorder, acute stress disorder, somatic symptom disorder, or major or mild neurocognitive disorder.

Specify if:
   With dissociative fugue: Apparently purposeful travel or bewildered wandering that is associated with amnesia for identity or for other important autobiographical information.

The prevalence of dissociative amnesia has been estimated at around 1%–3% in the general population; it affects more women than men. It has been reported to occur following severe physical or psychosocial stressors (e.g., natural disasters, war). In a study of combat veterans, between 5% and 20% were amnesic for their combat experiences. It has been estimated that from 5% to 14% of all military psychiatric casualties experience some degree of amnesia.

Dissociative fugue is a subtype of dissociative amnesia characterized by the inability to recall one's past and the assumption of a new identity, which may be partial or complete. The fugue usually involves sudden, unexpected travel away from home or one's workplace, is not due to a dissociative identity disorder, and is not induced by a substance or a general medical condition (e.g., temporal lobe epilepsy). Fugue states are reported to occur in psychologically stressful situations, such as natural disasters or war. Personal rejections, losses, or financial pressures are thought to have preceded the fugue in some cases. Fugues can last for months and lead to a complicated pattern of travel and identity formation.

The case of a woman who had a fugue state follows:

Carrie, a 31-year-old attorney from a small Midwestern town, was reported as missing for 4 days under mysterious circumstances. Carrie was known to have finished her day at work and to have exercised at a health spa but had failed to return home. Her car was found abandoned. A search was mounted, and it was assumed that she had been abducted or murdered, especially after a headless corpse was found. Candlelight vigils were held, psychics were consulted, and friends blanketed the community with posters offering rewards for help in locating her.

One month after her disappearance, Carrie called her father from Las Vegas, where she had been the entire time. She was at a local hospital and claimed to have had amnesia. Carrie reported that she had been physically assaulted while jogging on the night of her disappearance. During the struggle, she had been knocked unconscious: "When I came to, I was dazed, confused, and disoriented." She felt that the assault prompted the amnesia, leading her to forget her past. She later hitchhiked to Las Vegas, where she was found wandering aimlessly. The police took her to a nearby hospital, where she claimed a new identity.

With the help of a psychologist who used hypnosis, Carrie quickly recovered her memory and her identity. She returned home and resumed her legal practice. Her family and friends had described her as a "creature of habit" and were as baffled as was Carrie about her amnesia. She had no history of mental illness.

The differential diagnosis of dissociative amnesia includes many medical and neurological conditions that can cause memory impairment (e.g., a brain tumor, closed head trauma, dementia) as well as the effects of a substance (e.g., alcohol-related blackouts). A medical workup should include a physical examination, mental status examination, toxicological studies, an electroencephalogram, and other tests when indicated (e.g., magnetic resonance imaging brain scan).

As a general rule, the onset and termination of amnestic states due to a medical condition or a substance are unlikely to be associated with psychological stress. Memory impairment due to brain injury is likely to be more severe for recent than for remote events and to resolve slowly if at all; in these cases, memory only rarely recovers fully. Disturbances in attention, orientation, and affect are characteristic of many brain disorders (e.g., tumors, strokes, Alzheimer's disease) but are unlikely in dissociative amnesia. Memory loss from alcohol intoxication (i.e., blackouts) is characterized by impaired short-term recall and evidence of heavy substance abuse. *Malingering* involves reporting amnesia for behaviors that are alleged to be out of character when obvious reasons exist for secondary gain (e.g., claiming amnesia for a crime).

There is no established treatment for dissociative amnesia or fugue, and recovery tends to occur spontaneously. For some persons, a safe environment such as that found in a psychiatric hospital may foster recovery. As the name *fugue* implies, the condition involves psychological flight from overwhelming circumstances, and once these circumstances are resolved, the dissociative fugue resolves as well. In fugue states, recovery of past memories and the resumption of the individual's former identity may occur abruptly (i.e., over several hours) but can take much longer. Both conditions can recur, particularly when the precipitating stressors remain or return. Hypnosis has been reported to help patients recover missing memories. When memories return, patients should be helped to understand the reason for their memory loss and to reinforce healthy coping mechanisms.

Depersonalization/Derealization Disorder

Depersonalization/derealization disorder is characterized by feeling detached from oneself or one's surroundings, as though one were an outside observer; some patients experience a dreamlike state (see Box 10–8). A patient with depersonalization may feel as though he or she were cut off from his or her thoughts, emotions, or identity. Another may feel like a robot or automaton. Depersonalization may be accompanied by *derealization,* a sense of detachment, unreality, and altered relation to the outside world.

Box 10–8.   DSM-5 Diagnostic Criteria for Depersonalization/
Derealization Disorder

A. The presence of persistent or recurrent experiences of depersonalization, derealization, or both:
  1. **Depersonalization:** Experiences of unreality, detachment, or being an outside observer with respect to one's thoughts, feelings, sensations, body, or actions (e.g., perceptual alterations, distorted sense of time, unreal or absent self, emotional and/or physical numbing).
  2. **Derealization:** Experiences of unreality or detachment with respect to surroundings (e.g., individuals or objects are experienced as unreal, dreamlike, foggy, lifeless, or visually distorted).
B. During the depersonalization or derealization experiences, reality testing remains intact.
C. The symptoms cause clinically significant distress or impairment in social, occupational, or other important areas of functioning.
D. The disturbance is not attributable to the physiological effects of a substance (e.g., a drug of abuse, medication) or another medical condition (e.g., seizures).
E. The disturbance is not better explained by another mental disorder, such as schizophrenia, panic disorder, major depressive disorder, acute stress disorder, posttraumatic stress disorder, or another dissociative disorder.

In DSM-IV, depersonalization and derealization were separate disorders. With DSM-5, the two syndromes have been merged because research had shown little difference between persons with depersonalization alone and those with depersonalization accompanied by derealization.

The prevalence of depersonalization/derealization disorder is around 2% in the general population; it is equally common in men and women. Many people who are otherwise normal transiently experience mild depersonalization or derealization. For example, these symptoms can occur when a person is sleep deprived, travels to unfamiliar places, or is intoxicated with hallucinogens, marijuana, or alcohol. In a study of college students, one-third to one-half reported having experienced transient depersonalization/derealization. Persons exposed to life-threatening situations, such as traumatic accidents, may also experience these symptoms. For these reasons, depersonalization/derealization disorder is diagnosed only when it is persistent and causes distress.

The disorder typically begins in adolescence or early adulthood but rarely after age 40. Many persons vividly recall their first episode of depersonalization/derealization, which may begin abruptly. Some report a precipitating event, such as smoking marijuana. The duration of depersonalization/derealization episodes is highly variable, but they can last hours, days, or even weeks. Although depersonalization disorder is typically experienced as chronic and continuous, some people experience periods of remission. Exacerbations may follow psychologically stressful situations, such as the loss of an important relationship.

The cause of depersonalization/derealization disorder is unknown. The fact that depersonalization frequently accompanies several central nervous system disturbances (e.g., partial complex seizures, tumors, stroke, migraine) suggests a neurobiological basis. One recent theory holds that the state of increased alertness seen in depersonalization disorder results from activation of the prefrontal attentional systems combined with reciprocal inhibition of the anterior cingulate, causing "mind emptiness."

Mental disorders in which depersonalization/derealization symptoms sometimes occur must be ruled out, such as schizophrenia, major depression, phobias, panic disorder, obsessive-compulsive disorder, PTSD, and drug abuse. Medical conditions (e.g., partial complex seizures, migraine), sleep deprivation, and drug-induced states need to be ruled out as well.

There are no standard treatments for the disorder, but benzodiazepines may be helpful in reducing the accompanying anxiety (e.g., diazepam, 5 mg three times daily). SSRIs and clomipramine have been reported to relieve symptoms of depersonalization, although in a controlled trial fluoxetine proved ineffective. Patients also have been reported to benefit from hypnosis or CBT to help control their episodes of depersonalization/derealization. With CBT, patients learn to confront their distorted thoughts and challenge their feelings of unreality.

Clinical points for dissociative disorders

1. Medical conditions (e.g., tumors, temporal lobe epilepsy) must be ruled out as a cause of the amnesia, dissociation, or depersonalization/derealization.

2. The therapist should be patient and supportive. In most cases of amnesia, return of memory is rapid and complete.

3. Patients with dissociative identity disorder are especially challenging, and therapy may be long-term. The clinician may want to refer the patient to a therapist experienced in treating the disorder.

   - It may be best to help the patient gradually learn about the number and nature of his or her alters.

   - A goal with these patients should be to help them function better and to bring about better communication among the alters.

4. Medications have no proven benefit in treating dissociative disorders, although antidepressants may help some patients with depersonalization/derealization disorder.

   - Benzodiazepines may help to reduce the anxiety that often accompanies depersonalization.

■ Self-Assessment Questions

1. How is somatic symptom disorder diagnosed and what are its risk factors?
2. How does somatic symptom disorder differ from illness anxiety disorder?
3. Describe conversion disorder. What is the differential diagnosis?
4. How are the somatic symptom disorders managed?
5. How is factitious disorder distinguished from malingering?
6. Describe the dissociative disorders. What is the differential diagnosis for the dissociative disorders? Why are they controversial? What is a dissociative fugue?
7. What is a current etiological theory of dissociative identity disorder?
8. How are pseudohallucinations distinguished from true hallucinations?

9. What is depersonalization/derealization, and how common is it? What is its course and how is it treated?

Chapter 11

Feeding and Eating Disorders

O! that this too, too solid flesh would melt.

William Shakespeare, Hamlet

Feeding and eating disorders reflect dysfunctional appetitive drive and behavior and can span the entire age range. The chapter combines feeding disorders that are usually diagnosed in childhood with the classic eating disorders because of their shared phenomenology and pathophysiology. Added to the latter group is binge-eating disorder, new to DSM-5, an addition based on considerable research that has accumulated in the past decade. There are two residual categories for those with feeding or eating disorders who do not fit the criteria for a more specific disorder (other specified feeding and eating disorder and unspecified feeding and eating disorder). Table 11–1 lists the disorders included in this chapter.

TABLE 11–1.   DSM-5 feeding and eating disorders

Pica

Rumination disorder

Avoidant/restrictive food intake disorder

Anorexia nervosa

Bulimia nervosa

Binge-eating disorder

Other specified feeding or eating disorder

Unspecified feeding or eating disorder

■ Feeding Disorders

Pica

Pica is diagnosed when a person consumes nonnutritive substances on a persistent basis for a period of at least 1 month (Box 11–1). Described for centuries, historically pica has been considered an accompaniment to conditions such as pregnancy, to an intellectual disability, or as a symptom of medical disorders such as iron deficiency. Children up to age 24 months frequently mouth or even eat nonnutritive items, but this behavior does not suggest that the child has pica. Pica is not confined to children or to individuals with intellectual disabilities. To qualify for a diagnosis, the condition must have lasted at least 1 month. Because the mouthing of objects including nonnutritive, nonfood substances is developmentally normal in young infants, the minimum age of 2 years is required by the diagnosis.

Box 11–1.   DSM-5 Diagnostic Criteria for Pica

A. Persistent eating of nonnutritive, nonfood substances over a period of at least 1 month.
B. The eating of nonnutritive, nonfood substances is inappropriate to the developmental level of the individual.
C. The eating behavior is not part of a culturally supported or socially normative practice.
D. If the eating behavior occurs in the context of another mental disorder (e.g., intellectual disability [intellectual developmental disorder], autism spectrum disorder, schizophrenia) or medical condition (including pregnancy), it is sufficiently severe to warrant additional clinical attention.

Specify if:
   In remission: After full criteria for pica were previously met, the criteria have not been met for a sustained period of time.

Interestingly, people around the world eat clay or dirt (*geophagy*) for a variety of reasons. Commonly, geophagy is a traditional cultural activity that takes place during pregnancy, for religious ceremonies, or as a remedy for disease, particularly in Central Africa and the Southern United States. The indigenous Pomo of Northern California also include dirt in their diet. Although it is a cultural practice, it may also fill a physiological need (or perceived need) for nutrients.

There is no specific treatment for pica, though behavior therapy that rewards appropriate eating behavior or negatively reinforces nonnutritive food consumption has been described.

Rumination Disorder

Rumination disorder is characterized by the repeated regurgitation of food (Box 11–2). The disorder occurs across the age range and in both genders. Individuals with this disorder repeatedly regurgitate swallowed or partially digested food, which may then be re-chewed and either reswallowed or expelled. Adolescents and adults are less likely to re-chew regurgitated material than younger children. There is no retching, nausea, heartburn, odors, or abdominal pains associated with the regurgitation, as there is with typical vomiting. Although the disorder occurs more commonly in infants, young children, and people with developmental disabilities, it also occurs in otherwise healthy adolescents and adults. Unlike in typical vomiting, the regurgitation is commonly described as effortless and unforced. The regurgitation of food has to have lasted for at least 1 month.

Box 11–2. DSM-5 Diagnostic Criteria for Rumination Disorder

A. Repeated regurgitation of food over a period of at least 1 month. Regurgitated food may be re-chewed, re-swallowed, or spit out.
B. The repeated regurgitation is not attributable to an associated gastrointestinal or other medical condition (e.g., gastroesophageal reflux, pyloric stenosis).
C. The eating disturbance does not occur exclusively during the course of anorexia nervosa, bulimia nervosa, binge-eating disorder, or avoidant/restrictive food intake disorder.
D. If the symptoms occur in the context of another mental disorder (e.g., intellectual disability [intellectual developmental disorder] or another neurodevelopmental disorder), they are sufficiently severe to warrant additional clinical attention.

Specify if:
   In remission: After full criteria for rumination disorder were previously met, the criteria have not been met for a sustained period of time.

Not all individuals with rumination disorder, particularly older individuals and those with normal intelligence, re-chew the regurgitated food. Individuals with rumination disorder may have a history of reflux, and it may be difficult clinically to reliably parse out the medical and psychological components of the behavior. In recognition of this clinical difficulty, DSM-5 requires ruling out an associated gastrointestinal or other medical condition.

Rumination behavior is well documented to occur in persons with conventional eating disorders. This diagnosis requires that the rumination be more than a symptom of one of the eating disorders. If it occurs apart from the eating disorder, then it can be independently diagnosed. Rumination disorder commonly occurs in the context of developmental delays, often as a means of self-stimulation. In these cases, this behavior is more appropriately considered a symptom of these other conditions. If the rumination behavior is severe enough to warrant independent clinical attention, then the additional diagnosis of rumination disorder is appropriate.

As with pica, there are no specific treatments for the condition, but behavioral therapy that rewards nonrumination with parental attention and negatively reinforces nonrumination can be effective.

Avoidant/Restrictive Food Intake Disorder

Avoidant/restrictive food intake disorder is characterized by a disturbance of eating or feeding behavior that takes the form of avoiding or restricting food intake. Three main subtypes have been identified: individuals who do not eat enough or show little interest in feeding or eating; individuals who accept only a limited diet in relation to sensory features; and individuals whose food refusal is related to aversive experience (Box 11–3).

Box 11–3. DSM-5 Diagnostic Criteria for Avoidant/Restrictive Food Intake Disorder

---

A. An eating or feeding disturbance (e.g., apparent lack of interest in eating or food; avoidance based on the sensory characteristics of food; concern about aversive consequences of eating) as manifested by persistent failure to meet appropriate nutritional and/or energy needs associated with one (or more) of the following:

1. Significant weight loss (or failure to achieve expected weight gain or faltering growth in children).
2. Significant nutritional deficiency.
3. Dependence on enteral feeding or oral nutritional supplements.
4. Marked interference with psychosocial functioning.

B. The disturbance is not better explained by lack of available food or by an associated culturally sanctioned practice.

C. The eating disturbance does not occur exclusively during the course of anorexia nervosa or bulimia nervosa, and there is no evidence of a disturbance in the way in which one's body weight or shape is experienced.

D. The eating disturbance is not attributable to a concurrent medical condition or not better explained by another mental disorder. When the eating disturbance occurs in the context of another condition or disorder, the severity of the eating disturbance exceeds that routinely associated with the condition or disorder and warrants additional clinical attention.

Specify if:

In remission: After full criteria for avoidant/restrictive food intake disorder were previously met, the criteria have not been met for a sustained period of time.

Avoidance or restriction associated with insufficient intake or lack of interest in food usually develops in infancy or early childhood, although it can begin in adolescence; onset in adulthood is rare. This disorder does not include developmentally normal food avoidance, which is characterized by picky eating in childhood or reduced food intake associated with advanced age. Pregnant women may restrict intake or avoid certain foods due to altered sensory sensitivities, but this is a self-limited behavior and the diagnosis of avoidant/restrictive food intake disorder is not likely warranted unless the eating disturbance is extreme and full criteria are met.

Avoidant/restrictive food intake disorder appears equally common in males and females in infancy and childhood. Various functional consequences are associated with this disorder, such as impairments in physical development, relationship and social difficulties, caregiver stress, and problems in family functioning.

Because extreme poverty and cultural practices, such as religious fasting, can also result in significant weight loss, the diagnosis requires that the disorder is not better explained by lack of available food and that the disorder is not solely the result of a "culturally sanctioned" practice, such as particular religious or cultural observations, that might account for the disorder.

Restriction of energy intake relative to requirements, resulting in weight loss, is a core feature of anorexia nervosa and may be a compensatory behavior in bulimia nervosa. For older children or young adolescents, these disorders share a number of features such as low weight and food avoidance. Anorexia nervosa, however, is associated with fear of gaining weight and perceptual disturbances of one's body weight or shape. In the case of bulimia nervosa, the restriction or fasting is a compensatory behavior to the recurrent episodes of binge eating. It is necessary to make a distinction between restricted food intake in the context of eating disorders where there are weight or shape concerns and restricted food intake in the absence of such concerns.

Other conditions can cause feeding disturbances, including gastrointestinal (e.g., gastroesophageal reflux), endocrinological (e.g., diabetes), and neurological (e.g., those related to problems with oral/esophageal/pharyngeal structural or functional problems) conditions, and these disturbances need to be distinguished from avoidant/restrictive food intake disorder.

■ Eating Disorders

Anorexia nervosa and *bulimia nervosa,* the two major eating disorders, are each characterized by the presence of disturbed eating behaviors combined with an intense preoccupation with body weight and shape. To these, DSM-5 has added *binge-eating disorder,* which involves binge eating in the absence of compensatory behaviors. Many persons believe that these syndromes are a reflection of contemporary society's obsession with youth, beauty, and slimness. In fact, the disorders have been recognized for centuries. Richard Morton, an English physician, is generally credited with describing the syndrome of anorexia nervosa in 1694, although it was Sir William Gull who coined the term in 1873. Gull's patients were mostly emaciated young women with amenorrhea, constipation, and an abnormally slow pulse who were nonetheless remarkably overactive. His account is still noteworthy for its attention to detail.

Anorexia Nervosa

Anorexia nervosa is defined as a restriction of energy intake sufficient to cause significantly low body weight, and occurring in the presence of an intense fear of gaining weight or becoming fat (or persistent behavior that interferes with weight gain) and a disturbance in the perception of his or her body shape (see Box 11–4). The clinician should further specify whether the disorder is the restricting type (i.e., no bingeing or purging) or the binge-eating/purging type.

Body mass index (BMI; weight in kilograms/height in meters^2) is a useful measure; most adults with a BMI ≥18.5 would not be considered significantly underweight. A person whose BMI is <17 would be considered significantly underweight. People with anorexia nervosa are subtyped as mild, moderate, severe, or extreme on the basis of BMI.

The discrepancy between weight and perceived body image is key to the diagnosis of anorexia nervosa. Most underweight persons are concerned about their weight. They recognize when it is too low and express a desire to gain weight. By contrast, people with anorexia nervosa take delight in their weight loss and fear gaining weight. Bulimic persons often successfully hide their binge-eating and purging behaviors and often have normal weight. In practice, the two syndromes tend to overlap, so that patients often have a mixture of symptoms, such as Mary in the case vignette in the section "Epidemiology of the Eating Disorders."

Box 11–4.   DSM-5 Diagnostic Criteria for Anorexia Nervosa

A. Restriction of energy intake relative to requirements, leading to a significantly low body weight in the context of age, sex, developmental trajectory, and physical health. *Significantly low weight* is defined as a weight that is less than minimally normal or, for children and adolescents, less than that minimally expected.
B. Intense fear of gaining weight or of becoming fat, or persistent behavior that interferes with weight gain, even though at a significantly low weight.
C. Disturbance in the way in which one's body weight or shape is experienced, undue influence of body weight or shape on self-evaluation, or persistent lack of recognition of the seriousness of the current low body weight.

Specify whether:
   Restricting type: During the last 3 months, the individual has not engaged in recurrent episodes of binge eating or purging behavior (i.e., self-induced vomiting or the misuse of laxatives, diuretics, or enemas). This subtype describes presentations in which weight loss is accomplished primarily through dieting, fasting, and/or excessive exercise.
   Binge-eating/purging type: During the last 3 months, the individual has engaged in recurrent episodes of binge eating or purging behavior (i.e., self-induced vomiting or the misuse of laxatives, diuretics, or enemas).

Specify if:
   In partial remission: After full criteria for anorexia nervosa were previously met, Criterion A (low body weight) has not been met for a sustained period, but either Criterion B (intense fear of gaining weight or becoming fat or behavior that interferes with weight gain) or Criterion C (disturbances in self-perception of weight and shape) is still met.
   In full remission: After full criteria for anorexia nervosa were previously met, none of the criteria have been met for a sustained period of time.

Specify current severity:
The minimum level of severity is based, for adults, on current body mass index (BMI) (see below) or, for children and adolescents, on BMI percentile. The ranges below are derived from World Health Organization categories for thinness in adults; for children and adolescents, corresponding BMI per-

centiles should be used. The level of severity may be increased to reflect clinical symptoms, the degree of functional disability, and the need for supervision.

Mild: BMI ≥ 17 kg/m^2
Moderate: BMI 16–16.99 kg/m^2
Severe: BMI 15–15.99 kg/m^2
Extreme: BMI < 15 kg/m^2

Bulimia Nervosa

Bulimia nervosa consists of recurrent episodes of binge eating; a feeling of lack of control over eating during the binges; recurrent use of inappropriate compensatory behaviors to prevent weight gain, such as vomiting, use of laxatives or diuretics, strict dieting or fasting, or vigorous exercise; an average of at least one binge episode weekly for 3 months; and persistent overconcern with body shape and weight (see Box 11–5). Furthermore, the disturbance does not occur exclusively in the course of anorexia nervosa.

Box 11–5. DSM-5 Diagnostic Criteria for Bulimia Nervosa

A. Recurrent episodes of binge eating. An episode of binge eating is characterized by both of the following:

1. Eating, in a discrete period of time (e.g., within any 2-hour period), an amount of food that is definitely larger than what most individuals would eat in a similar period of time under similar circumstances.

2. A sense of lack of control over eating during the episode (e.g., a feeling that one cannot stop eating or control what or how much one is eating).

B. Recurrent inappropriate compensatory behaviors in order to prevent weight gain, such as self-induced vomiting; misuse of laxatives, diuretics, or other medications; fasting; or excessive exercise.

C. The binge eating and inappropriate compensatory behaviors both occur, on average, at least once a week for 3 months.

D. Self-evaluation is unduly influenced by body shape and weight.

E. The disturbance does not occur exclusively during episodes of anorexia nervosa.

Specify if:

In partial remission: After full criteria for bulimia nervosa were previously met, some, but not all, of the criteria have been met for a sustained period of time.

In full remission: After full criteria for bulimia nervosa were previously met, none of the criteria have been met for a sustained period of time.

Specify current severity:
The minimum level of severity is based on the frequency of inappropriate compensatory behaviors (see below). The level of severity may be increased to reflect other symptoms and the degree of functional disability.

Mild: An average of 1–3 episodes of inappropriate compensatory behaviors per week.

Moderate: An average of 4–7 episodes of inappropriate compensatory behaviors per week.

Severe: An average of 8–13 episodes of inappropriate compensatory behaviors per week.

Extreme: An average of 14 or more episodes of inappropriate compensatory behaviors per week.

Binge-Eating Disorder

Binge-eating disorder involves recurrent binge eating without compensatory behaviors (Box 11–6). The distinction between binge-eating disorder and bulimia nervosa is sometimes unclear, and the two diagnoses may represent different stages of the same underlying disorder. Compared with bulimia nervosa, people with binge-eating disorder are generally older, are more likely to be male, and have a later age at onset. Nearly two-thirds of individuals with binge-eating disorder have a history of using inappropriate compensatory behaviors, suggesting a past diagnosis of bulimia nervosa. Although weight and shape concerns are not required for the diagnosis, they are commonly part of the presentation.

Box 11–6. DSM-5 Diagnostic Criteria for Binge-Eating Disorder

---

A. Recurrent episodes of binge eating. An episode of binge eating is characterized by both of the following:

1. Eating, in a discrete period of time (e.g., within any 2-hour period), an amount of food that is definitely larger than what most people would eat in a similar period of time under similar circumstances.
2. A sense of lack of control over eating during the episode (e.g., a feeling that one cannot stop eating or control what or how much one is eating).

B. The binge-eating episodes are associated with three (or more) of the following:

1. Eating much more rapidly than normal.
2. Eating until feeling uncomfortably full.
3. Eating large amounts of food when not feeling physically hungry.
4. Eating alone because of feeling embarrassed by how much one is eating.
5. Feeling disgusted with oneself, depressed, or very guilty afterward.

C. Marked distress regarding binge eating is present.

D. The binge eating occurs, on average, at least once a week for 3 months.

E. The binge eating is not associated with the recurrent use of inappropriate compensatory behavior as in bulimia nervosa and does not occur exclusively during the course of bulimia nervosa or anorexia nervosa.

Specify if:

In partial remission: After full criteria for binge-eating disorder were previously met, binge eating occurs at an average frequency of less than one episode per week for a sustained period of time.

In full remission: After full criteria for binge-eating disorder were previously met, none of the criteria have been met for a sustained period of time.

Specify current severity:

The minimum level of severity is based on the frequency of episodes of binge eating (see below). The level of severity may be increased to reflect other symptoms and the degree of functional disability.

Mild: 1–3 binge-eating episodes per week.

Moderate: 4–7 binge-eating episodes per week.

Severe: 8–13 binge-eating episodes per week.

Extreme: 14 or more binge-eating episodes per week.

Epidemiology of the Eating Disorders

Estimates from high school– and college-age populations yield a prevalence among women of approximately 1% for anorexia nervosa and up to 4% for bulimia nervosa. For either disorder, the frequency in men is about one-tenth that for women. Isolated symptoms, such as binge eating, purging (e.g., self-induced vomiting), or fasting, are far more common than the disorders themselves. The gender difference is probably not artifactual, because population surveys confirm what clinicians have noted. Binge-eating disorder may be the most frequent eating disorder in the general population, affecting 3.5% of women and 2% of men; it is also common in those seeking weight loss treatment.

Eating disorders have an onset during adolescence or young adulthood. Anorexia nervosa typically has an earlier onset (early teens) than bulimia nervosa (late teens, early 20s). These disorders are found in all social strata, although in the past they were thought to be more common in the higher socioeconomic groups. Anorexia nervosa, however, is uncommon in nonindustrialized countries and is less frequent among African Americans in the United States. Eating disorders are overrepresented in occupations that require rigorous control of body shape (e.g., modeling, ballet). Male athletes—particularly wrestlers and jockeys—often develop eating disorders because they must meet strict weight criteria.

The following case vignette illustrates a patient who developed anorexia nervosa first and later achieved normal weight complicated by bulimia nervosa:

> Mary, a 36-year-old registered nurse, had a 16-year history of abnormal eating behaviors. Although she now maintained a normal weight and had regular periods, she had frequent binge/purge episodes.
>
> Mary grew up in a competitive, upper-middle-class family. The middle of five children, Mary felt unloved and ignored by her parents, who she believed favored the other children. Apart from occasional temper outbursts during her youth, Mary was well adjusted, performed well in school, was active in clubs, and had many friends.
>
> At age 20, she and a friend toured Europe together and would skip meals to save money. Both felt that they could afford to lose some weight. She lost about 25 pounds, and upon her return, her family became concerned with Mary's scarecrow-like appearance. Mary was happy with her weight loss and felt more attractive.
>
> Over the next 5 years, her weight fluctuated, but she remained underweight. Family members were concerned with her eating habits. She refused to eat meals with her family, adopted a vegetarian diet, and was often observed preparing high-calorie snacks. Mary eventually moved into her own apartment. Her brother remembers running into her at a grocery store and finding only diet soda, a single head of lettuce, and several bags of candy in the shopping cart. Early on, Mary had learned to induce vomiting, which later occurred spontaneously.
>
> Mary became obsessed with exercise. She jogged 10 miles each day and entered several marathons. She eventually cut back on her jogging when bone spurs and an old back injury flared up. Instead, she developed a new routine consisting of a 10-mile bicycle ride followed by a 45-minute swim. Mary was so busy with exercise that she had little time for friends and lost interest in dating.
>
> When Mary was 25, her mother talked her into seeing a physician for evaluation of her thinness, but the physician was not familiar with eating disorders and explained that Mary's thinness and abnormal eating behaviors were a harmless idiosyncrasy. Mary later sought help from a counselor for relationship problems but never sought help for her eating disorder.
>
> Nine years later, Mary continued to engage in occasional bingeing and purging but maintained a normal weight. She continued to work full-time, got married, and had two healthy children.

Clinical Findings

Anorexia nervosa is accompanied by a repertoire of behaviors designed to promote weight loss. Examples include extreme dieting, adoption of special diets (or vegetarianism), and refusal to eat meals with family members or to eat in restaurants. Anorexic persons often show an unusual preoccupation with food that belies their fear of gaining weight. The individual may clip and collect recipes or prepare elaborate meals for friends and relatives; some persons develop an interest in nutrition. At mealtime, the anorexic person may play with the food on his or her plate or cut meat into tiny pieces. Despite the concern of friends and family, persons with anorexia will insist that their weight is normal and, in fact, that they are overweight. Like Mary above, many anorexic persons develop an intense, obsessive interest in fitness and develop elaborate exercise routines. Abuse of laxatives, diuretics, or stimulants in an effort to enhance weight loss is relatively common.

Binge eating and purging typically occur in private. Enormous amounts of food can be consumed during a binge—for instance, an entire cake, a quart of ice cream, and a package of cookies. Binge eating may initially provide tension relief for the patient, but this relief is short-lived and generally leads to feelings of guilt and disgust. The person then induces vomiting, typically by placing the fingers in the throat; later, she or he may learn to vomit at will. Ipecac or other emetics are sometimes used to promote vomiting. Many bulimic persons, perhaps more than 10%, steal food by shoplifting or other means.

People with anorexia nervosa can experience profound weight loss. In addition to appearing emaciated, they can develop hypothermia, dependent edema, bradycardia, and hypotension. Some persons with anorexia nervosa develop sensitivity to temperature and report feeling cold much of the time. Near-chronic constipation leads many to become dependent on laxatives. Hormonal abnormalities can develop, including elevated growth hormone levels, increased plasma cortisol, and reduced gonadotropin levels. Thyroxin and thyroid-stimulating hormone can be normal even when triiodothyronine (T_3) is reduced. Men with anorexia nervosa generally have low levels of circulating testosterone and can show clinical signs of hypogonadism. For these reasons, many young people with anorexia have delayed sexual development and often have little interest in sex. Amenorrhea precedes the onset of obvious weight loss in one-fifth of female patients, though it is not required for the diagnosis.

Bulimic persons sometimes develop calluses on the dorsal surface of the hands (resulting from the irritation caused by placing fingers down the throat), dental erosion, and multiple caries. Rarely, esophageal erosion or tears occur. All are complications of frequent vomiting.

Medical complications caused by bulimic behavior include hypocalcemia or hypokalemic alkalosis (in those who engage in self-induced

---

TABLE 11–2. Medical complications of the eating disorders

Physical manifestations	**Laboratory abnormalities**
Amenorrhea	Dehydration[a]
Sensitivity to cold	Hypokalemia[a]
Constipation	Hypochloremia[a]
Low blood pressure	Alkalosis
Bradycardia	Leukopenia
Hypothermia	Elevated transaminases
Lanugo hair	Elevated serum cholesterol
Hair loss	Carotenemia
Petechia	Elevated BUN[a]
Carotenemic skin	Elevated amylase levels[a]
Parotid gland enlargement[a]	
Dental erosion, caries[a]	
Pedal edema	
Dry skin	

Endocrine abnormalities

Increased growth hormone levels

Increased plasma cortisol and loss of diurnal variation

Reduced gonadotropin levels (LH, FSH, impaired response to LHRH)

Low T_3, high T_3RU impaired TRH responsiveness[a]

Abnormal glucose tolerance test results

Abnormal dexamethasone suppression test results[a]

Note. BUN=blood urea nitrogen; FSH=follicle-stimulating hormone; LH=luteinizing hormone; LHRH=luteinizing hormone–releasing hormone; T_3=triiodothyronine; T_3RU= triiodothyronine reuptake; TRH=thyrotropin-releasing hormone.
[a]Seen in patients who binge and purge.

---

vomiting or who abuse laxatives and diuretics); electrolyte disturbances resulting in weakness, lethargy, or electrocardiographic changes such as depressed T waves; elevated serum transaminases, reflecting fatty degeneration of the liver; elevated serum cholesterol and carotenemia, reflecting malnutrition; and parotid gland enlargement and elevated serum amylase. The medical complications of the eating disorders are summarized in Table 11–2.

Course and Outcome

The long-term course of the eating disorders ranges from full recovery to malignant weight loss and rapid death. One study of patients with anorexia showed a death rate of 11% during a 12-year follow-up, a rate significantly higher than expected. From 25% to 40% of eating disorder patients have a good outcome, meaning that they eat normally, do not binge or purge, and are emotionally well adjusted. In the remaining patients, the characteristic symptoms of the illness (e.g., distorted body image, abnormal eating behaviors) persist. Poor outcome is associated with longer duration of illness, older age at onset, prior psychiatric hospitalizations, poor premorbid adjustment, and the presence of a comorbid personality disorder.

Etiology and Pathophysiology

The cause of eating disorders likely involves a combination of biological vulnerability, psychological predisposition, and societal influences. Genetic factors are probably important in anorexia nervosa, which has a concordance rate of nearly 70% for identical twins and only about 20% for nonidentical twins. Several studies have shown an increased frequency of bulimia nervosa among the relatives of bulimic persons.

Another factor may be a disturbance in serotonergic neurotransmission in the central nervous system (CNS). In the hypothalamus, serotonin helps to modulate feeding behavior by producing feelings of fullness and satiety. Patients with anorexia frequently report feeling "too full" after eating. Another effect of the CNS serotonin pathways involves regulation of mood, impulses, and obsessionality. Unsurprisingly, patients with anorexia nervosa are often rigid, inhibited, and perfectionistic.

Once dieting begins, psychological and physiological changes occur that perpetuate abnormal eating behavior. Anorexia nervosa often serves a positive function in the person's life by providing a refuge from upsetting life events or developmental issues involving relationships and sexuality. Some clinicians believe that anorexia nervosa represents an attempt to prolong childhood and escape the responsibilities of adulthood. Patients cling to their disorder and take comfort in their success with dieting. The tension relief gained from the avoidance of food or purging behavior is strongly reinforcing.

Physiological changes that occur in anorexia nervosa also reinforce the disorder. Corticotropin-releasing hormone secretion is enhanced in anorexia nervosa and may act to maintain abnormal eating behavior. Levels of vasopressin are high and oxytocin levels are low in the cerebrospinal fluid of underweight persons with anorexia. One hypothesis is that both hormones work together to promote distorted thinking patterns and obsessional concerns about food.

Diagnosis and Assessment

The diagnosis of an eating disorder is based on the patient's history and a careful mental status examination. A thorough physical examination should be part of the workup, with special attention given to vital signs, weight, skin quality and turgor, and the cardiovascular system. The patient's weight and height should be measured, and the appropriateness of weight for height, age, and gender should be determined according to his or her expected body weight or the BMI. This information can help guide decisions with respect to medical and nutritional management.

Laboratory studies can help to rule out alternative diagnoses. The workup should include a complete blood count, urinalysis, blood urea nitrogen, and serum electrolytes. For malnourished and severely symptomatic patients, other tests are indicated, including serum cholesterol and lipids; serum calcium, magnesium, phosphorus, and amylase; liver enzymes; and an electrocardiogram. Brain imaging with magnetic resonance or computed tomography is indicated in some patients to rule out a mass lesion. Thyroid function tests are indicated when hyperthyroidism is suspected as a cause of weight loss. Bone mineral densitometry is helpful in assessing and monitoring osteoporosis; bone-density measurements are more than two standard deviations below normal in about half of women with anorexia nervosa.

Other mental disorders need to be ruled out before making a diagnosis of anorexia nervosa or bulimia nervosa. Schizophrenia is sometimes accompanied by bizarre eating habits, but they are usually related to the patient's delusions. Major depression is frequently accompanied by poor appetite and significant weight loss, but this weight loss is not associated with a distorted body image and is unwanted. Ritualistic eating behaviors resulting in weight loss sometimes occur in patients with obsessive-compulsive disorder, but the weight loss is not accompanied by a distorted body image or fears of gaining weight.

Many patients with anorexia nervosa or bulimia nervosa have co-occurring major depression, an anxiety disorder, or a personality disorder. Obsessive-compulsive disorder, specific phobias, and agoraphobia are commonly diagnosed in patients with anorexia nervosa. Bulimic persons are at high risk for substance use disorders and "acting-out" personality disorders such as borderline personality disorder.

Medical illnesses also need to be ruled out as a cause of the eating disorder and weight loss. Conditions associated with severe weight loss include gastrointestinal disorders (e.g., a malabsorption syndrome) and endocrine disorders (e.g., hyperthyroidism). Midline tumors in the brain can be associated with anorexia and weight loss in the absence of localizing neurological abnormalities. Nevertheless, when the core features of an eating disorder are present—morbid fear of fatness and self-induced starvation—a medical cause is highly unlikely.

Clinical Management

The treatment of eating disorders has three main goals. The first goal is to restore a normal nutritional state. In patients with anorexia nervosa, this means restoring weight to within a normal range. In bulimic persons, this means ensuring that metabolic balance is achieved. The second goal is to modify the patients' disturbed eating behaviors. This will help the patient maintain his or her weight within a normal range and reverse (or lessen) binge eating, purging, and other abnormal eating behaviors. The third goal is to help change the patient's distorted and erroneous beliefs about the benefits of weight loss.

Treatment usually occurs on an outpatient basis, but some patients will need to be hospitalized. Severe starvation and weight loss, hypotension or hypothermia, and electrolyte imbalance are reasons for hospitalization. Depressed patients with eating disorders who have suicidal ideations or psychosis also require hospitalization. Failure of outpatient treatment, as indicated by the inability to gain weight or the inability to reverse severe binge/purge cycles, is another reason to hospitalize the patient. Partial hospital (or day treatment) programs are helpful to patients who need more supervision and support than can be obtained in an outpatient clinic but who do not require inpatient care. In these programs, patients attend the hospital during the day but live at home.

The treatment of anorexia nervosa or bulimia nervosa generally involves behavioral modification combined with individual and group psychotherapy. The purpose of behavior therapy is to restore normal eating behavior. In the hospital, this goal is accomplished by setting goals for both eating and weight gain and by targeting certain abnormal behaviors for correction (e.g., reducing the number of vomiting episodes for bulimic patients). Positive reinforcement is used to help patients achieve the goals outlined in a treatment contract that is agreed to by the patient. For example, patients who are able to achieve their weight goals are rewarded with special privileges, such as a pass with a family member. An example of a behavioral modification program is presented in Chapter 20 ("Behavioral, Cognitive, and Psychodynamic Treatments").

The patient should be weighed regularly, early in the morning after emptying the bladder and while wearing only a hospital gown. Daily fluid intake and output should be recorded. Patients should be observed for at least 2 hours after meals to prevent vomiting, even if attendants must accompany them to the bathroom. Patients are typically started on a diet providing about 500 calories more than the amount required to maintain their present weight; the caloric intake is gradually increased. At first, to prevent discomfort, it may be advisable to spread meals out over six feedings throughout the day. Those who are significantly underweight or are having trouble gaining weight may need tube feedings.

An electrocardiogram is essential for assessing palpitations or for evaluating changes consistent with hypokalemia. Prolongation of the QT interval contraindicates the use of tricyclic antidepressants and should lead to immediate medical intervention because it may increase the risk of ventricular tachycardia and sudden death. Gastric motility agents rarely relieve bloating sensations associated with refeeding. Stool softeners or bulk laxatives can help to alleviate the severe constipation associated with long-term use of stimulant laxatives or their withdrawal. The use of estrogen supplementation usually is not necessary, but patients should receive vitamins, including calcium, at a dosage of 1,000–1,500 mg/day and a multivitamin to ensure that vitamin D intake is adequate (400 IU/day).

Psychotropic medication can be helpful, particularly to those with bulimic behaviors. Several classes of antidepressant medications have been shown to decrease binge eating and purging behaviors, but they have no specific role in treating anorexia nervosa. The selective serotonin reuptake inhibitor (SSRI) fluoxetine (60 mg/day) is the only medication approved by the U.S. Food and Drug Administration for the treatment of bulimia nervosa. Other SSRIs are routinely prescribed and may be as effective. Tricyclic antidepressants and monoamine oxidase inhibitors are probably effective as well in reducing binge and purge cycles, but they are not considered first-line agents. Bupropion is contraindicated because it can lower seizure threshold in eating disorder patients with electrolyte disturbances. Antidepressants appear effective in the short term and may reduce binge/purge cycles by up to 70%. Less is known about their long-term effectiveness, as most studies have been of short duration. One study suggests that patients who respond in the short term should be treated for a minimum of 6 months. Second-generation antipsychotics (e.g., olanzapine) have been used in patients with anorexia nervosa and may promote weight gain and reduce cognitive distortions. Other drug therapies (e.g., mood stabilizers, antidepressants, anxiolytics) are indicated when the eating disorder is accompanied by psychosis, major depression, bipolar disorder, or an anxiety disorder.

Many patients with eating disorders will not seek treatment on their own and will deny their illness. They may resist treatment, and if hospitalized may leave against medical advice. For these reasons, the physician must use tact and skill to enlist the patient's cooperation. Once the patient is in treatment, the physician and patient should agree on a behavioral contract. The contract often becomes a focus of criticism, and the patient may make repeated requests of the physician to change it. The best approach is to stand firm with the contract so as to avoid repeated battles with the patient over additional changes that are sure to follow.

Individual psychotherapy should be practical and goal oriented. The therapy should focus on educating the patient about the illness, helping the patient to understand her or his symptoms, and explaining the need for treatment. Later, approaches that aim to promote insight can be used to help the patient resolve problems and conflicts that may have contributed to (or reinforced) the abnormal eating behavior. Family therapy is often helpful, especially when the patient is living at home and the disturbed eating behavior has been prompted by family interactions or when the disturbed eating behavior has created problems within the family. Intensive programs that emphasize a behavioral approach, such as nutritional education, cognitive restructuring techniques, and psychosocial support, seem to be the most effective.

Cognitive-behavioral therapy and interpersonal psychotherapy have both been shown to be effective in patients with bulimia nervosa. Cognitive-behavioral therapy has as its goal correcting inappropriate thoughts and beliefs that bulimic patients have about themselves and their disorder. With interpersonal psychotherapy, interpersonal sources of stress thought to precede or contribute to the person's disturbed eating behavior are addressed. Both therapies help to normalize eating behavior by reducing the number of binge/purge episodes. These therapies also are effective in patients with binge-eating disorder.

Clinical points for feeding and eating disorders

1. An empathic relationship should be encouraged. This goal may be hard to achieve because patients with anorexia can be oppositional and not sufficiently motivated to make the needed changes. Some will lack insight and refuse treatment.

2. The clinician should assess the patient carefully for psychiatric comorbidity.

   - The presence of psychiatric comorbidity complicates treatment and must be addressed. Eating disorder patients are highly likely to have comorbid major depression, anxiety disorders, substance abuse, or a personality disorder.

   - The presence of a personality disorder, particularly from Cluster B (e.g., borderline personality disorder), is common in bulimic persons and is associated with poor treatment outcome.

3. Clinicians should set a firm but nonpunitive behavioral contract with patients and have them sign it.

   - Reasonable targets for behavioral modification should be developed.

   - The goals should be set and changes avoided if possible.

4. Medication is of limited value in treating anorexia nervosa.

5. Medication is an important treatment adjunct in patients with bulimic behaviors.

   - SSRIs are the drugs of first choice; fluoxetine (20–60 mg/day) is the best researched, but others are likely to be effective as well (e.g., sertraline, 50–200 mg/day; paroxetine, 20–60 mg/day; escitalopram, 10–20 mg/day).

   - Tricyclic antidepressants and monoamine oxidase inhibitors are effective but are considered second-line choices because of their potential side effects and dangerousness in overdose.

   - Bupropion should be avoided because of its tendency to lower the seizure threshold.

6. Family therapy can be especially helpful with patients who still live at home or whose behavior has created problems within the family. Marital therapy will be helpful to those whose eating disorder has disrupted their marriage.

■ Self-Assessment Questions

1. What are the feeding disorders and how do they overlap with the eating disorders?

2. How do bulimia nervosa and anorexia nervosa differ? How do they overlap?
3. How is binge-eating disorder defined?
4. What are the social and demographic characteristics of eating disorder patients? Is the prevalence of eating disorders increasing?
5. What are some of the physiological and psychological theories about the cause of anorexia nervosa?
6. Describe typical clinical symptoms in anorexia nervosa and bulimia nervosa.
7. What potential medical complications may result from anorexia nervosa? Bulimia nervosa?
8. What is the natural history of the eating disorders? Do people die from eating disorders?
9. What are the major goals in the treatment of eating disorders?
10. Which medications are used in treating eating disorder patients?

Chapter 12

Sleep-Wake Disorders

The woods are lovely, dark and deep.
But I have promises to keep,
And miles to go before I sleep...

Robert Frost

The purpose of sleep remains a mystery, yet it occupies about one-third of our lives and is essential to survival. Prolonged sleep deprivation impairs thermal balance and energy regulation, causes cognitive impairment, and can contribute to death. It is no wonder that sleep complaints are among the most common that people report to their physicians.

The maintenance of a normal sleep-wake cycle is an important component of successful adaptation across the life cycle because our circadian rhythms help regulate mood and enhance cognitive performance. Up to 50% of patients seen in primary care practices report sleeping problems. Examples include the overweight attorney whose wife reports that he snores loudly at night and is drowsy during the day; the executive who falls asleep during important meetings; and the youth who sleepwalks and injures himself by tripping over furniture.

DSM-5 lists 12 sleep-wake disorders and several residual categories (see Table 12–1). This classification has been influenced by the second edition of the *International Classification of Sleep Disorders* (ICSD-2), published by the American Academy of Sleep Medicine. While DSM-5 does not include as many sleep disorders, the current diagnoses are compatible with ICSD-2.

TABLE 12–1.   **DSM-5 sleep-wake disorders**

Insomnia disorder

Hypersomnolence disorder

Narcolepsy

Breathing-related sleep disorders

     Obstructive sleep apnea hypopnea

     Central sleep apnea

     Sleep-related hypoventilation

Circadian rhythm sleep-wake disorders

Parasomnias

     Non–rapid eye movement sleep arousal disorders

     Nightmare disorder

     Rapid eye movement sleep behavior disorder

Restless legs syndrome

Substance/medication-induced sleep disorder

Other specified insomnia disorder

Unspecified insomnia disorder

Other specified hypersomnolence disorder

Unspecified hypersomnolence disorder

Other specified sleep-wake disorder

Unspecified sleep-wake disorder

■ Normal Sleep and Sleep Architecture

The average healthy adult requires about 7.5 to 8.5 hours of sleep per night, although some persons require more and some less to feel sufficiently rested. Normal sleep is influenced by many factors. For example, young people tend to sleep more than elderly persons, whose total sleep time tends to be decreased. The longer a person has been awake, the more quickly he or she will fall asleep.

Sleep stages in adults are divided into rapid eye movement (REM) and non-REM (NREM) sleep. These sleep stages alternate in a cycle that lasts between 70 and 120 minutes. Generally, three to six NREM/REM cycles occur nightly. The first REM period lasts 5–10 minutes; during the night, REM periods become longer and closer together and show progressively greater density of REM.

The normal sleep stages in adults are as follows:

- *Stage 0* is a period of wakefulness with eyes closed that occurs just before sleep onset. Electroencephalographic (EEG) recording mainly shows sinusoidal alpha waves over the occiput, which have a frequency of 8–13 cycles per second and a fairly low amplitude (or voltage). Muscle tone is increased. Alpha activity decreases as drowsiness increases.
- *Stage 1* is called the sleep-onset stage, or drowsiness, because it provides a brief transition from wakefulness to sleep. Alpha activity diminishes to less than 50% of the EEG recording. There is a low-amplitude, mixed-frequency signal, composed mainly of beta and the slower theta (4–7 cycles per second) activity. Stage 1 accounts for about 5% of the total sleep period.
- *Stage 2* is dominated by theta activity and the appearance of sleep spindles and K complexes. *Sleep spindles* are brief bursts of rhythmic (12–14 cycles per second) waves with a duration of 500–1,500 msec. *K complexes* are sharp, negative, high-voltage EEG waves, followed by slower, positive activity, with a duration of 500 msec. They are thought to represent a central nervous system (CNS) response to internal stimuli; they also can be elicited during sleep with external stimuli (e.g., a loud noise). Stage 2 usually accounts for about 45%–55% of the total sleep time.
- *Stage 3* is *slow-wave or deep sleep* characterized by high-voltage delta wave activity having a frequency of 1–2 cycles per second. As in Stage 2, muscle tone is increased, but eye movements are absent. This stage comprises about 15%–20% of the total sleep time.
- *REM sleep* is characterized by an EEG recording similar to that seen in Stage 1, along with a burst of rapid conjugate eye movements and reduced muscle tone. REM periods occur in phasic bursts and are accompanied by respiratory and cardiac rate fluctuations as well as penile and clitoral engorgement. This stage constitutes 20%–25% of the total sleep period and is also known as *desynchronized sleep.*

A normal young adult goes from waking into a period of NREM sleep lasting approximately 90 minutes before the first REM period; this portion of NREM sleep is referred to as *REM latency.* Most adults will transition through the several NREM sleep stages before entering REM sleep. REM sleep constitutes about 25% of the total sleep time in young adults but can exceed 50% in newborns. Infants can enter REM sleep directly, as do adults with narcolepsy.

Transitions from wakefulness to sleep are regulated by neurophysiological systems and controlled by reciprocal inhibition. Nuclei in the pons regulate REM sleep, and the perilocus ceruleus inhibits motor activity. At a biochemical level, increased acetylcholine activity promotes REM sleep. In addition, REM sleep is associated with decreased activity of monoamine—mostly adrenergic—neurotransmitters, such as dopamine, norepinephrine, and serotonin. NREM sleep, on the other hand, is associated with decreased adrenergic and cholinergic activity and is controlled primarily by the ventrolateral preoptic area.

■ Assessment of Sleep

Patients with sleep complaints should receive a thorough evaluation of their medical, psychiatric, and sleep history (see Table 12–2). The medical history should include a careful review of drug and medication use. Patients should be asked to maintain a sleep log, in which they record their bedtime, sleep latency (estimated time required to fall asleep), awake time, number of awakenings, daytime naps, and use of drugs or medications. Interviewing the patient's bed partner to learn about the presence of snoring, breathing difficulties, or leg jerks can be helpful.

Polysomnography is the principal diagnostic tool in sleep medicine and is a procedure in which electroencephalographic, electrooculographic, and electromyographic tracings are recorded during sleep. In fact, test results are critical to the assessment of several disorders, including narcolepsy, breathing-related sleep disorders, and rapid eye movement sleep behavior disorder. Polysomnography provides data on sleep continuity, sleep architecture, REM physiology, sleep-related breathing impairment, oxygen desaturation, cardiac arrhythmias, and periodic movements.

Another common laboratory procedure is the Multiple Sleep Latency Test (MSLT), which is used to measure excessive sleepiness. With the MSLT, the patient is given an opportunity to fall asleep in a darkened room for five 20-minute periods in 2-hour intervals across the patient's usual period of wakefulness. The average latency to sleep onset, assessed with polysomnography, is a measure of the tendency to fall asleep. An average sleep latency of less than 5 minutes indicates the presence of excessive sleepiness.

While many commonly encountered sleep complaints can be assessed and treated by nonspecialists, patients who have complicated sleep disorders, or who require specialized laboratory tests, should be referred to a sleep disorders clinic.

TABLE 12–2. Sleep history outline

Obtain data from patient, chart, and nursing staff. Review medication history, including illicit drugs, alcohol, and use of hypnotic medication. Obtain information on the following sleep characteristics:

- Usual sleep pattern
- Characteristics of disturbed sleep (for insomnia, difficulty falling asleep, difficulty staying asleep, or early-morning awakenings)
- The clinical course: onset, duration, frequency, severity, and precipitating and relieving factors
- 24-hour sleep-wake cycle (corroborate with staff and chart)
- History of sleep disturbances, including childhood sleep pattern and pattern of sleep when under stress
- Family history of sleep disorders
- Personal history of other sleep disorders
- Sleep pattern at home as described by bed partner
- Consumption of alcoholic beverages; over-the-counter caffeine tablets; coffee, tea, cola, and chocolate; herbals such as kava, which may be stimulating
- Use of prescription and over-the-counter medications

■ Insomnia Disorder

Insomnia disorder is characterized by difficulty initiating or maintaining sleep, or early morning awakening with an inability to return to sleep; the sleep difficulty occurs at least 3 nights a week for 3 months and is not due to another sleep disorder or the effects of a substance. It is not adequately explained by coexisting mental disorders or medical conditions (Box 12–1).

Box 12–1.   DSM-5 Diagnostic Criteria for Insomnia Disorder

A. A predominant complaint of dissatisfaction with sleep quantity or quality, associated with one (or more) of the following symptoms:

   1. Difficulty initiating sleep. (In children, this may manifest as difficulty initiating sleep without caregiver intervention.)
   2. Difficulty maintaining sleep, characterized by frequent awakenings or problems returning to sleep after awakenings. (In children, this may manifest as difficulty returning to sleep without caregiver intervention.)
   3. Early-morning awakening with inability to return to sleep.

B. The sleep disturbance causes clinically significant distress or impairment in social, occupational, educational, academic, behavioral, or other important areas of functioning.

C. The sleep difficulty occurs at least 3 nights per week.

D. The sleep difficulty is present for at least 3 months.

E. The sleep difficulty occurs despite adequate opportunity for sleep.

F. The insomnia is not better explained by and does not occur exclusively during the course of another sleep-wake disorder (e.g., narcolepsy, a breathing-related sleep disorder, a circadian rhythm sleep-wake disorder, a parasomnia).

G. The insomnia is not attributable to the physiological effects of a substance (e.g., a drug of abuse, a medication).

H. Coexisting mental disorders and medical conditions do not adequately explain the predominant complaint of insomnia.

Specify if:

With non–sleep disorder mental comorbidity, including substance use disorders
With other medical comorbidity
With other sleep disorder

Specify if:

Episodic: Symptoms last at least 1 month but less than 3 months.
Persistent: Symptoms last 3 months or longer.
Recurrent: Two (or more) episodes within the space of 1 year.

Note: Acute and short-term insomnia (i.e., symptoms lasting less than 3 months but otherwise meeting all criteria with regard to frequency, intensity, distress, and/or impairment) should be coded as an other specified insomnia disorder.

A patient's report of poor or nonrefreshing sleep may not accurately reflect the magnitude of any objective sleep disturbances that are present. The objective evidence is often relatively minor because subjective estimates of sleep latency and total sleep time tend to exaggerate the degree of any disturbance present.

Insomnia is a relatively common complaint in the general population and is even more common among psychiatric patients, although relatively few sufferers consult a physician. Insomnia occurs more frequently among the elderly, in women, among individuals with limited education and lower income, and in those with chronic (or multiple) medical problems.

The duration of insomnia is the most helpful factor in evaluating the patient's problem. Transient insomnia (no more than a few nights) typically occurs in people who usually sleep normally. This form of insomnia occurs at times of psychological stress, such as following the death of a loved one. Other situations associated with transient insomnia include a hospital admission, a public speaking engagement, or (for students) a scheduled examination. In these situations, the insomnia is rarely brought to medical attention because it is not seen as pathological and tends to self-correct.

"Sleep hygiene" measures have been developed for patients with chronic insomnia. These measures include the following:

- Waking up and going to bed at the same time every day, even on weekends
- Avoiding long periods of wakefulness in bed
- Not using the bed as a place to read, watch television, or work
- Leaving the bed and not returning until drowsy if sleep does not begin within a set period (e.g., 20–30 minutes)
- Avoiding napping
- Exercising at least three or four times a week (but not in the evening if this interferes with sleep)
- Discontinuing or reducing the consumption of alcoholic beverages, beverages containing caffeine, cigarettes, and sedative-hypnotic and anxiolytic drugs

Although these measures will be sufficient for many patients in improving their sleep quality, others will benefit from hypnotic medications (i.e., sleeping pills). While they may not cure insomnia, for many they can provide dramatic temporary relief. Hypnotics should be used mainly to treat transient and short-term insomnia, in combination with appropriate sleep hygiene. Long-term benefits are difficult to document, and these medications can be habit-forming. Traditionally, the benzodiazepines have been the first choice for reasons of safety and efficacy. Tolerance to their sleep-promoting effects appears to develop less often than it does with barbiturates, barbiturate-like compounds, and antihistamines. Several nonbenzodiazepine alternatives are available, such as zolpidem and eszopiclone. Compared with the benzodiazepines, these medications have less abuse potential, produce little tolerance, and tend not to cause daytime somnolence. Both benzodiazepine and nonbenzodiazepine hypnotics are listed in Table 12–3.

TABLE 12–3.   Medications used to treat insomnia

Drug (trade name)	Onset	Half-life, h	Dosage range, mg
Benzodiazepines			
Estazolam (ProSom)	Very fast	10–24	1–2
Flurazepam (Dalmane)	Very fast	50–100	15–30
Quazepam (Doral)	Very fast	15–35	7.5–15
Temazepam (Restoril)	Moderate	8–18	15–30
Triazolam (Halcion)	Very fast	2–3	0.125–0.5
Nonbenzodiazepines			
Eszopiclone (Lunesta)	Very fast	6	1–3
Ramelteon (Rozerem)	Very fast	1–3	8
Zaleplon (Sonata)	Very fast	1	5–20
Zolpidem (Ambien)	Very fast	2–3	5–10

Other drugs frequently used as sleeping aids include chloral hydrate (500–2,000 mg), a nonbarbiturate sedative-hypnotic known more for the fact that it is markedly potentiated by alcohol; the antihistamines diphenhydramine (25–100 mg) and doxylamine (25–100 mg), which are often used as hypnotic agents but are not as potent as the benzodiazepines; and the sedating antidepressant trazodone (50–200 mg), which appears to be effective. An alternative is a low-dose form of the tricyclic antidepressant doxepin (Silenor), which has recently gained U.S. Food and Drug Administration (FDA) approval for the treatment of insomnia characterized by difficulty with sleep maintenance.

■ Hypersomnolence Disorder

Excessive daytime somnolence affects about 5% of the adult population. With hypersomnolence disorder, the excessive sleepiness occurs at least 3 times a week for 3 months, as evidenced by prolonged sleep episodes, daytime sleep episodes, or difficulty being fully awake after abrupt awakening; the excessive sleepiness causes significant impairment or distress; and the excessive sleepiness is not accounted for by another sleep disorder, a medical condition or mental disorder, or the effects of a substance (Box 12–2).

Box 12–2.   DSM-5 Diagnostic Criteria for Hypersomnolence Disorder

---

A. Self-reported excessive sleepiness (hypersomnolence) despite a main sleep period lasting at least 7 hours, with at least one of the following symptoms:

   1. Recurrent periods of sleep or lapses into sleep within the same day.
   2. A prolonged main sleep episode of more than 9 hours per day that is nonrestorative (i.e., unrefreshing).
   3. Difficulty being fully awake after abrupt awakening.

B. The hypersomnolence occurs at least three times per week, for at least 3 months.

C. The hypersomnolence is accompanied by significant distress or impairment in cognitive, social, occupational, or other important areas of functioning.

D. The hypersomnolence is not better explained by and does not occur exclusively during the course of another sleep disorder (e.g., narcolepsy, breathing-related sleep disorder, circadian rhythm sleep-wake disorder, or a parasomnia).

E. The hypersomnolence is not attributable to the physiological effects of a substance (e.g., a drug of abuse, a medication).

F. Coexisting mental and medical disorders do not adequately explain the predominant complaint of hypersomnolence.

Specify if:

   With mental disorder, including substance use disorders
   With medical condition
   With another sleep disorder

Specify if:

   Acute: Duration of less than 1 month.
   Subacute: Duration of 1–3 months.
   Persistent: Duration of more than 3 months.

Specify current severity:

Specify severity based on degree of difficulty maintaining daytime alertness as manifested by the occurrence of multiple attacks of irresistible sleepiness within any given day occurring, for example, while sedentary, driving, visiting with friends, or working.

   Mild: Difficulty maintaining daytime alertness 1–2 days/week.
   Moderate: Difficulty maintaining daytime alertness 3–4 days/week.
   Severe: Difficulty maintaining daytime alertness 5–7 days/week.

Hypersomnolence disorder usually involves prolonged nocturnal sleep and continual daytime drowsiness. Nearly one-half of the patients report *sleep drunkenness* (i.e., excessive grogginess) on awakening, which may last several hours. Patients may report taking one or two naps daily (which can each last more than an hour), unlike the short naps typical of narcoleptic patients.

Polysomnographic studies have shown diminished delta sleep, increased number of awakenings, and reduced REM latency in patients with primary hypersomnia. The MSLT, described earlier, is used to document the short sleep latency. Hypersomnolence disorder is considered a diagnosis of exclusion, and other more specific disorders should be ruled out, such as narcolepsy or a breathing-related sleep disorder.

Treatment of hypersomnolence disorder involves a combination of sleep hygiene measures, stimulant drugs, and naps for some patients. Stimulants can help maintain wakefulness; both dextroamphetamine and methylphenidate have relatively short half-lives and are taken in multiple divided doses. Modafinil, which is used to treat narcolepsy (see section below), can be used to treat hypersomnolence disorder. Because stimulants have abuse potential, their use should be carefully monitored.

The following case describes a patient with hypersomnolence disorder treated in our clinic:

Chris, a 24-year-old college student, was being treated for obsessive-compulsive disorder (OCD) consisting mainly of intrusive and unwanted thoughts of harming others. His symptoms were well controlled with paroxetine, a serotonin reuptake inhibitor.

His mother, who usually accompanied him to the clinic, felt that his excessive sleeping and napping were even more of a problem than his OCD. She described how Chris would sleep 12–14 hours nightly and take afternoon naps. Chris admitted that he was frequently late for class and often fell asleep in class. He complained that he was too sleepy to study in the evening. All of these symptoms predated his treatment for OCD.

Chris was referred to a sleep disorders clinic; his polysomnography was unremarkable. Because there was no evidence of sleep attacks, cataplexy, sleep paralysis, or hypnagogic hallucinations, he received a diagnosis of primary hypersomnia and began treatment with methylphenidate. On this regimen, Chris was able to remain awake and alert during the day without napping. He was more alert in class, and his academic performance improved.

■ Narcolepsy

Narcolepsy is characterized by recurrent episodes of an irrepressible need to sleep. These sleep attacks occur with one or more of the following: episodes of cateplexy, cerebrospinal fluid hypocretin deficiency, nocturnal polysomnography showing a REM latency of 15 minutes or less, or MSLT showing a mean sleep latency of 8 minutes or less (Box 12–3).

Box 12–3.   DSM-5 Diagnostic Criteria for Narcolepsy

A. Recurrent periods of an irrepressible need to sleep, lapsing into sleep, or napping occurring within the same day. These must have been occurring at least three times per week over the past 3 months.

B. The presence of at least one of the following:

  1. Episodes of cataplexy, defined as either (a) or (b), occurring at least a few times per month:

    a. In individuals with long-standing disease, brief (seconds to minutes) episodes of sudden bilateral loss of muscle tone with maintained consciousness that are precipitated by laughter or joking.

    b. In children or in individuals within 6 months of onset, spontaneous grimaces or jaw-opening episodes with tongue thrusting or a global hypotonia, without any obvious emotional triggers.

  2. Hypocretin deficiency, as measured using cerebrospinal fluid (CSF) hypocretin-1 immunoreactivity values (less than or equal to one-third of values obtained in healthy subjects tested using the same assay, or less than or equal to 110 pg/mL). Low CSF levels of hypocretin-1 must not be observed in the context of acute brain injury, inflammation, or infection.

  3. Nocturnal sleep polysomnography showing rapid eye movement (REM) sleep latency less than or equal to 15 minutes, or a multiple sleep latency test showing a mean sleep latency less than or equal to 8 minutes and two or more sleep-onset REM periods.

Specify whether:

Narcolepsy without cataplexy but with hypocretin deficiency: Criterion B requirements of low CSF hypocretin-1 levels and positive polysomnography/multiple sleep latency test are met, but no cataplexy is present (Criterion B1 not met).

Narcolepsy with cataplexy but without hypocretin deficiency: In this rare subtype (less than 5% of narcolepsy cases), Criterion B requirements of cataplexy and positive polysomnography/multiple sleep latency test are met, but CSF hypocretin-1 levels are normal (Criterion B2 not met).

Autosomal dominant cerebellar ataxia, deafness, and narcolepsy:
This subtype is caused by exon 21 DNA (cytosine-5)-methyltransferase-1 mutations and is characterized by late-onset (age 30–40 years) narcolepsy (with low or intermediate CSF hypocretin-1 levels), deafness, cerebellar ataxia, and eventually dementia.

Autosomal dominant narcolepsy, obesity, and type 2 diabetes:
Narcolepsy, obesity, and type 2 diabetes and low CSF hypocretin-1 levels have been described in rare cases and are associated with a mutation in the myelin oligodendrocyte glycoprotein gene.

Narcolepsy secondary to another medical condition: This subtype is for narcolepsy that develops secondary to medical conditions that cause infectious (e.g., Whipple's disease, sarcoidosis), traumatic, or tumoral destruction of hypocretin neurons.

Specify current severity:

Mild: Infrequent cataplexy (less than once per week), need for naps only once or twice per day, and less disturbed nocturnal sleep.

Moderate: Cataplexy once daily or every few days, disturbed nocturnal sleep, and need for multiple naps daily.

Severe: Drug-resistant cataplexy with multiple attacks daily, nearly constant sleepiness, and disturbed nocturnal sleep (i.e., movements, insomnia, and vivid dreaming).

Narcolepsy affects about 1 in 2,000 persons; men and women are equally likely to develop narcolepsy. Narcolepsy may have a hereditary basis, for up to one-half of narcoleptic patients have a first-degree relative with the disorder.

Narcolepsy is one of the few DSM-5 disorders in which a biological mechanism has been identified and has been included in the criteria set. Narcolepsy nearly always results from the loss of hypothalamic hypocretin-producing cells, causing cerebrospinal fluid hypocretin-1 deficiency (less than or equal to one-third of control values, or 110 pg/mL in most laboratories). Hypocretin is a neurotransmitter that regulates arousal, wakefulness, and appetite.

Sleep attacks are the most striking feature of narcolepsy; these can last from seconds to 30 minutes or longer. Narcoleptic patients can experience sleep attacks at work, during conversations, or under other circumstances normally considered stimulating. Attacks may also occur while the person is engaged in sedentary and monotonous activities, such as watching television or using the computer.

Cateplexy is the presence of sudden bilateral loss of muscle tone precipitated by laughter or joking, or by spontaneous grimaces or jaw-opening episodes without an emotional trigger. About 70% of narcoleptic patients experience cataplexy.

A careful sleep history is helpful in making the diagnosis of narcolepsy, as are descriptions provided by parents, spouses, and bed partners. The diagnosis is relatively easy to make when auxiliary symptoms such as cataplexy are present. Polysomnography allows the clinician to rule out other sleep disorders such as a breathing-related sleep disorder (sleep apnea). People with narcolepsy tend to enter REM sleep quickly rather than after the more typical 90–120 minutes and during daytime naps. People with narcolepsy often develop psychological problems, most likely as a consequence of the adverse effects of the disorder on their family lives, job situations, and social interactions; these problems should be explored with the patient.

The clinical management of narcolepsy involves different treatments for the sleep attacks and the auxiliary symptoms. Stimulants are the preferred drugs for treating sleep attacks because of their rapid onset and relative lack of side effects. Methylphenidate is prescribed in multiple divided doses starting with 5 mg; the dosage may be gradually increased to a total of 60 mg/day. Dextroamphetamine can be prescribed in similar dosages. Modafinil (200–400 mg/day) is an effective alternative to the stimulants and is FDA approved. It is well tolerated and has minimal cardiovascular effects.

Sodium oxybate is FDA approved for the treatment of cataplexy associated with narcolepsy and has been shown to reduce the frequency of cataplexy episodes. The drug is administered as an oral solution in divided doses at bedtime and 2½–4 hours later in dosages ranging from 6 to 9 g/day. Because it is a CNS depressant, it can be dangerous if mixed with alcohol or other CNS depressants. Tricyclic antidepressants are sometimes used to treat cataplexy or sleep paralysis but have little effect on sleep attacks.

The physician should explain the nature of narcolepsy to the patient and his or her family. Social acquaintances and employers also may need education to understand that the disorder's symptoms are outside the patient's volitional control. The cooperation of an employer can be enormously helpful because one or two brief daily naps may reduce job difficulties and help lower the dosage requirement for stimulant medication. Patients should be warned about the potential danger of having a sleep attack while driving or engaging in activities requiring constant alertness.

■ Breathing-Related Sleep Disorders

Disturbed breathing mechanisms can disrupt sleep and lead to potentially serious medical, social, and psychological consequences. DSM-5 provides specific diagnostic criteria for a spectrum of breathing-related sleep disorders: obstructive sleep apnea hypopnea syndrome, central sleep apnea, and sleep-related hypoventilation. Although these disorders may share common underlying physiological risk factors (i.e., respiratory control instability), physiological and anatomical studies indicate differences in the pathogeneses of these disorders. Central sleep apnea is less dependent on structural airway abnormalities as compared to obstructive sleep apnea, which is more dependent on increased upper airway resistance. Sleep-related hypoventilation is often comorbid with other disorders that depress ventilation.

Obstructive Sleep Apnea Hypopnea

Obstructive sleep apnea hypopnea is the most common category of breathing-related sleep disorders. It is potentially serious because breathing repeatedly stops and starts during sleep. A pause in breathing is called an *apnea* episode. A decrease in airflow during breathing is called a *hypopnea* episode. Most people have brief apnea episodes during sleep, but the person with obstructive sleep apnea is rarely aware of having difficulty breathing, even upon awakening. When the muscles relax, a person's airway narrows or closes as he or she breathes in, and breathing may be inadequate for 10–20 seconds, lowering the level of blood oxygen. The brain senses this impaired breathing and briefly rouses the person from sleep.

Snoring is the most noticeable sign of obstructive sleep apnea. This is recognized as a problem by others witnessing the individual during sleep or is suspected by the person because of its effects on the body. Because the muscle tone of the body ordinarily relaxes during sleep, and the airway at the throat is composed of walls of soft tissue, which can collapse, it is not surprising that breathing can be obstructed during sleep. A minor degree of obstructive sleep apnea is considered to be within the bounds of normal sleep, and many individuals experience episodes of obstructive sleep apnea at some point during their life, but some are afflicted with chronic, severe obstructive sleep apnea.

Obstructive sleep apnea hypopnea (see Box 12–4) most commonly affects middle-aged and older adults and people who are overweight. Common signs and symptoms include excessive daytime sleepiness, loud snoring, observed episodes of breathing cessation during sleep, abrupt awakenings accompanied by shortness of breath, awakening with a dry mouth or sore throat, morning headache, difficulty staying asleep, and difficult-to-control high blood pressure. Disrupted breathing impairs the ability to achieve deep, restful sleep, resulting in the person feeling sleepy during waking hours. Importantly, snoring and daytime sleepiness may not be obvious because many patients with obstructive sleep apnea are not subjectively sleepy and may not snore. For instance, women may present with insomnia and fatigue.

Box 12–4.   DSM-5 Diagnostic Criteria for Obstructive Sleep Apnea Hypopnea

---

A. Either (1) or (2):

 1. Evidence by polysomnography of at least five obstructive apneas or hypopneas per hour of sleep and either of the following sleep symptoms:

    a. Nocturnal breathing disturbances: snoring, snorting/gasping, or breathing pauses during sleep.

    b. Daytime sleepiness, fatigue, or unrefreshing sleep despite sufficient opportunities to sleep that is not better explained by another mental disorder (including a sleep disorder) and is not attributable to another medical condition.

 2. Evidence by polysomnography of 15 or more obstructive apneas and/or hypopneas per hour of sleep regardless of accompanying symptoms.

Specify current severity:

 Mild: Apnea hypopnea index is less than 15.

 Moderate: Apnea hypopnea index is 15–30.

 Severe: Apnea hypopnea index is greater than 30.

Serious psychological consequences can include a general slowing of thought processes, memory impairment, and inattention. Patients often report anxiety, dysphoric mood, or multiple physical complaints.

A thorough medical assessment is necessary and may include a sleep laboratory evaluation with recording of respiration and monitoring of nocturnal oxygen desaturation. Initial treatment measures include weight loss, avoidance of sedative-hypnotics, and sleep position training (to encourage patients to avoid the supine position during sleep). In mild cases, some patients can be managed with custom made oral appliances that help keep the airway open.

Continuous positive airway pressure (CPAP) is the most widely used treatment. Room air is blown into the nose through a nasal mask or cushioned cannulae. Some patients do not tolerate CPAP well, but compliance can be enhanced by careful follow-up. Uvulopalatopharyngoplasty is a surgical alternative for patients with redundant oropharyngeal tissue. Tracheostomy is reserved for life-threatening situations in patients whose condition does not respond to CPAP or uvulopalatopharyngoplasty.

Central Sleep Apnea

Central sleep apnea is characterized by repeated episodes of apneas and hypopneas during sleep caused by variability in respiratory effort (see Box 12–5). These occur because the brain fails to send proper signals to the muscles that control breathing; in contrast, in obstructive sleep apnea hypopnea, a person cannot breathe normally because of upper airway obstruction.

Box 12–5.   DSM-5 Diagnostic Criteria for Central Sleep Apnea

A. Evidence by polysomnography of five or more central apneas per hour of sleep.
B. The disorder is not better explained by another current sleep disorder.

Specify whether:

Idiopathic central sleep apnea: Characterized by repeated episodes of apneas and hypopneas during sleep caused by variability in respiratory effort but without evidence of airway obstruction.

Cheyne-Stokes breathing: A pattern of periodic crescendo-decrescendo variation in tidal volume that results in central apneas and hypopneas at a frequency of at least five events per hour, accompanied by frequent arousal.

Central sleep apnea comorbid with opioid use: The pathogenesis of this subtype is attributed to the effects of opioids on the respiratory rhythm generators in the medulla as well as the differential effects on hypoxic versus hypercapnic respiratory drive.

Note: See the section "Diagnostic Features" in [DSM-5] text.

Specify current severity:

Severity of central sleep apnea is graded according to the frequency of the breathing disturbances as well as the extent of associated oxygen desaturation and sleep fragmentation that occur as a consequence of repetitive respiratory disturbances.

Central sleep apnea is a less common condition, accounting for fewer than 5% of sleep apnea cases. Common signs and symptoms of central sleep apnea are essentially the same as those seen in obstructive sleep apnea, described above. Although snoring indicates some degree of increased obstruction to airflow, snoring is not uncommon in people with central sleep apnea. Central sleep apnea is associated with several conditions, including heart failure and chronic opioid use. Importantly, central and obstructive sleep apneas may coexist (i.e., *complex sleep apnea*).

There are two main subtypes. *Idiopathic central sleep apnea* is characterized by sleepiness, insomnia, and awakenings due to dyspnea in association with five or more central apneas per hour of sleep. Central sleep apnea occurring in individuals with heart failure, stroke, or renal failure typically have a breathing pattern called *Cheyne-Stokes breathing,* which is characterized by a pattern of periodic crescendo-decrescendo variation in tidal volume that results in central apneas and hypopneas occurring at a frequency of at least five events per hour that are accompanied by frequent arousals.

The treatment of central sleep apnea is similar to that for obstructive sleep apnea. In some cases, medication (acetazolamide, theophylline) can be prescribed to stimulate breathing.

Sleep-Related Hypoventilation

Sleep-related hypoventilation is the result of a decreased response to high carbon dioxide during sleep and is characterized by frequent episodes of shallow breathing lasting longer than 10 seconds during sleep (see Box 12–6). Polysomnography shows episodes of decreased respiration associated with elevated carbon dioxide levels. Sleep-related hypoventilation is frequently associated with lung disease or neuromuscular or chest wall disorders.

Box 12–6.   DSM-5 Diagnostic Criteria for Sleep-Related
               Hypoventilation

A. Polysomnograpy demonstrates episodes of decreased respiration associated with elevated CO_2 levels. (**Note:** In the absence of objective measurement of CO_2, persistent low levels of hemoglobin oxygen saturation unassociated with apneic/hypopneic events may indicate hypoventilation.)

B. The disturbance is not better explained by another current sleep disorder.

Specify whether:

Idiopathic hypoventilation: This subtype is not attributable to any readily identified condition.

Congenital central alveolar hypoventilation: This subtype is a rare congenital disorder in which the individual typically presents in the perinatal period with shallow breathing, or cyanosis and apnea during sleep.

Comorbid sleep-related hypoventilation: This subtype occurs as a consequence of a medical condition, such as a pulmonary disorder (e.g., interstitial lung disease, chronic obstructive pulmonary disease) or a neuromuscular or chest wall disorder (e.g., muscular dystrophies, postpolio syndrome, cervical spinal cord injury, kyphoscoliosis), or medications (e.g., benzodiazepines, opiates). It also occurs with obesity (obesity hypoventilation disorder), where it reflects a combination of increased work of breathing due to reduced chest wall compliance and ventilation-perfusion mismatch and variably reduced ventilatory drive. Such individuals usually are characterized by body mass index of greater than 30 and hypercapnia during wakefulness (with a pCO_2 of greater than 45), without other evidence of hypoventilation.

Specify current severity:
Severity is graded according to the degree of hypoxemia and hypercarbia present during sleep and evidence of end organ impairment due to these abnormalities (e.g., right-sided heart failure). The presence of blood gas abnormalities during wakefulness is an indicator of greater severity.

Individuals with sleep-related hypoventilation present with complaints of insomnia or excessive sleepiness; feeling breathless when lying down (orthopnea); and having headaches upon awakening. During sleep, episodes of shallow breathing can be observed, and obstructive sleep apnea hypopnea or central sleep apnea may coexist. Consequences of ventilatory insufficiency, including pulmonary hypertension, cor pulmonale (right heart failure), polycythemia, and neurocognitive dysfunction, can be present. With progression of ventilatory insufficiency, blood gas abnormalities extend into wakefulness. Features of the medical condition causing sleep-related hypoventilation can also be present. Idiopathic sleep-related hypoventilation is a slowly progressive disorder of respiratory impairment. When comorbid with other disorders (e.g., chronic obstructive pulmonary disease, neuromuscular disorders, obesity), disease severity reflects the severity of the underlying condition.

The treatment of hypoventilation is directed at correcting the underlying disorder. For example, bronchodilators (e.g., albuterol, salmeterol) can be helpful in treating patients with obstructive lung disease. Theophylline may improve diaphragm muscle contractility and stimulate the respiratory center. Patients should refrain from using known respiratory depressants (e.g., alcohol, benzodiazepines). Some patients will need ventilatory assistance, including endotracheal intubation with mechanical ventilation or noninvasive bilevel positive-pressure ventilation. Weight loss should be encouraged in those who are overweight, since even modest loss improves minute ventilation; in refractory cases, bariatric surgery should be considered.

■ Circadian Rhythm Sleep-Wake Disorders

Circadian rhythm sleep-wake disorders are persistent or recurring patterns of sleep disruption that result from an altered sleep-wake schedule, or occur when the sleep-wake cycle is not correctly synchronized with a person's daily schedule. People with circadian rhythm sleep-wake disorders are generally able to get enough sleep if allowed to sleep and wake at the times dictated by their body clocks; sleep is usually of normal quality. (See Box 12–7 for the DSM-5 criteria.)

Box 12–7.   DSM-5 Diagnostic Criteria for Circadian Rhythm Sleep-Wake Disorders

---

A. A persistent or recurrent pattern of sleep disruption that is primarily due to an alteration of the circadian system or to a misalignment between the endogenous circadian rhythm and the sleep–wake schedule required by an individual's physical environment or social or professional schedule.
B. The sleep disruption leads to excessive sleepiness or insomnia, or both.
C. The sleep disturbance causes clinically significant distress or impairment in social, occupational, and other important areas of functioning.

Specify whether:

Delayed sleep phase type: A pattern of delayed sleep onset and awakening times, with an inability to fall asleep and awaken at a desired or conventionally acceptable earlier time.

> *Specify* if:
>
> **Familial:** A family history of delayed sleep phase is present.
>
> *Specify* if:
>
> **Overlapping with non-24-hour sleep-wake type:** Delayed sleep phase type may overlap with another circadian rhythm sleep-wake disorder, non-24-hour sleep-wake type.

Advanced sleep phase type: A pattern of advanced sleep onset and awakening times, with an inability to remain awake or asleep until the desired or conventionally acceptable later sleep or wake times.

> *Specify* if:
>
> **Familial:** A family history of advanced sleep phase is present.

Irregular sleep-wake type: A temporally disorganized sleep-wake pattern, such that the timing of sleep and wake periods is variable throughout the 24-hour period.

Non-24-hour sleep-wake type: A pattern of sleep-wake cycles that is not synchronized to the 24-hour environment, with a consistent daily drift (usually to later and later times) of sleep onset and wake times.

Shift work type: Insomnia during the major sleep period and/or excessive sleepiness (including inadvertent sleep) during the major awake period associated with a shift work schedule (i.e., requiring unconventional work hours).

Unspecified type

Specify if:

Episodic: Symptoms last at least 1 month but less than 3 months.

Persistent: Symptoms last 3 months or longer.

Recurrent: Two or more episodes occur within the space of 1 year.

Our body clocks (i.e., circadian cycles) are tightly linked to core body temperature, genetics, and light exposure. In constant darkness, they typically follow a 24.2-hour cycle, but they are reset to a 24-hour period by morning light exposure. For this reason, people sleep best by initiating sleep when "sleep debt"—which increases linearly while one is awake—is high and the alerting system starts to wane. We wake spontaneously when sleep debt—lowered by sleep—intersects with the rising alerting system, about 2.5 hours after our lowest core body temperature. It is difficult to sleep on a rising core body temperature, a problem experienced by night shift workers who try to sleep during the day. It is almost impossible to initiate sleep during the few hours before our core body temperature begins to fall, when alerting systems are most active.

The *delayed sleep phase type* of the disorder arises primarily from a history of a delay in the timing of the major sleep period (usually more than 2 hours) in relation to the desired sleep and wakeup times, resulting in symptoms of insomnia and excessive sleepiness. Symptoms include sleep-onset insomnia, difficulty waking in the morning, and excessive early day sleepiness. People with this pattern are "night owls" who are most alert at night and have difficulty waking in the morning. On the other hand, individuals with the *advanced sleep phase type* are "morning people" who prefer the early morning; their circadian biomarkers, such as melatonin levels and core body temperature rhythms, are "set" 2–4 hours earlier than usual.

One method for correcting the delayed sleep phase type is to have the affected person delay his or her sleep time by 30 minutes to 3 hours on successive nights. Whether through various activities, coffee and other stimulants, sunlight, or strong artificial light, the goal is to delay sleep onset by almost 24 hours. Patients will eventually fall asleep at a conventional time, such as 11 P.M.

The *shift work type* of the disorder affects people with unconventional work hours that interfere with maintaining a normal sleep-wake schedule (e.g., night shift workers or people who frequently change their work shift, such as nurses). Shift workers tend to have high rates of on-the-job sleepiness, tend to make more cognitive errors, and have high rates of drug use and divorce. They may never feel fully rested. When they want to sleep, they cannot, and when they are expected to be awake and alert, they are sleepy and drowsy. Of course, the best way to avoid these problems is to forgo shift work, but this may not be possible for some workers. The drug armodafinil (Nuvigil), a stimulant, is FDA approved for use in people with excessive sleepiness attributed to "shift work disorder" to improve wakefulness.

A related condition is *jet lag*, which affects people who travel frequently and cross multiple time zones. While this is not considered a DSM-5 sleep disorder because it is typically transient, travelers find it annoying and troublesome. The best way to deal with jet lag is to maintain one's usual sleep hours in the new time zone. Conventional wisdom is that most adults require about 1 day to adjust for each eastward time zone crossed and slightly less after westward travel. Alcohol and other substances that interfere with sleep should be avoided, and short-term use of hypnotic agents (e.g., zolpidem, 5–10 mg) can help.

■ Parasomnias

Parasomnias are disorders characterized by abnormal behavioral, experiential, or physiological events occurring in association with sleep, specific sleep stages, or sleep-wake transitions. NREM sleep arousal disorders and REM sleep behavior disorder are the most common. They serve as a reminder that sleep and wakefulness are not mutually exclusive.

Non–Rapid Eye Movement Sleep Arousal Disorders

The conditions comprising the *non–rapid eye movement sleep arousal disorders*—sleepwalking and sleep terrors—represent variations of the simultaneous admixture of elements of both wakefulness and NREM sleep, thereby resulting in the appearance of complex motor behavior without conscious awareness (sometimes called "state dissociation") (see Box 12–8).

Box 12–8.　DSM-5 Diagnostic Criteria for Non–Rapid Eye Movement Sleep Arousal Disorders

A. Recurrent episodes of incomplete awakening from sleep, usually occurring during the first third of the major sleep episode, accompanied by either one of the following:

　1. **Sleepwalking:** Repeated episodes of rising from bed during sleep and walking about. While sleepwalking, the individual has a blank, staring face; is relatively unresponsive to the efforts of others to communicate with him or her; and can be awakened only with great difficulty.

　2. **Sleep terrors:** Recurrent episodes of abrupt terror arousals from sleep, usually beginning with a panicky scream. There is intense fear and signs of autonomic arousal, such as mydriasis, tachycardia, rapid breathing, and sweating, during each episode. There is relative unresponsiveness to efforts of others to comfort the individual during the episodes.

B. No or little (e.g., only a single visual scene) dream imagery is recalled.

C. Amnesia for the episodes is present.

D. The episodes cause clinically significant distress or impairment in social, occupational, or other important areas of functioning.

E. The disturbance is not attributable to the physiological effects of a substance (e.g., a drug of abuse, a medication).

F. Coexisting mental and medical disorders do not explain the episodes of sleepwalking or sleep terrors.

Specify whether:
Sleepwalking type
　Specify if:
With sleep-related eating
With sleep-related sexual behavior (sexsomnia)
Sleep terror type

Sleepwalking consists of repeated episodes of arising from sleep and walking about, usually occurring in the first third of the sleep episode. The person typically has a blank stare and is relatively unresponsive to the efforts of others to communicate; he or she can only be awakened with great difficulty. On awakening, the person has amnesia for the episode and is alert and oriented within minutes. Both sleepwalking and sleep terrors generally occur within 3 hours of falling asleep. Electroencephalographic recordings show high-amplitude slow waves preceding the muscular activation that triggers the attack; sleepwalking occurs during Stage 3 NREM sleep.

Sleepwalking episodes are usually brief (less than 10 minutes). People walk about without purpose and are indifferent to their environment. Sleepwalkers have the ability to maneuver around objects and perform simple tasks such as opening doors or windows, a fact that makes sleepwalking dangerous.

The disorder is more common in children than in adults. Nearly 15% of children have had at least one episode of sleepwalking, but most will outgrow the disorder by late adolescence. In adults, sleepwalking is frequently associated with the presence of a mental disorder, such as major depression. The onset of sleepwalking in adults with no prior history of sleepwalking in childhood should prompt a search for specific etiologies, such as a breathing-related sleep disorder, nocturnal seizures, or the effect of medication. From 2% to 4% of adults have a postchildhood history of sleepwalking.

Sleep terrors (also known as *night terrors*) are a sudden partial arousal from delta sleep associated with screaming and frantic motor activity. These episodes occur during the first third of the sleep episode and often begin with a terrifying scream followed by intense anxiety and signs of autonomic hyperarousal (e.g., rapid breathing). Persons with sleep terrors may not fully awaken after an episode and usually have no detailed recall of the event the following morning. Sleep terrors are relatively uncommon and affect less than 3% of children.

The cause of sleep terrors is unknown, but, like sleepwalking, they appear to be familial. Most cases resolve by late adolescence.

Benzodiazepines (e.g., clonazepam, diazepam) may help to alleviate sleepwalking or sleep terrors through their suppression of Stage 3 sleep. Relapse is likely when the drugs are discontinued or at times of stress. Tricyclic antidepressants, selective serotonin reuptake inhibitors (SSRIs), and melatonin have been used and may be effective, although there has been little research to support these treatments. Better sleep hygiene may help in milder cases.

The most important consideration in managing patients with sleepwalking or sleep terror episodes is protection from injury. Attempts to actively interrupt episodes should be avoided because intervention may confuse or frighten the patient. Precautions may include placing latches on bedroom windows, installing alarms on doors, and having the patient sleep on the first level of the home. The bedroom floor should be free of objects, and there should be nothing breakable within reach of the person.

Nightmare Disorder

Nightmare disorder consists of repeated extended, extremely dysphoric, and well-remembered dreams that usually involve efforts to avoid threats to survival, security, or physical integrity. The nightmares can be lengthy and elaborate, with dream imagery that seems real inciting anxiety, fear, or other negative emotions (see Box 12–9). These generally occur during the second half of the sleep period. On awakening, the individual rapidly becomes alert and oriented. Mild autonomic arousal, including sweating, tachycardia, and tachypnea, may characterize the nightmares, but body movements and vocalizations are not typical. This condition may affect up to 6% of the general population and can become chronic.

Box 12–9. DSM-5 Diagnostic Criteria for Nightmare Disorder

A. Repeated occurrences of extended, extremely dysphoric, and well-remembered dreams that usually involve efforts to avoid threats to survival, security, or physical integrity and that generally occur during the second half of the major sleep episode.

B. On awakening from the dysphoric dreams, the individual rapidly becomes oriented and alert.

C. The sleep disturbance causes clinically significant distress or impairment in social, occupational, or other important areas of functioning.

D. The nightmare symptoms are not attributable to the physiological effects of a substance (e.g., a drug of abuse, a medication).

E. Coexisting mental and medical disorders do not adequately explain the predominant complaint of dysphoric dreams.

Specify if:
During sleep onset

Specify if:
With associated non–sleep disorder, including substance use disorders
With associated other medical condition
With associated other sleep disorder

Specify if:
Acute: Duration of period of nightmares is 1 month or less.
Subacute: Duration of period of nightmares is greater than 1 month but less than 6 months.
Persistent: Duration of period of nightmares is 6 months or greater.

Specify current severity:
Severity can be rated by the frequency with which the nightmares occur:
Mild: Less than one episode per week on average.

Moderate: One or more episodes per week but less than nightly.
Severe: Episodes nightly.

Nightmares tend to occur during REM sleep. They may occur at any time during the night but are more frequent during the second half, when REM cycles are increased in frequency and duration. In childhood, nightmares are often related to specific developmental phases and are particularly common during the preschool and early school years. In that age group, children may be unable to distinguish reality from dream content.

Nightmares also have been associated with febrile illness and delirium, particularly in elderly and chronically ill persons. Withdrawal from certain drugs, such as the benzodiazepines, also may result in nightmares. The increase in REM sleep after withdrawal of barbiturates or alcohol may be associated with a temporary increase in the intensity of dreaming and nightmares. More recently, the use of selective serotonin reuptake inhibitors (e.g., paroxetine, sertraline) and their withdrawal have been linked to vivid dreams or nightmares.

The main differential diagnosis for nightmare disorder includes major psychiatric illnesses that could lead to nightmares (e.g., major depression), the effects of a medication, and withdrawal from a drug or alcohol. When the mental illness is diagnosed and treated, the nightmares may resolve. Nightmares related to psychologically traumatic events (e.g., motor vehicle accident, sexual assault) may resolve with short-term counseling or the judicious use of sedative-hypnotics.

Rapid Eye Movement Sleep Behavior Disorder

Rapid eye movement sleep behavior disorder is defined by the presence of arousal during sleep associated with vocalization and/or complex motor behaviors. It has the potential to cause dramatic and potentially violent or injurious behavior arising from REM sleep (see Box 12–10).

Box 12–10.   DSM-5 Diagnostic Criteria for Rapid Eye
              Movement Sleep Behavior Disorder

A. Repeated episodes of arousal during sleep associated with vocalization and/or complex motor behaviors.

B. These behaviors arise during rapid eye movement (REM) sleep and therefore usually occur more than 90 minutes after sleep onset, are more frequent during the later portions of the sleep period, and uncommonly occur during daytime naps.

C. Upon awakening from these episodes, the individual is completely awake, alert, and not confused or disoriented.

D. Either of the following:
   1. REM sleep without atonia on polysomnographic recording.
   2. A history suggestive of REM sleep behavior disorder and an established synucleinopathy diagnosis (e.g., Parkinson's disease, multiple system atrophy).

E. The behaviors cause clinically significant distress or impairment in social, occupational, or other important areas of functioning (which may include injury to self or the bed partner).

F. The disturbance is not attributable to the physiological effects of a substance (e.g., a drug of abuse, a medication) or another medical condition.

G. Coexisting mental and medical disorders do not explain the episodes.

These behaviors may reflect motor responses to the content of action-filled or violent dreams of being attacked or trying to escape from a threatening situation, termed *dream enacting behaviors.* The vocalizations are often loud, emotion-filled, and profane. These behaviors may be very bothersome to the individual and the bed partner and may result in significant injury (e.g., falling or jumping out of bed, running, punching, thrusting, hitting, or kicking). REM sleep behavior disorder is one of the most important causes of sleep-related injurious or violent behavior. Upon awakening, the individual is immediately alert and oriented and can usually recall the dream content.

There is a relationship between REM sleep behavior disorder and neurodegenerative disorders (particularly Parkinson's disease, dementia with Lewy bodies, and multiple system atrophy). At least 50% of individuals with REM sleep behavior disorder presenting in sleep clinics will eventually develop one of these conditions. REM sleep behavior disorder occurs in less than 1% of the general population but is more prevalent in psychiatric populations. Tricyclic antidepressants, SSRIs, serotonin-norepinephrine reuptake inhibitors, and beta-blockers have been associated with REM sleep behavior disorders, but it is not known whether the medications cause the disorder or simply unmask an underlying predisposition.

The diagnosis of REM sleep behavior disorder requires clinically significant distress or impairment; the physiological effects of a substance (e.g., a drug of abuse, a medication) or another medical condition must be ruled out as causing the disturbance, and coexisting mental or medical disorders also must have been ruled out as a cause.

Clonazepam can be an effective treatment, but symptoms promptly return if the medication is discontinued. At least in the short term, both the dreamer and the bed partner should be protected by having them sleep in different rooms.

■ Restless Legs Syndrome

Restless legs syndrome, new to DSM-5, is a sensorimotor, neurological sleep disorder characterized by a desire to move the legs, usually associated with uncomfortable sensations typically described as creeping, crawling, tingling, burning, or itching (Box 12–11). Symptoms are worse when the individual is at rest, and frequent movements of the legs occur in an effort to relieve the uncomfortable sensations. Symptoms are worse in the evening or night, and in some individuals occur only in the evening or night.

Box 12–11.   DSM-5 Diagnostic Criteria for Restless Legs Syndrome

---

A. An urge to move the legs, usually accompanied by or in response to uncomfortable and unpleasant sensations in the legs, characterized by all of the following:

1. The urge to move the legs begins or worsens during periods of rest or inactivity.
2. The urge to move the legs is partially or totally relieved by movement.
3. The urge to move the legs is worse in the evening or at night than during the day, or occurs only in the evening or at night.

B. The symptoms in Criterion A occur at least three times per week and have persisted for at least 3 months.

C. The symptoms in Criterion A are accompanied by significant distress or impairment in social, occupational, educational, academic, behavioral, or other important areas of functioning.

D. The symptoms in Criterion A are not attributable to another mental disorder or medical condition (e.g., arthritis, leg edema, peripheral ischemia, leg cramps) and are not better explained by a behavioral condition (e.g., positional discomfort, habitual foot tapping).

E. The symptoms are not attributable to the physiological effects of a drug of abuse or medication (e.g., akathisia).

Restless legs syndrome is classified as a sleep-wake disorder because it interferes with sleep and may be associated with periodic limb movements during sleep. The syndrome affects about 5% of the general population. Patients report that symptoms begin in the evening and are relieved by moving the legs or walking. The sensations can delay sleep or waken the person from sleep.

The differentiation of restless legs syndrome from other conditions is important because many people report some urge or need to move the legs while at rest and do not have the disorder. The most important mimics of restless legs syndrome are leg cramps, positional discomfort, arthralgias or arthritis, myalgias, positional ischemia (numbness), leg edema, peripheral neuropathy, radiculopathy, and habitual foot tapping. Muscle "knots" or cramps, relief with a single postural shift, limitation in joints, soreness to palpation, and other abnormalities on physical exam are not characteristic of the syndrome. Worsening at night and periodic limb movements are more common in restless legs syndrome than in medication-induced akathisia or peripheral neuropathy.

Dopamine agonists such as pramipexole (0.125–0.5 mg/day) or ropinirole (0.25–4.0 mg/day) may be effective in treating restless legs syndrome. Dosages should be carefully titrated to the desired clinical effect.

■ Substance/Medication-Induced Sleep Disorder

The essential feature of *substance/medication-induced sleep disorder* is a prominent sleep disturbance judged to be primarily associated with the known effects of a substance of abuse or a medication. These disturbances are relatively common in clinical settings but are not always straightforward, and they depend on several factors, including the type of substance (or medication), the individual's response to the agent, and the substance's pharmacology. For example, caffeine is one of the most common causes of disrupted sleep and needs to be ruled out as a cause in any investigation of insomnia. Depending on the substance, one of four types of sleep disturbance may be reported, including insomnia disorder type, daytime sleepiness type, parasomnia type, and a mixed type for cases in which more than one type of sleep disturbance is present and none predominates.

Clinical points for sleep-wake disorders

1. A thorough sleep history is essential for accurate diagnosis and includes the recording of

   • Drug use pattern.

   • Use of alcohol, caffeine, and stimulant drugs.

   • An interview with the patient's bed partner.

2. For patients with insomnia, the sleep hygiene measures outlined in this chapter are the simplest and most overlooked strategy.

3. Complaints of disturbed sleep should alert the clinician to the possibility of a major psychiatric illness. Major depression and alcohol use disorders are probably the most common causes of disturbed sleep.

4. Prescribing hypnotics for patients with sleep complaints is inappropriate without having first made a diagnosis. For insomnia disorder, patients should be told that the sleeping pills are for temporary use only (e.g., days to weeks).

5. Temazepam and estazolam have probably the best therapeutic properties for a benzodiazepine hypnotic: rapid absorption, lack of metabolites, and an intermediate half-life that will allow a full night's sleep. The nonbenzodiazepine hypnotics are excellent alternatives.

6. Some clinicians consider methylphenidate the drug of choice for patients with narcolepsy or hypersomnolence disorder. It should be titrated up to 60 mg/day. The clinician should keep track of pill use because some patients may be tempted to abuse this medication. Modafinil is an effective alternative.

   • Sodium oxybate is available to treat narcolepsy complicated by cataplexy, although its usefulness is compromised by an awkward administration schedule.

7. If patients have unusual sleep complaints or disorders, a referral should be made to a sleep disorders clinic for a more thorough evaluation, which may include polysomnography and the Multiple Sleep Latency Test.

■ Self-Assessment Questions

1. What are the major sleep disorders?
2. What are sleep hygiene measures?
3. What are the REM and NREM stages? What is their significance?
4. Describe the appropriate use of hypnotic agents. Which are preferred?
5. How is hypersomnia managed?

6. What is hypocretin and what is its relationship with narcolepsy?
7. Describe the circadian rhythm sleep-wake disorders. What controls circadian rhythm? What is a "night owl?" A "morning type?" What is jet lag?
8. Distinguish between nightmare disorder and sleep terrors.
9. Does sleepwalking have the same significance in a child that it does in an adult? Describe simple measures that can be taken to reduce the chance of injury in the sleepwalker.
10. What are "dream enacting behaviors"?
11. What is the restless legs syndrome and how is it treated?

Chapter 13

Sexual Dysfunction, Gender Dysphoria, and Paraphilias

Lolita, light of my life, fire of my loins. My sin, my soul. Lo-lee-ta.

Vladimir Nabokov, Lolita

This chapter reviews the sexual dysfunctions, gender dysphoria, and paraphilic disorders. In DSM-5, each of these classes of disorder has its own chapter, although they are grouped together here for convenience.

■ Sexual Dysfunctions

DSM-5 identifies seven specific sexual dysfunctions that interfere with sexual interest, arousal, or functioning. In addition, there is a category for disorders that result from the effects of a substance or medication, *substance/medication-induced sexual dysfunction.* Two residual categories, *other specified sexual dysfunction* and *unspecified sexual dysfunction,* are available for sexual dysfunctions that do not meet the criteria for a more specific disorder, or when there is insufficient information to make a more specific diagnosis. All the sexual dysfunctions are listed in Table 13–1.

Sexual dysfunction is surprisingly common. The Global Study on Sexual Attitudes and Behaviors (GSSAB) found that among persons in North America, the prevalence of sexual dysfunctions occurring either periodically or frequently was 38% for women and 29% for men (see Table 13–2). Yet these conditions remain "off the radar screen" because

---

TABLE 13–1.   DSM-5 sexual dysfunctions

Delayed ejaculation

Erectile disorder

Female orgasmic disorder

Female sexual interest/arousal disorder

Genito-pelvic pain disorder

Male hypoactive sexual desire disorder

Premature (early) ejaculation

Substance/medication-induced sexual dysfunction

Other specified sexual dysfunction

Unspecified sexual dysfunction

---

few patients report them to their physicians, and fewer still seek treatment for them. Typical examples seen in everyday practice include the
postmenopausal woman who finds intercourse painful due to vaginal
dryness and the older man who finds it increasingly difficult to maintain an erection sufficient for sexual intercourse with his wife. The sexual dysfunctions tend to overlap, so that it is not uncommon for more
than one to be present. When this occurs, the clinician should diagnose
all of them.

The best known model of normal sexual functioning was developed
by William Masters and Virginia Johnson in the 1960s. Although recent
research has questioned some of its underlying assumptions, their
model remains valuable for understanding human sexual response.
Masters and Johnson described four phases:

1. The *desire phase* lasts minutes to hours. In this stage, sexual fantasies
   and the desire for sexual intimacy occur.
2. The *excitement phase* ("foreplay") consists of a subjective sense of
   pleasure and accompanying physiological changes that include penile tumescence and erection in men and vasocongestion of the pel-
   vis, vaginal lubrication and expansion, and swelling of the external
   genitalia in women.
3. The *orgasmic phase* consists of a peaking of sexual pleasure, with release of sexual tension and rhythmic contractions of the perineal
   muscles and reproductive organs. In men, there is a sensation of
   ejaculatory inevitability, which is followed by ejaculation of semen.
   In women, there are contractions (not always subjectively experi-

TABLE 13–2.   Frequency of self-reported sexual problems in North American men and women ages 40–80 years

Sexual dysfunction	%
Women	
Lack of sexual interest	33
Lubrication difficulties	27
Inability to reach orgasm	25
Pain during sex	14
Men	
Early ejaculation	27
Erectile difficulties	21
Lack of sexual interest	18
Inability to reach orgasm	15

Source. Adapted from Laumann et al. 2005.

enced as such) in the outer one-third of the vagina. In both men and women, the anal sphincter rhythmically contracts.

4. The *resolution phase* consists of a sense of muscular relaxation and general well-being. During this phase, men are physiologically refractory to further erection and orgasm for a variable period of time. In contrast, women may be able to respond to additional stimulation almost immediately.

One difficulty in evaluating sexual dysfunctions is that there are no widely accepted guidelines for determining what constitutes normal sexual functioning. As one might imagine, sexual functioning varies considerably by age, prior sexual experience, the availability of partners, and expectations based on cultural, ethnic, or religious affiliation.

DSM-5 requires that disorder-specific symptoms (e.g., delayed ejaculation) have persisted 6 months or longer and that the disorder causes clinically significant distress. Further, the disorder is not due to severe relationship stress; to another nonsexual mental disorder; or to the effects of a substance, medication, or medical condition (e.g., diabetes mellitus). The clinician can specify whether the symptoms are *lifelong* or *acquired*. If lifelong, the symptoms have been present since the person became sexually active. Further, the clinician can specify whether the disorder is *generalized* or *situational*. If generalized, the disorder is not limited to certain types of stimulation, situations, or partners.

Delayed Ejaculation

Delayed ejaculation occurs when a man achieves ejaculation during sexual activity only with great difficulty, if at all, despite adequate sexual stimulation (Box 13–1). This usually concerns partnered sexual activity, and not lone masturbation. There is little consensus as to the definition of "delay," and what constitutes a reasonable amount of time to reach orgasm differs among men and their sexual partners. Again, the clinician must take into account the man's age, sexual experience, and amount of sexual stimulation received.

Box 13–1.   DSM-5 Diagnostic Criteria for Delayed Ejaculation

A. Either of the following symptoms must be experienced on almost all or all occasions (approximately 75%–100%) of partnered sexual activity (in identified situational contexts or, if generalized, in all contexts), and without the individual desiring delay:

   1. Marked delay in ejaculation.
   2. Marked infrequency or absence of ejaculation.

B. The symptoms in Criterion A have persisted for a minimum duration of approximately 6 months.

C. The symptoms in Criterion A cause clinically significant distress in the individual.

D. The sexual dysfunction is not better explained by a nonsexual mental disorder or as a consequence of severe relationship distress or other significant stressors and is not attributable to the effects of a substance/medication or another medical condition.

Specify whether:

   Lifelong: The disturbance has been present since the individual became sexually active.

   Acquired: The disturbance began after a period of relatively normal sexual function.

Specify whether:

   Generalized: Not limited to certain types of stimulation, situations, or partners.

   Situational: Only occurs with certain types of stimulation, situations, or partners.

Specify current severity:

   Mild: Evidence of mild distress over the symptoms in Criterion A.

   Moderate: Evidence of moderate distress over the symptoms in Criterion A.

   Severe: Evidence of severe or extreme distress over the symptoms in Criterion A.

Some men may avoid sexual activity because of the frustration caused by their difficulty with ejaculation. Typically, the man and his partner report prolonged thrusting to the point of exhaustion or genital discomfort. Some sexual partners may feel responsible for the difficulty and blame themselves (i.e., for not being sufficiently attractive).

Erectile Disorder

Erectile disorder occurs when a man is unable to achieve an erection during partnered sexual activity as evidenced by one or more of three symptoms (Box 13–2). The disorder is relatively common, more so in older men. Erectile disorder is associated with low self-esteem, low self-confidence, and a compromised sense of masculinity. One result may be the avoidance of future sexual encounters because of a fear of failure and resultant embarrassment. Sexual satisfaction in the man's partner tends to be reduced.

Box 13–2.   DSM-5 Diagnostic Criteria for Erectile Disorder

A. At least one of the three following symptoms must be experienced on almost all or all (approximately 75%–100%) occasions of sexual activity (in identified situational contexts or, if generalized, in all contexts):

1. Marked difficulty in obtaining an erection during sexual activity.
2. Marked difficulty in maintaining an erection until the completion of sexual activity.
3. Marked decrease in erectile rigidity.

B. The symptoms in Criterion A have persisted for a minimum duration of approximately 6 months.

C. The symptoms in Criterion A cause clinically significant distress in the individual.

D. The sexual dysfunction is not better explained by a nonsexual mental disorder or as a consequence of severe relationship distress or other significant stressors and is not attributable to the effects of a substance/medication or another medical condition.

Specify whether:

Lifelong: The disturbance has been present since the individual became sexually active.

Acquired: The disturbance began after a period of relatively normal sexual function.

Specify whether:

Generalized: Not limited to certain types of stimulation, situations, or partners.

Situational: Only occurs with certain types of stimulation, situations, or partners.

Specify current severity:

Mild: Evidence of mild distress over the symptoms in Criterion A.

Moderate: Evidence of moderate distress over the symptoms in Criterion A.

Severe: Evidence of severe or extreme distress over the symptoms in Criterion A.

Erectile failure is associated with having sex with a previously unknown partner, the use of drugs or alcohol, or not wanting to have sex. Acquired erectile disorder is often associated with medical factors, such as diabetes and cardiovascular disease, and is likely to be persistent in most men. As might be expected, the incidence of erectile disorder increases with age. A minority of men diagnosed as having moderate erectile failure may experience spontaneous remission of symptoms without medical intervention.

Female Orgasmic Disorder

With *female orgasmic disorder,* the experience of orgasm is diminished, delayed, or even absent on almost all occasions of sexual activity (Box 13–3). Better known as anorgasmia, this disorder is sometimes difficult to assess because women's perceptions of orgasm are extremely varied, suggesting that it is experienced in very different ways, both across women and on different occasions by the same woman. Further, women show a wide range in the type or intensity of stimulation that elicits orgasm.

Box 13–3.   DSM-5 Criteria for Female Orgasmic Disorder

A. Presence of either of the following symptoms and experienced on almost all or all (approximately 75%–100%) occasions of sexual activity (in identified situational contexts or, if generalized, in all contexts):

   1. Marked delay in, marked infrequency of, or absence of orgasm.
   2. Markedly reduced intensity of orgasmic sensations.

B. The symptoms in Criterion A have persisted for a minimum duration of approximately 6 months.

C. The symptoms in Criterion A cause clinically significant distress in the individual.

D. The sexual dysfunction is not better explained by a nonsexual mental disorder or as a consequence of severe relationship distress (e.g., partner violence) or other significant stressors and is not attributable to the effects of a substance/medication or another medical condition.

Specify whether:

Lifelong: The disturbance has been present since the individual became sexually active.

Acquired: The disturbance began after a period of relatively normal sexual function.

Specify whether:

Generalized: Not limited to certain types of stimulation, situations, or partners.

Situational: Only occurs with certain types of stimulation, situations, or partners.

Specify if:

Never experienced an orgasm under any situation.

Specify current severity:

Mild: Evidence of mild distress over the symptoms in Criterion A.

Moderate: Evidence of moderate distress over the symptoms in Criterion A.

Severe: Evidence of severe or extreme distress over the symptoms in Criterion A.

Many women require clitoral stimulation to reach orgasm, and a relatively small proportion of women report that they always experience orgasm during penile-vaginal intercourse. Thus, a woman's experiencing orgasm through clitoral stimulation but not during intercourse does not meet criteria for a female orgasmic disorder. It is also important to consider whether orgasmic difficulties are the result of inadequate sexual stimulation; in these cases, a diagnosis of female orgasmic disorder is not made. Orgasmic difficulties in women often co-occur with problems related to sexual interest and arousal.

Women with female orgasmic disorder may have greater difficulty communicating about sexual issues than those without the disorder. Unlike men, overall sexual satisfaction in women tends not to be strongly correlated with orgasmic experience. Many women report high levels of sexual satisfaction despite rarely or never experiencing orgasm. Women report greater interest than men in the romantic aspects of a relationship, which does not depend on genital-to-genital contact.

Female Sexual Interest/Arousal Disorder

With *female sexual interest/arousal disorder,* the woman has either a lack of interest in sexual activity or arousal as evidenced by at least three of six symptoms (Box 13–4). The disorder occurs in up to one-third of all married women and is defined as the partial or complete failure to attain or maintain the lubrication-swelling response characteristic of the excitement stage or the complete lack of sexual excitement and pleasure. Women with this condition may experience painful intercourse, sexual avoidance, and disturbance of marital or sexual relationships. It is often associated with lack of sexual desire and anorgasmia. Before making a diagnosis of female sexual desire/arousal disorder, the clinician should take into account factors that affect sexual functioning, such as age, gender, and cultural background of the patient.

Box 13–4. DSM-5 Diagnostic Criteria for Female Sexual Interest/Arousal Disorder

---

A. Lack of, or significantly reduced, sexual interest/arousal, as manifested by at least three of the following:
   1. Absent/reduced interest in sexual activity.
   2. Absent/reduced sexual/erotic thoughts or fantasies.
   3. No/reduced initiation of sexual activity, and typically unreceptive to a partner's attempts to initiate.
   4. Absent/reduced sexual excitement/pleasure during sexual activity in almost all or all (approximately 75%–100%) sexual encounters (in identified situational contexts or, if generalized, in all contexts).
   5. Absent/reduced sexual interest/arousal in response to any internal or external sexual/erotic cues (e.g., written, verbal, visual).
   6. Absent/reduced genital or nongenital sensations during sexual activity in almost all or all (approximately 75%–100%) sexual encounters (in identified situational contexts or, if generalized, in all contexts).
B. The symptoms in Criterion A have persisted for a minimum duration of approximately 6 months.
C. The symptoms in Criterion A cause clinically significant distress in the individual.
D. The sexual dysfunction is not better explained by a nonsexual mental disorder or as a consequence of severe relationship distress (e.g., partner violence) or other significant stressors and is not attributable to the effects of a substance/medication or another medical condition.

Specify whether:
   Lifelong: The disturbance has been present since the individual became sexually active.

Acquired: The disturbance began after a period of relatively normal sexual function.

Specify whether:

Generalized: Not limited to certain types of stimulation, situations, or partners.

Situational: Only occurs with certain types of stimulation, situations, or partners.

Specify current severity:

Mild: Evidence of mild distress over the symptoms in Criterion A.

Moderate: Evidence of moderate distress over the symptoms in Criterion A.

Severe: Evidence of severe or extreme distress over the symptoms in Criterion A.

Low sexual interest can temporarily result from stressful situations such as overwork, from lack of privacy, or from a lack of opportunity for sexual activity. Women who are victims of domestic abuse may also report low sexual interest or arousal, which clinicians should keep in mind. Many women with this disorder are poorly informed about sexual matters, or are sexually inhibited because of their particular religious or cultural background.

Genito-Pelvic Pain/Penetration Disorder

Genito-pelvic pain/penetration disorder is diagnosed when a person has pain or discomfort, muscular tightening, or fear about pain when having sexual intercourse (Box 13–5). This disorder reflects a change from DSM-IV, wherein two disorders—dyspareunia and vaginismus—were used to diagnose sexual pain disorders. They are now merged into a single category because clinicians had difficulty in distinguishing between the two and their reliability was low.

Box 13–5.   DSM-5 Diagnostic Criteria for Genito-Pelvic Pain/Penetration Disorder

---

A. Persistent or recurrent difficulties with one (or more) of the following:

1. Vaginal penetration during intercourse.
2. Marked vulvovaginal or pelvic pain during vaginal intercourse or penetration attempts.
3. Marked fear or anxiety about vulvovaginal or pelvic pain in anticipation of, during, or as a result of vaginal penetration.

4. Marked tensing or tightening of the pelvic floor muscles during attempted vaginal penetration.

B. The symptoms in Criterion A have persisted for a minimum duration of approximately 6 months.

C. The symptoms in Criterion A cause clinically significant distress in the individual.

D. The sexual dysfunction is not better explained by a nonsexual mental disorder or as a consequence of a severe relationship distress (e.g., partner violence) or other significant stressors and is not attributable to the effects of a substance/medication or another medical condition.

Specify whether:

Lifelong: The disturbance has been present since the individual became sexually active.

Acquired: The disturbance began after a period of relatively normal sexual function.

Specify current severity:

Mild: Evidence of mild distress over the symptoms in Criterion A.

Moderate: Evidence of moderate distress over the symptoms in Criterion A.

Severe: Evidence of severe or extreme distress over the symptoms in Criterion A.

The diagnosis of genito-pelvic pain/penetration disorder requires the presence of one or more of the following problems: 1) difficulty having intercourse, 2) genito-pelvic pain, 3) fear of pain or vaginal penetration, and 4) tension of the pelvic floor muscles. Because major difficulty in any one of these symptom areas is often sufficient to cause clinically significant distress, a diagnosis can be made on the basis of marked difficulty in only one symptom area. Nonetheless, all four symptom areas should be assessed.

Genito-pelvic pain/penetration disorder may be associated with other sexual dysfunctions, for example female sexual interest/arousal disorder. The woman may have sufficient desire and interest in sexual activity, but only for those activities that are not painful or do not require penetration (e.g., oral sex). Yet even when sexual interest and desire are preserved, the woman may learn to avoid sexual situations and opportunities, and may even avoid or refuse gynecological examinations. It is not unusual for women who have not succeeded in having sexual intercourse to seek treatment only when they wish to conceive (i.e., the "unconsummated" marriage). Many women with genito-pelvic pain/penetration disorder experience considerable relationship or marital problems, but they may also report diminished feelings of femininity.

Women experiencing superficial pain during sexual intercourse often have a history of vaginal infections, although pain may persist following successful treatment. Pain during tampon insertion or the inability to insert tampons before any sexual contact has been attempted is an important risk factor for genito-pelvic pain/penetration disorder. Religious and cultural factors also predispose to the disorder, with some reports from Turkey, a Muslim country, showing strikingly high rates of the DSM-IV diagnosis of vaginismus.

Male Hypoactive Sexual Desire Disorder

Male hypoactive sexual desire disorder is diagnosed when a man has diminished desire for sexual activity and few if any sexual thoughts or fantasies (Box 13–6). Because DSM-5 has a new diagnosis for low sexual desire and arousal problems in women (i.e., female sexual interest/arousal disorder), male hypoactive sexual desire disorder was created to enable clinicians to diagnose a man's diminished sexual desire.

Box 13–6.   DSM-5 Diagnostic Criteria for Male Hypoactive Sexual Desire Disorder

---

A. Persistently or recurrently deficient (or absent) sexual/erotic thoughts or fantasies and desire for sexual activity. The judgment of deficiency is made by the clinician, taking into account factors that affect sexual functioning, such as age and general and sociocultural contexts of the individual's life.
B. The symptoms in Criterion A have persisted for a minimum duration of approximately 6 months.
C. The symptoms in Criterion A cause clinically significant distress in the individual.
D. The sexual dysfunction is not better explained by a nonsexual mental disorder or as a consequence of severe relationship distress or other significant stressors and is not attributable to the effects of a substance/medication or another medical condition.

Specify whether:
   Lifelong: The disturbance has been present since the individual became sexually active.
   Acquired: The disturbance began after a period of relatively normal sexual function.

Specify whether:
   Generalized: Not limited to certain types of stimulation, situations, or partners.

Situational: Only occurs with certain types of stimulation, situations, or partners.

Specify current severity:

Mild: Evidence of mild distress over the symptoms in Criterion A.

Moderate: Evidence of moderate distress over the symptoms in Criterion A.

Severe: Evidence of severe or extreme distress over the symptoms in Criterion A.

Male hypoactive sexual desire disorder may co-occur with erectile problems or abnormal ejaculation. In fact, it has been observed that persistent difficulties obtaining an erection can lead a man to lose interest in sexual activity. Men with this disorder often report that they no longer initiate sexual activity and are minimally receptive to a partner's attempt to initiate sexual activity. This doesn't mean that are not capable of engaging in sex, because engaging in some sexual activities may sometimes occur even in the presence of low sexual desire (e.g., masturbation or partnered sexual activity).

Premature (Early) Ejaculation

Premature (early) ejaculation occurs when a man ejaculates during partnered sexual activity within approximately 1 minute following vaginal penetration and before the individual wishes it (Box 13–7). Many men with this condition report a sense of lack of control over ejaculation and are apprehensive about their anticipated inability to delay ejaculation on future sexual encounters. From 20% to 30% of men age 18–70 express concern about how rapidly they ejaculate. Using the new definition in DSM-5, about 1%–3% of men would receive the diagnosis. Prevalence may increase with age.

Box 13–7.   DSM-5 Diagnostic Criteria for Premature (Early) Ejaculation

---

A. A persistent or recurrent pattern of ejaculation occurring during partnered sexual activity within approximately 1 minute following vaginal penetration and before the individual wishes it.

Note: Although the diagnosis of premature (early) ejaculation may be applied to individuals engaged in nonvaginal sexual activities, specific duration criteria have not been established for these activities.

B. The symptom in Criterion A must have been present for at least 6 months and must be experienced on almost all or all (approximately

75%–100%) occasions of sexual activity (in identified situational contexts or, if generalized, in all contexts).

C. The symptom in Criterion A causes clinically significant distress in the individual.

D. The sexual dysfunction is not better explained by a nonsexual mental disorder or as a consequence of severe relationship distress or other significant stressors and is not attributable to the effects of a substance/medication or another medical condition.

Specify whether:

Lifelong: The disturbance has been present since the individual became sexually active.

Acquired: The disturbance began after a period of relatively normal sexual function.

Specify whether:

Generalized: Not limited to certain types of stimulation, situations, or partners.

Situational: Only occurs with certain types of stimulation, situations, or partners.

Specify current severity:

Mild: Ejaculation occurring within approximately 30 seconds to 1 minute of vaginal penetration.

Moderate: Ejaculation occurring within approximately 15–30 seconds of vaginal penetration.

Severe: Ejaculation occurring prior to sexual activity, at the start of sexual activity, or within approximately 15 seconds of vaginal penetration.

For many, premature (early) ejaculation starts during the man's initial sexual experiences and persists throughout life. Some men may experience premature (early) ejaculation only during their initial sexual encounters, but gain ejaculatory control over time. In contrast, some men develop the disorder after a period of having a normal ejaculatory latency, a condition known as *acquired premature (early) ejaculation.* The acquired form likely has a later onset, usually appearing during or after the fourth decade of life. Reversal of medical conditions such as hyperthyroidism and prostatitis appears to restore ejaculatory latencies to baseline values.

Substance/Medication-Induced Sexual Dysfunction

Substance/medication-induced sexual dysfunction applies when a clinically significant sexual dysfunction is judged to result from the direct physiological effects of a medication or drug of abuse (Box 13–8). Acute intoxication with or chronic abuse of various substances (e.g., cocaine, opiates, amphetamines, sedatives, hypnotics) may decrease sexual interest and cause arousal difficulties or interfere with orgasm. In addition, many medications (e.g., antihypertensives, histamine H_2 receptor antagonists, antidepressants, anabolic steroids, stimulants, anxiolytics) can cause a decrease in sexual interest, cause erectile difficulties, or interfere with orgasm.

Box 13–8. DSM-5 Diagnostic Criteria for Substance/ Medication-Induced Sexual Dysfunction

A. A clinically significant disturbance in sexual function is predominant in the clinical picture.

B. There is evidence from the history, physical examination, or laboratory findings of both (1) and (2):

 1. The symptoms in Criterion A developed during or soon after substance intoxication or withdrawal or after exposure to a medication.

 2. The involved substance/medication is capable of producing the symptoms in Criterion A.

C. The disturbance is not better explained by a sexual dysfunction that is not substance/medication-induced. Such evidence of an independent sexual dysfunction could include the following:

 The symptoms precede the onset of the substance/medication use; the symptoms persist for a substantial period of time (e.g., about 1 month) after the cessation of acute withdrawal or severe intoxication; or there is other evidence suggesting the existence of an independent non-substance/medication-induced sexual dysfunction (e.g., a history of recurrent non-substance/medication-related episodes).

D. The disturbance does not occur exclusively during the course of a delirium.

E. The disturbance causes clinically significant distress in the individual.

Note: This diagnosis should be made instead of a diagnosis of substance intoxication or substance withdrawal only when the symptoms in Criterion A predominate in the clinical picture and are sufficiently severe to warrant clinical attention.

Specify if (see Table 1 in the [DSM-5] chapter "Substance-Related and Addictive Disorders" for diagnoses associated with substance class):

With onset during intoxication: If the criteria are met for intoxication with the substance and the symptoms develop during intoxication.

With onset during withdrawal: If criteria are met for withdrawal from the substance and the symptoms develop during, or shortly after, withdrawal.

With onset after medication use: Symptoms may appear either at initiation of medication or after a modification or change in use.

Specify current severity:
   Mild: Occurs on 25%–50% of occasions of sexual activity.
   Moderate: Occurs on 50%–75% of occasions of sexual activity.
   Severe: Occurs on 75% or more of occasions of sexual activity.

Etiology of the Sexual Dysfunctions

Sexual dysfunction can be caused by psychological factors, medical conditions, medications, or substances of abuse or, as often happens, a combination of several factors. For example, lack of sexual desire can result from chronic stress, anxiety, or depression, but it can also result from medications that either depress the central nervous system or decrease testosterone production. Prolonged sexual abstinence by itself can suppress desire. Physical illnesses or surgery can also depress sexual desire, especially when they affect body image (e.g., mastectomy, ileostomy).

Female orgasmic disorder—anorgasmia—can result from the effects of medication or surgery, or psychological factors, such as pregnancy fears, rejection by the sexual partner, or major depression. Cultural factors also may contribute. For example, in some authoritarian cultures, sexual intercourse is seen primarily as a marital duty meant to satisfy the man, rather than something for both partners to enjoy.

Erectile disorder can also be caused by medical conditions or psychological factors, or both (Table 13–3). Research shows that up to 75% of the men evaluated for erectile dysfunction have a medical cause for the disorder, such as cardiovascular disease (e.g., atherosclerotic disease), renal disorders (e.g., chronic renal failure), liver disease (e.g., cirrhosis), malnutrition, diabetes mellitus, multiple sclerosis, traumatic spinal cord injury, abuse of alcohol or other drugs, psychotropic medication, prostate surgery, or pelvic irradiation.

In determining the cause, it is important to determine whether spontaneous erections occur at times when the man does not plan to have intercourse (e.g., morning erections, erections with masturbation). If erections occur at these times, the disorder is more likely to have a psychological origin.

Because medications are so effective in treating erectile disorder, there is little reason for an extensive workup. A limited investigation should include fasting blood glucose to rule out diabetes, and a fasting lipid screen because erectile dysfunction is a known marker for cardiovascular disease. Some experts also recommend thyroid function tests to rule out hypo- or hyperthyroidism. Obtaining a serum testosterone

TABLE 13–3.   Causes of erectile disorder

Medical illness	Psychiatric illness
Acromegaly	Anxiety disorders
Addison's disease	Dementia
Diabetes	Major depression
Hyperthyroidism	Schizophrenia
Hypothyroidism	**Drugs**
Klinefelter's syndrome	Alcohol
Multiple sclerosis	Antiandrogens
Parkinson's disease	Anticholinergics
Pelvic surgery or irradiation	Antidepressants
Peripheral vascular disease	Antihypertensives (especially
Pituitary adenoma	centrally acting ones)
Spinal cord injury	Antipsychotics
Syphilis	Barbiturates
Temporal lobe epilepsy	Finasteride
	Marijuana
	Opioids
	Stimulants

level may be helpful in some patients to rule out hypogonadism associated with testosterone deficiency. If the assay is low, follow-up should include further endocrine testing such as luteinizing hormone, follicle-stimulating hormone, and prolactin levels.

Specialized tests can sometimes be helpful in assessing the cause of erectile disorder when treatment fails. This can begin with an injection of a vasoactive drug, such as alprostadil, into the corpus cavernosum to assess erectile potential. Obtaining an erection confirms the integrity of the penile vascular system. If the patient is unable to obtain an erection, additional investigations may include color Doppler ultrasonography of the penile vasculature, dynamic infusion cavernosumetry, and bulbocavernosus reflex latency times and somatosensory evoked potentials to assess the integrity of penile innervation. Penile angiography can be used to further explore the possibility of an isolated arterial occlusion if suggested by Doppler scanning. The latter procedure is for the rare patient who is a candidate for vascular reconstructive surgery.

Delayed ejaculation should be differentiated from *retrograde ejaculation*, in which ejaculation occurs but the seminal fluid passes backward into the bladder. Both delayed ejaculation and retrograde ejaculation can have a physiological cause, such as the effects of medication, genitourinary surgery (e.g., prostatectomy), or neurological disorders involving the lumbosacral section of the spinal cord. Centrally acting antihypertensives (e.g., guanethidine, α-methyldopa), tricyclic antidepressants (e.g., amitriptyline), or antipsychotics, particularly the phenothiazines (e.g., chlorpromazine, thioridazine), can be responsible for the disorder.

Antidepressants are a frequent cause of sexual dysfunction and may be responsible for low libido, orgasmic disorders in women, and ejaculation delay or failure in men. Up to 65% of persons taking one of the selective serotonin reuptake inhibitor (SSRI) antidepressants (e.g., fluoxetine, paroxetine, sertraline) report some degree of sexual dysfunction when carefully queried. In men, they can cause ejaculatory delay or failure. This is probably one of the most common reasons for treatment noncompliance.

Age itself must be taken into account as a cause of sexual dysfunction. Older persons are more likely to report lack of sexual desire, as well as other forms of sexual dysfunction itself. For example, older men may not ejaculate at every sexual encounter but perhaps only every second or third time.

Clinical Management of Sexual Dysfunctions

Treatment of the sexual dysfunctions was pioneered in the 1960s and 1970s by Masters and Johnson. When introduced, their brief "dual" sex therapy (e.g., 8–12 sessions) broke with tradition and was quickly embraced by the mental health community. Still widely employed, sex therapy is usually combined with cognitive-behavioral therapy that aims to correct irrational beliefs and dysfunctional thoughts held by one or both partners.

Treatment begins with educating the couple about normal sexual functioning and evaluating their ability to communicate about sex and intimacy. Once the problem has been identified, a series of graded assignments are given for specific sexual activities that the couple is expected to carry out in private. For example, with erectile disorder, the couple is assigned *sensate focus* exercises (i.e., nongenital caressing) to gradually increase awareness of the couple's erogenous zones, as they abstain from sexual intercourse. Genital stimulation is gradually included in the exercises. In time, the man is able to have erections without the pressure to perform and is able to successfully complete vaginal intercourse.

These methods can be used for many of the sexual dysfunctions and are modified depending on the presenting complaint. For example, in cases of female orgasmic disorder, therapy may involve training the woman to first have an orgasm by masturbation (sometimes with the aid of a vibrator) before treating the couple. With vaginismus, a form of genito-pelvic pain disorder in which muscular tightening can prevent intercourse, treatment may include individual therapy, meditation or other relaxation exercises, or the use of Hegar dilators, which are inserted into the vagina. (The size of the dilators is slowly increased over 3-5 days to gradually enlarge the vaginal opening.) If intercourse is painful because of vaginal dryness, topical estrogen may help, but the most simple solution is for the woman to use a lubricant.

The "squeeze method" can be used to treat premature (early) ejaculation. When the man feels he is about to ejaculate, the partner is instructed to squeeze the penis (for up to 5 seconds) by placing the thumb on the frenulum and the first and second fingers on the opposite side. This action effectively halts ejaculation so that the couple may prolong foreplay.

Medication has assumed an increasing role in the treatment of the sexual dysfunctions. SSRIs can be used to treat premature (early) ejaculation because a common side effect is ejaculatory delay (e.g., paroxetine, 20 mg/day). Men can also benefit from 1% dibucaine (Nupercaine) ointment applied to the coronal ridge and frenulum of the penis to reduce stimulation.

Testosterone has been used to treat both men and women with low sexual desire, although research on its use for this indication is inconsistent except in clear cases of hypogonadism. Furthermore, it has the potential to induce masculinizing side effects (e.g., hirsutism), which are problematic in women. Estrogen, either systemic or topical, has also been used to treat low sexual desire in women, but results are variable.

Three oral medications have been approved by the U.S. Food and Drug Administration (FDA) for the treatment of erectile disorder. Sildenafil, vardenafil, and tadalafil are each classified as phosphodiesterase-5 inhibitors. They enhance the effect of nitric oxide, which relaxes smooth muscles in the penis, increasing blood flow and allowing an erection to develop in response to sexual arousal. They differ in dosage, duration of effect, and adverse effects. Sildenafil (Viagra) works relatively quickly to produce an erection and is taken as needed in doses ranging from 25 to 100 mg. Vardenafil (Levitra), which lasts up to a day, is taken as needed at doses ranging from 5 to 20 mg. Tadalafil (Cialis) lasts up to 3 days and is taken in doses ranging from 5 to 20 mg/day. Each of these medications can cause headaches, upset stomach, nausea, and muscle aches. They have been used to treat female orgasmic disorder, but their effectiveness in women is not established.

Alprostadil, a synthetic version of the hormone prostaglandin E, is another drug approved for the treatment of erectile disorder. The drug either is injected directly into the base or side of the penis or is placed directly into the urethra with a special syringe. Either method of administration results in increased penile blood flow within minutes. The main drawback to this drug is the inconvenience and discomfort involved with its use.

Surgical treatments of erectile disorder are also available, but these are indicated only when medication is ineffective. The most common technique involves the insertion of a penile prosthesis. These devices are generally either semirigid or inflatable, and each has its advantages and disadvantages. A simple alternative is a vacuum pump device that produces an erection by increasing blood flow to the penis. Once an erection is achieved, a metal ring is placed around the base of the penis to maintain the erection for about 30 minutes.

Clinical points for sexual dysfunction
1. The clinician must learn to take a sexual history without shame or embarrassment. Patients will detect the clinician's anxiety, which will only serve to increase their own.
2. The clinician should not apologize for asking intimate questions. How a person behaves sexually is important to assess.   • Most people will be surprisingly forthcoming in describing their sex lives.
3. Couples and individuals can engage in sex therapy. The therapy may be used with equal success in opposite- or same-sex couples.
4. The principles of sex therapy are relatively simple to learn and emphasize education about sexual functioning, helping couples to communicate better, and correcting dysfunctional attitudes about sex that one or both partners may hold.
5. Therapy involves homework assignments, which assist the couple in learning to increase sensory awareness. This may include masturbation, sensate focus experiences, and special coital techniques or positions.   • This may help the couple learn to separate pleasure from physiological response (e.g., erection).
6. Erectile disorder can be effectively treated pharmacologically, whether the disorder is psychologically or medically based. Oral medications include sildenafil, vardenafil, and tadalafil. Another drug, alprostadil, is placed into the urethra with a special applicator or is injected directly into the penis.

Clinical points for sexual dysfunction *(continued)*
• Surgical techniques are available and involve the placement of a semirigid or an inflatable device.
• Vacuum pump devices that draw blood into the penis also are available.

■ Gender Dysphoria

Gender dysphoria refers to the distress that may accompany individuals' sense of incongruence between their own experience of gender and their assigned gender. In DSM-IV, the emphasis was on cross-gender identification, reflected by the term *gender identity disorder.* Another early term was *transsexualism,* which placed the focus on the transition from one gender to another. The new term places an emphasis on dysphoria, not identity per se, as the clinical problem. While not all individuals are distressed with their gender incongruence, some experience distress if the desired physical interventions (e.g., hormones, surgery) are unavailable to them.

In DSM-5, there are separate categories for children and for adolescents and adults. Two residual categories are available for those with gender dysphoria who do not meet the criteria for a more specific disorder. Table 13–4 lists the DSM-5 gender dysphoria diagnoses.

Gender dysphoria is relatively uncommon, with prevalence estimated at 1 in 30,000 men and 1 in 100,000 women. The disorder usually begins in childhood. In boys, early features include overidentification with the mother, overtly feminine behavior (e.g., playing with dolls), little interest in typical male pursuits (e.g., disliking sports), and peer relationships primarily with girls. Girls may show tomboyish behavior, but this is more acceptable in our society than is feminine behavior in boys and draws less attention.

The symptoms of gender dysphoria vary with age, as reflected in the DSM-5 criteria sets. A very young child may show signs of distress (e.g., intense crying) only when parents tell the child that he or she is not "really" a member of the other gender. If the parents and others are supportive of the child's desire to live in the role of the other gender, distress may be minimal and only emerge if the desire is interfered with. Adolescents and adults are much more likely to experience distress, but this tends to be lessened by a supportive environment (e.g., accepting family members) and knowledge that hormonal treatments and surgery are available. Impairment can vary from school refusal in

TABLE 13–4. DSM-5 gender dysphoria
Gender dysphoria in children
Gender dysphoria in adolescents and adults
Other specified gender dysphoria
Unspecified gender dysphoria

children to avoidance of social activities in adolescents and adults. Depression, anxiety, and substance use disorders can be a consequence of gender dysphoria.

In making the diagnosis, it is important to rule out other potential causes of gender dysphoria. With schizophrenia, a desire to change one's anatomical gender may be part of a complex delusion (e.g., the belief that the F.B.I. is conspiring to change the patient's sex). People with transvestic fetishism who cross-dress occasionally may come to feel that sex change surgery is a natural extension of their cross-dressing.

The following case describes a patient with gender dysphoria evaluated in our clinic:

> Will, a 25-year-old felon, was referred for evaluation of gender dysphoria. He had recently filed a lawsuit requesting that the state pay for gender reassignment surgery and allow him to wear women's clothing in prison.
>
> Will had never felt comfortable with his gender. He was effeminate as a child and enjoyed playing house, in which he would assume feminine roles such as playing the mother or sister. He also liked games associated with girls, such as hopscotch and jump rope, and was not very good at team sports. He began to cross-dress at age 9 and said that he felt more comfortable and natural when dressed as a girl.
>
> Will began to cross-dress full-time in his early 20s and for a 5-month period living as "Julie." Although Will was able to perform sexually with a woman, he would fantasize about being made love to by a man. He reported having sexual experiences with more than 100 male partners and several short-term same-sex relationships. Two months before his evaluation, Will lacerated his penis with a shard of glass.
>
> In addition to gender dysphoria, Will had a history of disciplinary and behavioral problems and as a young boy had been placed in detention. He had a history of misusing alcohol and marijuana and had run-ins with the law for minor offenses (e.g., shoplifting). He also had been hospitalized several times to treat depression and suicidal behavior.
>
> Although he clearly met criteria for gender dysphoria, Will's lawsuit ultimately failed and he remained at the men's prison.

DSM-5 subtypes people with gender dysphoria based on whether they have a disorder of sex development, such as a congenital adrenal disorder or androgen sensitivity syndrome. The clinician can also specify whether the person has transitioned to full-time living in the desired gender ("posttransition").

Many gender dysphoric persons will seek hormonal therapy and gender reassignment surgery. Gender dysphoria clinics in the United States and elsewhere may require that the person live as a member of the opposite sex for a year or longer before considering him or her for surgery.

In the transition from male to female, the individual is prescribed hormones (e.g., estradiol, progesterone) to promote the development of secondary female characteristics, including breast development; laser treatment and electrolysis are used to remove hair. Surgery is performed to remove the testes and penis and to create an artificial vagina (vaginoplasty). The female-to-male patient undergoes mastectomy, hysterectomy, and oophorectomy. Testosterone is prescribed to help develop muscle mass and deepen the voice. Some persons will choose to have an artificial penis constructed.

Most persons who undergo gender reassignment surgery are satisfied with the outcome. People who adjust well after surgery tend to have had a lifelong cross-gender identification, were able to "pass" convincingly as a member of the opposite sex before surgery, have good social support, have a college education, and have a steady job. Some patients will continue to benefit from psychotherapy following surgery to assist them in adjusting to their new gender role.

■ Paraphilic Disorders

In DSM-5, paraphilias are defined as involving "anomalous" sexual activity preferences and, in lay terms, include deviant patterns of sexual interests, fantasies, and behaviors. Further, DSM-5 distinguishes between *paraphilia* and *paraphilic disorder.* The former refers to the preferential sexual interest; the latter refers to the disorder that can result from the anomalous interest.

Diagnosis of a paraphilic disorder requires that, in addition to having a "recurrent and intense sexual arousal" from the anomalous preference, the person has acted on the urges and the urges have caused significant distress or impairment in social, occupational, or other im-

TABLE 13–5.	DSM-5 paraphilic disorders
Voyeuristic disorder	Pedophilic disorder
Exhibitionistic disorder	Fetishistic disorder
Frotteuristic disorder	Transvestic disorder
Sexual masochism disorder	Other specified paraphilic disorder
Sexual sadism disorder	Unspecified paraphilic disorder

portant areas of functioning—or, in the case of pedophilic disorder, "marked distress or interpersonal difficulty." (Obviously, "impairment" will sometimes involve legal problems that may arise in the wake of the behaviors.) The fantasies, urges, or behaviors must have lasted 6 months or more. For some, paraphilic fantasies or stimuli are obligatory for erotic arousal and are always included in sexual activity. In others, the paraphilic preferences occur only episodically, such as during periods of stress, whereas at other times the person is able to function sexually without paraphilic fantasies or stimuli.

Eight disorders are described in DSM-5 (see Table 13–5). They were selected for inclusion to maintain continuity with prior editions of DSM, because they are relatively common, or because they involve behaviors that have the potential to harm others and are classified as criminal offenses (e.g., pedophilic disorder). There are also two residual categories (*other specified paraphilia* and *unspecified paraphilia*) for disorders that fail to meet criteria for any of the specific paraphilias.

Some people meet criteria for more than one paraphilic disorder. In these cases, the sexual interests may be related (e.g., foot fetishism and shoe fetishism), but in other cases the link may not be obvious. In any event, comorbid diagnoses of separate paraphilic disorders may be warranted.

The eight disorders are not exhaustive of the types and varieties of possible paraphilic disorders (see Table 13–6). An example of an unusual paraphilic disorder, not listed in DSM-5, is *infantilism*, in which the person obtains sexual arousal and gratification by behaving like an infant. In one such case seen at our hospital, a 30-year-old former fighter pilot reported that he could function sexually only while wearing a diaper and sucking on a pacifier. He enjoyed having his partner change the diaper, apply baby powder, and bottle-feed him. Although the role-play initially was used for sexual gratification, he later found it comforting and generally wore a diaper under his clothing at all times.

TABLE 13–6. Paraphilic disorders

Preferential sexual act	Behaviors/objects of gratification
Disorders included in DSM-5	
Voyeurism	Observing unsuspecting persons ("window peeping")
Exhibitionism	Exposing one's genitals to unsuspecting persons
Frotteurism	Rubbing against nonconsenting persons
Sexual masochism	Inflicting pain and humiliation on oneself
Sexual sadism	Inflicting pain and suffering on others
Pedophilia	Prepubescent children
Fetishism	Nonliving objects or nongenital body parts
Transvestic fetishism	Cross-dressing
Non-DSM-5 paraphilias	
Coprophilia	Feces
Hypoxyphilia	Altered state of consciousness secondary to hypoxia
Infantilism	Behaving as though one is an infant
Klismania	Enemas
Necrophilia	Dead persons
Telephone scatologia	Obscene telephone calls
Urophilia	Urine
Zoophilia (bestiality)	Animal contacts

Etiology of Paraphilic Disorders

The systematic study of the paraphilic disorders began in the 1870s with the work of Krafft-Ebing, Hirschfeld, Ellis, and others. In 1886, Richard Krafft-Ebing, a Viennese psychiatrist, compiled the first systematic account of paraphilias in his book *Psychopathia Sexualis.* He considered sexual deviations to be hereditary and believed that they could be modified by social and psychological factors. Freud, also active at this time, explained sexual deviations as resulting from failures of the developmental processes during childhood. Learning theory has also been used to explain the paraphilias by linking deviant fantasies with the positive experience of orgasm. Once established, this process is reinforced through masturbation.

Some sexually deviant behaviors may have a neurobiological basis. For example, sexually inappropriate behaviors can occur in people with poor impulse control suggestive of a brain disorder (e.g., psychosis, major neurocognitive disorder). Research has shown that sex offenders have a high rate of abnormal electroencephalograms (EEGs). Also, abnormal brain computed tomography scans have been reported in pedophiles and other sexually aggressive men. Last, familial transmission and hypothalamic-pituitary-gonadal axis dysfunction have been reported in pedophilia.

People with antisocial personality disorder sometimes commit deviant sexual acts to gratify their immediate urges, although a true paraphilia may not exist.

Epidemiology of Paraphilic Disorders

The prevalence of the paraphilic disorders is unknown, but isolated incidences of exhibitionism or voyeurism were reported in 3% and 7% of the general population in Sweden, respectively. Nearly all persons with a paraphilic disorder are male. These disorders are relatively uncommon in psychiatric practice, and most cases come to attention only if treatment is sought or if there are forensic issues following an arrest (e.g., the person requires evaluation of competency). Many paraphilias would scarcely be reported at all because the activity takes place between consenting adults or by a lone individual. For example, the man who cross-dresses, is comfortable with his preference, and experiences no subjective distress is unlikely to come to clinical attention. Thus, people who are comfortable with their paraphilias are completely underrepresented in all samples.

Clinical Findings, Course, and Outcome

Paraphilias are generally established in adolescence, usually before age 18. They occur almost exclusively among men, although cases are described in women. Most people with paraphilias are heterosexual, not homosexual, contrary to commonly held views. These demographic features appear to hold true for fetishists, pedophiles, exhibitionists, and voyeurs. Co-occurring psychiatric disorders are common and include substance use disorders, mood and anxiety disorders, and personality disorders.

Paraphilias tend to be chronic but to vary in frequency of expression and severity depending on the individual's level of stress, opportunity for sexual activity, and sexual drive. Because sexual drive subsides with increasing age, they are probably less common in older adults. Many people with paraphilias have relatively normal sexual lives with their partner or spouse apart from the paraphilia. In fact, it is not uncommon for the partner to be unaware of the individual's paraphilic behavior.

Voyeuristic disorder involves looking at or observing ("peeping" at) unsuspecting persons, usually strangers, who are naked, are in the act of disrobing, or are engaging in sexual activity, for the purpose of achieving sexual arousal. Voyeurism is often an expression of sexual curiosity in adolescents and typically has an onset before age 15. To avoid pathologizing normative sexual interest and behavior that develops during puberty, DSM-5 requires that the person be age 18 or older. The course tends to be chronic.

The following case of voyeuristic disorder was reported in a local newspaper:

> A 27-year-old law student pleaded guilty to five counts of criminal trespass after admitting that he had repeatedly spied on women in dormitory showers. He was arrested near the dormitory one morning after students had caught him lying on the floor outside the women's shower and looking through the ventilation grate. He was chased out of the dormitory by the women who had found him there.
>
> Residents of the dormitory had banded together and would watch for him daily from 5:00 A.M. to 9:00 A.M., believing that he would repeat his act. The "peeper" was well known at the dorm for his voyeurism and for making a nuisance of himself.

Exhibitionistic disorder involves the exposure of one's genitals to an unsuspecting person. This disorder accounts for about one-third of the sexual offenders referred for treatment. The person, usually a man, typically masturbates when exposing his genitals, and there is usually no attempt at having sexual activity with the other person. When exhibitionism begins in older adults, the behavior may indicate the presence of a neurocognitive disorder, such as Alzheimer's disease. Fewer arrests are made for exhibitionism in older age groups suggesting that the condition becomes less severe with age, or that the individual has better control.

Frotteuristic disorder involves touching or rubbing against a nonconsenting person. This behavior tends to occur in crowded places from which the person can readily escape, such as a busy sidewalk or a subway car. The person, usually a man, may rub his genitals against the other person's thighs or buttocks, or touch her genitals or breasts with his hands. Frotteurism is most common in the 15- to 25-year age group.

Sexual masochism disorder involves sexual fantasies, urges, or behaviors of being humiliated, bound, or otherwise made to suffer that cause clinically significant distress or impairment in social, occupational, or other important areas of functioning. *Sexual sadism disorder* involves sexual fantasies, urges, or behaviors in which the psychological or physical suffering (including humiliation) of a victim is sexually arousing to the person. In addition, the person has acted on the urges with a nonconsenting person, or the urges or fantasies cause marked distress or interpersonal difficulty.

Pedophilic disorder involves sexual activity with a prepubescent child, generally age 13 or younger. By definition, the individual with pedophilic disorder must be 16 years or older and at least 5 years older than the child. People with this condition generally report an attraction to children of a particular age range. Some individuals prefer boys, some prefer girls, and some are aroused by both boys and girls. Activity may be limited to undressing the child or exposing one's genitals and masturbating in front of the child. Others will have oral, anal, or vaginal sex with the child. Importantly, experiencing distress about having sexual fantasies, urges, or behaviors involving children is not required for the diagnosis mainly because many people with pedophilic disorder are comfortable with their behavior. They may justify their sexual activity with children by claiming that the behavior is educational, or that the child enjoyed (or wanted) the experience. The disorder tends to begin in adolescence and is chronic, more so among those who have a preference for boys.

The person with *fetishistic disorder* is aroused by nonliving objects (e.g., rubber garments, women's underclothing, high-heeled shoes) or through a highly specific focus on a nongenital body part (e.g., feet). The diagnosis is not made if the fetish objects are limited to articles of female clothing used in cross-dressing or devices such as a vibrator designed for the purpose of tactile genital stimulation. Typically, contact with the object produces sexual arousal, which is followed by masturbation. People with a fetish may spend considerable time seeking their desired objects.

The following vignette describes a man with fetishistic disorder who was seen in our clinic:

> Daniel, a 41-year-old attorney, had his law license suspended after admitting to breaking into and entering more than 100 homes to obtain women's underwear for sexual gratification. He entered the houses through unlocked doors or would sometimes jimmy a lock with a credit card or knife. Once inside the house, he would seek undergarments to use later in solitary acts of masturbation. He was finally caught after he entered a neighbor's home, where he was found searching for the

woman's underwear. He was apprehended and charged with criminal trespass. Daniel was later convicted and placed on probation. He denied subsequent episodes of pilfering undergarments at a follow-up 5 years later, but he admitted that the urges remained. He believed that a renewed interest in religion was responsible for improved self-control.

Transvestic disorder involves cross-dressing that typically begins at puberty. The diagnosis is no longer limited to men as it was in DSM-IV. Early on, the person experiences the cross-dressing as sexually stimulating. As the person gains confidence, the clothes may be worn in public and the individual may become part of a transvestic subculture. The disorder tends to be chronic, although the urge to cross-dress may decline as the sexual drive lessens. In some cases, the cross-dressing will be accompanied by gender dysphoria.

Clinical Management of Paraphilic Disorders

Cognitive-behavioral therapy has become the mainstay of treatment of the paraphilic disorders, and its elements are widely incorporated into programs for sex offenders. For example, cognitive-behavioral methods are used to help restructure the faulty cognitions that people with paraphilias use to justify their behavior (e.g., erroneously interpreting a child's docility as an expression of sexual desire). This treatment may be combined with relaxation training to help reduce the anxiety and stress that frequently precede paraphilic behavior. Methods to reduce deviant arousal patterns include *masturbatory satiation* (satiating or boring the patient with his own deviant fantasies) and *covert sensitization* (replacing fantasies with unpleasant images). *Masturbatory conditioning* is used to generate arousal to nondeviant themes. Social skills training is used to help the patient learn to communicate more effectively with appropriate adult partners. A follow-up study of 194 child molesters treated with behavior modification (including some of the methods just described) showed success (i.e., no recidivism) in 82% at 12 months posttreatment. Although these results are encouraging, it is not known whether they can generalize to other paraphilias or to persons not motivated by threats of arrest or incarceration.

There are no FDA-approved medications for the treatment of paraphilias. Research has mainly focused on testosterone-lowering drugs, the SSRIs, and naltrexone.

Both medroxyprogesterone and leuprolide act peripherally to reduce serum testosterone levels and centrally to reduce sexual drive. The aim is to decrease paraphilic fantasies and their associated behaviors while avoiding erectile dysfunction. Medroxyprogesterone is given orally at dosages ranging from 100 to 400 mg/day. A long-acting preparation (Depo-Provera) may be given intramuscularly at dosages of 200–400 mg every 7–10 days. Leuprolide, a luteinizing hormone–releasing hormone agonist, has been used at a dose of 7.5 mg/month by depot injection. The long-term risks of these medications have not been adequately studied, and for that reason they should be used with caution. The gonadotropin-releasing hormone analogue triptorelin was found effective in a controlled trial, but the drug is unavailable in the United States.

The following patient with exhibitionistic disorder and compulsive masturbation treated at our hospital illustrates the use of medroxyprogesterone and, later, an SSRI to curb anomalous sexual urges and behaviors:

> Frank, a 38-year-old mechanic, presented to the outpatient department seeking help. He had left his wife 3 days earlier, fearing that another arrest for indecent exposure would humiliate his family and friends.
>
> Frank's story soon unfolded. At age 10, he had lost a testicle in an accident and was teased endlessly by his classmates, leading to feelings of insecurity and inadequacy. He started to masturbate at age 12 and was soon masturbating up to five times daily. Although he could not remember when it first occurred, he began to masturbate in public settings, which he found sexually exciting. The masturbation had a compulsive quality, and he felt powerless to stop.
>
> The masturbatory behavior continued over a 25-year period, leading to several arrests for indecent exposure. Frank sought psychotherapy after each arrest, but he would soon drop out. He denied other paraphilic behaviors but admitted having had two episodes of exhibitionism, first at age 18 to a girl sitting next to him in class and once during his honeymoon. Frank had married at age 23 and described the marriage as stable and his sexual relationship with his wife as satisfying.
>
> Frank was admitted to the hospital for further evaluation. Physical examination confirmed the absence of the right testicle, but results of the examination were otherwise normal. His serum testosterone level was 288 ng/dL (normal serum level is 200–800 ng/dL). Treatment was begun with medroxyprogesterone. At a follow-up visit 1 month later, his serum testosterone had fallen to 41 ng/dL. He had resisted masturbating in public places and no longer had spontaneous erections. He was back with his wife, who was happy with his progress. Six months later, he chose to discontinue the medication and within 1 month had relapsed.
>
> Frank presented for follow-up 10 years later after an arrest for soliciting a prostitute. He had continued to compulsively masturbate and to expose himself to unsuspecting women. He had divorced in the meantime and had not sought treatment. Paroxetine (40 mg/day) was pre-

scribed, and over the next year, Frank reported that the drug helped him to control his sexual urges and behaviors. He also had become involved in a support group for "sex addicts."

SSRIs have also been used to reduce paraphilic fantasies and behavioral impulsivity. An open-label study with sertraline showed that individuals with various paraphilias seemed to benefit. Naltrexone, an opioid receptor blocker, may be effective in curbing paraphilic fantasies and behavior as well.

Testosterone-lowering drugs should be reserved for patients whose symptoms do not respond to SSRIs or naltrexone or for those whose hypersexuality is uncontrolled or dangerous. Other drug therapy, including antipsychotic or antidepressant medication, is indicated when the paraphilia is associated with schizophrenia, major depression, or an anxiety disorder.

In addition to individual therapy and medication, some patients will benefit from couples therapy when the paraphilia has disrupted the relationship. Twelve-step programs are available in many locations that provide an opportunity for people to seek support from others with similar problems (e.g., Sex Addicts Anonymous).

Clinical points for paraphilic disorders

1. The history is of utmost importance in treating paraphilic disorders. The therapist must learn where and when the behavior occurs and whether the focus of desire is a person or an object.

    - Most persons with a paraphilic disorder have a variety of deviant sexual interests and behaviors, and the therapist is safe in assuming that more is present than initially meets the eye.

2. Paraphilic disorders are challenging to treat, but cognitive-behavioral therapy may offer the best hope for success. The purpose of treatment is to reduce deviant arousal patterns and to generate new arousal in response to nondeviant themes.

    - Methods may include masturbatory satiation and conditioning, social skills training, and cognitive restructuring.

3. Medications may help to reduce paraphilic fantasies and inappropriate sexual behaviors, but none are FDA approved for this purpose.

    - SSRIs and naltrexone have been used with some success.

    - Testosterone-lowering agents are generally reserved for repeat offenders whose actions are uncontrolled or potentially dangerous.

4. Difficult cases should be referred to clinicians experienced in treating these disorders.

■ Self-Assessment Questions

1. What are the three major types of sexual disorders discussed in this chapter?
2. Describe the four stages of Masters and Johnson's sexual response cycle.
3. What are the medical causes of erectile disorder (impotence)?
4. Describe "dual" sex therapy. What are "sensate focus" exercises?
5. What medications are used to treat erectile disorder?
6. What are the antecedent behavioral characteristics of persons with gender dysphoria?
7. What are the treatments for gender dysphoria? What factors predict a good outcome to gender reassignment surgery?
8. How can learning theory help explain paraphilic behavior?
9. How are the paraphilic disorders treated? Describe cognitive-behavioral therapy for a person with a paraphilic disorder. What medications can be used to curb unwanted sexual behaviors?

Chapter 14

Disruptive, Impulse-Control, and Conduct Disorders

Kleptomaniac, *n*.: a rich thief.

Ambrose Bierce, The Devil's Dictionary

Impaired self-regulation is the hallmark of the disruptive, impulse-control, and conduct disorders. These disorders are usually multidetermined and associated with physical or verbal injury to self, others, or objects, or with violating the rights of others. All can cause considerable emotional distress and social or occupational impairment, and yet, while common, they are frequently underappreciated and ignored. Many experts refer to these conditions as *externalizing disorders* because they place a person into conflict with others. On the other hand, *internalizing disorders*—such as the mood and anxiety disorders—are inwardly directed and, although causing distress, are less likely to affect society.

This chapter reflects the approach taken by the authors of DSM-5 to group related disorders together based on clinical and biological evidence. Included are oppositional defiant disorder, intermittent explosive disorder, conduct disorder, antisocial personality disorder (although its criteria and text remain with the personality disorders in DSM-5), pyromania, and kleptomania. Both oppositional defiant disorder and conduct disorder were included in the DSM-IV chapter "Disorders Usually First Diagnosed in Infancy, Childhood, or Adolescence." Two residual categories exist for those whose disruptive behavior does not fit one of the more specific categories. The disorders are listed in Table 14–1.

TABLE 14–1. DSM-5 disruptive, impulse-control, and conduct disorders

Oppositional defiant disorder

Intermittent explosive disorder

Conduct disorder

Antisocial personality disorder

Pyromania

Kleptomania

Other specified disruptive, impulse-control, and conduct disorder

Unspecified disruptive, impulse-control, and conduct disorder

■ Oppositional Defiant Disorder

Oppositional defiant disorder (ODD) is a diagnosis for children and adolescents with difficult and challenging behaviors that, while defiant, are not generally dangerous or illegal (see Box 14–1). The disorder is diagnosed on the basis of angry or irritable, defiant, or vindictive behavior of at least 6 months' duration, with a minimum of four out of eight symptoms in three categories: angry/irritable mood, argumentative/defiant behavior, and vindictiveness.

Box 14–1. DSM-5 Diagnostic Criteria for Oppositional Defiant Disorder

A. A pattern of angry/irritable mood, argumentative/defiant behavior, or vindictiveness lasting at least 6 months as evidenced by at least four symptoms from any of the following categories, and exhibited during interaction with at least one individual who is not a sibling.

Angry/Irritable Mood

1. Often loses temper.
2. Is often touchy or easily annoyed.
3. Is often angry and resentful.

Argumentative/Defiant Behavior

4. Often argues with authority figures or, for children and adolescents, with adults.
5. Often actively defies or refuses to comply with requests from authority figures or with rules.

6. Often deliberately annoys others.
7. Often blames others for his or her mistakes or misbehavior.

Vindictiveness

8. Has been spiteful or vindictive at least twice within the past 6 months.

Note: The persistence and frequency of these behaviors should be used to distinguish a behavior that is within normal limits from a behavior that is symptomatic. For children younger than 5 years, the behavior should occur on most days for a period of at least 6 months unless otherwise noted (Criterion A8). For individuals 5 years or older, the behavior should occur at least once per week for at least 6 months, unless otherwise noted (Criterion A8). While these frequency criteria provide guidance on a minimal level of frequency to define symptoms, other factors should also be considered, such as whether the frequency and intensity of the behaviors are outside a range that is normative for the individual's developmental level, gender, and culture.

B. The disturbance in behavior is associated with distress in the individual or others in his or her immediate social context (e.g., family, peer group, work colleagues), or it impacts negatively on social, educational, occupational, or other important areas of functioning.

C. The behaviors do not occur exclusively during the course of a psychotic, substance use, depressive, or bipolar disorder. Also, the criteria are not met for disruptive mood dysregulation disorder.

Specify current severity:

Mild: Symptoms are confined to only one setting (e.g., at home, at school, at work, with peers).

Moderate: Some symptoms are present in at least two settings.

Severe: Some symptoms are present in three or more settings.

Typically, in addition to temper outbursts, these children argue with their parents, refuse to clean their rooms, or fail to obey a curfew. While most children are occasionally naughty, children with ODD are more frequently naughty, and more so than most children at the same mental age. Clearly, there is a fine line between normal misbehavior and ODD, and there is great variation in the definition of "more frequent," depending on who is rendering the judgment. For instance, religiously conservative or authoritarian families are likely to be less tolerant of opposition and defiance than are families with other types of backgrounds. Thus, to some extent, the appearance of children with this diagnosis in child psychiatry clinics may partially reflect a given family's threshold for accepting defiant behavior, which must be considered in treatment planning.

Oppositional defiant disorder has a prevalence of around 3%, and before adolescence it is more frequent in boys; the gender ratio appears to even out after puberty. ODD first appears during the preschool years and rarely later, and may precede the onset of conduct disorder, particularly for those with the childhood-onset type. However, many children and adolescents with ODD do not develop conduct disorder, but remain at risk for mood and anxiety disorders. The defiant, argumentative, and vindictive symptoms carry most of the risk for conduct disorder, whereas the angry-irritable mood symptoms carry most of the risk for emotional disorders.

Other disorders need to be ruled out. Unlike conduct disorder (described later in the chapter), which specifies that the child must have violated personal rights and social rules (thereby making it more likely that the child's deviant behavior has come to the attention of people outside the immediate family), ODD is defined almost totally on the basis of annoying, difficult, and disruptive behavior. Attention-deficit/hyperactivity disorder (ADHD) is often comorbid with ODD, but the child's failure to conform to requests of others does not occur solely in situations that demand sustained effort and attention or demand that the child sit still. ODD shares many features with the new diagnosis *disruptive mood dysregulation disorder,* such as negative mood and temper outbursts, but the severity, frequency, and chronicity of temper outbursts are more severe in children with disruptive mood dysregulation disorder than in those with ODD. (In DSM-5, the diagnosis of disruptive mood dysregulation disorder takes precedence over ODD, if the criteria for both disorders are met.) Intermittent explosive disorder also involves high rates of anger, but people with this disorder show serious aggression toward others that is not part of the definition of ODD.

Common sense dictates that management of ODD should emphasize individual and family counseling, with treatment of co-occurring ADHD or other disorders with medications as needed. Most work in targeting ODD has been cognitively based, with the goal of helping the child manage anger, improve problem-solving ability, develop techniques to delay impulsive responses, and improve social interactions. With parental management training, parents learn to better manage their child's behavior as well as to promote desired behaviors. School-based programs, such as those aimed at resisting negative peer influences and reduction of bullying and antisocial behavior, may be helpful in this age group.

■ Intermittent Explosive Disorder

Intermittent explosive disorder (IED) is diagnosed when a person has verbal aggression or behavioral outbursts representing a failure to control aggressive impulses (see Box 14–2). These episodes are out of proportion to the provocation or to the psychosocial stressor. The diagnosis is used for persons in whom the loss of control is out of character and not merely part of a pattern of overreacting to life's problems. Therefore, mental disorders in which assaultive behaviors occur as a matter of course, such as antisocial or borderline personality disorder, psychotic disorders, mania, or alcohol or drug use disorders, need to be ruled out. A sudden behavioral change accompanied by outbursts in an otherwise healthy person suggests a neurocognitive disorder, which also needs to be ruled out.

Box 14–2.   DSM-5 Diagnostic Criteria for Intermittent Explosive Disorder

---

A. Recurrent behavioral outbursts representing a failure to control aggressive impulses as manifested by either of the following:

  1. Verbal aggression (e.g., temper tantrums, tirades, verbal arguments or fights) or physical aggression toward property, animals, or other individuals, occurring twice weekly, on average, for a period of 3 months. The physical aggression does not result in damage or destruction of property and does not result in physical injury to animals or other individuals.
  2. Three behavioral outbursts involving damage or destruction of property and/or physical assault involving physical injury against animals or other individuals occurring within a 12-month period.

B. The magnitude of aggressiveness expressed during the recurrent outbursts is grossly out of proportion to the provocation or to any precipitating psychosocial stressors.

C. The recurrent aggressive outbursts are not premeditated (i.e., they are impulsive and/or anger-based) and are not committed to achieve some tangible objective (e.g., money, power, intimidation).

D. The recurrent aggressive outbursts cause either marked distress in the individual or impairment in occupational or interpersonal functioning, or are associated with financial or legal consequences.

E. Chronological age is at least 6 years (or equivalent developmental level).

F. The recurrent aggressive outbursts are not better explained by another mental disorder (e.g., major depressive disorder, bipolar disorder, disruptive mood dysregulation disorder, a psychotic disorder, antisocial personality disorder, borderline personality disorder) and are not attributable to another medical condition (e.g., head trauma, Alzheimer's disease) or to the physiological effects of a substance (e.g., a drug of abuse, a medication). For children ages 6–18 years, aggressive behavior that occurs as part of an adjustment disorder should not be considered for this diagnosis.

Note: This diagnosis can be made in addition to the diagnosis of attention-deficit/hyperactivity disorder, conduct disorder, oppositional defiant disorder, or autism spectrum disorder when recurrent impulsive aggressive outbursts are in excess of those usually seen in these disorders and warrant independent clinical attention.

People with IED tend to be primarily young men with relatively low frustration tolerance. A recent study suggested a 7% lifetime prevalence, but some suggest that "pure" cases of IED are rare—that is, cases unaccompanied by any indication of a brain disorder (e.g., abnormal electroencephalographic findings, neurological soft signs, presence of abnormal personality traits). Comorbid mood and anxiety disorders are common.

Medication to reduce or eliminate aggressive impulses may be helpful, although none are approved by the U.S. Food and Drug Administration for this purpose. Both the selective serotonin reuptake inhibitor (SSRI) fluoxetine and the antiepileptic drug oxcarbazepine have been found superior to placebo in reducing impulsive aggression in people with IED. Other SSRIs, mood stabilizers (e.g., lithium carbonate, carbamazepine), and β-blockers (e.g., propranolol) have been used to treat IED, but their use is supported mainly by case studies or small case series. Second-generation antipsychotics (e.g., risperidone) have been used to dampen aggressive impulses in other clinical populations (e.g., dementia patients, patients with borderline personality disorder) and may be helpful in treating IED. Benzodiazepines should be avoided because of their tendency to cause behavioral disinhibition.

Cognitive-behavioral therapy (CBT) may be helpful. With CBT, patients can learn to recognize when they are becoming angry and to identify and defuse the triggers that lead to outbursts. One study showed that CBT was superior to a wait list in reducing anger and hostility in persons with IED.

■ Conduct Disorder

Conduct disorder is a pattern of behavioral problems in children or adolescents and is considered a forerunner of antisocial personality disorder in adults. The DSM-5 criteria require the presence of at least 3 of 15 antisocial behaviors in the past 12 months (with at least 1 criterion present in the past 6 months) (see Box 14–3). The criteria define four major domains of relevant behavior: aggression toward people and animals, destruction of property, deceitfulness or theft, and serious violations of rules. Individuals who manifest this delinquent behavior are further subdivided into two different subtypes. The *childhood-onset type* begins before age 10 years and probably has a more guarded prognosis, whereas the *adolescent-onset type* begins after age 10 years and is more likely to have a better outcome.

Box 14–3.   DSM-5 Diagnostic Criteria for Conduct Disorder

A. A repetitive and persistent pattern of behavior in which the basic rights of others or major age-appropriate societal norms or rules are violated, as manifested by the presence of at least three of the following 15 criteria in the past 12 months from any of the categories below, with at least one criterion present in the past 6 months:

Aggression to People and Animals

1. Often bullies, threatens, or intimidates others.
2. Often initiates physical fights.
3. Has used a weapon that can cause serious physical harm to others (e.g., a bat, brick, broken bottle, knife, gun).
4. Has been physically cruel to people.
5. Has been physically cruel to animals.
6. Has stolen while confronting a victim (e.g., mugging, purse snatching, extortion, armed robbery).
7. Has forced someone into sexual activity.

Destruction of Property

8. Has deliberately engaged in fire setting with the intention of causing serious damage.
9. Has deliberately destroyed others' property (other than by fire setting).

Deceitfulness or Theft

10. Has broken into someone else's house, building, or car.
11. Often lies to obtain goods or favors or to avoid obligations (i.e., "cons" others).
12. Has stolen items of nontrivial value without confronting a victim (e.g., shoplifting, but without breaking and entering; forgery).

Serious Violations of Rules

13. Often stays out at night despite parental prohibitions, beginning before age 13 years.

14. Has run away from home overnight at least twice while living in the parental or parental surrogate home, or once without returning for a lengthy period.
15. Is often truant from school, beginning before age 13 years.

B. The disturbance in behavior causes clinically significant impairment in social, academic, or occupational functioning.

C. If the individual is age 18 years or older, criteria are not met for antisocial personality disorder.

Specify whether:

Childhood-onset type: Individuals show at least one symptom characteristic of conduct disorder prior to age 10 years.

Adolescent-onset type: Individuals show no symptom characteristic of conduct disorder prior to age 10 years.

Unspecified onset: Criteria for a diagnosis of conduct disorder are met, but there is not enough information available to determine whether the onset of the first symptom was before or after age 10 years.

Specify if:

With limited prosocial emotions: To qualify for this specifier, an individual must have displayed at least two of the following characteristics persistently over at least 12 months and in multiple relationships and settings. These characteristics reflect the individual's typical pattern of interpersonal and emotional functioning over this period and not just occasional occurrences in some situations. Thus, to assess the criteria for the specifier, multiple information sources are necessary. In addition to the individual's self-report, it is necessary to consider reports by others who have known the individual for extended periods of time (e.g., parents, teachers, co-workers, extended family members, peers).

Lack of remorse or guilt: Does not feel bad or guilty when he or she does something wrong (exclude remorse when expressed only when caught and/or facing punishment). The individual shows a general lack of concern about the negative consequences of his or her actions. For example, the individual is not remorseful after hurting someone or does not care about the consequences of breaking rules.

Callous—lack of empathy: Disregards and is unconcerned about the feelings of others. The individual is described as cold and uncaring. The person appears more concerned about the effects of his or her actions on himself or herself, rather than their effects on others, even when they result in substantial harm to others.

Unconcerned about performance: Does not show concern about poor/problematic performance at school, at work, or in other important activities. The individual does not put forth the effort necessary to perform well, even when expectations are clear, and typically blames others for his or her poor performance.

Shallow or deficient affect: Does not express feelings or show emotions to others, except in ways that seem shallow, insincere, or superficial (e.g., actions contradict the emotion displayed; can turn emotions "on" or "off" quickly) or when emotional expressions are used for gain (e.g., emotions displayed to manipulate or intimidate others).

Specify current severity:

Mild: Few if any conduct problems in excess of those required to make the diagnosis are present, and conduct problems cause relatively minor harm to others (e.g., lying, truancy, staying out after dark without permission, other rule breaking).

Moderate: The number of conduct problems and the effect on others are intermediate between those specified in "mild" and those in "severe" (e.g., stealing without confronting a victim, vandalism).

Severe: Many conduct problems in excess of those required to make the diagnosis are present, or conduct problems cause considerable harm to others (e.g., forced sex, physical cruelty, use of a weapon, stealing while confronting a victim, breaking and entering).

Children who are especially difficult can be further designated as having *limited prosocial emotions* on the basis of their symptoms. This subtype is considered the childhood equivalent of the adult with psychopathy (an extreme form of antisocial personality disorder that is associated with callous behavior and lack of remorse).

Children or adolescents with conduct disorder typically are angry, sullen, and resentful when placed in the context of the adult world with its pressures to conform, stay in school, and persist in conspicuously dull activities. School performance usually is average to poor. These children or adolescents typically consider their schoolwork irrelevant or uninteresting, do not complete homework, and are often truant. When they are with their peers, their anger and sullenness often disappear and they seem to be having a good time. Beneath the veneer of anger, toughness, and rebellion, however, they often have profound feelings of self-doubt and worthlessness, although they may be reluctant to discuss these feelings with either adults or their peers. Some children with conduct disorder have been either physically or sexually abused by their parents.

The following is the case history of a girl with conduct disorder seen in one of our clinics:

Heather, a 14-year-old girl, was brought to the child psychiatry clinic by her mother with the complaint that "Heather is getting out of hand. I just can't seem to discipline her anymore." Heather was the youngest of four children and the only girl in the family. She was the product of a normal pregnancy and delivery and had completed her developmental milestones on schedule. She had been an average student but had taken a particular interest in sports as a child.

Heather's parents had separated and divorced 3 years earlier. This appeared to bother Heather much more than her brothers, because she had always been "her father's little girl." Her father had developed a relationship with a woman in another city, had moved away, saw the children infrequently, and was not dependable in child support payments.

Heather's behavior problems began when she entered junior high school. She began to enter puberty in sixth grade, and by seventh grade her body was markedly feminized. Her mother reported that she seemed to react to this by "acting tougher instead of more like a girl." She started to hang out more with boys her own age or slightly older and began to smoke cigarettes secretly (although the evidence could be smelled all over the house and on her clothes). Her grades, previously average, began to drop steadily. She also showed signs of increasingly devious behavior, lying to her mother about where she was going, returning at night well past predefined deadlines, and staying home "sick" without telling her mother. Items that Heather could not afford, such as expensive costume jewelry and cosmetics, began to appear in the house. Whenever Heather's mother confronted her, Heather became angry and ran out of the house, several times staying away overnight.

When interviewed alone, Heather was initially evasive and defensive, looking at the floor and answering questions very briefly. She was an attractive, slightly overweight, dark-haired girl attired in conventional teenage garb with a slightly punk touch (multiple earrings in her ears, leather boots, sleeveless T-shirt bearing an obscene logo and showing a nude couple embracing). Eventually she admitted to most of the conduct abnormalities that her mother had described.

It was concluded that Heather was having difficulties but that she had many strengths as well: a relatively intact childhood, normal intelligence, a history of adequate school performance, and a mother who appeared to genuinely care about her. Heather was seen in individual therapy on a weekly basis for 3–4 months, with a primary emphasis on supportive and relationship approaches. Heather began to talk freely about her difficulties in adjusting to the loss of her father, her experience of entering puberty, and her confusion about whether it was better to relate to her male peers (from whom she desperately desired love and approval) as a "tough girl" or a "sexy girl." With Heather's permission, she was also seen jointly with her mother in family therapy. Heather responded well to therapy, and it was possible to terminate the therapy successfully at the end of the school year.

About 8% of boys and 3% of girls meet criteria for conduct disorder. Research shows that an estimated 40% of boys and 25% of girls with conduct disorder will eventually qualify for a diagnosis of antisocial personality disorder. Children who are able to form relationships and to internalize social norms have a better outcome, as do children who are less aggressive. Age at onset may also affect outcome. Children who develop conduct problems at a very early age (e.g., 5 years) are more likely to have an enduring pattern of antisocial behavior than are children who develop behavioral problems linked to teenage peer pressure.

The etiology of conduct disorder is almost certainly multifactorial and involves genetics and psychosocial factors. Family studies indicate that children with conduct disorder tend to come from families with high prevalence rates of antisocial personality disorder, mood disorders, substance use disorders, and learning disorders. Adopted children may have higher rates of conduct disorder, consistent with reports that the adopted offspring of female felons have a high rate of antisocial behavior, such as traffic violations or arrests for robbery, which suggests that there may be at least some genetic component to conduct disorder. Psychosocial factors probably play a major role in the development of conduct disorders. These include parental separation or divorce; parental substance abuse; forms of poor parenting such as rejection, abandonment, abuse, inadequate supervision, and inconsistent or excessively harsh discipline; and association with a delinquent peer group.

Conduct disorder is highly comorbid with ADHD and mood and anxiety disorders. At least 10% of children with conduct disorder have specific learning disorders. In general, the greater the comorbidity, the more complicated the case and the worse the outcome.

The clinical management of conduct disorder varies greatly, depending on the age of the child, the symptoms with which he or she presents, the extent of comorbidity, the availability of family supports, and the child's intellectual and social assets. A relatively mild case, such as was represented by Heather, typically is treated with individual and family therapy. At the opposite extreme are those cases in which the child comes from a highly deviant family and engages in repeated antisocial acts that bring him or her to legal attention; such cases may require removal from the home and placement in a group home or perhaps even in a juvenile detention facility. In some situations, an important part of managing the child with a conduct disorder involves teaching the parents more effective parenting skills. With parental management training, parents learn to communicate more effectively with their child, to apply appropriate and consistent discipline, to monitor the child's whereabouts, and to steer the child away from bad peers. Research suggests that this approach may offer the best hope for the errant child.

Children and adolescents with conduct disorder and a co-occurring disorder (e.g., ADHD) can benefit from medication to treat the co-occurring disorder. Apart from such indications, however, medications are not typically used to treat conduct disorder. Nevertheless, lithium carbonate, psychostimulants, haloperidol, and second-generation antipsychotics are sometimes used "off label" to reduce aggression in children who are out of control. The use of these medications should be closely monitored because of their potential for serious adverse effects.

■ Pyromania

Pyromania is defined as deliberate and purposeful fire setting on more than one occasion; tension or affective arousal before the act; fascination with, interest in, curiosity about, or attraction to fire and its contents and characteristics; and pleasure, gratification, or relief when setting fires or when witnessing or participating in their aftermath (Box 14–4). Based on this definition, the arsonist who sets fires for monetary gain or for political or criminal purposes does not qualify for the diagnosis. People with antisocial personality disorder, conduct disorder, or mania sometimes set fires but do not have a sense of fascination with fire, nor do they experience the tension and relief with fire setting that people with pyromania describe. Deliberate fire setting is probably motivated most frequently by anger or revenge.

Box 14–4.　DSM-5 Diagnostic Criteria for Pyromania

A. Deliberate and purposeful fire setting on more than one occasion.
B. Tension or affective arousal before the act.
C. Fascination with, interest in, curiosity about, or attraction to fire and its situational contexts (e.g., paraphernalia, uses, consequences).
D. Pleasure, gratification, or relief when setting fires or when witnessing or participating in their aftermath.
E. The fire setting is not done for monetary gain, as an expression of sociopolitical ideology, to conceal criminal activity, to express anger or vengeance, to improve one's living circumstances, in response to a delusion or hallucination, or as a result of impaired judgment (e.g., in major neurocognitive disorder, intellectual disability [intellectual developmental disorder], substance intoxication).
F. The fire setting is not better explained by conduct disorder, a manic episode, or antisocial personality disorder.

There are few data on prevalence, but a study of psychiatric inpatients found that about 6% had a lifetime history of pyromania. Although pyromania was once thought to occur primarily in boys or men, a recent report suggests that gender distribution may be equal. Onset tends to be in the late teens or early 20s. Mood, substance use, and other impulsive behaviors are common in people with pyromania. Fire setting is considered a poor prognostic sign for children with conduct disorders and correlates with adult aggression.

Clinicians should begin by identifying other co-occurring mental disorders that can be a focus of treatment (e.g., major depression). Treatment of the coexisting disorder may itself reduce fire-setting behavior. There is no clear role for medication in the treatment of pyromania itself. If the patient is a child or adolescent, the parents should be taught consistent but nonpunitive methods of discipline. Family therapy may help in dealing with the broader issue of family dysfunction often found in patients with pyromania. The patient needs to understand the dangerousness and significance of the fire setting. With fire safety education, a visit to a burn unit or scene of a fire may help to make patients aware of the consequences of their behavior. Patients also need to learn alternative ways of coping with stressful situations to decrease reliance on fire setting as an outlet.

■ Kleptomania

Kleptomania involves the recurrent failure to resist impulses to steal objects not needed for personal use or for their monetary value; an increasing sense of tension immediately before committing the theft; and pleasure, gratification, or relief at the time of the theft (Box 14–5). The stealing is not committed to express anger or vengeance, is not in response to hallucinations or delusions, and is not better accounted for by antisocial personality disorder, conduct disorder, or a manic episode.

Box 14–5.   DSM-5 Diagnostic Criteria for Kleptomania

A. Recurrent failure to resist impulses to steal objects that are not needed for personal use or for their monetary value.
B. Increasing sense of tension immediately before committing the theft.
C. Pleasure, gratification, or relief at the time of committing the theft.
D. The stealing is not committed to express anger or vengeance and is not in response to a delusion or a hallucination.
E. The stealing is not better explained by conduct disorder, a manic episode, or antisocial personality disorder.

The prevalence of kleptomania is uncertain, but a survey of the U.S. general population showed shoplifting to have a lifetime prevalence of 11%. While most shoplifters do not have kleptomania, the data suggest that kleptomania may be more common than once thought. Mood and anxiety disorders frequently co-occur with kleptomania. Stealing impulses and behaviors often change along with the patient's mood.

Kleptomania begins in adolescence or early adulthood and tends to be chronic. Nearly three-quarters of persons with kleptomania are women. One of us (D.W.B.) followed clinically an 88-year-old woman with a history of impulsive stealing since age 16. Only the humiliation of an arrest at age 78, and the resultant publicity, kept her from stealing again, despite her nearly continuous urges.

There are no standard treatments, but medication may be helpful in some patients. One approach is to start by prescribing an SSRI antidepressant. If the patient fails to benefit from a trial of the SSRI, this can be followed by a trial of naltrexone (50–150 mg/day), which has specifically been found to be more effective than placebo in a randomized controlled trial but requires careful monitoring and can cause nausea and vomiting. Targeting treatment of a comorbid disorder (e.g., major depression) may also help reduce the stealing behaviors, particularly if they are prompted by dysphoric moods.

Individual psychotherapy that is cognitively based may help. The goal is to help steer the individuals away from stealing, to help them avoid cues that trigger stealing, and to teach them to substitute other, more benign behaviors to replace the stealing (e.g., socializing with friends rather than shopping alone).

As with the elderly woman described above, many persons with kleptomania are arrested for shoplifting and are processed through the legal system. The embarrassment and shame they experience may keep some from acting on their urges, but this tends not to last. Probation may help some by providing a regular reminder of what might occur if the person is caught stealing again. A self-imposed ban on shopping to head off potential thefts is probably the most common approach to managing the urges, but this is seldom sustainable in the long run.

■ Other Disruptive, Impulse-Control, and Conduct Disorders

Compulsive shopping and Internet addiction are two examples of disorders that, although not listed as diagnoses in DSM-5, would fall within the category *other specified disruptive, impulse-control, and conduct disorder.*

Compulsive Shopping

Compulsive shopping is characterized by an irresistible urge to buy items that are either unneeded or unwanted. The person usually has a feeling of tension before buying, followed by a sense of gratification or relief with buying. Compulsive shopping behavior can lead to serious financial problems, including bankruptcy, and can contribute to marital and family strife.

The disorder is chronic and typically has an onset in the late teens or early 20s, corresponding to the age when most persons become emancipated from their families and first obtain credit cards. Most compulsive shoppers are young women who spend excessive amounts on clothing, shoes, and makeup.

There is no standard treatment, although cognitive-behavioral therapy appears effective. SSRIs may be helpful in reducing the compulsive behaviors, particularly in depressed or anxious patients.

Internet Addiction

Internet addiction involves excessive or poorly controlled computer use that leads to impairment or distress. The disorder has attracted increasing attention that has paralleled the growth in computer use and Internet access. Internet addicts describe urges to use the computer when offline, to have a sense of tension or arousal before logging on, and to feel guilty or depressed when spending too much time online. There is no consensus regarding its treatment, but limiting a person's Internet access may help. *Internet gaming disorder* is a variant of Internet addiction but is focused on those who are preoccupied with computer-based games and is listed in the DSM-5 chapter "Conditions for Further Study."

Clinical points for disruptive, impulse-control, and conduct disorders

1. Oppositional defiant disorder needs to be distinguished from normal defiant behavior that typically occurs in young children (ages 2–4) and adolescents. Treatment will necessarily target both the child and the family.

2. Intermittent explosive disorder may respond to the SSRI fluoxetine, a mood stabilizer (e.g., oxcarbazepine), propranolol, or a second-generation antipsychotic.

    - CBT may help patients learn to identify stressors that trigger outbursts, which patients can then defuse.

> **Clinical points for disruptive, impulse-control, and conduct disorders (continued)**
>
> - Patients must know that they are responsible for the consequences of their behavior.
>
> 3. Conduct disorder is very difficult to treat, but mild cases may respond to a combination of psychotherapy and medication to reduce anger and irritability.
>
>   - Family therapy is essential because parents need help in understanding and managing their misbehaving child.
>
> 4. The child with pyromania may benefit from fire safety training.
>
>   - A visit to a burn center may be a graphic reminder of the harm he or she might cause others.
>
> 5. Persons with kleptomania may benefit from naltrexone or one of the SSRIs (e.g., fluoxetine, paroxetine).
>
>   - A self-imposed shopping ban may be the best short-term strategy to forestall stealing.
>
>   - Consumer credit counseling may be beneficial.
>
> 6. The Internet addict who lives at home should have his or her computer access monitored.
>
>   - Parents should consider canceling Internet service or limiting computer use.

■ Self-Assessment Questions

1. Describe oppositional defiant disorder and discuss its relationship to conduct disorder. Can ODD lead to adult antisocial personality disorder?
2. Define *intermittent explosive disorder*. Which disorders exclude this diagnosis?
3. Describe the symptoms of conduct disorder. What are the prevalence and gender ratio for conduct disorder? What are "limited prosocial emotions"?
4. Discuss pyromania and its differential diagnosis. What is its course and outcome? How can it be treated?
5. How does the person with kleptomania differ from the ordinary shoplifter?
6. Describe two examples of an "other specified disruptive, impulse-control, and conduct disorder."

Chapter 15

Substance-Related and Addictive Disorders

> I persevered in my abstinence for ninety hours.... Then I took—ask me not how much; say, ye severest, what would ye have done?
>
> *Thomas De Quincey,* Confessions
> of an English Opium Eater

Acornucopia of psychoactive substances is readily available with the potential for abuse and addiction. Alcohol is perhaps the oldest and most important example, but other substances of abuse also have been around since antiquity. Many others are a product of modern chemistry, and additional drugs continue to be synthesized at a dizzying pace.

The problems resulting from the misuse of alcohol or other substances appear more extensive today than in the past, probably because of increased availability. One consequence has been the rapid growth in arrests and incarceration for drug-related offenses, contributing to prison overcrowding. At the same time, the disease concept of addiction has taken hold, encouraging problem drinkers and drug abusers alike to seek help in a humane and nonjudgmental way. Nonetheless, receiving appropriate treatment in an overburdened and poorly funded system is an ongoing challenge.

Substance use disorders are widespread. The Epidemiologic Catchment Area survey in the 1980s found that the lifetime prevalence of alcohol use disorders ranged from 11.5% to 15.7%, drug use disorders from 5.5% to 5.8%, and any substance use disorder from 15% to 18.1%. The more recent National Epidemiological Study of Alcohol-Related Conditions reported 12-month prevalence rates of 8.5% for any alcohol use disorder and 2% for any drug use disorder. In these surveys, these disorders were more common in men, younger individuals, and those with low income.

Unfortunately, the true extent of substance use and abuse is much greater. Nearly two-thirds of adult Americans occasionally drink alcoholic beverages, and 12% drink almost every day and become intoxicated several times a month. Marijuana has been used by more than one-quarter of Americans and is regularly smoked by about 20 million Americans. A 2007 household survey found that nearly 6 million Americans admitted to using cocaine in the prior year. Patterns of use change, however, reflecting the fluctuating popularity of drugs, and their availability and cost.

■ Diagnosis of Substance-Related Disorders

Ten substance-related disorder classes are reviewed in this chapter: alcohol; caffeine; cannabis; hallucinogens (with separate categories for phencyclidine and other hallucinogens); inhalants; opioids; sedatives, hypnotics, and anxiolytics; stimulants; tobacco; and other (or unknown) substances (Table 15–1). DSM-IV's pathological gambling, now renamed *gambling disorder,* has been moved to this class, reflecting evidence that gambling activates the brain's reward system similarly to drugs of abuse. Although the term *addiction* appears in the title of the chapter, it is not used as a diagnostic term in DSM-5 because of its uncertain definition. Nonetheless, some clinicians choose to use the word as a form of shorthand—as do we—to describe severe problems related to alcohol or drug use (e.g., *addict, addictive, addiction*).

Substance use disorders involve the inappropriate use of a substance. In the past, problematic use was diagnosed as either *abuse* or *dependence,* distinguished mainly on the basis of severity. In DSM-5, abuse and dependence are merged so that each class of drug has its own criteria set for a "use" disorder. Research had shown that abuse and dependence diagnoses overlapped and that clinicians had trouble distinguishing one from the other. Also, intoxication and withdrawal are now separate disorders for most of the substances: *intoxication* is a reversible syndrome due to the recent use of a substance, whereas *withdrawal* consists of a cluster of symptoms with an onset closely following cessation of the drug (or reduction in dose) that is relatively specific to a drug (or drugs).

The substance use disorders follow a set of standard criteria. In each case 2 or more of 11 problematic behaviors must occur within a 12-month period leading to clinically significant impairment or distress. The 11 symptoms involve overall groupings of impaired control, social

---

TABLE 15–1. DSM-5 substance-related and addictive disorders

Alcohol-related disorders

Alcohol use disorder
Alcohol intoxication
Alcohol withdrawal

Caffeine-related disorders

Caffeine intoxication
Caffeine withdrawal

Cannabis-related disorders

Cannabis use disorder
Cannabis intoxication
Cannabis withdrawal

Hallucinogen-related disorders

Phencyclidine use disorder
Other hallucinogen use disorder
Phencyclidine intoxication
Other hallucinogen intoxication
Hallucinogen persisting perception disorder

Inhalant-related disorders

Inhalant use disorder
Inhalant intoxication

Opioid-related disorders

Opioid use disorder
Opioid intoxication
Opioid withdrawal

Sedative-, hypnotic-, or anxiolytic-related disorders

Sedative, hypnotic, or anxiolytic use disorder
Sedative, hypnotic, or anxiolytic intoxication
Sedative, hypnotic, or anxiolytic withdrawal

Stimulant-related disorders

Stimulant use disorder
Stimulant intoxication
Stimulant withdrawal

Tobacco-related disorders

Tobacco use disorder
Tobacco withdrawal

Other (or unknown) substance-related disorders

Other (or unknown) substance-induced disorders

Non-substance-related disorders

Gambling disorder

impairment, risky use, and pharmacological criteria (i.e., evidence of tolerance or withdrawal). **Because these criteria sets are so similar, only that for alcohol use disorder is reproduced in this chapter** (see Box 15–1 in section "Alcohol-Related Disorders" below). As a general rule, the use of one substance greatly increases the chance that a person will use another. In DSM-5, if criteria are met for more than one substance use disorder, all are diagnosed (e.g., severe alcohol use disorder, mild cannabis use disorder).

Substance use disorders are rated for severity: mild requires the presence of two or three symptoms; moderate, four or five symptoms; and severe, six or more symptoms. In addition, clinicians can specify if the disorder is in "early remission" (i.e., no symptom criteria met for the past 3 months), or "sustained remission" (i.e., no symptom criteria met for the past 12 months).

■ Assessment of Substance-Related Disorders

The assessment of substance-related disorders requires a careful history, a thorough physical examination, and a detailed mental status examination. Few addicted persons will spontaneously report their alcohol or drug use. More commonly, these individuals will present for evaluation of a medical complaint or for emotional distress. Some will be brought in by concerned family members seeking assessment for their loved one.

A detailed interview may help to uncover social, marital, occupational, or legal problems that may have contributed to the substance use. The clinician should remember that misuse of a substance—alcohol, drugs, or both—can lead to the development of depression, mania, or psychoses. Likewise, many addicted persons will have co-occurring mental disorders, such as major depression, bipolar disorder, or an anxiety disorder, that should be diagnosed and treated. Personality disorders—particularly antisocial and borderline personality disorders—are common in addicted persons and may contribute to continued substance misuse.

Additional history obtained from relatives or friends, or from other physicians, will help fill in the gaps. Even patients who are straightforward about their misuse of substances may minimize its extent. Once the physician's suspicion has been raised, he or she should inquire specifically about each class of commonly misused substances and record the patient's pattern of use.

A physical examination can offer signs of intoxication and withdrawal, depending on when the individual presents at a hospital or clinic. The clinician should be forthright and nonjudgmental and help these patients obtain needed services.

Laboratory testing for substances of abuse has become a routine part of the work-up in emergency departments for patients who are unresponsive or confused; tests are also routinely used now during insurance examinations, in the workplace, in the military, and in the criminal justice system. Intoxication and overdosage are the most common indications to test for drugs of abuse, but such testing should be considered when assessing a patient who presents with alterations in mood or behavior. Most testing involves sampling blood or urine. Urine drug screenings are easily performed and are generally reported as positive or negative for a particular substance. Blood alcohol levels (discussed later) are easily obtained. Most screenings cover the major substances of abuse. Due to contamination, morning urine sampling should be avoided, and if sample dilution or substitution is suspected, direct observation of voiding may be indicated. Cannabis, which is fat soluble, can be detected in urine up to 3 weeks after the last use.

The following patient treated at our hospital illustrates many of the symptoms that beset substance abusers, as well as some of the factors that lead to the abuse. Laura's story also points to the dilemma that caregivers face with uncooperative patients and our imperfect solutions:

> Laura, a 21-year-old American Indian nursing assistant, was referred to the hospital for evaluation of substance abuse. She was adopted at an early age, and her adoptive parents took care to ensure that she was adequately clothed and fed but provided little emotional nurturing. Laura was sexually molested for several years by one of her adoptive brothers, and at age 12 she became pregnant by him. She carried the baby to term and gave it up for adoption.
>
> Laura started using marijuana and drinking alcoholic beverages at age 12; she was using "uppers" by age 14 and later turned to inhaled cocaine and crack. She also admitted to having tried an assortment of other drugs, including PCP, lysergic acid diethylamide (LSD), and heroin. To pay for her drug use, Laura sold drugs and later engaged in prostitution.
>
> In the 6 months before her hospitalization, she had begun to inject cocaine intravenously, sometimes in combination with heroin (a "speedball") and reported that she enjoyed the sexual feelings she received from the injections. Laura admitted using unclean needles despite knowing that they could transmit HIV. Her boyfriend was a drug dealer with an extensive prison record and worked as her pimp.
>
> Laura had received prior mental health treatment for depression and had had several admissions for drug detoxification, one after a suicide attempt. She usually left against medical advice.

Laura was referred under a court order and told us she had no plans to stop using drugs. She was eventually transferred to a drug rehabilitation center. The referral was based on our hope that at some point the treatment would "take." Our alternative was to do nothing.

■ Etiology of Substance-Related Disorders

The combination of genetics and individual biology, the person's environment, and the substance itself leads to addictive disorders. No single factor determines whether a person will abuse drugs or alcohol.

Some people appear to have an inherited vulnerability to substance abuse. Research strongly supports a role for genetics in the etiology of alcohol and other substance use disorders (e.g., tobacco, opioids), including family, twin, and adoption studies. Genetic factors are estimated to contribute to 40%–60% of the variability in the risk for addiction. The neurobiological mechanisms by which environmental factors interact with genes to create vulnerability to addiction are just beginning to be understood.

Molecular genetic techniques are being used to search for an alcohol use disorder gene (or genes). The best-replicated findings are genes encoding for the alcohol-metabolizing enzymes that are protective against the development of alcoholism. An example is the *ADH2*2* allele, which is common among Asian populations and may help to explain their lower prevalence of alcohol use disorders. It is likely that multiple genes conferring vulnerability interact with multiple environmental risk factors.

Research has begun to identify the neurobiological substrates of addiction. Dopamine pathways that form part of the central nervous system (CNS) "reward system" have been identified in the ventral tegmental region of the forebrain and in the nucleus accumbens. All drugs of abuse appear to target the brain's reward system by flooding the circuit with dopamine. In another example, the opioids bind with μ opioid receptors that imitate the action of β-endorphin with these same receptors, triggering a cascade of biochemical brain processes associated with normal activities that promote pleasure (e.g., eating, sex). The association of drug-induced pleasurable experiences likely results in strong conditioning, which may account for the enhanced excitement reported by substance users.

The pharmacological properties of the drug itself may contribute to abuse. Some agents (e.g., alcohol, opioids, anxiolytics) can produce rapid relief of anxiety. Stimulants generally relieve boredom and fatigue and provide a sensation of energy and increased mental alertness. Hallucinogens provide a temporary escape from reality. These properties all contribute to misuse. Substances that do not give pleasure to the user (e.g., haloperidol) are rarely abused. In general, drugs with rapid onset and briefer action (e.g., cocaine, alprazolam) are preferred. Methods of administration that enhance the rapidity of onset—for example, sniffing, smoking, or intravenous use—are often exploited to provide an added kick. Tolerance and withdrawal symptoms also contribute to abuse. Users quickly learn that higher doses of some substances are needed to get the same effect and that the drug itself can be used to prevent unpleasant withdrawal symptoms.

Other medical and psychiatric disorders have been linked with substance misuse, including chronic pain, anxiety disorders, and depression. Many patients experiencing physical or emotional pain often seek relief through drugs or alcohol and are at high risk for substance misuse. And while no single personality pattern has been associated with substance misuse, the frequency of personality disorders among substance abusers is very high. Other psychological characteristics seen in substance abusers include hostility, low frustration tolerance, inflexibility, and inability to delay gratification. Several longitudinal studies have shown that many of these traits (e.g., aggressiveness, childhood rebellion) predict the development of substance misuse.

Societal and family values influence the use of illicit drugs. When parents smoke cigarettes, drink alcoholic beverages, or use drugs, their offspring are more prone to use these substances, perhaps through learning that their use is socially acceptable. People whose friends use alcohol or drugs are more likely to use them as well, which suggests that peers influence a person's choices. Susceptibility to peer influence has been associated with the lack of a close bond with one's parents, a large amount of time spent away from home, and increased reliance on peers as opposed to parents.

■ Alcohol-Related Disorders

Alcohol is the most commonly abused substance in most parts of the world and is associated with significant morbidity and mortality. While common in the general population, alcohol use disorders are even more frequent in hospital patients, including 25%–50% of medical-surgical patients and up to 50%–60% of psychiatric inpatients in some settings. People who misuse alcohol are commonly referred to as "alcoholic" by the lay public.

There are two to three men for each woman with an alcohol use disorder, and the usual age at onset is between ages 16 and 30. Onset is earlier in men than women, although the medical complications progress more rapidly in women. People in certain occupations are prone to alcohol use disorder, including bartenders, construction workers, and writers. Other groups prone to alcoholism include individuals who use tobacco; those with mood and anxiety disorders; those with antisocial personality disorder; and those with a gambling disorder.

Diagnosis and Assessment

Alcohol use disorder is a problematic pattern of alcohol use leading to clinically significant impairment or distress. Two or more of 11 problematic behaviors must occur within a 12-month period for the diagnosis to be made (Box 15–1). Depending on the number of symptoms present, the disorder is specified as *mild, moderate,* or *severe.* Separate categories are used for *alcohol intoxication* and *alcohol withdrawal.* The clinician should record all diagnoses that are present (e.g., alcohol intoxication, moderate alcohol use disorder).

Box 15–1. DSM-5 Diagnostic Criteria for Alcohol Use Disorder

A. A problematic pattern of alcohol use leading to clinically significant impairment or distress, as manifested by at least two of the following, occurring within a 12-month period:

1. Alcohol is often taken in larger amounts or over a longer period than was intended.
2. There is a persistent desire or unsuccessful efforts to cut down or control alcohol use.
3. A great deal of time is spent in activities necessary to obtain alcohol, use alcohol, or recover from its effects.
4. Craving, or a strong desire or urge to use alcohol.
5. Recurrent alcohol use resulting in a failure to fulfill major role obligations at work, school, or home.
6. Continued alcohol use despite having persistent or recurrent social or interpersonal problems caused or exacerbated by the effects of alcohol.
7. Important social, occupational, or recreational activities are given up or reduced because of alcohol use.
8. Recurrent alcohol use in situations in which it is physically hazardous.
9. Alcohol use is continued despite knowledge of having a persistent or recurrent physical or psychological problem that is likely to have been caused or exacerbated by alcohol.

10. Tolerance, as defined by either of the following:
    a. A need for markedly increased amounts of alcohol to achieve intoxication or desired effect.
    b. A markedly diminished effect with continued use of the same amount of alcohol.
11. Withdrawal, as manifested by either of the following:
    a. The characteristic withdrawal syndrome for alcohol (refer to Criteria A and B of the criteria set for alcohol withdrawal, [DSM-5] pp. 499–500).
    b. Alcohol (or a closely related substance, such as a benzodiazepine) is taken to relieve or avoid withdrawal symptoms.

Specify if:

In early remission: After full criteria for alcohol use disorder were previously met, none of the criteria for alcohol use disorder have been met for at least 3 months but for less than 12 months (with the exception that Criterion A4, "Craving, or a strong desire or urge to use alcohol," may be met).

In sustained remission: After full criteria for alcohol use disorder were previously met, none of the criteria for alcohol use disorder have been met at any time during a period of 12 months or longer (with the exception that Criterion A4, "Craving, or a strong desire or urge to use alcohol," may be met).

Specify if:

In a controlled environment: This additional specifier is used if the individual is in an environment where access to alcohol is restricted.

Specify current severity:

Mild: Presence of 2–3 symptoms.
Moderate: Presence of 4–5 symptoms.
Severe: Presence of 6 or more symptoms.

---

[a]Criteria for alcohol use disorder are shown to represent the similar criteria sets for all the DSM-5 substance use disorders.

The four-question CAGE test is a simple screen that can be used to assess the presence of an alcohol use disorder (see Table 15–2). Problematic use is suggested by any positive response or overly defensive answer.

Blood alcohol concentration roughly correlates with level of intoxication. The following levels apply to persons who are not tolerant to alcohol:

0–100 mg/dL: A sense of well-being, sedation, tranquility
100–150 mg/dL: Incoordination, irritability
150–250 mg/dL: Slurred speech, ataxia
>250 mg/dL: Passing out, unconsciousness

TABLE 15–2. CAGE: screening test for an alcohol use disorder

C   Have you felt the need to CUT DOWN on your drinking?

A   Have you felt ANNOYED BY CRITICISM of your drinking?

G   Have you felt GUILTY (or had regrets) about your drinking?

E   Have you felt the need for an EYE-OPENER in the morning?

Source.   Adapted from Ewing 1984.

Higher concentrations—greater than 350 mg/dL—can lead to coma and death. The presence of few clinical symptoms of intoxication in a person with a level of 150 mg/dL or higher is strong evidence of an alcohol use disorder.

In many jurisdictions, a motor vehicle operator is considered legally under the influence at a blood alcohol concentration of 0.08 g per 100 mL, equivalent to 80 mg/dL. In hospitals and clinics, blood samples are used to test for blood alcohol levels, but breath testing for alcohol has become a standard part of the roadside assessment for driving impairment.

Other laboratory measures can be useful. People with alcohol use disorder can develop increased high-density lipoprotein cholesterol, increased lactate dehydroxygenase, decreased low-density lipoprotein cholesterol, decreased blood urea nitrogen, decreased red blood cell volume, and increased uric acid level. Mean corpuscular volume is increased in up to 95% of individuals with an alcohol use disorder. Liver enzymes are frequently abnormal, including an increase in γ-glutamyltransferase (GGT) level, which may be an early sign of alcohol misuse. Transaminase (aspartate aminotransferase and alanine aminotransferase) levels also are increased.

Clinical Findings

There is no standard or general clinical picture of people who misuse alcohol. In its earliest stages, alcohol misuse can be difficult to identify. With the person in denial, family members and coworkers are often in the best position to identify early symptoms. These can include lowered work productivity, lateness or unexplained absences, and irritability or moodiness.

As the disorder progresses, physical changes can occur, such as the development of acne rosacea; palmar erythema; or painless enlargement of the liver consistent with fatty infiltration. Other early manifestations include respiratory or other infections, unexplained bruises, periods of amnesia, minor accidents (e.g., unexplained falls at home), and concerns about the person's driving skills or an arrest or accident related to driving while intoxicated. As the disorder advances, jaundice or ascites can develop, as can testicular atrophy, gynecomastia, and Dupuytren's contractures. At this point the misuse of alcohol has probably disrupted the person's life, contributing to job loss, loss of friendships, and both marital discord and family problems.

The following case illustrates the many types of problems that developed in a man with an alcohol use disorder:

> Ed, a 66-year-old attorney, was brought to an alcohol rehabilitation unit by his wife and son. On arrival, he smelled of alcohol and was mildly disheveled. In a belligerent manner, and slurring his words, Ed said that he would not stay. His wife intervened and told him firmly that she would file for divorce if he refused to stay and get help. He stayed.
>
> Ed had a 20-year history of excessive drinking. He had started drinking socially while in the Army. After his military service he had married, obtained his law degree, and established a successful career as a trial attorney. Although he sometimes enjoyed a single beer or cocktail after work, the drinking never progressed. In his mid-40s, Ed's alcohol consumption began to escalate. He would drink several beers or cocktails in the evening and then fall asleep. He and his wife began to fight, mainly about his drinking, which he denied was a problem.
>
> A series of personal crises followed. Ed had an affair with a divorcée, separated from his wife, and eventually sought a divorce. He had a falling-out with his law partners and withdrew from his longtime friends. His drinking took a more serious turn. His caseload decreased as lawyers in his town became aware of his impairment. He began to drink in the morning, had several cocktails at lunch, and continued his drinking in the evening, finally passing out on the sofa. He continued to deny his alcoholism, even when confronted by his new wife and all his children.
>
> His doctor became concerned. Ed was overweight and hypertensive and had developed the stigmata of alcoholism: spider angiomata, acne rosacea, and palmar erythema. The progression of his alcoholism was so gradual that by the time of hospital admission, no one could remember what Ed's personality had once been like.
>
> The inpatient program consisted of individual, group, and family therapy sessions following an uneventful withdrawal. By the end of his 30-day stay, he was noticeably happier, was more optimistic, and looked forward to the future. Three years later, he was still abstinent, had developed a more satisfying relationship with his wife and children, and had reestablished his law practice.

Medical Complications

Alcohol use disorders can affect a person's medical and emotional health and lead to a broad range of social problems (Table 15–3). Medical problems range from benign fatty infiltration of the liver to fulminant liver failure. Almost all organ systems are affected by the heavy use of alcohol. The gastrointestinal tract is particularly affected, with consequences including gastritis, diarrhea, and peptic ulcers. Other effects include fatty infiltration of the liver, cirrhosis in about 10% of heavy drinkers, and pancreatitis. Cardiomyopathy, thrombocytopenia, anemia, and myopathy have all been reported.

The CNS and peripheral nervous system may be damaged by the direct and indirect effects of alcohol. Peripheral neuropathy commonly occurs in a stocking-and-glove distribution, probably the result of an alcohol-induced vitamin B deficiency. Cerebellar damage can cause dysarthria and ataxia. Wernicke's encephalopathy can result from thiamine deficiency and consists of nystagmus, ataxia, and mental confusion (which may reverse with an injection of thiamine). The Wernicke-Korsakoff syndrome occurs when cognitive and memory impairment endures, although it may be reversible in one-third of patients. This syndrome involves an anterograde amnesia characterized by the presence of *confabulation,* in which a patient invents stories to fill in memory gaps. The syndrome is associated with necrotic lesions of the mamillary bodies, thalamus, and other brain stem regions.

A major neurocognitive disorder (dementia) can develop as a result of either vitamin deficiency or the direct effects of alcohol, although the exact mechanism is unknown. Chronic alcohol misuse also has been associated with enlarged cerebral ventricles and widened cortical sulci, effects that may be partially reversible when the individual stops drinking. Neuropsychological testing of alcoholic persons generally reveals mild to moderate cognitive deficits that, like structural abnormalities, partially reverse with sobriety.

The *fetal alcohol syndrome* (FAS) has been described in children whose mothers are alcoholic. This syndrome is related to excessive maternal consumption of alcohol during pregnancy, especially when binge drinking produces a surge in blood alcohol levels. Abnormalities associated with this disorder include facial anomalies (i.e., small head circumference, epicanthic folds, indistinct philtrum, small midface), low IQ, and behavior problems. FAS affects about one to two infants per 100,000 live births. Women should be warned that FAS can result from alcohol consumption during pregnancy.

TABLE 15–3. **Medical and psychosocial hazards associated with alcohol use disorders**

Drug interactions

Gastrointestinal
  Esophageal bleeding
  Mallory-Weiss tear
  Gastritis
  Intestinal malabsorption

Pancreatitis

Liver disease
  Fatty infiltration
  Hepatitis
  Cirrhosis

Nutritional deficiency
  Malnutrition
  Vitamin B deficiency

Neuropsychiatric
  Wernicke-Korsakoff syndrome
  Cortical atrophy/ventricular dilation
  Alcohol-induced dementia
  Peripheral neuropathy
  Myopathy
  Depression
  Suicide

Endocrine system
  Testicular atrophy
  Increased estrogen levels

Alcohol withdrawal
  Uncomplicated withdrawal (the "shakes")
  Seizures
  Hallucinosis
  Withdrawal delirium (delirium tremens)

Infectious disease
  Pneumonia
  Tuberculosis

Cardiovascular
  Cardiomyopathy
  Hypertension

Cancer
  Oral cavity
  Esophagus
  Large intestine/rectum
  Liver
  Pancreas

Birth defects
  Fetal alcohol syndrome

Psychosocial
  Accidents
  Crime
  Spouse and child abuse
  Job loss
  Divorce, separation

Alcohol consumption is a frequent cause of traumatic injuries and contributes to more than 50% of all motor vehicle deaths each year. Household injuries also are common. Subdural hematomas occur in many elderly persons who fall and sustain head injuries when intoxicated.

Cancer rates of the mouth, tongue, larynx, esophagus, stomach, liver, and pancreas are increased. The precise role that alcohol plays in these cancers is uncertain because its effects are confounded by those of smoking and tobacco use. Alcohol interferes with male sexual function and can cause impotence and affect fertility by lowering serum testosterone levels. Increased circulating levels of estrogen can cause breast enlargement (gynecomastia) and a female escutcheon (pubic hair pattern) in men.

Psychiatric complications include intoxication and withdrawal disorders, amnestic syndromes such as Wernicke-Korsakoff syndrome, and/or alcohol-related neurocognitive disorders. Major depression occurs in up to 60% of alcoholic patients. Suicide rates are high among those who misuse alcohol; at greatest risk are those with a history of interpersonal loss within the past year, best defined as the loss of an intimate relationship.

Course and Outcome

In a review of 10 large studies, researchers concluded that 2%–3% of people with an alcohol use disorder become abstinent each year and about 1% return to asymptomatic or controlled drinking. These findings were true for both treated and untreated samples, supporting the hypothesis that alcohol use disorders are self-limiting for some persons. In the 10 studies, 46%–87% of the subjects continued to misuse alcohol at follow-up; 0%–33% were asymptomatic drinkers; and 8%–39% had achieved abstinence.

Clinical Management

Alcohol-related disorders often require medical intervention. Intoxication is the most common disorder and rarely requires more than simple supportive measures, such as decreasing external stimuli and removing the source of alcohol. When respiration is compromised by excessive alcohol intake, intensive care may be required.

Treatment of alcohol withdrawal depends on the syndrome that develops. Importantly, while withdrawal symptoms typically follow the abrupt cessation of alcohol consumption, they can also develop when users simply reduce their usual high intake.

- *Uncomplicated alcohol withdrawal* (the "shakes") begins 12–18 hours after the cessation of drinking and peaks at 24–48 hours, then subsides within 5–7 days, even without treatment. Minor symptoms include anxiety, tremors, and nausea and vomiting; heart rate and blood pressure may be increased.
- *Alcoholic withdrawal seizures* ("rum fits") occur 7–38 hours after the cessation of drinking and peak between 24 and 48 hours. The patient may have a single burst of one to six generalized seizures; status ep-

ilepticus is rare. Withdrawal seizures occur primarily as a consequence of severe, long-term alcohol misuse.

- *Alcoholic hallucinosis*—vivid and unpleasant auditory, visual, or tactile hallucinations—begins within 48 hours of cessation of drinking and occurs in the presence of a clear sensorium. The hallucinations typically last about 1 week but can become chronic. Like withdrawal seizures, they are a sign of severe alcohol misuse.

- *Alcohol withdrawal delirium* (delirium tremens, or "DTs") occurs in about 5% of hospitalized alcoholic patients but in about one-third of those with withdrawal seizures. Symptoms include confusion, agitation, perceptual disturbance mild fever, and autonomic hyperarousal. The delirium begins 2–3 days after the drinking stops or after a significant reduction of intake and peaks 4 or 5 days later. Death is rare, although mortality rates of 15% were reported in the past.

Clinicians should always ask patients to describe their past symptoms that had developed when they either stopped drinking or cut back from their usual heavy drinking. The most common symptoms reported are mild tremors; far fewer will have had seizures, hallucinations, or delirium tremens. Some patients will misidentify their shakes as "DTs"; however, few people truly understand delirium tremens (including physicians!). Further, a patient would be unlikely to recall an episode of delirium tremens. For that reason, students might ask patients whether a doctor had ever told them that they had been agitated or confused, or required seclusion or restraint, during withdrawal.

The following case illustrates the dramatic nature of an alcohol withdrawal delirium and its management:

Dave, a 34-year-old unemployed veteran, requested admission for alcohol withdrawal treatment. He had a 10-year history of alcoholism and had experienced delirium tremens, blackouts, and withdrawal seizures. He had been admitted many times for alcohol withdrawal and rehabilitation services and was well known at the hospital for his unpleasant and critical attitude.

Dave had been drinking heavily—about 1 quart of liquor daily—since his last inpatient stay 3 months earlier, particularly during the week before seeking help. He was tremulous, hypertensive, and diaphoretic. The "Librium protocol" (i.e., chlordiazepoxide taper, described later) was instituted. To the chagrin of the treatment team, Dave insisted on leaving against medical advice the next day.

Dave was brought back to the hospital the following day by the police. He had been found wandering aimlessly in the nearby town. He was noticeably paranoid and thought that he was being plotted against. He was also disoriented; he knew where he was but was unable to give the date or the year. By the next morning, Dave was febrile, had very high diastolic blood pressure, and was diaphoretic. Because of his belligerence and physical restlessness, he was placed in seclusion, and restraints were used for his protection. Over the next 2 days, he received nearly 1,200 mg of chlordiazepoxide, but he remained loud and agitated. Intravenous hydration was required because of his poor oral intake. The nurses observed him playing an imaginary game of chess with unseen partners.

On the third day of hospitalization, Dave awakened and was fully oriented. He remained suspicious but was no longer hallucinating. He gradually returned to his baseline over the next week and was discharged.

The management of alcohol withdrawal consists of general support (i.e., adequate food and hydration, careful medical monitoring), nutritional supplementation, and the use of benzodiazepines. People who have a history of uncomplicated withdrawal and have a physician who is familiar with the patient can be managed as outpatients. Treatment may include chlordiazepoxide (25–50 mg four times daily), tapered slowly over the next 4–5 days.

Those with comorbid medical conditions or mental disorders, impaired ability to follow instructions, inadequate or absent social support, or a history of severe withdrawal symptoms will require careful monitoring and may need to be hospitalized. Patients should receive an adequate diet plus oral thiamine (100 mg), folic acid (1 mg), and multivitamins. Thiamine (100–200 mg intramuscularly) can be administered if oral intake is not possible and should be given before any situation in which glucose loading is required, because glucose can deplete thiamine stores. Chlordiazepoxide should be administered in dosages ranging from 25 to 100 mg orally four times daily on the first day, with a 20% per day decrease in dosage over 4–5 days. (A specific protocol is recommended in Table 15–4.) Additional doses can be given for breakthrough signs or symptoms (e.g., tremors or diaphoresis). The 10-item Clinical Institute Withdrawal Assessment is an objective rating scale that can be used to monitor the withdrawal state.

Chlordiazepoxide and the other benzodiazepines are the preferred drugs for withdrawal because of their safety and cross-tolerance with alcohol. Chlordiazepoxide is most often recommended because of its long half-life and low cost, but other benzodiazepines work just as well. Intermediate- or short-acting benzodiazepines (e.g., lorazepam, oxazepam) are generally preferred in patients with liver damage or in elderly patients because these benzodiazepines lack metabolites and are renally excreted. Diazepam can be given to interrupt seizures should status epilepticus occur. Other drugs, including carbamazepine, clonidine, propranolol, and valproate, have been used to treat alcohol withdrawal, but their role in treating the disorder is not yet clear.

TABLE 15–4. Management of alcohol withdrawal syndromes

---

1. Chlordiazepoxide protocol

    - 50 mg every 4 hours × 24 hours, then
    - 50 mg every 6 hours × 24 hours, then
    - 25 mg every 4 hours × 24 hours, then
    - 25 mg every 6 hours × 24 hours

The protocol should be started when 3 of the following 7 parameters are met: systolic blood pressure >160 mm Hg, diastolic blood pressure >100 mm Hg, pulse >110 beats/min, temperature >38.3°C, nausea, vomiting, or tremors. The dose should be held if any of the following signs are present: nystagmus, sedation, ataxia, slurred speech, or the patient is asleep.

2. Thiamine: 50–100 mg orally or intramuscularly × 1; folic acid: 1 mg/day orally

3. Haloperidol: 2–5 mg/day; or risperidone: 2–6 mg/day for patients with alcoholic hallucinosis

4. For delirium tremens:

    - 10 mg of intravenous diazepam (or 2–4 mg of lorazepam), followed by 5-mg doses (or 1–2 mg of lorazepam) every 5–15 minutes until calm; once stabilized, the dosage may be tapered slowly over 4 or 5 days
    - Seclusion and restraints as necessary
    - Adequate hydration and nutrition

Delirious patients require additional care; this may include seclusion and restraints. To facilitate patient care, 10 mg of intravenous diazepam (or 2–4 mg of lorazepam) may be given, followed by 5-mg doses every 5–15 minutes (or 1–2 mg of lorazepam) thereafter until the patient is calm. Once the patient has stabilized, the benzodiazepine dosage should be tapered slowly over the next 4 or 5 days. Intravenous hydration also may be necessary, although most alcoholic patients are overhydrated, not dehydrated, as is commonly believed. Any electrolyte disturbance should be corrected, and the patient should be examined for injuries or evidence of a physical illness (e.g., pneumonia).

Haloperidol (2–5 mg/day) or one of the second-generation antipsychotics (e.g., risperidone, 2–6 mg/day) may help relieve the frightening hallucinations of the patient with alcoholic hallucinosis. The medication usually is discontinued when the hallucinations stop.

Rehabilitation

Rehabilitation follows the alcohol detoxification process. There are two goals: 1) that the patient remain sober, and 2) that coexisting disorders be identified and treated. Perhaps two-thirds of these patients have additional mental disorders (including mood or anxiety disorders) and will benefit from their treatment. Because an alcohol use disorder itself can cause depression and most alcohol-induced depressions lift with sobriety, antidepressants are probably needed only for patients who remain depressed after 2–4 weeks of sobriety.

As a first step, the patient should be told that his or her disorder is significant and potentially life-threatening. Receiving a diagnosis may be the single most important step in leading to change.

Patients should be encouraged to attend Alcoholics Anonymous (AA), a worldwide self-help group for recovering alcoholic persons founded in 1935. AA uses a program of 12 steps; new members are asked to admit their problems, to give up a sense of personal control over the disease, to make personal amends, and to help others to achieve sobriety. The meetings provide a blend of acceptance, belonging, forgiveness, and understanding.

A team approach is used for hospitalized patients. Group therapy enables patients to see their own problems mirrored in others and to learn better coping skills. With individual therapy, the person can learn to identify triggers that prompt drinking and learn more effective coping strategies. Family therapy is often important because the family system that has been altered to accommodate the person's drinking may end up reinforcing it. These issues can be addressed in family therapy. Inpatient programs also provide education about the harmful effects of alcohol.

Motivational interviewing is being increasingly used to help persuade patients to make their own case for change (i.e., to abandon alcohol). Avoiding confrontation, the therapist seeks to achieve clarity about the patient's motivation for change, impediments that stand in the way of making needed change, and possible actions that might bring about change.

The U.S. Food and Drug Administration (FDA) has approved the use of three drugs—disulfiram, naltrexone, and acamprosate—for the treatment of DSM-IV alcohol dependence (which roughly corresponds to DSM-5's moderate or severe alcohol use disorder). Disulfiram inhibits aldehyde dehydrogenase, an enzyme necessary for the metabolism of alcohol. Inhibiting this enzyme leads to the accumulation of acetaldehyde when alcohol is consumed. Acetaldehyde is toxic and induces noxious symptoms, such as nausea, vomiting, palpitations, and hypotension. Disulfiram should be prescribed only after careful consideration and with the full cooperation of the patient. The usual dosage is 250 mg once daily. Because patients taking disulfiram are aware of the potential adverse reaction, they are motivated to avoid alcohol.

Naltrexone, a μ-opioid antagonist, appears to reduce the pleasurable effects of and craving for alcohol. The recommended daily dosage is 50 mg. The drug is generally well tolerated but can produce nausea, headache, anxiety, or sedation. A black box warning advises that naltrexone not be given to people with severe liver disease and that its use requires periodic monitoring of liver enzymes. Acamprosate, a glutamate receptor modulator, also reduces craving. Acamprosate is generally well tolerated, although some patients report headache, diarrhea, flatulence, and nausea. The recommended dosage is two 333-mg tablets three times a day, a dosing schedule that may limit its acceptance.

Both naltrexone and acamprosate help patients to maintain abstinence, thereby reducing the risk of relapse. For those who are chronically noncompliant, naltrexone is also available in an extended-release injectable formulation that is administered monthly.

A large government-supported multicenter trial, the COMBINE study, found that naltrexone, when given with a modest program of medical management, was as effective as specialized behavioral treatment in preventing relapse. The researchers concluded that naltrexone along with medical management could be easily delivered in most health care settings, thus serving alcohol-abusing persons who might otherwise not receive treatment.

Rehabilitation programs usually take place in residential or outpatient settings. In general, the patients most likely to benefit have a stable marriage and home life, are employed, have fewer co-occurring psychiatric disorders (especially antisocial personality disorder), and have no family history of alcoholism. Nearly 50% of treated alcoholic persons relapse, most commonly during the first 6 months following treatment. Even though relapse is common, treatment should be viewed as beneficial and cost-effective, with the potential to reduce the medical and social complications of alcohol use disorders.

Clinical points for management of alcohol-related disorders

1. People who misuse alcohol need acceptance and not blame.

2. Even if the person has failed to benefit from rehabilitation efforts, the clinician must not give up!

3. Treatment of alcohol withdrawal should take place in an inpatient setting if the patient has a history of severe "shakes," hallucinations, seizures, or delirium tremens. Other patients—perhaps the majority— can be treated on an outpatient basis.

Clinical points for management of alcohol-related disorders _(continued)_
•   Chlordiazepoxide is standard treatment, but other benzodiazepines (e.g., lorazepam, clonazepam) work just as well.
4.   The clinician should manage the patient's other comorbid disorders (e.g., panic disorder, major depression); when untreated, these disorders can contribute to relapse.
5.   The patient should be referred to AA to provide ongoing social support and encouragement from persons similarly affected.
6.   The family should be included in the treatment process.
•   Alcohol use disorders affect every member of the family, and unresolved issues may lead to relapse.
•   Family members should be encouraged to attend Al-Anon, a support group for relatives of people who misuse alcohol.

■ Other Substance-Related Disorders

Caffeine-Related Disorders

Caffeine is by far the most commonly used psychoactive substance in the world. The most potent source of caffeine is coffee, with tea and soft drinks providing smaller amounts. Caffeine is also available in nonprescription products such as analgesics and many over-the-counter pain and cold remedies. Research evidence supports the diagnoses of both _caffeine intoxication_ and _caffeine withdrawal._ While some caffeine users appear to have symptoms consistent with problematic use, there is no "use" disorder category in DSM-5.

The mild stimulant effects of caffeine occur at doses of 50–150 mg (i.e., one cup of coffee). These effects include increased alertness and improved verbal and motor performance. At higher dosages, unless tolerance has been achieved, signs of intoxication occur, including restlessness, irritability, and insomnia. Massive doses can lead to seizures and coma. Withdrawal from caffeine can induce headaches, lethargy, irritability, and depression. Higher daily dosages are more likely to lead to withdrawal.

Because caffeine is well known to aggravate anxiety syndromes such as panic disorder and generalized anxiety disorder, clinicians should always ask patients about their caffeine intake. Chronic use can itself cause excessive anxiety; in DSM-5, this condition is called _caffeine-induced anxiety disorder._ Caffeine intake can contribute to excess gastric acidity, and thereby worsen esophageal and gastric disorders, and can exacerbate fibrocystic breast disease in women. Caffeine also is probably the most common and underrecognized cause of insomnia.

Once caffeine intoxication is diagnosed, treatment consists of reducing or gradually eliminating caffeine from the diet. Decaffeinated cola drinks, tea, and coffee are widely available.

Cannabis-Related Disorders

Cannabis-related disorders can result from use of *Cannabis sativa*, commonly referred to as marijuana, weed, pot, herb, grass, and reefer. The active ingredient is delta-9-tetrahydrocannabinol (THC). *Cannabis sativa* contains varying amounts of THC, but in general plants today have much higher THC concentrations than in the past. *Cannabis* is a generic term that also refers to other forms including synthetic cannabinoid compounds. Synthetic oral formulations are available by prescription for medical indications in some areas, and there is a growing movement in the United States to decriminalize possession of small amounts of marijuana, or even to legalize its use.

In DSM-5, diagnoses include cannabis intoxication, cannabis withdrawal, and cannabis use disorder. *Cannabis withdrawal* is a new diagnosis based on research showing that the syndrome can be reliably identified and has a time course typical of other substance withdrawal syndromes. Diagnosis of a cannabis use disorder requires 2 or more of 11 problematic behaviors occurring within a 12-month period. The symptoms include a pattern of use; craving; and impaired social, occupational, or recreational functioning, as well as evidence of tolerance or withdrawal.

Marijuana achieved popularity in the drug subculture in the 1960s and 1970s and remains the most widely used illicit drug in the United States. Although marijuana use is often thought of as relatively benign, it is common in people with other mental disorders and is associated with an increased risk for developing schizophrenia. Use of cannabis is also associated with increased risk of cigarette smoking and abuse of other drugs.

Cannabis has diverse effects on the brain, prominent among which are actions on CB_1 and CB_2 cannabinoid receptors found throughout the central nervous system. Commonly smoked (in the form of a "joint"), cannabis is sometimes ingested orally by mixing it into food. Also, devices have been developed in which cannabis is vaporized. When marijuana is smoked, intoxication occurs within 10–30 minutes. THC and its metabolites are lipid soluble and accumulate in fat cells; the half-life is approximately 50 hours. Intoxication can last 2–4 hours, depending on the dosage, although behavioral changes may continue for many hours. Oral ingestion (e.g., from adding marijuana to baked goods) produces a slower onset of action but leads to more powerful intoxicant effects.

Cannabis intoxication can lead users to feel a sense of euphoria and serenity. Users develop increased appetite and thirst, feel that their senses are heightened, and report improved self-confidence. Users also report feeling that time has slowed. Unwanted effects include conjunctivitis (red eyes), tachycardia, dry mouth (cotton mouth), and coughing fits. Many psychological effects reported by marijuana users are similar to those reported by LSD users, such as the development of perceptual distortions, sensitivity to sound, and a feeling of oneness with the environment. But users can also develop feelings of anxiety and paranoia (e.g., hypervigilance, suspiciousness), impaired attention, and decreased motor coordination. Marijuana rarely causes dangerous psychological or physical reactions.

Marijuana has been shown to impair the transfer of material from immediate to long-term memory. Electroencephalographic studies show a suppression of rapid eye movement (REM) sleep and diffuse slowing of background activity. It is often difficult to isolate the effects of marijuana because many of its regular users also take other drugs.

Cannabis withdrawal is characterized by irritability and nervousness, insomnia, poor appetite, restlessness, and depressed mood. Physical signs can include tremors, sweating, fever, chills, and headache.

Professional help usually is not needed to treat the adverse effects of marijuana. Benzodiazepines (e.g., diazepam) may help to calm highly anxious users. There is no specific treatment for withdrawal, but supportive measures (e.g., temporary use of an anxiolytic, hypnotic, or nonsteroidal anti-inflammatory drug) can help.

Hallucinogen-Related Disorders

Hallucinogens have been used for thousands of years and in multiple cultures. They are a diverse group of compounds, most synthetic, but two (peyote, mescaline) of botanical origin. The best known are probably LSD (lysergic acid diethylamide), mescaline, MDMA (3,4-methylenedioxymethamphetamine), and psilocybin. In DSM-5, phencyclidine (PCP), known as angel dust or crystal, is included in the class because it is a commonly used drug of abuse with hallucinogenic properties.

These drugs can induce hallucinations, perceptual disturbances, and feelings of unreality. Some persons believe that hallucinogens bring them closer to God or can expand their minds. The drugs became popular in the late 1960s and early 1970s when "psychedelic" experiences were romanticized and self-styled drug gurus such as the late Timothy Leary advocated their use. Because they are sympathomimetics, hallucinogens can cause tachycardia, hypertension, sweating, blurry vision, pupillary dilation, and tremors. They affect several neurotransmitter systems, including the dopamine, serotonin, acetylcholine, and γ-aminobutyric acid (GABA) systems. Tolerance develops rapidly to the euphoric and psychedelic effects of hallucinogens.

The hallucinogens differ in quality and duration of their subjective effects. As the prototype, LSD is short acting and rapidly absorbed. Onset of action occurs within an hour of ingestion, and effects last between 6 and 12 hours. In addition to autonomic hyperarousal, the drug causes varied psychological effects, including profound alterations in perception (e.g., colors may be experienced as brighter and more intense), and senses appear heightened. Emotions seem to intensify, and many users report becoming more introspective. Many users claim that their use leads to spiritual and philosophical insight. In fact, these properties led psychiatrists to experiment with LSD and other hallucinogens in the early 1960s for therapeutic purposes, such as to facilitate communication, improve insight, and increase self-esteem.

"Bad trips" occasionally occur, in which patients become markedly anxious or paranoid. Another undesirable outcome is the *flashback,* a brief reexperiencing of the drug's effects that occurs in situations unrelated to taking the drug. Flashbacks consist of visual distortions, geometric hallucinations, and misperceptions. Flashbacks that cause marked distress are diagnosed as *hallucinogen persisting perception disorder.* The disorder is usually self-limiting, but it may become chronic in rare cases.

Chronic psychosis has been reported in some hallucinogen users, and it was once thought that these drugs could induce schizophrenia. Although these drugs can cause psychotic episodes in some people, it is likely that users who develop schizophrenia probably would have developed the illness regardless of their hallucinogen use.

Several new "designer" drugs have grown in popularity during the past decade, including methylenedioxymethamphetamine (MDMA), better known as Ecstasy. Mainly used by youth and young adults, it first appeared at "raves" around 1995. Its use has grown dramatically, perhaps because of its acute reinforcing effects. It induces an intense feeling of attachment and connection to others and high energy, which makes users feel that they can dance all night or for days on end. Other effects include altered time perception, a sense of peacefulness, euphoria, increased desire for sex, and heightened sensory perceptions. The drug can also lead to anxiety, depression, and psychosis. Cognitive and memory deficits have been described in chronic users.

Although there is no known withdrawal syndrome for hallucinogens, benzodiazepines have been used to help calm users who experience an adverse reaction when "talking them down" (i.e., explaining that their reaction is due to the drug and providing reassurance) does not work. Overdose can result in a medical emergency. Hyperpyrexia, tachycardia, arrhythmias, stroke, dehydration, or even death can result.

PCP can be administered in several different ways (e.g., orally, intravenously, intranasally). Onset of action occurs in as little as 5 minutes and peaks in about 30 minutes. Users report euphoria, derealization, tingling sensations, and a feeling of warmth. With moderate dosages, bizarre behavior can occur, along with myoclonic jerks, confusion, and disorientation. Higher dosages can produce coma and seizures. Death can result from respiratory depression. Unlike hallucinogen users, who tend to have dilated pupils, PCP users have normal or small pupils. Chronic psychotic episodes can follow its use. PCP can also cause long-term cognitive deficits.

Treatment may be required for adverse reactions. Diazepam can be used to treat agitation, but severe behavioral disturbances may require use of a short-term antipsychotic, preferably one with a relative lack of anticholinergic side effects (e.g., haloperidol, risperidone). Phentolamine or other antihypertensive drugs can be used to reduce elevated blood pressure. Ammonium chloride can be used to acidify the urine to promote the drug's elimination, although its use is generally unnecessary.

Inhalant-Related Disorders

Inhalants are the cheapest and most readily available of the various substances of abuse. Paint thinner, airplane glue, and typewriter correction fluid are just a few of the inhalants that are commonplace. The active substances in the inhalants include toluene, acetone, benzene, and other organic hydrocarbons. Methods of inhalation may vary, but usually a substance is sprayed into a plastic bag and inhaled. Inhalants are dangerous because they can damage the CNS, liver, kidneys, and bone marrow. They enter the bloodstream quickly and have rapid onset of action.

An inhalant use disorder is defined by the problematic use of a hydrocarbon-based inhalant. Diagnosis requires 2 or more of 11 problematic behaviors occurring within a 12-month period. The symptoms include a pattern of use; craving; and impaired social, occupational, or recreational functioning, as well as evidence of tolerance or withdrawal. DSM-5 also recognizes other inhalant substances that may produce inhalant use disorder: nitrous oxide gas, which is available as a propellant in whipped cream dispensers or diverted from medical or dental sources, and amyl, butyl, and isobutyl nitrate gases, which are sold as room deodorizers and are inhaled to enhance sexual experience. Inhalation of these gases produces peripheral vasodilatation, lightheadedness, and headache. The disorder is common in adolescents, perhaps because the inhalants are widely available and inexpensive.

The use of volatile solvents is widespread, and it is estimated that 1 in 10 persons younger than age 17 has experimented with them. Because they are widely available and cheap, inhalants are mostly used by young persons who have trouble gaining access to other psychoactive substances.

Most users of inhalants are male. Latinos and American Indians are overrepresented among inhalant users. Although experimentation with inhalants is extremely common, regular use is found primarily among the low-income groups, children of alcoholic parents, and children from abusive or chaotic homes.

Inhalants are CNS depressants and produce intoxication similar to that of alcohol but of shorter duration. Effects can last 5–45 minutes and include feelings of excitation, disinhibition, and euphoria. Adverse effects include dizziness, slurred speech, and ataxia. Inhalants also may induce an acute delirium characterized by impaired concentration and disorientation. Hallucinations and delusions have been reported with their use. Other effects include loss of appetite, lateral nystagmus, hypoactive reflexes, and double vision. At higher dosages, patients may become stuporous or comatose.

Inhalants do not cause a specific withdrawal syndrome. Because inhalants often contain high concentrations of heavy metals, permanent neuromuscular and brain damage can occur, along with serious risk of damage to the kidneys, liver, and other organs from benzene and other hydrocarbons.

Opioid-Related Disorders

The opioids include natural and synthetic substances with morphine-like actions that are full agonists to the μ opioid receptor. They include morphine, heroin, hydrocodone, oxycodone, codeine, tramadol, and meperidine. Opioids are prescribed as analgesics, anesthetics, antidiarrheal agents, and cough suppressants. Buprenorphine, a drug that has both opiate agonist and antagonist effects, is also included in this class. Besides heroin, opium is the most widely consumed illegal opiate in the world. In the United States, the nonmedical use of prescription opioids is a significant problem. Opioid users have a high likelihood of developing an opioid use disorder and have an increased risk for HIV, as well as hepatitis B and C viruses.

Opioid abuse is more common in urban settings and more prevalent in men and in African Americans. Among those who misuse prescription pain relievers, there is a slight female preponderance. Opioid abuse is more common among health care professionals than among other occupations, probably because of the availability of these drugs in medical settings. More than five times as many people misuse prescription opioid pain relievers as use heroin. Many persons addicted to opioids have other mental illnesses, including other substance addictions, a mood or anxiety disorder, or antisocial personality disorder. Many users turn to crime because of the relatively high cost of their drug addiction.

The course and outcome of an opioid addiction is variable and depends on availability of the drug and exposure to its use. In a 12-year follow-up of opioid-addicted patients treated in a federal treatment center, 98% returned to using opioids within 12 months of release. A follow-up study in London found a relapse rate of 53% within 6 months. A 24-year follow-up of persons addicted to narcotics in California confirmed that substance abuse and criminal involvement continued over the years and that cessation of drug use was uncommon. However, a study of military veterans who had used opioids in Vietnam found that fewer than 2% continued their use after returning home. These discrepant findings suggest that there may be more than one type of opioid user. Opioid addiction is associated with high mortality rates because of inadvertent fatal overdoses, accidental deaths, and suicide.

Opioid users need to be carefully evaluated because they are likely to have comorbid medical illness. Opioid users also are at high risk for developing medical conditions resulting from malnutrition and use of dirty needles—for example, hepatitis B and C infection, HIV infection, pneumonia, skin ulcers at injection sites, and cellulitis.

Opioids can be injected, snorted, or smoked, producing both euphoria and a sense of well-being. Drowsiness, inactivity, psychomotor retardation, and impaired concentration follow. Physical signs that occur after a heroin-addicted person "shoots up" (which may occur three or more times a day) include flushing, pupillary constriction, slurred speech, respiratory depression, hypotension, hypothermia, and bradycardia. Constipation, nausea, and vomiting are also frequent.

Tolerance eventually develops to most of these drug effects, including the initial euphoria. Sexual interest diminishes, and in women, menstruation may cease. In chronic users, depending on dosage and drug potency, withdrawal symptoms begin approximately 10 hours after the last dose with short-acting opioids (e.g., morphine, heroin) or after a longer period with longer-acting substances (e.g., methadone). Minor withdrawal symptoms include lacrimation, rhinorrhea, sweating, yawning, piloerection, hypertension, and tachycardia. Symptoms that indicate more severe withdrawal include hot and cold flashes, muscle and joint pain, nausea, vomiting, and abdominal cramps. Seizures sometimes occur during meperidine withdrawal. Psychological symptoms of withdrawal include severe anxiety and restlessness, irritability, insomnia, and decreased appetite.

Patients addicted to opioids can be gradually withdrawn under medical supervision using methadone, a long-acting opioid. Importantly, methadone can be administered only in inpatient or outpatient settings federally licensed for methadone detoxification. The initial methadone dosage is determined by the presenting signs and symptoms of withdrawal (see Table 15–5). The dose is then repeated in 12 hours, and supplemental doses of 5 mg or 10 mg are given as needed if withdrawal symptoms are not suppressed. Once the 24-hour dosage is determined, the dosage is tapered at the rate of 20% per day for short-acting opioids or 10% per day for long-acting opioids. Methadone can be given in two to three divided doses daily, and the patient's vital signs should be recorded before each dose. It is unusual for a starting dose to exceed 40 mg during the initial 24 hours of withdrawal. Withdrawal from short-acting substances (e.g., heroin, morphine) typically takes 7–10 days. Withdrawal from longer-acting substances (e.g., methadone) proceeds more slowly (e.g., 2–3 weeks).

TABLE 15–5. **Methadone withdrawal dosing schedule**

Signs and symptoms	Initial methadone dose, mg
Lacrimation, rhinorrhea, diaphoresis, yawning, restlessness, insomnia	5
Dilated pupils, piloerection, muscle twitching, myalgias, arthralgias, abdominal pain	10
Tachycardia, hypertension, tachypnea, fever, anorexia, extreme restlessness, nausea	15
Diarrhea, vomiting, dehydration, hyperglycemia, hypotension	20

Source. Adapted from Perry et al. 2006.

Another drug used to withdraw patients from opioids is clonidine, which suppresses the autonomic signs of withdrawal. Patients do better with an abrupt switch to clonidine when the methadone dosage is first stabilized at 20 mg or less daily. At the first sign of opioid withdrawal, the patient is given 0.3–0.5 mg (0.006 mg/kg) of clonidine, which is repeated at bedtime. For the next 4 days, the patient receives 0.9–1.5 mg/day in three to four divided doses. The dose should be withheld if the diastolic blood pressure falls below 60 mm Hg or marked sedation occurs. On days 6–8, the dosage can be decreased by 50%, and on day 9, clonidine can be discontinued altogether. For long-acting opioids, clonidine reduction should occur on days 11–14, with discontinuation on day 15.

Benzodiazepines can be used to treat mild cases of withdrawal and have the advantage of relieving anxiety and promoting needed sleep. Mild analgesics, such as the nonsteroidal anti-inflammatory drugs, can relieve muscle aches and pain. Gastrointestinal distress can be treated with dicyclomine.

If the patient is also addicted to a sedative, hypnotic, or anxiolytic drug in addition to an opioid, it is safest to stabilize the patient on a dosage of methadone and then withdraw the sedative, hypnotic, or anxiolytic first, because withdrawal from such drugs is potentially the more dangerous syndrome.

Participation in a federally licensed methadone maintenance program continues to be the major alternative to complete cessation of use. In such a program, methadone is administered orally (e.g., 60–100 mg/day). Because of its long half-life (22–56 hours) and its wide distribution in the body, the drug is well tolerated and produces almost no withdrawal symptoms. The rationale for methadone maintenance is that by switching addicted persons to methadone, their drug hunger is alleviated so that they are less preoccupied with drug-seeking behavior. This approach has been successful, and most people enrolled in these programs have significant decreases in opioid and nonopioid drug use, criminal activity, and depressive symptoms. They also show increases in gainful employment and stability in social relationships. Many programs espouse the view that methadone is a transitional treatment that will eventually lead to total abstinence, and at least one well-designed study has shown that methadone maintenance programs produce better results than detoxification. Methadone programs also emphasize ongoing individual and group psychotherapy. This helps keep addicted persons in the program and provides new skills to help them cope with day-to-day problems without resorting to drugs.

There are now several alternatives to methadone maintenance. Naltrexone, a long-acting opioid antagonist, is FDA approved to treat opioid dependence. The drug is usually started following drug withdrawal, at dosages of 50–100 mg/day, or 100–150 mg three times weekly. Its use is intended to block the pleasurable effects of opioid drugs thereby making their use less attractive. Buprenorphine (Subutex), a mixed opioid agonist–antagonist, and a combination of buprenorphine and naloxone (Suboxone) are FDA approved to treat opioid dependence. The prescription use of these agents is limited to specially trained physicians who meet certain requirements.

Sedative-, Hypnotic-, and Anxiolytic-Related Disorders

Sedative, hypnotic, and anxiolytic substances include benzodiazepines, benzodiazepine-like drugs, carbonates, barbiturates, and barbiturate-like hypnotics. This class includes all prescription sleeping medications and almost all prescription antianxiety medications. Nonbenzodiazepine antianxiety drugs (e.g., buspirone) are not included in this class because they are not associated with significant misuse. At high doses, these drugs can be lethal, particularly if mixed with alcohol. Sedative, hypnotic, and anxiolytic substances are available both by prescription and on the black market. All sedatives, hypnotics, and anxiolytics are cross-tolerant with one another and with alcohol. (Cross-tolerance refers to the phenomenon of tolerance to a drug that develops because of exposure to a pharmacologically similar substance.)

The first barbiturate, barbital, was introduced in 1903. Later, other sedative-hypnotics (e.g., meprobamate) came along, and the first benzodiazepines became available in the 1960s. Because of their wide margin of safety, the benzodiazepines have largely displaced barbiturates and the earlier nonbarbiturate sedative-hypnotics from the market. An overdose of barbiturates is potentially fatal, but the benzodiazepines produce almost no respiratory depression, and the ratio of lethal to effective dosage is extraordinarily high.

The benzodiazepines are among the most widely prescribed medications in the United States; about 15% of the general population is prescribed a benzodiazepine in any given year. Research shows that most prescriptions for benzodiazepines are appropriate, and only a small percentage of patients abuse the drugs. Nonetheless, prescribing practices contribute to the problem of sedative-hypnotic abuse, and physicians have an obligation to monitor and, if necessary, limit the use of these drugs (see box below). Further information about the rational use of sedative-hypnotics is found in Chapter 21 ("Psychopharmacology and Electroconvulsive Therapy").

Rational prescribing of sedative-hypnotic drugs

1. Avoid or limit prescriptions to patients if risk for substance abuse is suggested by
  • A history of alcohol misuse
  • A history of drug misuse
  • The presence of an antisocial or borderline personality disorder
  • A strong family history of substance misuse
2. Learn to recognize "red flag" presentations by patients seeking prescription drugs, as suggested by
  • Dramatic claims of need for a scheduled drug
  • Reports of lost prescriptions
  • Frequent requests for early refills
  • Requests for a specific scheduled drug, reports of allergies to other drugs, or use of nonscheduled drugs for pain relief or anxiety
  • Obtaining prescriptions from many physicians ("doctor-shopping")

Source. Courtesy of William R. Yates, M.D.

Sedative, hypnotic, and anxiolytic misuse can lead to medical and social complications, occupational problems (e.g., job loss), impaired relationships, and even crime. Not much is known about the natural history of sedative, hypnotic, and anxiolytic misuse, but as with an alcohol use disorder, the course probably is chronic and relapsing.

Sedative, hypnotic, and anxiolytic intoxication and withdrawal vary little from drug to drug, although withdrawal symptoms may be more intense with the shorter-acting drugs (e.g., alprazolam) and more prolonged with the longer-acting ones (e.g., diazepam). The syndromes are similar to those seen with alcohol use disorders, which is not surprising because these drugs are cross-tolerant.

Intoxication symptoms are dose related. Lethargy, impaired mental functioning, poor memory, irritability, self-neglect, and emotional disinhibition all may occur. As intoxication progresses, slurred speech, ataxia, and impaired coordination can develop. With higher dosages, death can result from respiratory depression, a complication that rarely occurs with the benzodiazepines.

Withdrawal needs to be carefully monitored. Conservative management consists of very slow taper of the drug over days or even weeks. Some patients will need formal detoxification in the hospital to forestall the development of significant withdrawal symptoms.

TABLE 15–6. **Pentobarbital-diazepam tolerance test**

---

1. Pentobarbital 200 mg (or diazepam 20 mg) is administered orally. Evaluate in 2 hours:

   • No tolerance—the patient is asleep but arousable

   • Tolerance to 400–500 mg of pentobarbital (or 40–50 mg of diazepam)—the patient is grossly ataxic and has a coarse tremor or lateral nystagmus

   • Tolerance to 600 mg of pentobarbital (or 60 mg of diazepam)—the patient is mildly ataxic

   • Tolerance to 800 mg of pentobarbital (or 80 mg of diazepam)—the patient has slight nystagmus

   • Tolerance to 1,000 mg of pentobarbital (or 100 mg of diazepam)—the patient is asymptomatic

2. If the patient remains asymptomatic, an additional oral dose of pentobarbital 200 mg (or diazepam 20 mg) is given.

   • Failure to become symptomatic at this dose suggests a daily tolerance of >1,600 mg of pentobarbital (or 160 mg of diazepam)

Abrupt drug discontinuation leads to anxiety, restlessness, and a feeling of apprehension in the first 24 hours. Coarse tremors soon develop, and deep tendon reflexes become hyperactive. Weakness, nausea and vomiting, orthostatic hypotension, sweating, and other signs of autonomic hyperarousal occur. On the second or third day after discontinuation, grand mal seizures can occur. The seizures generally consist of a single convulsion or burst of several convulsions; status epilepticus rarely develops. A withdrawal delirium, associated with confusion, disorientation, and visual and somatic hallucinations, sometimes develops. Barbiturate withdrawal can be especially serious, and without medical intervention can result in death.

The patient should be slowly tapered off the drug. If the patient's usual maintenance dose is known, that can serve as the starting point. A pentobarbital (or diazepam) tolerance test can be performed in those who are unreliable or in whom the dose is difficult to determine (see Table 15–6). The test should be administered to a patient who is not currently intoxicated and who can be medically monitored in the hospital.

Once the level of tolerance has been established, the patient is withdrawn using diazepam or another long-acting benzodiazepine (e.g., clonazepam). Long-acting barbiturates such as phenobarbital can also be used, but their use is now relatively uncommon. With diazepam, the daily dosage is decreased by 10 mg from an initial level equal to the intoxicating dosage. If phenobarbital is used, the initial dose is determined by substituting 30 mg of phenobarbital for every 100 mg of pentobarbital administered during the tolerance test. For example, if the patient is tolerant to 400 mg of pentobarbital, the starting dose of phenobarbital is 120 mg. During withdrawal, the daily dosage of phenobarbital is decreased by 30 mg. On these schedules, the patient will be somewhat uncomfortable during the withdrawal period. If signs of withdrawal worsen or if the patient becomes somnolent or intoxicated, the schedule can be adjusted and the patient can be given more diazepam (or phenobarbital), or the schedule can be stretched out. Some patients will present at the hospital already experiencing withdrawal symptoms, in which case pentobarbital or diazepam should be administered in sufficient dosages to make them comfortable before withdrawal is initiated.

Certain general rules apply to patients given these drugs. The drugs should be targeted at specific symptoms or syndromes (e.g., generalized anxiety disorder), and their use should be limited to weeks or months when possible. The drugs should be prescribed at the minimum dosage necessary to control the patient's symptoms. Because of the proven safety and efficacy of benzodiazepines, there is no reason to prescribe the more dangerous barbiturates or the other nonbarbiturate sedative-hypnotics.

Stimulant-Related Disorders

Stimulants include dextroamphetamine, methylphenidate, methamphetamine, cocaine, and several other substances that share similar pharmacological activity. They elevate mood, increase energy and alertness, decrease appetite, and improve task performance. These drugs also cause autonomic hyperarousal, which leads to tachycardia, elevated blood pressure, and pupillary dilation. Amphetamines were first used in the 1930s and have been prescribed to treat depression, obesity, sleep disorders, and attention-deficit/hyperactivity disorder.

The abuse potential of stimulants was recognized relatively early. Because of their overuse in the 1970s as diet pills, changes in the regulation of their legitimate distribution were made to stem the tide of abuse. More recently, their use has increased along with the rise in the cases of diagnosed attention deficit/hyperactivity disorder, which is commonly treated with stimulants. In addition to recreational use, students also use these drugs to boost academic performance. Their use is now widespread on college campuses.

Cocaine differs structurally from the amphetamines but has similar effects. Derived from the coca plant, cocaine has legitimate medical use as a

TABLE 15–7. Common psychological and physical symptoms in 32 freebase cocaine abusers

Psychological symptoms	%	Physical symptoms	%
Paranoia	63	Blurred vision	34
Visual hallucinations	50	Coughing	34
Craving	47	Muscle aches	34
Asocial behavior	41	Dry skin	28
Impaired concentration	38	Tremors	28
Irritability	31	Weight loss	25
Bad dreams	31	Chest pains	22
Hyperexcitability	28	Episodic unconsciousness	16
Violence	28	Difficult urination	16
Auditory hallucinations	25	Respiratory problems	9
Lethargy	25	Edema	9
Depression	25	Seizures	3

Source. Adapted from Vereby and Gold 1988.

local anesthetic. Cocaine is a popular recreational drug, although its use has generally been restricted to affluent groups because of its high cost.

In addition to a use disorder, stimulants are also associated with intoxication and withdrawal syndromes. Stimulant intoxication is diagnosed on the basis of recent use, maladaptive behavior, and evidence of autonomic hyperarousal. Cocaine intoxication also has the potential to induce tactile hallucinations (e.g., "coke bugs"); in DSM-5 this can be specified as a "perceptual disturbance."

Psychological symptoms of cocaine intoxication include a sense of euphoria, disinhibition, sexual arousal, enhanced feelings of mastery, and improved self-esteem. Depending on how the drug is administered (e.g., intranasally, intravenously), users may experience a rapid onset of euphoria, or "rush." Users smoking a purified cocaine base freed from its salts and cutting agents (i.e., freebasing) report an even more rapid but short-lived high. Table 15–7 presents a list of common psychological and physical symptoms seen in freebase cocaine abusers.

Stimulant intoxication can induce aggression, agitation, and impaired judgment. A paranoid psychosis similar to those seen in patients with schizophrenia can develop but usually subsides 1–2 weeks after the drug use stops. If a stimulant-induced psychosis persists, a diagnosis of schizophrenia should be considered if it is clear that there is no continuing source of the drug. Delirium is a rare complication that gradually resolves once the drug has been discontinued. Cocaine also has been associated with serious medical complications, such as acute myocardial infarction due to coronary artery constriction and anoxic brain damage due to cocaine-induced seizures.

Cessation or reduction of a stimulant drug can lead to symptoms of withdrawal commonly referred to as a "crash." Symptoms include fatigue and depression, nightmares, headache, profuse sweating, muscle cramps, and hunger. Symptoms usually peak in 2–4 days. Intense dysphoria can occur, peaking between 48 and 72 hours after the last dose of the stimulant.

Because intoxication and stimulant-induced psychotic disorder are generally self-limiting, no specific treatment is necessary. Benzodiazepines (e.g., diazepam, lorazepam) can be used to treat agitation or anxiety. Antipsychotics have been used to treat stimulant-induced psychoses but are usually unnecessary because the psychosis is short-lived once the offending drug has been stopped. Elimination of the drug can be accelerated by acidifying the urine with ammonium chloride, but this step is rarely necessary. A withdrawal depression that persists longer than 2 weeks can be treated with antidepressants, although their use in these cases has not been systematically evaluated.

No medications have been consistently effective in treating stimulant dependence. Desipramine and other antidepressants, the dopamine agonists bromocriptine and amantadine, and even disulfiram have been used to treat cocaine dependence, but their success has been mixed. Cognitive-behavioral therapy has also been used and appears promising.

Tobacco-Related Disorders

Nicotine is a highly addictive drug found in cigarettes, chewing tobacco and snuff, and other tobacco products. About 20% of adult Americans smoke, although smoking is even more frequent in certain groups (e.g., minority groups, low-income persons, less-educated persons). Rates among psychiatric patients are also very high. For example, alcohol- or drug-abusing patients are highly likely to smoke, and nearly 90% of schizophrenic patients smoke.

Smoking is well known to cause lung cancer, emphysema, and cardiovascular disease. Snuff and chewing tobacco have been associated with oropharyngeal cancers. Secondary smoke has been associated with respiratory and cardiovascular diseases.

Nicotine addiction develops quickly and is often reinforced by peer pressure. In the past few decades, society has changed its views on smoking, and fewer people now take up smoking.

Nicotine withdrawal usually begins within 1 hour after the last cigarette is smoked and peaks within 24 hours. Withdrawal may last weeks or months and consists of nicotine craving, irritability, anxiety, restlessness, and decreased heart rate. Weight gain and depression often follow smoking cessation.

Because the consequences of tobacco use are so potentially harmful, all physicians have a responsibility to urge their patients not to use tobacco products and to assist patients who do use them to quit. There are several FDA-approved treatments for smoking cessation. These options include nicotine transdermal patches and nicotine-containing gum, lozenges, and inhalers; bupropion, an antidepressant marketed as Zyban; and varenicline (Chantix), a newer option that may be more effective than nicotine replacement or bupropion. The combination of nicotine-replacement patches or gum with bupropion or varenicline may work even better.

Other Specified Substance-Related and Addictive Disorders

This diagnostic class includes substances that do not fit any of the above categories such as anabolic steroids; nonsteroidal anti-inflammatory drugs; cortisol; antiparkinsonian medications; antihistamines; nitrous oxide; amyl-, butyl-, or isobutyl-nitrites; betel nut (chewed in many cultures to produce mild euphoria); kava (from a South Pacific pepper plant); or cathinones (including *khât* plant agents and synthetic chemical derivatives) that produce stimulant effects. This category is also used for patients who have been misusing drugs but the specific compound is unknown. Anabolic steroids, nitrate inhalants, and nitrous oxide are discussed below.

Anabolic Steroids

Anabolic steroids are widely abused by athletes who believe that their performance and muscle mass will be enhanced by their use. Although these drugs may initially produce a sense of well-being, this feeling is later replaced by anergy, dysphoria, and irritability. Frank psychosis can develop, as can serious medical problems, including liver disease.

Nitrate Inhalants

Nitrate inhalants ("poppers") produce an intoxicated state characterized by a feeling of fullness in the head, mild euphoria, a change in time perception, relaxation of the smooth muscles, and possibly an increase in sexual feelings. These drugs carry the possible risk of immune system impairment, respiratory system irritation, and a toxic reaction that may lead to vomiting, severe headaches, and hypotension.

Nitrous Oxide

Nitrous oxide ("laughing gas") can cause intoxication characterized by light-headedness and a floating sensation that quickly clear once the administration of gas stops. Temporary confusion or paranoia can occur when this substance is used regularly.

■ Clinical Management of Substance-Related Disorders

Treatment of drug use disorders can be thought of as having two phases. Detoxification is the major goal of the first phase. Continuation treatment or "rehabilitation" is the second phase.

Detoxification may be difficult to achieve in some patients, such as those with potentially serious withdrawal syndromes (e.g., users of barbiturates or opioids) but may be easier with others whose drugs of abuse (e.g., hallucinogens) have no specific withdrawal syndrome. Hospitalization is necessary for safe detoxification in some patients so that tolerance can be determined and a slow drug taper can be monitored under medical supervision. The circumstances of detoxification should be determined by the patient and physician working together.

Many persons addicted to drugs have serious medical conditions that the physician also must address during this phase of treatment. For example, a heroin-addicted person may have an antecubital cellulitis and be seropositive for HIV; a cocaine-addicted person may have an eroded nasal septum (from sniffing the drug) that has become secondarily infected.

Psychiatric comorbidity is important to assess during the first phase of treatment. Many, if not most, substance abusers have additional mental disorders that can have a profound effect on their treatment outcome. Abuse of other substances is the most common comorbidity, followed by mood disorders, anxiety disorders, and personality disorders. Comorbidity complicates treatment efforts and reduces the likelihood of success. Examples include the amphetamine abuser who develops a suicidal depression during withdrawal and the heroin-addicted person with an antisocial personality disorder whose use seems, in part, motivated by his membership in a street gang that celebrates drug use.

The continuation phase of treatment consists of efforts to rehabilitate the patient and to prevent future drug abuse. The success of this phase is almost completely dependent on the motivation of the patient because there is no way to truly assess or enforce compliance—except, of course, by frequent and random drug screening tests and threats of punishment for noncompliance. Such strict enforcement is neither possible nor desirable, except in the military, in certain professions (e.g., pilots), and in authoritarian societies.

Multimodal approaches are necessary for rehabilitation. Individual psychotherapy is important to help patients learn about their motivation for using drugs and to learn alternative methods for handling stressful situations. Group therapy, especially in the hospital or outpatient programs, is useful in confronting patients with the seriousness of their problem and how the drug significantly affects their lives. Peer groups are unequaled in their ability to achieve confrontation. Among cocaine-dependent persons, the combination of individual and group psychotherapy works best at preventing relapse, as one study has shown.

Among other approaches, cognitive-behavioral therapy may help the patient reverse habits that lead to or promote drug use or may correct cognitive distortions (e.g., "If I don't use drugs, I won't be popular"). Social skills training may help some patients break a cycle of getting in with the wrong crowd and learn to meet and be accepted by more appropriate peers. Family therapy and marital counseling are necessary adjuncts in other patients. Examples include the teenager whose inhalant use has disrupted his family life and the young man whose marriage is coming apart because of his cocaine addiction.

Contingency management, a form of behavior therapy, is used in some programs to encourage a drug-free lifestyle. With contingency management, people are "rewarded" (or positively reinforced) for appropriate behavior. For example, each time a person submits a clean urine sample, he or she receives a voucher that can be exchanged for retail goods or services. Research shows that low-cost rewards can be effective in reducing drug use.

Medical approaches for the continuation phase of treatment can be important. Methadone maintenance has an established role in the treatment of opioid addiction. The user is given a carefully monitored substitute addiction that allows him or her to function in society. Buprenorphine is another recent alternative for the maintenance phase of treatment. Patients with comorbid psychiatric disorders may, of course, benefit from ongoing treatment of anxiety, depression, or psychosis.

Self-help groups have become an integral part of a comprehensive treatment approach to substance use disorders. AA has led the way for the creation of sister groups, such as Cocaine Anonymous, Narcotics Anonymous, and Drugs Anonymous; all follow a 12-step model. These groups are now available in many parts of the United States. They provide an atmosphere of mutual support in which recovering addicted persons can share their experiences.

Clinical points for substance-related disorders

1. The clinician should not allow his or her personal beliefs and attitudes about drug abuse to interfere with the care of the addicted patient.

   • Patients need a consistent yet firm approach.

   • The clinician should neither condemn addicted persons nor condone their behavior.

2. The clinician should assess the patient for medical and psychiatric comorbidity. Many addicted persons have potentially serious medical problems that require treatment, significant addictions to other substances, and co-occurring mood and anxiety disorders, or a personality disorder.

3. The clinician should be prepared for relapses during the continuation phase of treatment. Relapse is nearly inevitable, but it does not represent failure of the treatment program. The clinician must be there to help the patient get back on the wagon.

4. Support groups can be very helpful to the patient, and referral to community-based organizations is essential.

■ Non–Substance-Related Disorders

There are several conditions that do not involve ingestion of substances yet have similarities to alcohol and drug addictions. These are the so-called *behavioral addictions,* and several have been described, including sex addiction, compulsive shopping, and Internet addiction. The authors of DSM-5 concluded that only one—gambling disorder—had sufficient supporting data to be included in this section.

Gambling Disorder

Gambling has occurred in almost all cultures and throughout human history. Most individuals gamble responsibly, yet some become preoccupied with gambling and experience its many negative consequences. Officially recognized in DSM-III as "pathological gambling," the disorder was classified an impulse-control disorder. Renamed *gambling disorder* in DSM-5, it has been moved to this chapter because of research showing its close connection to the substance-related disorders. The DSM-5 diagnostic criteria are listed in Box 15–2.

Box 15–2. DSM-5 Diagnostic Criteria for Gambling Disorder

A. Persistent and recurrent problematic gambling behavior leading to clinically significant impairment or distress, as indicated by the individual exhibiting four (or more) of the following in a 12-month period:

1. Needs to gamble with increasing amounts of money in order to achieve the desired excitement.
2. Is restless or irritable when attempting to cut down or stop gambling.
3. Has made repeated unsuccessful efforts to control, cut back, or stop gambling.
4. Is often preoccupied with gambling (e.g., having persistent thoughts of reliving past gambling experiences, handicapping or planning the next venture, thinking of ways to get money with which to gamble).
5. Often gambles when feeling distressed (e.g., helpless, guilty, anxious, depressed).
6. After losing money gambling, often returns another day to get even ("chasing" one's losses).
7. Lies to conceal the extent of involvement with gambling.
8. Has jeopardized or lost a significant relationship, job, or educational or career opportunity because of gambling.
9. Relies on others to provide money to relieve desperate financial situations caused by gambling.

B. The gambling behavior is not better explained by a manic episode.

Specify if:

Episodic: Meeting diagnostic criteria at more than one time point, with symptoms subsiding between periods of gambling disorder for at least several months.

Persistent: Experiencing continuous symptoms, to meet diagnostic criteria for multiple years.

Specify if:

In early remission: After full criteria for gambling disorder were previously met, none of the criteria for gambling disorder have been met for at least 3 months but for less than 12 months.

In sustained remission: After full criteria for gambling disorder were previously met, none of the criteria for gambling disorder have been met during a period of 12 months or longer.

Specify current severity:

Mild: 4–5 criteria met.

Moderate: 6–7 criteria met.

Severe: 8–9 criteria met.

Gambling disorder affects 0.4%–2% of the general population. The prevalence is lower in areas with limited gambling opportunities. Two-thirds of people with gambling disorder are male; they typically begin to gamble in adolescence, and some become "hooked" almost from their first bet. Women take up gambling later than men but tend to develop a gambling disorder more quickly. Mood and anxiety disorders, substance use disorders, and personality disorders are common in people with gambling disorder.

The following case is that of a woman who suffered the damaging effects of gambling disorder:

> Mary, a 42-year-old accountant, had gambled recreationally for years. At age 38, for reasons she could not explain, she became hooked on casino slot machines. Her interest in gambling gradually escalated, and within a year Mary was gambling during most business days. She also gambled most weekends, telling her husband she was at work. To acquire money for gambling, Mary created a fake company to which she transferred nearly $300,000 from her accounting firm. The embezzlement was eventually detected and Mary was arrested. Following her arrest, and the associated public humiliation, Mary became severely depressed and attempted suicide by drug overdose. After a brief hospital stay, Mary entered counseling and was prescribed paroxetine. In the plea bargain, she agreed to perform 400 hours of community service.

Gambling disorder runs in families and may be genetically related to the substance use disorders and antisocial personality disorder. Brain imaging research shows that gambling activates the brain's "reward" circuitry, but also that reduced activity occurs in areas mediating planning and decision making.

The use of medications to treat gambling disorder is being actively researched. The opioid antagonist naltrexone (50–200 mg/day) has been shown to be more effective than placebo. Nalmefene, another opioid antagonist, has also been shown to reduce gambling urges and behaviors, but it is unavailable in the United States. The selective serotonin reuptake inhibitors are being studied and may be helpful, particularly in depressed or anxious patients.

Referral to Gamblers Anonymous, a 12-step program similar to Alcoholics Anonymous, may be helpful, although dropout rates are high. Inpatient treatment and rehabilitation programs similar to those for substance use disorders may be helpful for selected patients.

Other patients can benefit from individual psychotherapy geared toward helping them understand why they gamble and assisting them in dealing with feelings of hopelessness, depression, and guilt. Cognitive-behavioral theory (CBT) can be used to address the irrational thoughts and beliefs associated with pathological gambling ("I'll win big with the next bet!"). CBT is often combined with motivational interviewing. With motivational interviewing, therapists encourage the patient to make needed changes in his or her behavior. Relapse prevention methods can help patients identify the triggers that promote gambling and teach them how to deal more effectively with these triggers. Family therapy offers the addicted gambler an opportunity to make amends, to learn better communication skills, and to repair the rifts that gambling inevitably creates in families.

■ Self-Assessment Questions

1. What is the benefit to the disease concept of addiction?
2. How is an alcohol use disorder diagnosed? Intoxication? Withdrawal?
3. What are the clinical findings in alcohol use disorder?
4. List the medical complications of alcohol use disorder. What are the associated laboratory abnormalities?
5. What are the major alcohol withdrawal syndromes, and how are they treated?
6. Discuss the role of disulfiram, naltrexone, and acamprosate in the treatment of alcohol use disorders.
7. What are the predictors of good outcome in alcohol treatment programs? Describe motivational interviewing.
8. How widespread are drug use disorders, and what are their risk factors?
9. What are the symptoms of PCP intoxication?
10. Why are the inhalants potentially dangerous?
11. Describe opioid withdrawal. How is it treated?
12. What medications are used to treat opioid dependence?
13. Describe the withdrawal syndrome from sedatives, hypnotics, and anxiolytics.
14. Why are barbiturates dangerous? Describe the pentobarbital-diazepam tolerance test.
15. What are the psychological effects of cocaine use?
16. What are the approved treatments for smoking cessation?
17. What is contingency management?
18. Describe the treatment of gambling disorder.

Chapter 16

Neurocognitive Disorders

When age has crushed the body with its might,
The limbs collapse with weakness and decay,
The judgment limps, and mind and speech give way.

Lucretius

eurocognitive disorders include delirium and the syndromes of major neurocognitive disorder, mild neurocognitive disorder, and their etiological subtypes (e.g., Alzheimer's disease, Lewy bodies, Parkinson's disease). They involve structural or functional disturbances of brain function leading to impairments in memory, abstract thinking, or judgment. They are acquired and are associated with a clinically significant decline from a previous level of functioning. The neurocognitive disorders are unique among DSM-5 classes because their underlying pathology—and their etiology—is often known. This is in contrast with most disorders (e.g., schizophrenia, bipolar disorder) in which the etiology is unknown. The neurocognitive disorders are listed in Table 16–1.

DSM-5 has transformed the classification of the neurocognitive disorders by introducing two new categories—*major neurocognitive disorder* and *mild neurocognitive disorder*—that are distinguished on the basis of severity. Diagnostic criteria are provided for each condition, followed by criteria for specific etiological subtypes (e.g., major neurocognitive disorder due to Alzheimer's disease). Mild neurocognitive disorder is an important new category because it acknowledges less severe levels of impairment that can also be a focus of care. The term *dementia* has been replaced with *neurocognitive disorder,* although the former may still be used to describe the etiological subtypes. The word dementia had been used mainly to describe degenerative conditions that mostly affect

TABLE 16–1. DSM-5 neurocognitive disorders

Delirium

 Other specified delirium

 Unspecified delirium

Major neurocognitive disorder

Mild neurocognitive disorder

Subtypes of major or mild neurocognitive disorder

 Due to Alzheimer's disease

 Frontotemporal neurocognitive disorder

 With Lewy bodies

 Due to traumatic brain injury

 Substance/medication-induced

 Due to traumatic brain injury

 Due to HIV infection

 Due to prion disease

 Due to Parkinson's disease

 Due to Huntington's disease

 Due to another medical condition

 Due to multiple etiologies

 Unspecified neurocognitive disorder

older adults. In contrast, the terms major and mild neurocognitive disorder have broader application and also are preferred in describing younger individuals with cognitive impairment resulting from traumatic brain injury or HIV infection.

The criteria for major and mild neurocognitive disorder are based on six defined key cognitive domains. They are:

1. *Complex attention:* sustained attention, divided attention, selective attention, processing speed
2. *Executive function:* planning, decision making, working memory, responding to feedback/error correction, overriding habits, mental flexibility
3. *Learning and memory:* immediate memory, recent memory (including free recall, cued recall, and recognition memory)
4. *Language:* expressive language (including naming, fluency, grammar and syntax) and receptive language

5. *Perceptual motor ability:* construction and visual perception
6. *Social cognition:* recognition of emotions, theory of mind (i.e., ability to understand another person's mental state), behavioral regulation

■ Delirium

Delirium is one of the most important neurocognitive disorders and is characterized by a disturbance of attention, awareness, and cognition that develops over a short period of time (hours to days). Its defining feature is a reduced orientation to the environment that may fluctuate during the course of the day. Delirium results from the direct physiological consequences of a medical condition, substance intoxication or withdrawal, exposure to a toxin, or multiple etiologies. DSM-5 subtypes include substance intoxication delirium, substance withdrawal delirium, medication-induced delirium, delirium due to another medical condition, and delirium due to multiple etiologies. (See Box 16–1 for the DSM-5 criteria.)

Box 16–1.   DSM-5 Diagnostic Criteria for Delirium

A. A disturbance in attention (i.e., reduced ability to direct, focus, sustain, and shift attention) and awareness (reduced orientation to the environment).
B. The disturbance develops over a short period of time (usually hours to a few days), represents a change from baseline attention and awareness, and tends to fluctuate in severity during the course of a day.
C. An additional disturbance in cognition (e.g., memory deficit, disorientation, language, visuospatial ability, or perception).
D. The disturbances in Criteria A and C are not better explained by another preexisting, established, or evolving neurocognitive disorder and do not occur in the context of a severely reduced level of arousal, such as coma.
E. There is evidence from the history, physical examination, or laboratory findings that the disturbance is a direct physiological consequence of another medical condition, substance intoxication or withdrawal (i.e., due to a drug of abuse or to a medication), or exposure to a toxin, or is due to multiple etiologies.

Specify whether:

   Substance intoxication delirium: This diagnosis should be made instead of substance intoxication when the symptoms in Criteria A and C predominate in the clinical picture and when they are sufficiently severe to warrant clinical attention.

Substance withdrawal delirium: This diagnosis should be made instead of substance withdrawal when the symptoms in Criteria A and C predominate in the clinical picture and when they are sufficiently severe to warrant clinical attention.

Medication-induced delirium: This diagnosis applies when the symptoms in Criteria A and C arise as a side effect of a medication taken as prescribed.

Delirium due to another medical condition: There is evidence from the history, physical examination, or laboratory findings that the disturbance is attributable to the physiological consequences of another medical condition.

Delirium due to multiple etiologies: There is evidence from the history, physical examination, or laboratory findings that the delirium has more than one etiology (e.g., more than one etiological medical condition; another medical condition plus substance intoxication or medication side effect).

Specify if:

Acute: Lasting a few hours or days.

Persistent: Lasting weeks or months.

Specify if:

Hyperactive: The individual has a hyperactive level of psychomotor activity that may be accompanied by mood lability, agitation, and/or refusal to cooperate with medical care.

Hypoactive: The individual has a hypoactive level of psychomotor activity that may be accompanied by sluggishness and lethargy that approaches stupor.

Mixed level of activity: The individual has a normal level of psychomotor activity even though attention and awareness are disturbed. Also includes individuals whose activity level rapidly fluctuates.

Delirium is especially common in hospital settings, affecting an estimated 10%–15% of medical patients. Elderly patients, especially those older than 80 years, are at high risk. Additional risk factors include a preexisting dementia, recent surgery, bone fractures, systemic infections, and recent use of narcotics or antipsychotics. An estimated 40%–50% of the patients with delirium die within 1 year.

Clinical Findings

The hallmark of delirium is the rapid development of disorientation, confusion, and global cognitive impairment. Characteristic features include a disturbance of consciousness evidenced by reduced clarity of awareness of the environment; difficulty focusing, sustaining, or shifting attention; impaired cognition; and perceptual disturbances (e.g., illusions). The patient's mental status tends to fluctuate; he or she can appear normal at one point, yet minutes later is disoriented and hallucinating. Other symptoms include sleep-wake cycle disturbances with worsening at night ("sundowning"); disorientation to place, date, or person; incoherence; restlessness; agitation; and excessive somnolence.

The following vignette illustrates a relatively typical case of delirium:

> An 84-year-old retired police chief was brought to the emergency department because of a 4- to 5-day history of lassitude, lower-extremity weakness, bladder incontinence, and mental confusion. The patient had fallen 4 weeks earlier and had sustained a scalp laceration that required suturing. He had no history of recent alcohol use.
>
> The patient was cooperative but drowsy and distractible. He was oriented to person but not to date or place. His memory for recent events was poor, and he could not recall three objects either immediately or at 3 minutes. He thought that Franklin Roosevelt was the current president. Interestingly, the patient had known the paternal grandfather of one of the authors (D.W.B.) and was able to speak at length of this remote relationship.
>
> A presumptive diagnosis of delirium was made, and a medical workup was begun. A computed tomography (CT) scan showed the presence of bilateral subdural hematomas. The patient was transferred to the neurosurgery service and burr hole evacuation was performed. The delirium cleared, but the patient had a residual dementia. He was transferred to a long-term nursing facility.

Etiology

Delirium is considered an emergency, and its presence should lead to an immediate search for a medical cause. Because delirium is a *syndrome* and not a disease, it is best seen as the final common pathway of many potential causes. These include metabolic disturbances from infection, febrile illness, hypoxia, hypoglycemia, drug intoxication or withdrawal states, or hepatic encephalopathy. Potential causes that lie *within* the central nervous system (CNS) include brain abscesses, stroke, traumatic injuries, and postictal states. Other causes that may be seen particularly in the elderly are new-onset arrhythmias (e.g., atrial fibrillation) and cardiac ischemia.

Assessment

Evaluation should begin by gathering a thorough history and conducting a detailed physical examination. Informants should be interviewed because it is unlikely that the patient will be able to provide information. Close attention should be given to the presence of focal neurological signs, such as weakness or sensory loss, papilledema, and frontal lobe release signs (e.g., suck, snout, palmomental, rooting reflexes) that indicate global brain dysfunction. Laboratory tests should include routine blood and urine studies (e.g., complete blood count, urinalysis), chest X-ray, a brain CT or magnetic resonance imaging (MRI) scan, an electrocardiogram, lumbar puncture (in selected patients), toxicology screen, blood gases, and an electroencephalogram. Test results will vary depending on the underlying cause of the delirium.

Serum urine toxicology is essential in patients presenting in emergency departments to evaluate for illicit drug use. Delirious patients frequently have temperature elevations that probably represent autonomic instability or an underlying infection. Generalized diffuse slowing is often found on the electroencephalogram.

The major problem in differential diagnosis is distinguishing delirium from a confusional state due to schizophrenia or a mood disorder. Delirious patients tend to have a more acute presentation, are globally confused, and have greater impairment in attention. Hallucinations, when present, are fragmentary and disorganized and tend to be visual or tactile, as opposed to the auditory hallucinations seen in patients with psychotic disorders. Delirious patients are less likely to have a personal or family history of mental illness. However, the presence of a prior mental illness does not preclude the possibility of developing a delirium.

Clinical Management

The underlying medical condition must be corrected if possible. In many cases, the cause will remain unknown. Measures taken to maintain the patient's health and safety should include constant observation, consistent nursing care, and frequent reassurance with repeated simple explanations. Restraints may be necessary in agitated patients. External stimulation should be minimized. Because shadows or darkness may be frightening, delirious patients tend to do better in quiet, well-lit rooms.

Unnecessary medication should be discontinued, including sedatives or hypnotics (e.g., benzodiazepines). Not only are delirious patients sensitive to drug side effects, but the drugs may contribute to the delirium. Agitated patients may be calmed with low doses of high-potency antipsychotics (e.g., haloperidol, 1–2 mg every 2–4 hours as needed) or a second-generation antipsychotic. Older drugs with significant anticholinergic activity (e.g., chlorpromazine) should be avoided because they can worsen or prolong the delirium.

If sedation is necessary, low doses of short-acting benzodiazepines (e.g., oxazepam, lorazepam) can be helpful. Unrecognized alcohol withdrawal can manifest as delirium, particularly in postsurgical patients. This problem is common in hospitals: a patient presents for surgery, fails to disclose his or her history of alcohol misuse, and within days of the surgery develops a delirium. Benzodiazepines can be helpful in these cases because they will treat the alcohol withdrawal symptoms. (See Chapter 15, "Substance-Related and Addictive Disorders," for information on the treatment of alcohol withdrawal.)

Clinical points for delirium

1. In the hospital, a quiet, restful setting that is well lighted is best for the confused patient.

2. Consistency of personnel is less likely to upset the delirious patient.

3. Reminders of day, date, time, place, and situation should be prominently displayed in the patient's room.

4. Medication for behavioral management should be limited to those cases in which behavioral interventions have failed.

   - Only essential drugs should be prescribed, and polypharmacy should be avoided.

   - Sedatives, hypnotics, and anxiolytics should be avoided; the exception is where the delirium is due to alcohol withdrawal.

   - Unmanageable behavior may require the use of antipsychotics (e.g., haloperidol) or, alternatively, benzodiazepines with short half-lives (e.g., lorazepam).

■ Major and Mild Neurocognitive Disorders

Major and *mild neurocognitive disorder* lie along a spectrum of severity in terms of cognitive and functional impairment. They are acquired, with multiple or overlapping causes. In contrast, intellectual developmental disorder, also characterized by cognitive impairment, is either congenital or occurs in the early developmental period. Level of impairment distinguishes major and mild neurocognitive disorder from the mild memory changes that occur during normal aging, which are often called *benign senescent forgetfulness*. Major neurocognitive disorder corresponds to the condition referred to in DSM-IV as *dementia*. The diagnosis *mild neurocognitive disorder* corresponds to the older term *mild cognitive impairment,* applied to a condition that was not recognized in DSM-IV. The new diagnosis was introduced in DSM-5 because it had become increasingly clear that many people with milder degrees of impairment could benefit from diagnosis and referral for treatment and community services. Further, mild cognitive impairment had been recognized as a prodromal state that can progress to dementia (in about 12% of such persons each year).

There are important distinctions between the two syndromes. Major neurocognitive disorder causes "significant" cognitive decline and "substantial" impairment in cognitive performance; in addition, deficits "interfere" with independence in everyday living. With mild neurocognitive disorder, cognitive decline and impairment in cognitive function are "modest," and the deficits do not interfere with capacity for independence in everyday activities. Box 16–2 presents the DSM-5 criteria for major neurocognitive disorder. Because the criteria for mild neurocognitive disorder are so similar—except for the distinctions just noted—they are not reproduced here.

Box 16–2.   DSM-5 Diagnostic Criteria for Major Neurocognitive
Disorder

A. Evidence of significant cognitive decline from a previous level of performance in one or more cognitive domains (complex attention, executive function, learning and memory, language, perceptual-motor, or social cognition) based on:

1. Concern of the individual, a knowledgeable informant, or the clinician that there has been a significant decline in cognitive function; and
2. A substantial impairment in cognitive performance, preferably documented by standardized neuropsychological testing or, in its absence, another quantified clinical assessment.

B. The cognitive deficits interfere with independence in everyday activities (i.e., at a minimum, requiring assistance with complex instrumental activities of daily living such as paying bills or managing medications).
C. The cognitive deficits do not occur exclusively in the context of a delirium.
D. The cognitive deficits are not better explained by another mental disorder (e.g., major depressive disorder, schizophrenia).

Specify whether due to:
Alzheimer's disease
Frontotemporal lobar degeneration
Lewy body disease
Vascular disease
Traumatic brain injury

> **Substance/medication use**
> **HIV infection**
> **Prion disease**
> **Parkinson's disease**
> **Huntington's disease**
> **Another medical condition**
> **Multiple etiologies**
> **Unspecified**
>
> *Specify:*
>> **Without behavioral disturbance:** If the cognitive disturbance is not accompanied by any clinically significant behavioral disturbance.
>> **With behavioral disturbance** *(specify disturbance):* If the cognitive disturbance is accompanied by a clinically significant behavioral disturbance (e.g., psychotic symptoms, mood disturbance, agitation, apathy, or other behavioral symptoms).
>
> *Specify* current severity:
>> **Mild:** Difficulties with instrumental activities of daily living (e.g., housework, managing money).
>> **Moderate:** Difficulties with basic activities of daily living (e.g., feeding, dressing).
>> **Severe:** Fully dependent.

The core feature of both major and mild neurocognitive disorder is a decline in one or more cognitive domains based on 1) the patient's history (reported by the patient and/or knowledgeable informants) and 2) performance on an objective assessment that falls below expectation or has declined over time. Reports of cognitive decline and objective evidence should be seen as complementary and mutually reinforcing. If a clinician is overly focused on objective testing, a disorder may go undetected in high-functioning people whose currently "normal" performance actually represents a substantial decline in abilities. Likewise, a neurocognitive disorder may be incorrectly diagnosed in people whose currently "low" performance does not represent a change from their own baseline or results from other factors such as test conditions.

Major neurocognitive disorders are relatively uncommon in people younger than age 65. The percentage of those affected is linear: between ages 65 and 75 about 10% will be affected; at age 90 about 50% will be affected. The rates of major neurocognitive disorder are even higher among elderly hospitalized patients and physically ill persons. Because the growth in the United States population of those older than 65 years is outstripping the growth in the general population, it is clear that the problem of major neurocognitive disorder will be even greater in the future. Providing for the care of large numbers of patients will be one of the major tasks that American society will need to address as "baby boomers" age.

Clinical Findings

Apart from major and mild neurocognitive disorders that develop fairly abruptly, such as those resulting from a stroke, most typically develop insidiously, and in fact preliminary signs may be overlooked or misattributed to normal aging. In its earliest stages, the only symptom of a neurocognitive disorder may be a subtle change in the patient's personality, a decrease in the range of the patient's interests, the development of apathy, or the development of labile or shallow emotions. Intellectual skills are gradually affected and may be noticed initially in work settings where high performance is required. The patient may be unaware of (or deny) the loss of his or her intellectual sharpness.

As the disorder advances, cognitive impairment becomes more pronounced, mood and personality changes become exaggerated, and psychotic symptoms can develop. The patient may lack insight and remain unconcerned even though family members have noticed substantial deficits. Sometimes caregivers need to intervene and restrict activities such as driving.

When the neurocognitive disorder is advanced, the patient may be unable to perform basic tasks such as self-feeding or caring for personal hygiene, may become incontinent, and may develop extreme emotional lability. Patients frequently forget names of friends and are sometimes unable to recognize close relatives. In the end stages of a neurocognitive disorder, a patient may be mute and unresponsive. At that point, death usually follows within 1 year.

The noncognitive symptoms are often the most troublesome, especially from the family member's viewpoint (see Table 16–2). About one-half of patients with Alzheimer's disease will develop psychotic symptoms such as hallucinations and/or delusions. Nearly 20% of Alzheimer patients also develop clinical depression, and perhaps an equal number will have milder depressive symptoms. Depression is even more common in patients with vascular forms of neurocognitive disorder. A co-occurring depression can intensify both cognitive and memory disturbance.

Diagnosis and Assessment

Patients concerned about their cognitive performance (or family members who may bring their relative to medical attention) should be asked

TABLE 16–2. Behavior problems identified by family members of 55 dementia patients

Behavior	Families reporting problems, %
Memory disturbance	100
Temper outbursts	87
Demanding or critical behavior	71
Night awakening	69
Hiding things	69
Communication difficulties	68
Suspiciousness	63
Making accusations	60
Poor mealtime behavior	60
Daytime wandering	59
Poor hygiene	53
Hallucinations	49
Delusions	47
Physical violence	47
Incontinence	40
Difficulty with cooking	33
Hitting or assaults	32
Problems driving	20
Problems smoking	11
Inappropriate sexual behavior	2

Source. Adapted from Rabins et al. 1982.

about specific symptoms that the patient may have. For example, memory concerns include difficulty remembering a short grocery list or keeping track of the plot of a television program; executive concerns include difficulty resuming a task when interrupted, organizing tax records, or planning a holiday meal. At the mild neurocognitive disorder level, the person is likely to describe these tasks as being more difficult or as requiring extra time or effort or even compensatory strategies. Further, the person and his or her family members may not notice such symptoms or may view them as normal, particularly in the elderly. At the major neurocognitive disorder level, such tasks may only be completed with assistance or may be abandoned altogether. The difficulties must represent changes rather than lifelong patterns: the individual or informant may clarify this issue, or the clinician can infer change from prior experience with the patient or from occupational or other clues. It is also critical to determine that the difficulties are related to cognitive loss rather than to motor or sensory limitations (e.g., vision or hearing loss).

Besides the history, the physical examination and mental status examination are the best tools to detect neurocognitive disorders. To supplement a formal mental status examination, the Mini-Mental State Examination (MMSE), a quick, at-the-bedside test, can be used to obtain a rough index of cognitive impairment. The quick screener assesses orientation, memory, constructional ability, and the ability to read, write, and calculate. Thirty points are possible: a score of less than 25 is suggestive of impairment, and a score of less than 20 usually indicates definite impairment. There are other bedside tests, but the MMSE is the most widely used.

Laboratory testing will help in the search for treatable causes of the neurocognitive disorder, even though most causes are irreversible; only about 3% will fully resolve. All patients with a new-onset dementia should have a complete blood count; liver, thyroid, and renal function tests; serologic tests for syphilis and HIV; urinalysis; electrocardiogram; and chest X-ray. Serum electrolytes, serum glucose, and vitamin B_{12} and folate levels should be measured. Most of the readily reversible metabolic, endocrine, vitamin deficiency, and infectious states, whether causal or complicating, will be uncovered with these simple tests when combined with the history and physical examination findings. Other laboratory tests are helpful in carefully selected patients. For example, a CT or an MRI brain scan is appropriate in the presence of a history suggestive of a mass lesion, focal neurological signs, or a rapid onset of neurocognitive disorder. Electroencephalograms are appropriate for patients with altered consciousness or suspected seizures. Pulse oximetry is indicated when compromised respiratory function is evident. Single-photon emission computed tomography (SPECT) or positron emission tomography (PET) imaging can help to distinguish Alzheimer's disease from other forms of neurocognitive disorder. In fact, fluorodeoxyglucose PET imaging has been approved by Medicare as a diagnostic tool for distinguishing Alzheimer's disease from other dementias. In Alzheimer's dementia, there is characteristic temporal and parietal hypometabolism. The medical workup for neurocognitive disorders is summarized in Table 16–3.

Neuropsychological testing can be helpful as part of the overall evaluation of the patient. Testing can be done to obtain baseline data by which to measure change both before and after treatment; to evaluate highly ed-

---

TABLE 16–3. Medical workup for neurocognitive disorders

---

1. Complete history
2. Thorough physical examination, including neurological examination
3. Mental status examination
4. Laboratory studies
   - Complete blood count, with differential
   - Serum electrolytes
   - Serum glucose
   - Blood urea nitrogen
   - Creatinine
   - Liver function tests
   - Serology for syphilis and HIV
   - Thyroid function tests
   - Serum vitamin B_{12}
   - Folate
   - Urinalysis and urine drug screen
   - Electrocardiogram
   - Chest X-ray
   - Pulse oximetry
   - Brain computed tomography or magnetic resonance imaging
5. Neuropsychological testing (e.g., attention, memory, cognitive function)
6. Optional tests
   - Functional neuroimaging (e.g., positron emission tomography, single-photon emission computed tomography)
   - Lumbar puncture

---

ucated individuals suspected of developing an early dementia when brain imaging or other test results are ambiguous; and to help in distinguishing delirium from dementia and depression. These tests also can be repeated serially to track changes in attention, memory, and cognition.

Because symptoms of major neurocognitive disorders (dementia) and delirium overlap, it is important to separate the two syndromes. In some cases, both will be present, or the delirium may present first, not clear entirely, and leave the patient cognitively impaired. Because delirium is considered a medical emergency and will prompt a search for a cause, it needs to be carefully distinguished from dementia. Characteristics that help to separate dementia from delirium are highlighted in Table 16–4.

It is equally important to separate major neurocognitive disorder (dementia) from *pseudodementia,* a condition that sometimes accompanies depressive disorders. With pseudodementia, the depressed patient appears to have dementia. He or she may be unable to remember correctly, cannot calculate well, and complains—often bitterly—of lost cognitive abilities and skills. The importance of this distinction is obvious: the patient with pseudodementia has a treatable illness (depression) and does not have a dementia. That said, pseudodementia is increasingly being recognized as a condition that occurs in people at high risk of progressing to dementia.

Most patients with neurocognitive disorders can be evaluated on an outpatient basis. In practice, hospital admissions involving these patients are usually for the evaluation and treatment of behavioral and psychological disturbances such as aggression, violence, wandering, psychosis, or depression. Other reasons for hospitalization include suicidal threats or behaviors, rapid weight loss, and acute worsening without an apparent cause.

Etiological Subtypes of Major or Mild Neurocognitive Disorder

Due to Alzheimer's Disease

Alzheimer's disease is the most common cause of dementia, accounting for 50%–60% of cases and affecting approximately 2.5 million Americans. In DSM-5, Alzheimer's disease is divided into probable and possible types. With major neurocognitive disorder due to *probable* Alzheimer's disease, there is evidence of either 1) a causative genetic mutation from family history or genetic testing and/or 2) decline in memory and learning and at least one other cognitive domain; progressive decline; and no evidence of mixed etiology. If neither is present, possible Alzheimer's disease is diagnosed.

For *mild neurocognitive disorder due to Alzheimer's disease,* given the lesser degree of certainty, a *probable* diagnosis requires evidence of a causative Alzheimer's disease gene, from either genetic testing or a positive family history; otherwise, the diagnosis is only *possible* (see Box 16–3). If the etiology appears mixed, mild neurocognitive disorder due to multiple etiologies should be diagnosed. In any case, for both mild and major neurocognitive disorder due to Alzheimer's disease, the clinical features must not suggest another primary etiology for the disorder.

TABLE 16–4.   Clinical features differentiating dementia from delirium

Dementia	Delirium
Chronic or insidious	Acute onset
Sensorium unimpaired early on	Sensorium clouded
Normal level of arousal	Agitation or stupor
Progressive and deteriorating	Often reversible
Common in nursing homes and psychiatric hospitals	Common on medical, surgical, and neurological wards

---

Box 16–3.   DSM-5 Diagnostic Criteria for Major or Mild Neurocognitive Disorder Due to Alzheimer's Disease

A. The criteria are met for major or mild neurocognitive disorder.
B. There is insidious onset and gradual progression of impairment in one or more cognitive domains (for major neurocognitive disorder, at least two domains must be impaired).
C. Criteria are met for either probable or possible Alzheimer's disease as follows:

For major neurocognitive disorder:

Probable Alzheimer's disease is diagnosed if either of the following is present; otherwise, **possible Alzheimer's disease** should be diagnosed.

1. Evidence of a causative Alzheimer's disease genetic mutation from family history or genetic testing.
2. All three of the following are present:
   a. Clear evidence of decline in memory and learning and at least one other cognitive domain (based on detailed history or serial neuropsychological testing).
   b. Steadily progressive, gradual decline in cognition, without extended plateaus.
   c. No evidence of mixed etiology (i.e., absence of other neurodegenerative or cerebrovascular disease, or another neurological, mental, or systemic disease or condition likely contributing to cognitive decline).

For mild neurocognitive disorder:

Probable Alzheimer's disease is diagnosed if there is evidence of a causative Alzheimer's disease genetic mutation from either genetic testing or family history.

Possible Alzheimer's disease is diagnosed if there is no evidence of a causative Alzheimer's disease genetic mutation from either genetic testing or family history, and all three of the following are present:

1. Clear evidence of decline in memory and learning.
2. Steadily progressive, gradual decline in cognition, without extended plateaus.
3. No evidence of mixed etiology (i.e., absence of other neurodegenerative or cerebrovascular disease, or another neurological or systemic disease or condition likely contributing to cognitive decline).

D. The disturbance is not better explained by cerebrovascular disease, another neurodegenerative disease, the effects of a substance, or another mental, neurological, or systemic disorder.

Alzheimer's disease usually has an insidious onset, leading to death within 8–10 years after symptoms are first recognized. Estimates of its prevalence range from 5% at age 65 to 40% by age 90. Symptoms worsen progressively, eventually resulting in near collapse of cognitive functioning. Physical findings are generally absent, or they are present only in later stages: hyperactive deep tendon reflexes, Babinski's sign, and frontal lobe release signs. The presence of illusions, hallucinations, or delusions is associated with accelerated cognitive deterioration. Cortical atrophy and enlarged cerebral ventricles are typically seen on CT or MRI scans.

The case of composer Maurice Ravel illustrates the tragedy of Alzheimer's disease:

Ravel, a leader of the French musical impressionist movement, excelled at piano composition and orchestration. At age 56, after completing his most famous work, Concerto in G Minor, he began to complain of fatigue and lassitude, symptoms that were in keeping with his chronic insomnia and lifelong hypochondriasis. His symptoms continued to progress, and his creative energy waned.

The following year, after a minor automobile accident, Ravel's cognitive abilities began to erode. His capacity to remember names, to speak spontaneously, and to write became impaired. An eminent French neurologist noted that Ravel's ability to understand verbal speech was superior to his ability to speak or to write. Tragically, Ravel also developed *amusia*, the inability to comprehend musical sounds. His last public performance occurred shortly thereafter. He was no longer capable of the coordination, cognition, and speech necessary to lead an orchestra.

Ravel's friends made futile attempts to help him, trying to stimulate him intellectually any way they could, but gradually his speech and intellectual functions declined further. Within 4 years of the onset of dementia, Ravel was mute and incapable of recognizing his own music.

Ravel died at age 62 after a neurosurgical procedure, the indications for which remain unclear. No autopsy was done, but his neurologist had suspected a cerebral degenerative disease. Syphilis, a common illness of the day, had been ruled out.

Traditionally, Alzheimer's disease cases have been divided into those that have an early onset (age 65 and younger) and those with a late onset (over age 65). Early-onset patients often have an onset in the fifth decade, and the disorder has been linked to mutations on chromosomes 1, 14, and 21. The early-onset variant is relatively rare, however, and nearly all cases seen in the community are late-onset (or sporadic).

While new neuroimaging techniques are evolving rapidly toward the capability of an accurate diagnosis during life, the definitive diagnosis of Alzheimer's disease is largely still considered a diagnosis made at autopsy. Two primary abnormalities characterize the histopathological features of Alzheimer's disease: amyloid plaques and neurofibrillary tangles. Amyloid plaques in the brain are generated from amyloid precursor protein (APP), which is cleaved by enzymes called secretases to form β-amyloid. The β-amyloid of the 42 amino acid type has been found to accumulate in excess in the brains of persons with Alzheimer's disease, and the β-amyloid-42 protein is known to aggregate into plaques that are associated with inflammation and neuronal death. The second characteristic histopathological feature is the presence of neurofibrillary tangles. These are comprised of hyperphosphorylated tau protein that folds within the intracellular cytoplasm of neurons and is also associated with cell death.

In contrast to neuronal plaques, neurofibrillary tangles are seen more commonly in a variety of neurodegenerative diseases, such as frontotemporal dementia, as well as in persons with closed head injuries. To utilize these abnormalities as an in vivo marker, there has been research examining cerebrospinal fluid (CSF) levels of amyloid and tau proteins. Alzheimer's disease has been associated with a reduction in CSF amyloid levels compared with those in healthy subjects, which is thought to be due to sequestration of the amyloid within the neuronal plaques. Conversely, tau protein is elevated in the CSF of Alzheimer's patients compared to controls. This finding likely reflects that tau protein increases in the context of neuronal damage.

Risk factors include a history of head injury, Down syndrome, low educational and occupational level, and having a first-degree relative with Alzheimer's disease. In fact, up to 50% of the first-degree relatives of persons with Alzheimer's disease are affected with the disorder by age 90 years. A genetic polymorphism on chromosome 19, apolipoprotein E (*APOE*), has been found to influence the risk of Alzheimer's disease. The *APOE* ε4 allele increases risk and decreases age at onset, and the *APOE* ε2 allele has a protective effect.

Frontotemporal

Frontotemporal neurocognitive disorder, originally called *Pick's disease,* accounts for about 5% of all cases of dementia in unselected autopsy series and is a relatively common cause of dementia in persons under age 65. There are a behavioral variant and three language variants that have distinct patterns of brain atrophy and some distinctive neuropathology. Individuals with behavioral-variant subtype present with varying degrees of apathy or disinhibition. They may lose interest in socialization, self-care, and personal responsibilities, or display socially inappropriate behaviors. Insight is usually impaired. Formal neuropsychological testing may show relatively few deficits in the early stages. Individuals with language-variant subtypes present with primary progressive aphasia with gradual onset.

In general, this disorder is characterized by tau-positive inclusions and a subgroup of cases with parkinsonian features linked to chromosome 17. The disease is gradually progressive, with median survival being 6–11 years after symptom onset and 3-4 years after diagnosis.

With Lewy Bodies

Neurocognitive disorder with Lewy bodies may account for up to 25% of neurocognitive disorder cases and is progressive. In addition to changes in the brain parenchyma typical for Alzheimer's disease, Lewy bodies—eosinophilic inclusion bodies—are present in the cerebral cortex and brainstem. The disorder includes not only progressive cognitive impairment with early changes in complex attention and executive function rather than learning and memory, but also visual hallucinations, hallucinations in other sensory modalities, depression, and delusions. There may be a concurrent rapid eye movement sleep behavior disorder. Autonomic dysfunction, such as orthostatic hypotension and urinary incontinence, may occur. Another core feature is spontaneous parkinsonism, which begins after the onset of cognitive decline. A diagnostically suggestive feature is low striatal dopamine transporter uptake on SPECT or PET scans.

Up to 50% of individuals with this disorder have significant sensitivity to antipsychotic drugs. For that reason, these medications should be used with extreme caution in managing the psychotic symptoms. Second-generation antipsychotics are better tolerated if medication is needed for behavioral control

Vascular

Vascular neurocognitive disorder is the second most common cause of dementia after Alzheimer's disease, accounting for about 15%–30% of dementia cases; in many cases the two forms are combined. The diagnosis requires the presence of a neurocognitive disorder and the conclusion that cerebrovascular disease is the primary (if not exclusive) pathology that accounts for the cognitive deficits. Vascular etiology may range from large-vessel stroke to microvascular disease. For that reason, the presentation is heterogeneous because of the many types of vascular lesions and their extent and location. Lesions may be focal, multifocal, or diffuse and occur in various combinations.

Commonly associated symptoms are personality and mood changes, loss of motivation (abulia), depression, and emotional lability. The development of late-onset depressive symptoms accompanied by psychomotor slowing and executive function deficits is a common presentation in older adults with progressive small-vessel ischemic disease ("vascular depression").

Neurocognitive disorder caused by multiple infarcts probably accounts for the bulk of the cases and results from accumulation of cerebral infarcts in persons with atherosclerotic disease of the major vessels or heart valves; it may be accompanied by focal neurological deficits. A history of rapid onset and a stepwise deterioration occurring in patients in their 50s or 60s help to distinguish vascular from degenerative forms of neurocognitive disorder. Assessing for the presence of cerebrovascular disease relies on history, physical examination, and neuroimaging. Clinical evidence of cerebrovascular disease includes documented history of stroke, with cognitive decline temporally associated with the event, or physical signs consistent with stroke (e.g., hemiparesis; pseudobulbar syndrome; visual field defect).

Patients with vascular forms of dementia often have a history of high blood pressure or diabetes, and many will have had prior strokes, many of them "silent" or asymptomatic. Atherosclerosis in major arteries may be surgically correctable, but because atherosclerosis occurs diffusely among smaller intracranial vessels, there is no specific treatment for most forms of the disorder. As preventive measures, blood pressure can be controlled in those with hypertension and anticoagulants or aspirin can be administered to help prevent thrombus formation, thereby decreasing the risk of myocardial infarction and stroke.

Due to Traumatic Brain Injury

Traumatic brain injury is caused by an impact to the head, or other events that cause rapid movement or displacement of the brain within the skull, for example blast injuries that are commonly seen in wartime. Traumatic brain injuries are relatively common, and an estimated 2% of the general population lives with such injuries.

Characteristics include at least one of the following: loss of consciousness, posttraumatic amnesia, disorientation and confusion, or, in more severe cases, neurological signs (e.g., positive neuroimaging, a new onset of seizures or a marked worsening of a preexisting seizure disorder, visual field cuts, anosmia, hemiparesis). To be attributable to traumatic brain injury, the neurocognitive disorder must present either immediately after the brain injury occurs or immediately after the individual recovers consciousness after the injury and must persist past the acute postinjury period.

Traumatic brain injuries may be accompanied by disturbances in emotional function (e.g., irritability, easy frustration, tension and anxiety, affective lability); personality changes (e.g., disinhibition, apathy, suspiciousness, aggression); and physical disturbances (e.g., headache, fatigue, sleep disorders, vertigo or dizziness, tinnitus or hyperacusis, photosensitivity, anosmia, reduced tolerance to psychotropic medications). In more severe cases, neurological signs and symptoms (e.g., seizures, hemiparesis) can occur. The cognitive presentation is variable. Difficulties in the domains of complex attention, executive ability, learning, and memory are common as well as slowing in speed of information processing and disturbances in social cognition. If there is a brain contusion, intracranial hemorrhage, or penetrating injury, there may be additional neurocognitive deficits, such as aphasia, neglect, and constructional dyspraxia.

Substance/Medication-Induced

Major or mild neurocognitive disorder due to substance/medication use needs to be distinguished from the cognitive impairments commonly seen with substance intoxication or withdrawal. The impairments seen in intoxication or withdrawal are usually reversible, whereas substance/medication-induced neurocognitive disorder is a persisting condition.

While nonspecific decrements in a range of cognitive abilities can occur with nearly any substance of abuse and a variety of medications, some patterns occur more frequently with selected drug classes. For example, a neurocognitive disorder due to sedative, hypnotic, or anxiolytic drugs (e.g., benzodiazepines, barbiturates) may show greater disturbances in memory than in other cognitive functions. A neurocognitive disorder induced by alcohol frequently manifests with a combination of impairments in executive-function and memory and learning domains.

With alcohol, the neurocognitive disorder is usually mild except when there is a *Wernicke's encephalopathy*, a clinical syndrome characterized by ophthalmoplegia, ataxic gait, nystagmus, and mental confusion caused by thiamine deficiency associated with chronic alcohol misuse. The term *Wernicke-Korsakoff* (or *Korsakoff's*) syndrome is used when cognitive and memory impairment endures. (See Chapter 15, "Substance-Related and Addictive Disorders," for a more complete discussion of these syndromes.)

Due to HIV Infection

People with HIV infections are at increased risk of developing a neurocognitive disorder. HIV infects several types of cells, most particularly immune cells. Over time, the infection can cause severe depletion of "T-helper" (CD4) lymphocytes, resulting in an immunocompromised state, and may lead to opportunistic infections and neoplasms. This advanced form of HIV infection is termed *acquired immune deficiency syndrome* or *AIDS*. Diagnosis of HIV is confirmed by established laboratory methods such as enzyme-linked immunosorbent assay for HIV antibody with Western blot confirmation and/or polymerase chain reaction-based assays for HIV.

Depending on stage of HIV disease, about one-third to over one-half of HIV-infected individuals have at least mild neurocognitive disturbance. An estimated 25% of individuals with HIV will have signs and symptoms that meet criteria for mild neurocognitive disorder; fewer than 5% would meet criteria for major neurocognitive disorder.

HIV-related neurocognitive disorders could result from direct HIV infection of the CNS, intracranial tumors, infections (e.g., toxoplasmosis, cryptococcosis), or the indirect effects of systemic disease (e.g., septicemia, hypoxia, electrolyte imbalance). The diagnosis of a major or mild neurocognitive disorder due to HIV infection should only be given when cognitive impairment is judged to be due to the direct CNS effects of HIV. Because neurocognitive disorders can occur in the early stages of HIV infection, evaluation for HIV seropositivity is indicated for persons at high risk for infection (e.g., gay men, drug-addicted persons) who develop cognitive, mood, or behavior changes.

Due to Prion Disease

Neurocognitive disorders due to prion disease include those resulting from a group of subacute spongiform encephalopathies such as Creutzfeldt-Jakob disease, variant Creutzfeldt-Jakob disease, kuru, Gerstmann-Sträussler- Scheinker syndrome, and fatal insomnia. They are caused by small proteinaceous particles called *prions*, once called "slow viruses."

Creutzfeldt-Jakob disease is the best-known example of a prion disease. It is a rare and rapidly fatal condition that causes death within months. There is no known treatment. The incubation period can last months to years. It has a peak incidence between age 50 and 70. Severe cerebellar and/or extrapyramidal signs are present, along with myoclonus. Akinetic mutism and cortical blindness sometimes occur. Triphasic complexes are found on electroencephalograms in about 80% of the cases. Histopathology shows spongiform changes consisting of fine vacuolation of the neuropil of the gray matter, associated with astrocytosis and neuronal loss.

Creutzfeldt-Jakob disease occurs sporadically and may be inherited or transmitted by intracerebral electrodes, grafts of dura mater, corneal transplants, and human-derived growth hormone and gonadotropin. A new variant recently has been described that has an earlier onset (27 years vs. 60 years), more psychiatric symptoms, a longer course (14 months vs. 4 months), and an absence of triphasic complexes on electroencephalography.

Due to Parkinson's Disease

Up to three-quarters of people with *Parkinson's disease* will develop a major neurocognitive disorder during the course of their disease. A mild neurocognitive disorder will occur in another quarter. People with Parkinson's disease who are older and have more severe disease appear more likely to develop cognitive problems. The essential feature is cognitive decline following the onset of Parkinson's disease. The disturbance must occur in the setting of established Parkinson's disease, and deficits must have developed gradually. Features can include apathy, depressed mood, anxious mood, hallucinations, delusions, personality changes, rapid eye movement sleep behavior disorder, and excessive daytime sleepiness.

Parkinson's disease is more common in men than women. Onset is typically between the sixth and ninth decades of life, with most expression in the early 60s. Mild neurocognitive disorder often develops relatively early in the course of Parkinson's disease; major impairment typically occurs late.

Due to Huntington's Disease

Huntington's disease is a neuropsychiatric disorder with autosomal-dominant inheritance. Genetic testing shows a CAG trinucleotide repeat expansion in the *HTT* gene, located on chromosome 4. Progressive cognitive impairment is a core feature, with early changes in executive function (i.e., processing speed, organization, and planning) rather than learning and memory. Cognitive and associated behavioral changes often precede the emergence of the typical motor abnormalities of brady-kinesia and choreiform movements. Depression, irritability, anxiety, obsessive-compulsive symptoms, and apathy are common symptoms and psychosis less so. These emotional and behavioral symptoms often precede the onset of motor symptoms.

The average age at diagnosis of Huntington's disease is approximately 40 years, although this varies widely. Age at onset is inversely correlated with CAG expansion length. Juvenile Huntington's disease (onset before age 20) may present more commonly with bradykinesia, dystonia, and rigidity than with the choreic movements characteristic of the adult-onset disorder. The disease is gradually progressive, with median survival approximately 15 years after motor symptom diagnosis.

Other behavioral disturbances may include pronounced apathy, disinhibition, impulsivity, and impaired insight, with apathy often becoming more progressive over time. Early movement symptoms may involve the appearance of fidgetiness of the extremities as well as mild apraxia (i.e., difficulty with purposeful movements), particularly with fine motor tasks. As the disorder progresses, other motor problems include impaired gait (ataxia) and postural instability. Motor impairment eventually affects speech production (dysarthria) such that the speech becomes very difficult to understand, which may result in significant distress resulting from the communication barrier in the context of comparatively intact cognition. Advanced motor disease severely affects gait with progressive ataxia, and eventually people become unable to walk. End-stage motor disease impairs motor control of eating and swallowing, typically a major contributor to death from aspiration pneumonia.

Due to Another Medical Condition

The diagnosis *neurocognitive disorder due to another medical condition* is used when an individual has a cause other than those listed specifically in DSM-5. Potential causes include brain tumors, subdural hematomas, normal-pressure hydrocephalus, multiple sclerosis, neurosyphilis, hypoglycemia, renal or hepatic failure, childhood and adult storage diseases, and vitamin deficiencies.

Subdural hematomas are large blood clots caused by a disruption of the veins that bridge the brain parenchyma and the meninges, and they usually result from blunt trauma. They are capable of producing a dementia, or they may complicate other forms of dementia. Risk factors include being older than age 60 and having a history of alcoholism, epilepsy, or renal dialysis. Treatment involves surgical evacuation of the clot through a burr hole in the skull.

Normal-pressure hydrocephalus is caused by excessive accumulation of CSF, which gradually dilates the ventricles of the brain in the presence of normal CSF pressure. The flow of CSF from the ventricles to its usual site of absorption becomes obstructed, so that fluid collects within the ventricles, resulting in the triad of dementia, gait disturbance, and urinary incontinence. Normal-pressure hydrocephalus can result from brain trauma, but the cause usually is unknown. Some patients respond dramatically to surgical placement of a shunt to remove the excess fluid buildup.

Infections that involve the brain are capable of producing a dementing illness. Many cases of dementia are prevented by the effective treatment of meningitis and encephalitis, whether caused by bacteria, fungi, protozoa, or viruses. Chronic infectious processes—for example, those caused by bacteria (e.g., Whipple's disease), fungi (e.g., *Cryptococcus*), or other microorganisms (e.g., syphilis)—may cause a dementia but are potentially reversible to some extent, depending on appropriate diagnosis and treatment. A postinfectious encephalomyelitis occurring after a viral exanthem may produce sufficient brain damage to result in a dementia.

Metabolic and pulmonary diseases can cause neurocognitive disorders. Metabolic diseases of the thyroid, parathyroid, adrenal, and pituitary glands can cause a dementia and usually are readily identified. Pulmonary diseases can produce a dementia as a result of hypoxia or hypercapnia, as can chronic or acute renal failure and liver failure (i.e., hepatic encephalopathy). Dementia is common in patients with diabetes as a result of either hypoglycemia or hyperosmolar coma. All are partially or completely reversible depending on the early diagnosis and treatment of the underlying condition.

Nutritional disorders can cause or contribute to dementia in some cases. Pernicious anemia (B12 deficiency), folate deficiency, and pellagra (niacin deficiency) are all capable of causing a dementia, and are not always reversible. Pellagra is a major problem in underdeveloped countries and typically shows a dramatic response to niacin, even when mental changes have been present for a long time.

Other rare causes of dementia include diseases of the cerebellum (cerebellar, spinocerebellar, and olivopontocerebellar degeneration), and motor neurons (amyotrophic lateral sclerosis); herpes simplex encephalitis; and the dementia of multiple sclerosis. Numerous hereditary metabolic diseases are associated with dementia, including Wilson's disease (hepatolenticular degeneration), metachromatic leukodystrophy, the adrenoleukodystrophies, and the neuronal storage diseases (e.g., Tay-Sachs disease).

Clinical Management of Major and Mild Neurocognitive Disorders

Cholinergic therapies address the well-known deficit of acetylcholine in Alzheimer's disease. Three cholinesterase inhibitor drugs are commonly used: donepezil, rivastigmine, and galantamine. These drugs are equally effective and work to slow the rate of cognitive decline. Another drug, tacrine, is also U.S. Food and Drug Administration (FDA) approved but is used less frequently because of poor tolerability and the need to monitor liver enzymes. There is a marked variation in response—some patients show tremendous improvement, whereas others show very little improvement. These drugs do not alter the course of the disease and work best in persons in the earliest stages of the disease (i.e., mild neurocognitive disorder). Side effects across this class of drugs include nausea, emesis, diarrhea, anorexia, and weight loss, all of which tend to be mild and temporary. Dosages are titrated slowly to the target.

Memantine is the first of a new generation of cognitive enhancers, and it blocks the N-methyl-D-aspartate (NMDA) receptor, one of two receptors that normally bind glutamate. This receptor is thought to mediate certain aspects of learning and memory. The drug is approved by the FDA to treat moderate to severe Alzheimer's disease. Like the cholinesterase inhibitors, the main benefit of the drug is to slow the inevitable decline in cognitive functioning. (See Table 16–5 for a list of the cognitive enhancers.) A recent study suggests that vitamin E (2,000 IU/day) may slow functional decline in people with mild to moderate Alzheimer's disease.

Other medications are used for the symptomatic treatment of associated anxiety, psychosis, or depression, including the anxiolytics, antipsychotics, and antidepressants, respectively. The physician should use the lowest effective dosage, because patients with dementia often poorly tolerate drug side effects. In treating depression in patients with dementia, physicians should avoid tricyclic antidepressants and use the better-tolerated selective serotonin reuptake inhibitors (SSRIs). Whatever drug is used, patients with dementia require lower dosages than do people without dementia.

Irritability, hostility, aggression, uncooperativeness, and assaultiveness are the most difficult and vexing problems to manage in patients with major neurocognitive disorder. Disturbing and disruptive symptoms may make it difficult to keep the patient within his or her family or social situation and can lead to institutionalization. Second-generation antipsychotics (SGAs) are frequently prescribed to help

TABLE 16–5.   Cognitive enhancement medications

Drug	Trade name	Dosage range (mg/day)
Donepezil	Aricept	5–10
Galantamine	Reminyl	8–24
Memantine	Namenda	10–20
Rivastigmine	Exelon	1.5–6
Tacrine	Cognex	40–160

control behavioral problems in these patients and are at least moderately effective (e.g., olanzapine, 2.5–10 mg/day; quetiapine, 25–200 mg/day; risperidone, 0.25–3 mg/day), but they need to be carefully titrated. Recent warnings by the FDA have emphasized the importance of careful monitoring of SGAs due to an increased mortality risk associated with their use in dementia patients. The older, conventional low-potency antipsychotics (e.g., chlorpromazine) should be avoided because of their anticholinergic activity that can worsen confusion. Trazodone, given as a bedtime dose (25–100 mg), may be helpful in relieving nighttime agitation or sundowning. Benzodiazepines should be avoided except for the occasional treatment of bouts of acute agitation in persons who otherwise have no need for ongoing anti-agitation medication. Low doses of lorazepam (0.25–1 mg) may be helpful in these situations. Lithium carbonate, valproate, carbamazepine, and other agents have been tried for long-term management of behavioral problems, but their role in treating dementia patients is unclear.

Behavioral strategies can be enormously helpful. Simple adjustments to the physical environment, talking calmly with patients, and encouraging appropriate socialization can help relieve problem behaviors. A regular and predictable daily schedule, structured activities, and avoidance of alcohol, caffeine, and diuretics are important. *Reminiscence group therapy* may help patients to maintain their social skills and improve mood and morale. With reminiscence therapy, patients are encouraged to discuss past activities, events, and experiences, often with the aid of photographs, familiar household items, and music. Even severely impaired patients can react to familiar social activities and to music. Self-help groups for family members provide educational and psychological support. Day care centers may provide needed relief for caregivers. A useful manual is *The 36-Hour Day* by Mace and Rabins.

Clinical points for major and mild neurocognitive disorders

1. Both at home and in care facilities, patients usually respond better to low-stimulus environments than to high-stimulus situations.

   • Patients with dementia have difficulty interpreting sensory input and easily become overwhelmed.

2. Consistency and routine are important for reducing confusion and agitation.

3. Families are often overwhelmed by caring for their cognitively impaired relative. The clinician should

   • Recommend that family members attend support groups (available in most communities).

   • Recommend appropriate reading material.

   • Counsel relatives to minimize confrontational or critical comments.

4. Families will need psychological support if the patient requires institutionalization, to lessen the guilt they almost inevitably feel.

5. Cognitive enhancers may slow the rate of cognitive decline but will not reverse decline. They are most effective in those with mild disorders. Accompanying depression generally responds to antidepressants, and acute agitation or psychosis may respond to a second-generation antipsychotic.

   • Use an SSRI to treat depression.

   • Conventional low-potency antipsychotics should be avoided because of their anticholinergic activity that can worsen confusion.

   • High-potency conventional antipsychotics are generally safe (e.g., haloperidol) but may cause pseudoparkinsonism.

   • Second-generation antipsychotics may increase mortality risk, so should be used with care.

   • Trazodone given as a bedtime dose may help to relieve nighttime agitation.

■ Self-Assessment Questions

1. What are the differences between major and mild neurocognitive disorders? What are the six cognitive domains?
2. How are delirium and major neurocognitive disorder (dementia) alike? How do they differ?
3. What constitutes a medical workup for the neurocognitive disorders?

4. Describe Alzheimer's disease. What are its histopathological findings?
5. List some of the different causes of dementia.
6. How does Alzheimer's disease differ from frontotemporal dementia?
7. Describe pseudodementia. What are its signs and symptoms?
8. What are prions? Describe Creutzfeldt-Jakob disease.
9. Describe the cognitive and behavioral symptoms of a neurocognitive disorder due to Huntington's disease.
10. What is the "symptom triad" in normal-pressure hydrocephalus?
11. Describe Wernicke's encephalopathy. What is its relationship to the Wernicke-Korsakoff syndrome? What is the treatment?
12. Describe the cognitive enhancers. What is their proposed mechanism of action? What else can clinicians recommend for the management of dementia?

Chapter 17

Personality Disorders

All is caprice, they love without measure those whom they will soon hate without reason.

Thomas Sydenham

aladaptive character traits have been recognized since Cain killed his brother Abel. In ancient Greece, Hippocrates observed and classified many of the mental illnesses that are recognized today. Although he had no category for personality disorders, he described four temperaments believed to embody the elements of earth, air, fire, and water: the optimistic sanguine, the irritable choleric, the sad melancholic, and the apathetic phlegmatic. Variations of this simple classification of temperament were used right up to the twentieth century; the German psychiatrist Emil Kraepelin, in fact, described the personalities he found in manic-depressive patients and their relatives as depressive, hypomanic, or irritable, terms that correspond to the melancholic, sanguine, and choleric temperaments.

Formal attempts to list the variety of personality types took root with the publication of DSM-I in 1952, in which seven different types of personality disturbances were described. With the arrival of DSM-III in 1980, criteria for 11 different personality disorders were enumerated, including several new disorders created in response to clinical and research observations. The list of personality disorders was pared to 10 in DSM-IV and has not changed in DSM-5 (see Table 17–1). In addition, the diagnosis *personality change due to another medical condition* can be used in cases where an individual has personality changes that result from a medical condition (e.g., a tumor, stroke, or head injury). Residual categories are available for use in situations in which the person clearly has a personality disorder but the criteria for any specific disorder are not met, or in which the personality pattern is not described by the DSM-5 classification (e.g., immature personality disorder).

TABLE 17–1.   DSM-5 personality disorders

Cluster A (the "eccentric" disorders)

  Paranoid

  Schizoid

  Schizotypal

Cluster B (the "dramatic" disorders)

  Antisocial

  Borderline

  Histrionic

  Narcissistic

Cluster C (the "anxious" disorders)

  Avoidant

  Dependent

  Obsessive-compulsive

Personality change due to another medical condition

Other specified personality disorder

Unspecified personality disorder

Personality disorders are defined as an enduring pattern of inner experience and behavior that deviates markedly from the expectations of the individual's culture, is pervasive and inflexible, has an onset in adolescence or early adulthood, is stable over time, and leads to distress or impairment. As a general rule, personality disorders are representative of long-term functioning and are not limited to episodes of illness. A personality disorder is not diagnosed, for instance, in a person who develops transient personality changes during an episode of major depression.

The 10 disorders are divided among three clusters. Each cluster is characterized by phenomenologically similar disorders, or disorders whose criteria overlap.

- Cluster A consists of the eccentric disorders—paranoid, schizoid, and schizotypal personality disorders. They are characterized by a pervasive pattern of abnormal cognition (e.g., suspiciousness), self-expression (e.g., odd speech), or relating to others (e.g., reclusiveness).
- Cluster B consists of the dramatic disorders—borderline, antisocial, histrionic, and narcissistic personality disorders. They are character-

ized by a pervasive pattern of violating social norms or the rights of others (e.g., criminal behavior), impulsivity, excessive emotionality, grandiosity, or "acting out" (e.g., tantrums, self-abusive behavior, angry outbursts).

- Cluster C consists of the anxious disorders—avoidant, dependent, and obsessive-compulsive personality disorders. They are characterized by a pervasive pattern of abnormal fears involving social relationships, separation, and need for control.

Many psychiatrists and psychologists believe that the DSM approach to diagnosis has little relevance to clinical reality and is not helpful in treating patients. These clinicians generally prefer a *dimensional* approach in which personality traits are described along a continuum from no dysfunction to severe dysfunction. There is growing consensus that the major share of differences in personality among individuals can be described by four or five major traits. In the best-known model, the traits (or factors) are extraversion, agreeableness, conscientiousness, neuroticism, and openness to experience. In this context, *neuroticism* refers to a tendency to worry, to feel nervous, and to be self-conscious, temperamental, and high-strung.

While dimensional assessment models have many advantages, they can be complicated and time-consuming to use. During the process that led to DSM-5, the committee tasked with revising the personality disorders developed a proposal to dimensionally rate up to five broad personality domains and 25 specific trait facets. The model was not included in the DSM-5 diagnostic criteria section and was thought by many to be overly complex. However, it remains available for clinicians and researchers to use and study, and can be found in Section III of DSM-5, "Emerging Measures and Models."

◼ Epidemiology

Epidemiological surveys show that personality disorders are common in the general population, with between 9% and 16% of respondents meeting criteria for one or more personality disorders. The prevalence is even greater in psychiatric samples. In some studies, 30%–50% of outpatients have a personality disorder, although the frequency and types differ depending on the mental disorders assessed. For example, in one study, 51% of persons with major depression, 64% of persons with generalized anxiety disorder, and 56% of persons with panic disorder had a comorbid personality disorder. Incarcerated persons have an even higher frequency of personality disorder.

The frequency of specific personality disorder differs by gender. Antisocial personality disorder occurs more frequently in men, whereas borderline personality disorder, histrionic personality disorder, and dependent personality disorder are more frequent in women. Others have a fairly equal gender distribution (schizoid, schizotypal, and obsessive-compulsive personality disorders). Younger persons are at greater risk for a personality disorder than older individuals, as prevalence diminishes with advancing age. Other general risk factors include lower levels of education and lower socioeconomic status. Substance misuse and cigarette smoking are more frequent among those with a personality disorder than those without.

Personality disorders tend to have an onset in adolescence and are established by young adulthood. Personality changes that appear later in life strongly suggest the presence of another mental disorder (e.g., early stages of schizophrenia), a neurocognitive disorder, or a disorder caused by a medical condition or the effects of a substance. If a personality disorder is to be diagnosed in a person younger than age 18, DSM-5 requires that the maladaptive personality features be present for at least 1 year. The exception is antisocial personality disorder, in which an age requirement is specified (18 years), as is the requirement that certain childhood behaviors be present along with the adult traits. Although no other personality disorders have child or adolescent criteria, research suggests that behavioral precursors such as affective lability or impulsivity can sometimes be traced back to childhood. Furthermore, personality pathology in childhood or adolescence is often predictive of adult maladjustment and the development of a personality disorder.

Personality disorders can cause enormous problems for individuals and society and are frequently associated with impaired social, interpersonal, and occupational adjustment. Family life, marriages, and academic and work performance suffer. Rates of unemployment, homelessness, divorce and separation, domestic violence, and substance misuse are high. These disorders also are associated with increased rates of health care utilization (e.g., emergency department visits, hospitalizations) and excessive rates of traumatic accidents. As a group, individuals with personality disorders are at risk for early death from suicide or accidents. The risk of suicide is about the same as that seen for major depression.

Personality disorders are generally thought to be stable and enduring, yet several recent follow-up studies show a more subtle and complex picture. Over varying lengths of follow-up, fewer people will meet criteria for a personality disorder, yet most remain impaired in interpersonal, occupational, and other important life domains. For example, in one large study, 668 patients at five sites were followed. By 2 years, around 40% of persons initially found to meet criteria for the schizotypal, borderline, avoidant, or obsessive-compulsive types still met criteria for the personality disorder. Persons with the poorest functioning initially tended to have the poorest functioning at follow-up. This study tends to confirm what psychiatrists have long held to be true—that is, that many persons with personality disorder become less symptomatic as they age, and although some may experience remission, most continue to have impaired functioning in important life domains. With regard to antisocial personality disorder and borderline personality disorder, this phenomenon has been called "burnout," a term implying that the disturbance diminishes over time like a light bulb dimming until its glow fades. Which symptoms lessen in severity is a matter of conjecture, but at least for borderline personality disorder, diminished impulsivity is one such symptom. Follow-up studies also suggest that personality disorders, like other mental illnesses, tend to wax and wane in severity over time, often in response to significant life events.

Nearly all persons with a personality disorder have one or more comorbid mental disorders, with major depression being the most frequent. Other mood, anxiety, substance use, and eating disorders are all commonly diagnosed in persons with a personality disorder. Comorbidity among the personality disorders is also very common, with persons with one disorder frequently meeting criteria for another. As mentioned earlier, few persons have a "pure" case in which they meet criteria for only one personality disorder.

The presence of a personality disorder affects the course and outcome of a comorbid mental disorder. For example, depressed patients with a personality disorder tend to be younger, are more likely to be female, are more likely to have a history of marital instability, are more likely to report precipitating stressors for the depression, and are more likely to have a history of nonserious suicide attempts. Importantly, the presence of a personality disorder is often associated with a poorer response to treatment, as has been shown for several mental disorders, including major depression, panic disorder, and obsessive-compulsive disorder.

■ Etiology

Various potential causes have been proposed for the personality disorders. Psychoanalysts have long suggested that early life events are causative factors and that personality disorders occur when a person fails to progress through appropriate stages of psychosexual development. In fact, several of the DSM-5 disorders derive from the oral, anal, and phallic character types that were described by Freud and others. Fixation at the oral stage was thought to result in a personality characterized by demanding and dependent behavior (i.e., dependent personality disorder). Fixation at the anal stage was thought to lead to a personality characterized by obsessionality, rigidity, and emotional aloofness (i.e., obsessive-compulsive personality disorder). Fixation at the phallic stage was believed to cause shallowness and an inability to engage in intimate relationships (i.e., histrionic personality). These broad character types do, in fact, show some correlation with the five-factor model of personality disorder described earlier, but little evidence shows that they are related to developmental fixations early in life.

Research evidence suggests that childhood abuse or maltreatment is associated with risk for personality disorder in general and perhaps borderline and antisocial personality disorders specifically. The resulting trauma is thought to cause difficulty in developing trust and intimacy. An early home environment in which domestic abuse, divorce, separation, or parental absence is found also can contribute to the risk of developing a personality disorder.

Genetic factors help to explain some of the personality disorders. Family, twin, and adoption studies suggest that schizotypal personality disorder is genetically related to schizophrenia. Family and adoption studies also have confirmed a strongly genetic factor in the etiology of antisocial and borderline personality disorders. Less evidence is available for the heritability of the other personality disorders. Some evidence suggests that basic dimensions of personality (e.g., callousness, intimacy problems) are inherited along a continuum with normality.

The neurobiology of personality disorders is being actively studied. Schizotypal personality disorder has been associated with impaired smooth pursuit eye movement, impaired performance on tests of executive function, and increased ventricular-brain ratio on computed tomography. Aberrant serotonin neurotransmission has been linked to impulsive and aggressive behaviors typical of both borderline and antisocial personality disorders. As a group, antisocial persons have low resting pulse, low skin conductance, and increased amplitude on event-related potentials. These findings suggest to some that people with antisocial personality disorder are chronically underaroused and seek out potentially risky situations to raise their arousal to more optimal levels.

Abnormal brain structure and function have been associated with borderline personality disorder and antisocial personality disorder.

With the former, positron emission tomography has shown altered metabolism in prefrontal regions, including the anterior cingulate cortex; reduced frontal and orbitofrontal volume also has been reported. One study of antisocial persons found them to have reduced prefrontal gray matter, while another identified specific abnormalities in the processing of emotions in psychopathic criminals. On functional magnetic resonance imaging scans, the criminals showed less affect-related activity in important limbic structures and increased activity in the frontotemporal cortex. Because these brain regions help regulate mood and behavior, impulsive aggression or emotional instability could stem from functional abnormalities in these areas.

Cultural factors may affect the development and expression of a personality disorder. The best evidence for this comes from cross-cultural research showing very low rates of antisocial personality disorder in Taiwan, China, and Japan. Possibly, the family structure in East Asian cultures helps to maintain high levels of cohesion. Similarly low rates of antisocial personality disorder occur in Jewish families, presumably because of their strong family structures. Yet at the same time, the repressive style seen in these same families may have an association with Cluster C disorders.

■ Diagnosis

Individuals with a personality disorder often have little insight into the difficulties their maladaptive traits create, and thus are prone to view others as the source of their problems. For that reason, only rarely does the presence of a personality disorder itself lead the individual to seek help. More likely, the consequences of the person's ongoing troubles— chronic depression, poor work performance, relationship difficulties— lead him or her to seek help. The clinician's task is to assist the patient to understand how the maladaptive personality traits contribute to his or her ongoing problems. The clinician can then help the patient to develop new skills to modify the maladaptive traits that contribute to the individual's difficult life situations.

The diagnosis of a personality disorder requires a thorough personal and social history and a careful mental status examination. Several structured interviews and self-report instruments are available to help with diagnosis but are mainly used in research. More typically, the clinician's inquiries will lead to the conclusion that a personality disorder may be present. When this is suspected, the clinician should inquire about the kinds of symptoms found in these patients. We have observed that one clue to the presence of a personality disorder is that the patient's immediate problem and his or her social history often intertwine.

As with other psychiatric or behavioral disorders, the patient's history forms the most important basis for diagnosing a personality disorder. The clinician's initial goal is to define the extent of the disorder through relatively nonintrusive inquiries; he or she should then move on to more detailed and specific questions regarding the patient's attitudes and behaviors. For general screening purposes, a clinician might ask about problems in the following domains: interpersonal relationships, sense of self, work, affect, impulse control, and reality testing. Suggested questions include the following:

- Do you often have days when your mood is constantly changing?
- How do you feel when you are not the center of attention?
- Do you frequently insist on having what you want right now?
- Are you concerned that certain friends or co-workers are not really loyal or trustworthy?
- Are you concerned about saying the wrong things in front of other people?
- How often do you avoid getting to know someone because you are worried he or she may not like you?

Once the clinician forms his or her initial impression, detailed inquiries can be made guided by the core features of the suspected personality disorder. Because of great overlap among the different personality disorders, inquiries may need to be fairly broad.

Collateral information also is important when a personality disorder is suspected but the patient denies or seems unaware of his or her maladaptive traits. A person with antisocial personality disorder may deny criminal activity or minimize its significance ("He deserved to be mugged!"). Information from relatives, the police, or a parole officer can be helpful in confirming the severity and extent of the behavior. An informant also can be helpful in determining whether an observed behavior is characteristic of the patient's long-term functioning or whether the trait has been sufficiently severe to cause recurrent problems in how the person interacts with others. Of course, confidentiality must be preserved, so informants can only be contacted with the patient's consent.

It is important not to make a personality disorder diagnosis prematurely. Patients with major depression are often socially anxious and dependent on others, traits that tend to recede or disappear when the depression is successfully treated. For that reason, caution needs to be used in making the diagnosis, particularly when the patient has a disorder like major depression that can distort one's normal personality or exaggerate preexisting personality traits. Long-term observation may be necessary with some patients to confirm the diagnosis of personality disorder.

The concept of a personality disorder also needs to be separated from normal personality. Most people have minor personality quirks or idiosyncrasies, but these rarely rise to the level of a disorder. A key distinction is that the trait in question is inflexible, maladaptive, and leads to distress or impairment in one or more life domains. Most people learn to adapt to changing circumstances and learn from experience. People with a personality disorder often persist with their maladaptive behaviors regardless of the consequences. The clinician should also be aware of cultural issues that may affect a personality disorder diagnosis because certain traits may be considered normal in some societies but not others. For example, in some societies, belief in magic and sorcery is widespread and culturally accepted; in contemporary American society, such beliefs may be viewed as magical thinking associated with a schizotypal personality disorder.

■ Treatment

It is difficult to generalize about the treatment of the various personality disorders. First, few of the 10 personality disorders have been studied sufficiently to recommend specific treatments. For this reason, recommendations made below are often based on clinical experience, not research evidence. Second, the disorders are sufficiently different that treatment recommendations for one disorder may not apply to another. For example, the person with avoidant personality disorder has symptoms of extreme anxiety and inhibition; the person with borderline personality disorder, on the other hand, has difficulty with anger, moodiness, and impulsivity. That said, contrary to assumptions that persons with personality disorder cannot benefit from treatment, reviews of outcome studies have shown that treatment results are largely positive.

Treatment of the personality disorders can be divided into pharmacologic or psychological interventions. Although many drug treatment studies of personality disorder have been conducted over the past few decades, the pace of progress has been slow compared with the major mental disorders such as major depression or schizophrenia. There are currently no medications approved by the U.S. Food and Drug Administration for *any* personality disorder. Furthermore, some disorders have been studied extensively (e.g., borderline personality disorder) and others almost not at all (e.g., histrionic personality disorder). The same is true for psychotherapy (mainly involving individual and group treatments): borderline personality disorder has been actively studied, and several evidence-based psychotherapies now exist, whereas schizoid personality disorder, for example, has been virtually ignored. Other forms of psychological treatment for personality disorder, including family therapy and marital (or couples) therapy, have such a small data base that it is difficult to make sound recommendations for these forms of treatment.

■ The DSM-5 Personality Disorders

Cluster A Disorders

Paranoid Personality Disorder

Paranoid personality was first described by Adolf Meyer in the early twentieth century. These patients are chronically suspicious, distrust others, and fulfill their suspicious prophecies by leading others to be overly cautious and deceptive (see Box 17–1). Frank delusions are absent. Persons with paranoid personality disorder rarely seek treatment, most likely because of their general suspiciousness of others, including psychiatrists and therapists. The disorder has an estimated prevalence of 1%–4% in the general population. It is often first recognized when the patient seeks treatment for a mood or anxiety disorder.

Box 17–1.   DSM-5 Diagnostic Criteria for Paranoid Personality Disorder

---

A. A pervasive distrust and suspiciousness of others such that their motives are interpreted as malevolent, beginning by early adulthood and present in a variety of contexts, as indicated by four (or more) of the following:

 1. Suspects, without sufficient basis, that others are exploiting, harming, or deceiving him or her.
 2. Is preoccupied with unjustified doubts about the loyalty or trustworthiness of friends or associates.

3. Is reluctant to confide in others because of unwarranted fear that the information will be used maliciously against him or her.
4. Reads hidden demeaning or threatening meanings into benign remarks or events.
5. Persistently bears grudges (i.e., is unforgiving of insults, injuries, or slights).
6. Perceives attacks on his or her character or reputation that are not apparent to others and is quick to react angrily or to counterattack.
7. Has recurrent suspicions, without justification, regarding fidelity of spouse or sexual partner.

B. Does not occur exclusively during the course of schizophrenia, a bipolar disorder or depressive disorder with psychotic features, or another psychotic disorder and is not attributable to the physiological effects of another medical condition.

Note: If criteria are met prior to the onset of schizophrenia, add "premorbid," i.e., "paranoid personality disorder (premorbid)."

Apart from diagnosing and managing the patient's primary problem, the clinician should take care to be supportive and to listen patiently to their accusations and complaints while being open, honest, and respectful. When rapport has been established, alternative explanations for the patient's misperceptions can be suggested. Group therapy should be avoided because patients with paranoid personality disorder tend to misinterpret statements and situations that arise in the course of the therapy. Antipsychotics may help to reduce their suspiciousness, although these drugs have not been specifically studied for this condition.

Schizoid Personality Disorder

The term *schizoid* was originally used to characterize the premorbid seclusiveness of schizophrenic patients and their eccentric relatives. The concept of schizoid personality disorder was narrowed in DSM-III and became restricted to persons with a profound defect in the ability to form personal relationships and to respond to others in a meaningful way (see Box 17–2). The following case from our hospital illustrates the disorder:

Box 17–2. DSM-5 Diagnostic Criteria for Schizoid Personality Disorder

A. A pervasive pattern of detachment from social relationships and a restricted range of expression of emotions in interpersonal settings, beginning by early adulthood and present in a variety of contexts, as indicated by four (or more) of the following:

1. Neither desires nor enjoys close relationships, including being part of a family.
2. Almost always chooses solitary activities.
3. Has little, if any, interest in having sexual experiences with another person.
4. Takes pleasure in few, if any, activities.
5. Lacks close friends or confidants other than first-degree relatives.
6. Appears indifferent to the praise or criticism of others.
7. Shows emotional coldness, detachment, or flattened affectivity.

B. Does not occur exclusively during the course of schizophrenia, a bipolar disorder or depressive disorder with psychotic features, another psychotic disorder, or autism spectrum disorder and is not attributable to the physiological effects of another medical condition.

Note: If criteria are met prior to the onset of schizophrenia, add "premorbid," i.e., "schizoid personality disorder (premorbid)."

Michael, a 24-year-old man, was transferred to the psychiatric inpatient unit after receiving treatment for a self-inflicted gunshot wound to the head. The bullet grazed his scalp but did not cause a brain injury. According to his family, he had been depressed for several weeks before shooting himself. After transfer, Michael denied feeling depressed and believed that there was no reason for him to be in the hospital.

Michael had always been considered shy by his relatives, he was socially isolated, and he had no friends that his family was aware of. He had done poorly in school and had dropped out before graduating from high school. Michael had never dated and had no interest in sexual activity, apart from masturbation. Michael admitted that he was not emotionally close to any of his family members, and although he lived with his elderly father, he showed little interest or affection in describing their relationship. Despite having average intelligence, Michael had never persisted with a job and was currently unemployed. He preferred to stay home and watch television or play computer games. He had never bothered to obtain a driver's license.

Michael believed that his only problem was episodic depression. He neither complained about his social isolation and emotional aloofness nor accepted the fact that these symptoms could reflect an underlying disorder. He had no interest in changing his ways and refused referral for psychotherapy.

Like Michael, patients with schizoid personality disorder have no close relationships and choose solitary activities. They rarely experience strong emotions, express little desire for sexual experience with another person, are indifferent to praise or criticism, and display a constricted affect.

Schizoid personality disorder has a prevalence of 3%–5% in the general population. It is relatively uncommon in clinical settings because persons with this disorder rarely seek psychiatric care. When people with this disorder come to clinical attention, it is generally because of a co-occurring disorder such as major depression. They tend to lack the insight and motivation necessary for individual psychotherapy and would probably find the intimacy of traditional group therapy threatening. That said, these individuals may be candidates for the types of day programs or drop-in centers that are often affiliated with community mental health centers. If the patient expresses a strong desire for social contact, it may be that avoidant personality disorder is the more appropriate diagnosis.

Schizotypal Personality Disorder

Schizotypal personality disorder was conceptualized during the development of DSM-III in response to observations that the relatives of schizophrenic patients often had a cluster of schizophrenic-like traits. Schizotypal personality disorder now is considered part of the schizophrenia spectrum, along with schizophreniform disorder, schizoaffective disorder, and schizophrenia.

Schizotypal personality disorder is characterized by a pattern of peculiar behavior, odd speech and thinking, and unusual perceptual experiences. Schizotypal patients are frequently socially isolated and have "magical" beliefs, mild paranoia, inappropriate or constricted affect, and social anxiety (see Box 17–3).

Box 17–3. DSM-5 Diagnostic Criteria for Schizotypal
Personality Disorder

A. A pervasive pattern of social and interpersonal deficits marked by acute discomfort with, and reduced capacity for, close relationships as well as by cognitive or perceptual distortions and eccentricities of behavior, beginning by early adulthood and present in a variety of contexts, as indicated by five (or more) of the following:

1. Ideas of reference (excluding delusions of reference).
2. Odd beliefs or magical thinking that influences behavior and is inconsistent with subcultural norms (e.g., superstitiousness, belief in clairvoyance, telepathy, or "sixth sense"; in children and adolescents, bizarre fantasies or preoccupations).
3. Unusual perceptual experiences, including bodily illusions.
4. Odd thinking and speech (e.g., vague, circumstantial, metaphorical, overelaborate, or stereotyped).

5. Suspiciousness or paranoid ideation.
6. Inappropriate or constricted affect.
7. Behavior or appearance that is odd, eccentric, or peculiar.
8. Lack of close friends or confidants other than first-degree relatives.
9. Excessive social anxiety that does not diminish with familiarity and tends to be associated with paranoid fears rather than negative judgments about self.

B. Does not occur exclusively during the course of schizophrenia, a bipolar disorder or depressive disorder with psychotic features, another psychotic disorder, or autism spectrum disorder.

Note: If criteria are met prior to the onset of schizophrenia, add "premorbid," e.g., "schizotypal personality disorder (premorbid)."

Surveys show that schizotypal personality disorder has a prevalence of around 4%–5%, and there is no gender difference. Comorbidity with mood, substance use, and anxiety disorders is common.

The treatment of schizotypal personality disorder often centers on issues that led the person to seek treatment, such as feelings of alienation or isolation, paranoia, or suspiciousness. Exploratory and group psychotherapies may be overly threatening to these patients, but social skills training can be helpful. The goal is to help the individual to develop an awareness of what behaviors others (e.g., coworkers, store clerks) may consider odd or eccentric and to develop a repertoire of social skills that will assist him or her in making interactions with others more productive and satisfying.

Although not well studied, antipsychotics are sometimes prescribed to these patients. Second-generation antipsychotics (e.g., risperidone, 1–6 mg/day; olanzapine, 5–20 mg/day) are well tolerated and may help to reduce the intense anxiety, paranoia, and unusual perceptual experiences these individuals experience.

Cluster B Disorders

Antisocial Personality Disorder

Antisocial personality disorder has been clinically recognized for more than 200 years. Antisocial patients typically report a history of childhood behavior problems (e.g., fighting with peers, conflicts with adults) that fulfill criteria for conduct disorder. Fire setting and cruelty to animals and other children are particularly worrisome symptoms. As the antisocial youth reaches adulthood, other problems develop reflecting age-appropriate responsibilities, such as uneven job performance or domestic abuse. Unreliability, reckless behavior, and inappropriate aggression are frequent problems. Criminal behavior, pathological lying, and the use of aliases are also characteristic of the disorder (Box 17–4). Marriages are often marked by instability or emotional and physical abuse of the spouse; separation and divorce are common.

Box 17–4.   DSM-5 Diagnostic Criteria for Antisocial Personality Disorder

A. A pervasive pattern of disregard for and violation of the rights of others, occurring since age 15 years, as indicated by three (or more) of the following:

1. Failure to conform to social norms with respect to lawful behaviors, as indicated by repeatedly performing acts that are grounds for arrest.
2. Deceitfulness, as indicated by repeated lying, use of aliases, or conning others for personal profit or pleasure.
3. Impulsivity or failure to plan ahead.
4. Irritability and aggressiveness, as indicated by repeated physical fights or assaults.
5. Reckless disregard for safety of self or others.
6. Consistent irresponsibility, as indicated by repeated failure to sustain consistent work behavior or honor financial obligations.
7. Lack of remorse, as indicated by being indifferent to or rationalizing having hurt, mistreated, or stolen from another.

B. The individual is at least age 18 years.
C. There is evidence of conduct disorder with onset before age 15 years.
D. The occurrence of antisocial behavior is not exclusively during the course of schizophrenia or bipolar disorder.

The following case is of a patient treated at our hospital and illustrates the lifelong difficulties that arise from antisocial personality disorder:

> Russell, age 18, was admitted for evaluation of antisocial behavior. His early childhood was chaotic and abusive. His alcoholic father had married five times and abandoned his family when Russell was 6. Because his mother had a history of incarceration and was unable to care for him, Russell was placed in foster care until he was adopted at age 8.
>
> Russell had a criminal streak from early childhood. He lied, cheated at games, shoplifted, and stole money from his mother's purse. Because of continued law-breaking, he was sent to a juvenile reformatory for 2 years at age 16. While in the reformatory, he slashed another boy with a razor blade in a fight. Russell had his first sexual experience before his peers and after leaving the reformatory had several different sexual partners.

Russell's IQ was measured at 112. He was discharged after a 16-day stay and was considered unimproved. He was poorly cooperative with attempts at both individual and group therapy.

Russell was followed up 30 years later. He used an alias and lived in an impoverished area of a small Midwestern community. Now 48, Russell looked physically ill and was haggard in appearance. He admitted to over 20 arrests and five felony convictions on charges ranging from attempted murder and armed robbery to driving while intoxicated. He had spent more than 17 years in prison. While in prison, Russell had escaped with the help of his biological mother, with whom he then had a sexual relationship. He was returned to prison 2 months later. His most recent arrest occurred within the past year and was for public intoxication and simple assault.

Russell reported at least nine hospitalizations for alcohol detoxification, the latest occurring earlier that year. He admitted to past use of marijuana, amphetamines, tranquilizers, cocaine, and heroin.

He had never held a full-time job in his life; the longest job he had held lasted 60 days. He was currently doing bodywork on cars in his own garage to earn a living but had not done any work for several months. He had lived in six different states and in the past 10 years had moved more than 20 times.

Russell reported that his common-law wife took tranquilizers for emotional problems and that the marriage was unsatisfactory. He reported occasionally attending Alcoholics Anonymous at a local church but otherwise did not socialize.

Russell admitted that he had not yet settled down and told us that he still spent money foolishly, was frequently reckless, and got into frequent fights and arguments. He said that he got a "charge out of doing dangerous things."

Antisocial personality disorder has a prevalence of 2%–4% in men and 0.5%–1% in women. The percentages are much higher in psychiatric hospitals and clinics, among the homeless and the incarcerated, and among substance-abusing persons. The disorder is worse early in its course, and antisocial symptoms tend to recede with advancing age.

Comorbid substance use disorders, mood and anxiety disorders, attention-deficit/hyperactivity disorder, other personality disorders (e.g., borderline personality disorder), and gambling disorder are common. Antisocial persons frequently attempt suicide, and mortality studies show high rates of death from natural causes as well as accidents, suicides, and homicides.

The disorder has no standard treatments. Several drugs reduce aggression, the chief problem for many antisocial persons, but are not routinely prescribed; they include lithium carbonate, valproate, and the antipsychotics. Benzodiazepines should be avoided because of their abuse potential and tendency to cause behavioral dyscontrol. Medication should target comorbid mood or anxiety disorders or attention-deficit/hyperactivity disorder because treating these may help to reduce antisocial behavior.

Antisocial patients can be very difficult; they tend to blame others, have a low tolerance for frustration, are impulsive, and rarely form trusting relationships. There is some evidence that cognitive-behavioral therapy may be helpful to those with mild symptoms who have insight into their problems.

Borderline Personality Disorder

Borderline personality disorder was introduced in DSM-III, although the concept has a much longer history. The disorder is characterized by a pervasive pattern of mood instability, unstable and intense interpersonal relationships, impulsivity, inappropriate or intense anger, lack of control of anger, recurrent suicidal threats and gestures, self-mutilating behavior, marked and persistent identity disturbance, chronic feelings of emptiness, and frantic efforts to avoid real or imagined abandonment (see Box 17–5). Patients also may experience transient paranoid ideation or dissociative symptoms. Thomas Sydenham, an English physician best known for describing Saint Vitus' dance, captures the essence of borderline personality in his quotation at the beginning of this chapter.

Box 17–5.   DSM-5 Diagnostic Criteria for Borderline Personality Disorder

---

A pervasive pattern of instability of interpersonal relationships, self-image, and affects, and marked impulsivity, beginning by early adulthood and present in a variety of contexts, as indicated by five (or more) of the following:

1. Frantic efforts to avoid real or imagined abandonment. (**Note:** Do not include suicidal or self-mutilating behavior covered in Criterion 5.)
2. A pattern of unstable and intense interpersonal relationships characterized by alternating between extremes of idealization and devaluation.
3. Identity disturbance: markedly and persistently unstable self-image or sense of self.
4. Impulsivity in at least two areas that are potentially self-damaging (e.g., spending, sex, substance abuse, reckless driving, binge eating). (**Note:** Do not include suicidal or self-mutilating behavior covered in Criterion 5.)
5. Recurrent suicidal behavior, gestures, or threats, or self-mutilating behavior.
6. Affective instability due to a marked reactivity of mood (e.g., intense episodic dysphoria, irritability, or anxiety usually lasting a few hours and only rarely more than a few days).
7. Chronic feelings of emptiness.

8. Inappropriate, intense anger or difficulty controlling anger (e.g., frequent displays of temper, constant anger, recurrent physical fights).
9. Transient, stress-related paranoid ideation or severe dissociative symptoms.

Borderline personality disorder is one of the more common personality disorders among psychiatric patients. Its frequency in the general population has been estimated to be as high as 6%. More than three-quarters of borderline patients engage in deliberate self-harm (e.g., cutting, overdoses), and about 10% commit suicide.

Better long-term outcome is associated with higher intelligence, self-discipline, and social support from friends and relatives. Hostility, antisocial behavior, suspiciousness, and vanity are traits associated with poor outcome. These patients frequently have comorbid major depression, dysthymia, anxiety disorders, and substance abuse or dependence.

The following case example describes a patient with borderline personality disorder seen at our hospital:

Diane, a 50-year-old divorced woman, had a history of emotional instability dating to age 10, when she made her first suicide attempt. By her early 20s, she had the onset of episodes of depression, and frequent hospitalizations that had amounted to about 3–4 months per year. From her 20s to her mid-40s, she made several serious suicide attempts, including jumping from a building (and breaking both legs in the process) and taking several drug overdoses.

Diane had a history of alcohol abuse but had been sober for nearly 25 years with the help of Alcoholics Anonymous, which she attended regularly. Diane also had a history of problem gambling and continued to have sporadic gambling episodes. In the past, gambling behaviors had led her to steal money from her boyfriend or to write bad checks, resulting in legal charges and, on one occasion, a short jail sentence.

Anger dyscontrol and turbulent interpersonal relationships had also been problematic for her. Diane completed a significant number of college courses but failed to graduate because of her behavioral problems. In the past, her disorder had interfered with maintaining consistent employment. Abandonment issues and feelings of emptiness were also present. Her intense, frequently shifting moods often resulted in poor management of her diabetes.

Diane was referred for group therapy, which she later credited with giving her a better understanding of the disorder. The therapy targeted her poor medication compliance, her impulsivity, and her emotional intensity. For each problem area, she learned new skills to increase her range of alternative responses and to increase her awareness of the consequences of each alternative. She was also prescribed risperidone (4 mg/day) to help stabilize her mood.

There were no suicide attempts in the subsequent 5 years, and hospital stays were limited to a few days per year. She developed a stable relationship, volunteered regularly at her church, and pursued several hobbies.

In the past few decades, several group treatment programs have been developed that appear to reduce the overall severity of the disorder and lessen the associated mood instability, impulsivity, and social disability. Several employ cognitive-behavioral methods to help correct accompanying maladaptive thoughts, beliefs, and behaviors. Dialectical behavior therapy (DBT) is the best-known program and involves intensive year-long treatment that includes both individual and group therapy. An alternative is the less intensive 20-week Systems Training for Emotional Predictability and Problem Solving (STEPPS) program, which combines psychoeducation and skills training. There are several other evidence-based programs, but they may have limited availability.

Pharmacotherapy for borderline personality disorder tends to focus on the patients' target symptoms. Selective serotonin reuptake inhibitors (SSRIs) such as fluoxetine may be helpful in reducing depressive symptoms and suicidal ideations and behaviors. Antipsychotics can help to treat perceptual distortions, anger dyscontrol, suicidal behavior, and mood instability. Because suicide attempts are frequent in these patients, physicians should be cautious about prescribing any medication that could be dangerous in overdose. Benzodiazepine tranquilizers should be avoided, except perhaps for short-term use (e.g., days to weeks), because they can cause behavioral disinhibition or may be abused.

Patients with borderline personality disorder have the potential to cause intense feelings of frustration, guilt, or anger in their caregivers. The unfortunate irony is that these individuals fear abandonment from others and yet they react to perceived signs of it in a manner that alienates those who try to be supportive. Students are well advised to seek guidance from experienced clinicians in order to set boundaries that strike an appropriate balance between being overly distant and overly involved.

Histrionic Personality Disorder

Histrionic personality disorder takes its name from *hysteria,* first described in the nineteenth century and associated with conversion, somatization, and dissociation. Self-dramatizing behaviors were observed to be associated with hysteria. People with histrionic personality disorder show a pattern of excessive emotionality and attention-seeking behavior. Typical symptoms include excessive concern with appearance and wanting to be the center of attention (see Box 17–6). Histrionic persons are often gregarious and superficially charming but can be manipulative, vain, and demanding.

Box 17–6.   DSM-5 Diagnostic Criteria for Histrionic Personality
            Disorder

A pervasive pattern of excessive emotionality and attention seeking, beginning by early adulthood and present in a variety of contexts, as indicated by five (or more) of the following:

1. Is uncomfortable in situations in which he or she is not the center of attention.
2. Interaction with others is often characterized by inappropriate sexually seductive or provocative behavior.
3. Displays rapidly shifting and shallow expression of emotions.
4. Consistently uses physical appearance to draw attention to self.
5. Has a style of speech that is excessively impressionistic and lacking in detail.
6. Shows self-dramatization, theatricality, and exaggerated expression of emotion.
7. Is suggestible (i.e., easily influenced by others or circumstances).
8. Considers relationships to be more intimate than they actually are.

The disorder has a prevalence of nearly 2% in the general population. Histrionic persons tend to seek out medical attention and to make frequent use of available health services. Some experts suggest that histrionic personality disorder is a gender-biased diagnosis that merely describes a caricature of stereotypical femininity because it is frequently diagnosed among women in clinical samples. The cause of histrionic personality disorder is unknown, although it has been linked through family studies to somatization disorder (now somatic symptom disorder) and antisocial personality disorder.

Some experts recommend a supportive, problem-solving approach or cognitive-behavioral therapy to help patients counter their distorted thinking, such as the inflated self-image that many histrionic patients have. With interpersonal psychotherapy, the patient can focus on conscious (or unconscious) motivations for seeking out disappointing partners and being unable to commit oneself to a stable, meaningful relationship. Group therapy may be useful in addressing provocative and attention-seeking behavior. Patients may not be aware of their annoying behaviors, and it may be helpful to have others point them out.

Narcissistic Personality Disorder

Narcissistic personality disorder was introduced in DSM-III and is named after Narcissus from Greek mythology. Narcissus, it should be recalled, fell in love with his own reflection. Freud used the term to describe persons who were self-absorbed; it was later expanded to describe the more general concept of excessive self-love and grandiosity.

The disorder is characterized by grandiosity, lack of empathy, and hypersensitivity to evaluation by others (see Box 17–7). Narcissistic persons are egotistical, inflate their accomplishments, and often manipulate or exploit those around them to achieve their own aims. They have an exaggerated sense of entitlement and believe that they deserve special treatment. They expect to receive love and admiration but have little empathy for others. Narcissistic individuals are often irritating, haughty, or difficult; although they appear outwardly charming, relationships tend to be superficial and cold. They tend to have little insight into their own narcissism. Some narcissistic individuals may view themselves as extraordinarily caring and selfless while making it clear that they believe they deserve a great deal of praise and special treatment because they are so giving to others.

Box 17–7. DSM-5 Diagnostic Criteria for Narcissistic Personality Disorder

---

A pervasive pattern of grandiosity (in fantasy or behavior), need for admiration, and lack of empathy, beginning by early adulthood and present in a variety of contexts, as indicated by five (or more) of the following:

1. Has a grandiose sense of self-importance (e.g., exaggerates achievements and talents, expects to be recognized as superior without commensurate achievements).
2. Is preoccupied with fantasies of unlimited success, power, brilliance, beauty, or ideal love.
3. Believes that he or she is "special" and unique and can only be understood by, or should associate with, other special or high-status people (or institutions).
4. Requires excessive admiration.
5. Has a sense of entitlement (i.e., unreasonable expectations of especially favorable treatment or automatic compliance with his or her expectations).
6. Is interpersonally exploitative (i.e., takes advantage of others to achieve his or her own ends).
7. Lacks empathy: is unwilling to recognize or identify with the feelings and needs of others.

8. Is often envious of others or believes that others are envious of him or her.
9. Shows arrogant, haughty behaviors or attitudes.

The following case illustrates many of the symptoms of narcissistic personality disorder:

> Dr. Smith, a 53-year-old physician, was known for having an expansive and grandiose attitude and for belittling the accomplishments of his colleagues.
>
> While seeking the admiration and adulation of others, he rarely reciprocated, displaying superficial charm without a genuine capacity for empathy. His nurse remarked to a colleague, "When you talk to him, it's like you're not even really there as a person. It's like he can't connect."
>
> Dr. Smith's sense of entitlement led him to bill Medicare and other insurance carriers for services that he had never rendered or that were inflated on the bills. He believed that changes in the reimbursement system penalized him and that he was entitled to a higher level of payment because of his training, experience, and keen intelligence.
>
> At the urging of his colleagues in practice, and after being repeatedly caught and confronted about his billing fraud, Dr. Smith entered therapy with a well-known psychoanalyst and psychiatrist, Dr. Brown. Dr. Smith told a colleague, months into therapy: "I think Dr. Brown envies me; he knows how much money I make. I can tell the size of my practice, and my success, bothers him."
>
> Dr. Smith eventually was investigated, indicted on multiple criminal fraud counts, and tried in federal court. Many of his colleagues testified against him in federal court. "I can't believe they would *do* this to me," he was heard to say. Convicted on all counts, Dr. Smith was sentenced to 5 years in a federal penitentiary.

Narcissistic personality disorder has been considered uncommon, although a recent survey reported a prevalence of around 6%. Some experts argue that the disorder is not a valid syndrome because narcissistic traits are common in the general population, as well as in people with other personality disorder types. The criteria also overlap with those of other disorders, such as borderline personality disorder, leading some to question its distinctiveness. Like other personality disorders, narcissistic personality disorder is generally viewed as stable over time, although research suggests that it may vary under the influence of significant life events, such as achievement and new relationships.

There are few data on the treatment of persons with narcissistic personality disorder. When these individuals seek help, it is likely for the anger or depression they feel when deprived of something they feel entitled to, such as a promotion. This is sometimes referred to as a "narcissistic injury." Treatment recommendations have ranged from intensive psychodynamic psychotherapy to interpersonal or cognitive-behavioral psychotherapy. Narcissistic patients can be very difficult to treat because their narcissism can interfere with the process of psychotherapy. For example, their grandiosity can lead them to resist admitting personal responsibility for their problems, while their sense of entitlement can lead them to make unreasonable demands on the therapist.

Cluster C Disorders

Avoidant Personality Disorder

Avoidant personality disorder was introduced in DSM-III to describe people who are inhibited, introverted, and anxious. These individuals tend to have low self-esteem, are hypersensitive to rejection, are apprehensive and mistrustful, are socially awkward and timid, are uncomfortable and self-conscious, and fear being embarrassed or acting foolish in public (see Box 17–8).

Box 17–8. DSM-5 Diagnostic Criteria for Avoidant Personality Disorder

---

A pervasive pattern of social inhibition, feelings of inadequacy, and hypersensitivity to negative evaluation, beginning by early adulthood and present in a variety of contexts, as indicated by four (or more) of the following:
1. Avoids occupational activities that involve significant interpersonal contact because of fears of criticism, disapproval, or rejection.
2. Is unwilling to get involved with people unless certain of being liked.
3. Shows restraint within intimate relationships because of the fear of being shamed or ridiculed.
4. Is preoccupied with being criticized or rejected in social situations.
5. Is inhibited in new interpersonal situations because of feelings of inadequacy.
6. Views self as socially inept, personally unappealing, or inferior to others.
7. Is unusually reluctant to take personal risks or to engage in any new activities because they may prove embarrassing.

Some experts have questioned the independence of the disorder, which they see as lying along a spectrum with the anxiety disorders. In fact, many features of avoidant personality disorder are indistinguishable from those of social anxiety disorder, and the two disorders frequently overlap. Avoidant personality disorder may involve a genetic predisposition to chronic anxiety.

Several psychotherapeutic strategies have been developed for the treatment of avoidant personality disorder. Group therapy may help the person to overcome his or her social anxiety and to develop interpersonal trust. Assertiveness and social skills training can be helpful, as can systematic desensitization to treat anxiety symptoms, shyness, and introversion. Cognitive-behavioral therapy can help to correct dysfunctional attitudes (e.g., "I had better not open my mouth because I'll probably say something stupid"). Benzodiazepines can be useful while the patient is attempting to enter previously avoided social situations. It is best to limit the use of these drugs to short periods (e.g., weeks to months), although some patients will benefit from long-term use. SSRIs also may be helpful because they are effective in treating social anxiety disorder.

Dependent Personality Disorder

Dependent personality disorder is characterized by a pattern of relying excessively on others for emotional support (see Box 17–9). Psychoanalysts have linked dependency to fixation at the oral stage of development, which focuses on the biological gratification that arises from feeding. Other theorists have tied dependent personality to the disruption of attachments early in life. Others view dependency as stemming from overprotectiveness and parental authoritarianism experienced in childhood. The disorder has a prevalence of around 0.5% in the general population.

Box 17–9.   DSM-5 Diagnostic Criteria for Dependent Personality Disorder

---

A pervasive and excessive need to be taken care of that leads to submissive and clinging behavior and fears of separation, beginning by early adulthood and present in a variety of contexts, as indicated by five (or more) of the following:

1. Has difficulty making everyday decisions without an excessive amount of advice and reassurance from others.
2. Needs others to assume responsibility for most major areas of his or her life.
3. Has difficulty expressing disagreement with others because of fear of loss of support or approval. (**Note:** Do not include realistic fears of retribution.)
4. Has difficulty initiating projects or doing things on his or her own (because of a lack of self-confidence in judgment or abilities rather than a lack of motivation or energy).
5. Goes to excessive lengths to obtain nurturance and support from others, to the point of volunteering to do things that are unpleasant.
6. Feels uncomfortable or helpless when alone because of exaggerated fears of being unable to care for himself or herself.

7. Urgently seeks another relationship as a source of care and support when a close relationship ends.
8. Is unrealistically preoccupied with fears of being left to take care of himself or herself.

The following patient, in whom dependency issues were important, was seen at our hospital:

> Bob, a 45-year-old farm laborer, presented for evaluation of major depression, which had been chronic for several years. He also reported a long-standing eating disorder, which had resulted in significant weight loss. For 10 years, Bob had feared becoming fat like his father, who had died unexpectedly of a myocardial infarction.
>
> In addition to these problems, Bob described a dull and passive lifestyle. The third of eight children, Bob had left school after eighth grade to work on the family farm, as had his siblings. The family remained close because there were few opportunities for outside friendships. Bob reported that he had rarely dated, although he had once been "sweet on a girl." He denied any current interest in developing a relationship.
>
> Bob lived with his mother until she insisted he move out at age 44, which he did reluctantly. Although he lived alone, he remained in close contact with his mother, eating meals with her twice daily and phoning her 10–20 times a day. He relied on her to make decisions for him, even minor ones about day-to-day activities.
>
> Bob had no interests or hobbies apart from his farm chores. He admitted that he was uncomfortable being alone in his mobile home, which prompted him to call his mother.
>
> Although Bob gained weight steadily on a refeeding protocol, it became clear that he would need supervision outside the hospital. Because his mother was too old to help (and it was felt that her supervision would only worsen his dependency on her), a decision was made by his family to place Bob in a residential care facility.

Considerable research on the psychology of dependency has been done, yet there have been few empirical studies of dependent personality disorder. One criticism of the disorder is that it is not sufficiently distinctive to stand alone and that dependency on others commonly occurs in people with other personality disorder types; it is also common in persons with chronic medical or psychiatric disorders. Comorbid mood and anxiety disorders are common. People with dependent personality have poor social and family ties, in part because their dependency on others accentuates and promotes interpersonal conflicts.

There is little consensus on the treatment of dependent personality disorder. Cognitive-behavioral therapy is recommended as a way to encourage emotional growth, assertiveness, effective decision making, and independence. The therapist might have the patient set goals for each session and challenge his or her assumptions related to dependency (e.g., "I won't be able to make up my mind without Mother's input"). Some patients benefit from more focused assertiveness training or social skills training. Marital counseling is indicated when the patient's dependence on his or her spouse is adversely affecting their relationship.

Obsessive-Compulsive Personality Disorder

Obsessive-compulsive personality disorder is characterized by perfectionism and inflexibility associated with overconscientiousness and constricted emotions (see Box 17–10). It has an estimated prevalence of 1%–2% in the general population. Unlike other personality disorders, this disorder appears to be more common in those with higher levels of education and those in higher income brackets. Comorbidity with mood and anxiety disorders is frequent.

Box 17–10.   DSM-5 Diagnostic Criteria for Obsessive-Compulsive Personality Disorder

---

A pervasive pattern of preoccupation with orderliness, perfectionism, and mental and interpersonal control, at the expense of flexibility, openness, and efficiency, beginning by early adulthood and present in a variety of contexts, as indicated by four (or more) of the following:

1. Is preoccupied with details, rules, lists, order, organization, or schedules to the extent that the major point of the activity is lost.
2. Shows perfectionism that interferes with task completion (e.g., is unable to complete a project because his or her own overly strict standards are not met).
3. Is excessively devoted to work and productivity to the exclusion of leisure activities and friendships (not accounted for by obvious economic necessity).
4. Is overconscientious, scrupulous, and inflexible about matters of morality, ethics, or values (not accounted for by cultural or religious identification).
5. Is unable to discard worn-out or worthless objects even when they have no sentimental value.
6. Is reluctant to delegate tasks or to work with others unless they submit to exactly his or her way of doing things.
7. Adopts a miserly spending style toward both self and others; money is viewed as something to be hoarded for future catastrophes.
8. Shows rigidity and stubbornness.

For many years it was thought that this disorder led to the development of obsessive-compulsive disorder (OCD). Although research shows that some patients with OCD have a comorbid obsessional-compulsive personality, most do not. Individuals with OCD are generally more willing to identify their symptoms as pathological, whereas individuals with obsessive-compulsive personality disorder tend to view many of their symptoms (e.g., collecting, perfectionism) as desirable.

There have been few studies on the treatment of obsessive-compulsive personality disorder. Some experts recommend psychodynamic psychotherapy; however, although these patients tend to intellectualize and may be insightful, they develop little feeling or emotion. Cognitive-behavioral therapy may help these individuals understand that the world is not made up of clearly defined black and white lines of rigidly held beliefs. SSRIs may be helpful in reducing the need for perfectionism and the unnecessary ritualizing that sometimes develops.

Clinical points for personality disorders
1. Patients have enduring, long-term problems, and therapy may be long-term as well. Years of maladaptive behavior cannot be easily understood or reversed.
2. Have a positive attitude! Personality disorders cause a great deal of pain and suffering to patients and those in their lives. Have empathy for them.
3. Avoid becoming overinvolved, such as giving out your home telephone number or relating your personal problems to the patient. These behaviors are called "boundary" issues, which indicate that the lines separating the relationship between doctor and patient have become blurred.
4. Ground rules for therapy must be established (e.g., that the therapist is willing to see the person regularly, at a specified time).   • Spell out what the patient should do or whom the patient should call when he or she is in a crisis.   • Spell out the consequences of self-damaging acts (e.g., hospitalization, referral to another therapist).
5. Seek support for yourself from peers or supervisors. Some patients with personality disorders can be a handful, and the therapist may need advice or consultation from time to time.
6. Support groups can be enormously helpful to the patient, and referral to community-based organizations is essential.

■ Self-Assessment Questions

1. What are the Greek temperaments, and why are they still useful descriptively?
2. How are the personality disorders defined?
3. How common are the personality disorders? Which ones are more common in men? Which ones are more common in women? Are the disorders stable over time?
4. What evidence is there for genetic or biological origin for the personality disorders? Which personality disorders?
5. Describe the three personality disorder clusters.
6. How do schizoid and schizotypal personality disorders differ? How do these two categories differ from avoidant personality disorder?
7. Are medications useful in treating Cluster A disorders? Which medications?
8. For which disorders might social skills training or assertiveness training be useful?
9. What is the childhood precursor of antisocial personality disorder? What biological abnormalities have been found in these patients? Are medications of any value?
10. What features characterize the Cluster C disorders? What are the general treatment recommendations for these disorders? How does obsessive-compulsive personality disorder differ from OCD?

PART III

SPECIAL TOPICS

Chapter 18

Psychiatric Emergencies

*The thought of suicide is a great consolation; by means of it one gets success-
fully through many a bad night.*

Friedrich Nietzsche

Dangerous or violent situations are relatively common in busy
emergency departments, psychiatric units, and even general medical
wards. Examples include the agitated and out of control manic patient
requiring sedation; the patient with borderline personality disorder
who has cut her wrists and says she has no reason to live; and the patient high on methamphetamine threatening bodily harm to emergency
personnel. These scenarios are typical of those that physicians encounter in the course of their clinical duties, particularly psychiatrists and
those who work in emergency departments. For this reason, students
and residents should understand how to assess and clinically manage
psychiatric emergencies.

■ Violent and Assaultive Behaviors

Violence is all too common in society. Daily news reports of senseless
killings and assaults, drive-by shootings, and domestic violence document these events. People fear the possibility of becoming victims of violent crime, even as crime rates have steadily dropped in the past two
decades. Too often, the media have exaggerated the link between violence and mental illness, contributing to the fear felt by many of us, but
also to the stigma experienced by psychiatric patients.

Most mentally ill persons are law-abiding and nonviolent. Nonetheless, research shows that patients with schizophrenia, mania, neurocognitive disorders (e.g., dementia, delirium), and substance use disorders

are more likely to become violent than are patients with other diagnoses or persons who are not mentally ill. Moreover, psychotic persons are more likely to commit violent acts than are nonpsychotic individuals. Brain-injured and intellectually disabled persons also are at higher risk for committing violent acts.

The following vignette describes the unfortunate but rather typical case of an aggressive patient with a dementia seen in our hospital:

> Donald, a 71-year-old man with advanced Alzheimer's disease, was admitted for evaluation of violent and unpredictable behavior. His wife and family had cared for him at home during the 7-year illness. As the illness progressed, Donald became more confused and made more frequent misinterpretations of external stimuli. For example, his wife had a deep voice, which led him at times to conclude that a strange man was in the house. This was especially frightening to him and led him to threaten his wife with a knife.
>
> Donald was observed to be disoriented and confused. He did not know the date, his location, or the situation. He required considerable assistance with his grooming and dress. At times, without apparent provocation, he would strike his nurses or would make threatening gestures, such as karate chops. This behavior was frightening because of its unpredictability.
>
> He was given a high-potency antipsychotic (haloperidol, 2 mg/day) to reduce his paranoia and agitation. He was placed in a nursing home familiar with the care of patients with Alzheimer's disease.

The public—and often the courts—expect psychiatrists and other mental health professionals to be especially skilled in predicting violent behavior. In truth, while they are no more skilled than laypersons in making long-term predictions about violence, mental health professionals *are* in a position to predict violence in clinical settings. Certain elements of the clinical situation, including the patient's diagnosis and past behavior, can give an indication of the patient's potential for imminent violence, thereby allowing appropriate interventions to be made. A patient's history of violent behavior is probably the single best predictor of future dangerousness. Clinical wisdom suggests that past behavior predicts future behavior. The accuracy of predictions is improved in clinical populations that have high base rates for violence, such as patients on a locked psychiatric inpatient unit.

Etiology and Pathophysiology

Much of the violence in society appears to be related to the misuse of alcohol and other drugs, either indirectly through activities involved in obtaining these substances or directly through their use. In clinical settings, the contribution to violence from substance misuse is well known; alcohol use disorders in particular are strongly associated with violence due to their tendency to cause disinhibition, to decrease perceptual and cognitive alertness, and to impair judgment. Other substances of abuse, including cocaine and other stimulants, hallucinogens, phencyclidine (PCP), and sedative-hypnotics, have also been associated with violence and aggression.

One of the strongest predictors of adult violence is childhood aggression. This may be evident from a history of childhood behavioral problems or delinquent behavior, or a past diagnosis of conduct disorder. Of special concern is the triad of fire setting, animal cruelty, and enuresis during childhood that is especially predictive of violence. Many adult perpetrators of abuse are themselves victims of childhood abuse (emotional, physical, or sexual). For some, violence has its roots in a chaotic home environment, but for others there may be a biological predisposition toward violence.

Other risk factors are associated with a tendency to violence. People with low incomes are more likely to be both perpetrators and victims of violence, perhaps because of the alienation, discrimination, family breakdown, and general sense of frustration that the poor experience. Antisocial and borderline personality disorders are associated with violent behavior, a fact that is reflected by their high prevalence among incarcerated persons. With advancing age and maturity, people with these disorders are less likely to act out. The presence of readily available firearms in our society also has contributed to the general level of violence because they can turn what would be an assault into a murder. This has become tragically apparent in the growing number of mass killings that have occurred in the past decade, many in schools, such as the 2012 shooting in Newtown, Connecticut.

At a neurophysiological level, aggressive behavior has been associated with disturbed central nervous system serotonin function. Low cerebrospinal fluid (CSF) 5-hydroxyindoleacetic acid (5-HIAA) levels are correlated with impulsive violence, one of the best-replicated laboratory findings in psychiatry. (5-HIAA is a metabolite of serotonin.) Serotonin has been hypothesized to act as the central nervous system's natural policing mechanism, helping to keep impulsive and violent behavior in check.

Violence is sometimes related to a brain injury or disorder (e.g., tumors, strokes) or to a seizure disorder (e.g., partial complex seizures). People with traumatic brain injuries are more likely than noninjured persons to become violent or aggressive, but aggressive acts by patients with epilepsy are relatively uncommon.

Assessing Risk for Violence

Risk assessment for violent behavior involves a review of pertinent clinical variables and requires a thorough psychiatric history and careful mental status examination. Even in routine assessments, patients should be asked the following questions:

- Have you ever thought of harming someone else?
- Have you ever seriously injured another person?
- What is the most violent thing you have ever done?

The prediction of violence can be compared to weather forecasting. Like weather forecasting, assessment of violence risk becomes less accurate beyond the short term (i.e., 24–48 hours). Furthermore, like weather forecasts, risk assessments should be updated frequently. Clinical variables associated with violence are summarized in Table 18–1.

A differential diagnosis should be based on the patient's history, physical examination, and mental status examination, and in some cases laboratory findings. Interventions are generally based on the diagnosis. For example, a violent schizophrenic patient will need treatment with antipsychotic medication. A manic patient will probably require a combination of a mood stabilizer and an antipsychotic to adequately control his or her behavior.

When interviewing the violent or threatening patient, the clinician should remain calm and speak softly. Comments or questions should appear nonjudgmental, such as "You seem upset; perhaps you can tell me why you feel that way." The interviewer should always have an easy escape route in case the patient becomes aggressive and should avoid towering over the patient. If possible, both patient and clinician should be seated, allowing personal distance between the two. Direct eye contact should be avoided, and the interviewer should try to project a sense of empathy and concern. Family members, friends, police, and others who have pertinent information on the patient should be interviewed.

Managing the Violent Patient

In the hospital or clinic setting, the violent patient presents an emergency. To ensure the safety of the patient and others, it is important that staff be sufficient in number and well trained in seclusion and restraint techniques. Students and residents should remember that seclusion or restraint is considered an emergency safety measure that aims to pre-

---

TABLE 18–1. Clinical variables associated with violence

A history of violent acts

Inability to control anger

A history of impulsive behavior (e.g., recklessness)

Paranoid ideation or frank psychosis

Lack of insight in psychotic patients

Command hallucinations in psychotic patients

The stated desire to hurt or kill another person

Presence of an acting-out personality disorder (e.g., antisocial personality disorder, borderline personality disorder)

Presence of a dementia, delirium, or alcohol or drug intoxication

---

vent injury to the patient and others and is never used as punishment or for the convenience of the staff.

Once a decision has been made to restrain or to seclude the patient, a staff member—backed up by at least four other team members—should approach the patient after first clearing the area of other patients. The patient should be told that he or she is being secluded or restrained because of uncontrolled behavior and should be asked to walk quietly to the seclusion area with or without underarm support. If the patient does not cooperate, staff members should each take a limb in a plan agreed to beforehand. The patient is brought to the ground, with his or her head controlled to avoid biting. Restraints should be applied. If the patient is taken to the seclusion room, staff members should grasp the patient's legs at the knee and the patient's arms around the elbow with underarm support. Specific techniques will vary by institution, but all aim to provide for the safety of the patient and others.

Once secluded, the patient should be searched. Belts, pins, and other potentially dangerous items should be removed, and the patient should be dressed in a hospital gown. If tranquilizing medication is needed, it can be injected (or taken orally if the patient is cooperative). With agitated patients, the best strategy is to combine a high-potency antipsychotic with a benzodiazepine (e.g., haloperidol, 2–5 mg; lorazepam, 1–2 mg). The dose of both agents can be repeated every 30 minutes until the patient has sufficiently calmed. One-on-one observation of the patient by nursing staff is generally mandatory in these situations.

Although rules differ from hospital to hospital, the clinician should carefully document the reasons for seclusion or restraint (e.g., harm to self or others, threatening gestures), the condition of the patient, laboratory investigations being pursued (e.g., urine drug screen), medication being administered, type of restraint used, and the criteria for discontinuation of restraints.

Clinical points about violent patients

1. Predicting violent behavior is difficult, even under the best of circumstances, but violence is often associated with the following:

   - Alcohol or other drug intoxication.

   - Neurocognitive disorders, such as Alzheimer's disease, delirium, or traumatic brain injury.

   - Psychotic disorders.

   - "Acting out" personality disorders (e.g., antisocial personality disorder, borderline personality disorder).

2. The patient should be approached in a slow and tactful manner.

   - The clinician should not appear threatening or provocative.

   - The clinician should use a soft voice, appear passive, and maintain interpersonal distance.

   - Allow for ready escape: never let the patient get between you and the door.

3. The clinician should ask the patient what is wrong or why he or she feels angry.

   - Most patients are willing to disclose their feelings.

4. Violent psychiatric patients need to be in the hospital, where their safety and the safety of others can be assured.

5. Orders for violence precautions and seclusion or restraint orders should be written, when applicable.

   - The risk of violence and the presence of assaultive behaviors should be carefully monitored.

   - The clinician should document the assessment and plan and review them frequently.

6. The underlying condition should be vigorously treated.

7. For outpatients, the risk of violent behaviors should be monitored at each contact; the patient (or family) should remove all firearms from the home.

   - Family members should be instructed to contact the local police (i.e., call 911) if violence erupts.

■ Suicide and Suicidal Behavior

Suicide is the tenth most frequent cause of death for adults and the third leading cause of death for persons between ages 15 and 24. Over 34,000 suicides occur each year in the United States—about one every 18 minutes. A suicide affects not only surviving friends and family members but also the victim's physician, because most people who commit suicide communicate their suicidal intentions to and see physicians before they die. For this reason, clinicians must familiarize themselves with suicide and be prepared to educate patients and family members about risk for suicide, assess risk for suicide in their patients, and intervene when appropriate to prevent a suicide.

Epidemiology

Nearly 1% of the United States general population ultimately commits suicide, a rate of about 11.3 suicides per 100,000 persons. Suicide rates are specific for age, gender, and race. Rates for men tend to increase steadily with age and reach a peak after age 75 years. Rates for women tend to peak in the late 40s or early 50s (see Figure 18–1). Nearly three times as many men take their lives as women, and whites are more likely than blacks to kill themselves. An alarming trend has been the rise in the suicide rate among young men and women, possibly as a result of increasing rates of drug abuse or perhaps attributable to the cohort effect (discussed later in this chapter).

Suicide rates differ by geographic region as well. In the United States, rates are highest in the western states and lowest in the mid-Atlantic states. Rates are very high in central European countries and in Scandinavia. For example, in Hungary, the rate hovers around 40 suicides per 100,000 persons. Rates are low in countries with large Catholic or Muslim populations.

About two-thirds of suicide completers are men. Most are more than 45 years old, white, and separated, widowed, or divorced. Psychiatric diagnosis tends to vary with age. Suicide completers younger than age 30 are more likely to have a substance use disorder or antisocial personality disorder. Suicide completers older than age 30 are more likely to have a mood disorder.

Suicide rates tend to peak during the late spring and have a smaller secondary peak in the fall. Rates are affected by economic conditions and were very high during the Great Depression of the 1930s; they are typically low during times of war. Certain occupations are associated with a high risk for suicide. Professionals, including physicians, are at high risk.

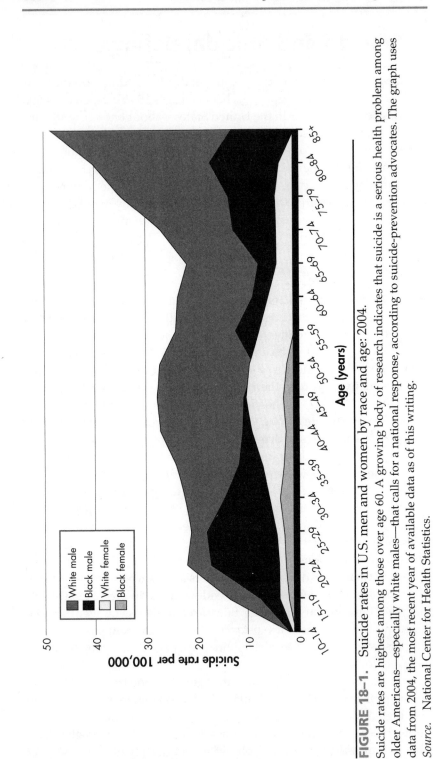

FIGURE 18–1.   Suicide rates in U.S. men and women by race and age: 2004.

Suicide rates are highest among those over age 60. A growing body of research indicates that suicide is a serious health problem among older Americans—especially white males—that calls for a national response, according to suicide-prevention advocates. The graph uses data from 2004, the most recent year of available data as of this writing.

Source.   National Center for Health Statistics.

Etiology and Pathophysiology

Over 90% of suicide completers had a major psychiatric disorder at the time of the act, and more than half were clinically depressed. Substance use disorders affect nearly one-half of suicide completers, while schizophrenia, anxiety disorders, and other mental illnesses are less common.

The risk for suicide is much higher among psychiatric patients than in the general population. Research shows that certain psychiatric disorders are associated with high rates of suicide. For example, 10%–15% of persons hospitalized with mood disorders and around 10% of persons with schizophrenia will commit suicide. Risk for suicide is further increased by the presence of a personality disorder, particularly in persons with a mood or substance use disorder. Thus, although psychiatric and/or medical illnesses usually are necessary for suicide to occur, their presence is not a sufficient explanation, because most mentally ill persons do not kill themselves.

About 5% of suicide completers have serious physical illnesses at the time of suicide. Suicide rates are reported to be high in persons who have traumatic brain injuries, epilepsy, multiple sclerosis, Huntington's disease, Parkinson's disease, cancer, and AIDS.

A small number of persons committing suicide appear to have no evidence of mental or physical illness. Many have argued that these suicides are rational and based on a logical appraisal of the need for death. An example is an elderly widower with terminal cancer who is not clinically depressed but has no hope for the future and wishes to end his physical pain. Many of these so-called rational suicides are probably irrational, but information was unavailable to confirm the presence of a mental illness because the person who died was socially isolated and informants were not available for interview.

Suicide runs in families and may have a genetic component. Examination of large kindreds, such as the Old Order Amish in Pennsylvania, shows that suicide tends to cluster in certain pedigrees—pedigrees also filled with mood disorders. Twin studies have reported higher concordance for suicide among identical twins than nonidentical twins. One large adoption study found a higher prevalence of suicide among biological relatives of probands who had killed themselves than among the relatives of control probands, providing further evidence of a hereditary contribution to suicide. The acid cystein proteinase inhibitor (*ACPI*) gene on chromosome 2 was recently identified as conferring risk for suicidal behavior.

At a physiological level, suicide—like impulsive violence—has also been associated with low levels of CSF 5-HIAA and with other findings that suggest disturbed serotonin neurotransmission. Follow-up studies have shown that many suicide completers had abnormal dexamethasone suppression test results, suggesting the presence of hypothalamic-pituitary-adrenal axis hyperactivity. Suicide completers also have been found to have high levels of urinary metabolites of cortisol and to have enlarged adrenal glands. All of these measures are abnormal in severe depression; therefore, they may indicate depression rather than risk for suicide.

Suicide Methods

Firearms are the most common method used to commit suicide in the United States, perhaps because firearms are readily available and can be immediately lethal. Firearms are followed in frequency by poisoning (i.e., a drug overdose), hanging, cutting, jumping, and other methods. Men are more likely than women to use violent methods, such as firearms or hanging, a tendency that may explain why men are more successful in killing themselves. Women tend to use less violent means, such as poisoning by overdose. Women are beginning to choose more lethal methods, a trend that may ultimately lead to higher suicide rates.

Clinical Findings

Suicide is an act of desperation. Nearly two-thirds of suicidal persons communicate their suicidal intentions to others. Their communication may be as direct as reporting their plan and the date they intend to carry it out. Other communications are less obvious; for instance, the patient may say to his relatives, "You won't have to put up with me much longer!"

Suicide can occur during all phases of a depressive episode. It is commonly believed that suicide risk is highest during the recovery phase, when a patient has regained sufficient energy to carry out the suicide. Because the suicidal urge waxes and wanes during the course of a depressive episode, the clinician should not be lulled into a false sense of security based on the phase of a patient's illness.

Suicide completers tend to be socially isolated. Nearly 30% of suicide completers have a history of suicide attempts, and about one in six leaves a suicide note. Clinicians should be alert to behaviors that suggest suicidal intent: preparing a will, giving away possessions, or purchasing a burial plot. One of the strongest correlates of suicidal behavior is hopelessness, a finding independent of psychiatric diagnosis.

Patients remain at high risk for suicide after hospital discharge. Although depressed patients may appear to be significantly improved at the time of discharge, relapse can occur quickly. In a follow-up of depressed patients, nearly 42% of 36 suicides occurred within 6 months of hospital discharge, 58% by 1 year, and 70% by 2 years. Therefore, recently discharged patients need close follow-up.

Triggering events in adolescents or young adults often include academic problems or troubled relationships with parents. In older persons, the event may be poor finances or health. More than 50% of alcoholic persons who commit suicide have a history of relationship loss (usually of an intimate relationship) within the year before suicide. This is not the case among persons with major depressive disorder.

Youth Suicide

Suicide rates have been climbing in both males and females between ages 15 and 24 years. In fact, studies have shown that recent cohorts (i.e., groups of persons in the population with similar characteristics, such as being born in the same decade) have higher suicide rates than older cohorts. Why rates are increasing in younger age groups is a mystery, but other data seem to show that the prevalence of depression also is increasing in each successive cohort. Drug abuse has become a serious problem for society, especially young persons, and may be contributing to the higher rates of suicide.

Teenagers are more prone to the effects of peer pressure than are adults, and this may be reflected in suicide clusters. It has been suggested that media portrayals of suicide, such as those in television movies or documentaries, are followed by an increased rate of both suicide attempts and suicides, often by the method depicted.

Suicide Attempters
Versus Suicide Completers

Suicide attempts are intentional acts of self-injury that do not result in death. They are 5–20 times as frequent as suicides—perhaps more so, because most suicide attempts go unreported and many persons who attempt suicide do not seek medical attention. Although suicide completers usually have a diagnosis of major depression or alcohol use disorder, suicide attempters are less likely to have these conditions. They may instead have other conditions, such as a personality disorder.

Suicide completers carefully plan their act, use effective means (e.g., firearms, hanging), and carry out the suicide in private or make provisions to avoid discovery. They are serious about ending their lives. In contrast, suicide attempters, who are three times more likely to be women and usually younger than 35 years, act impulsively, make provisions for rescue, and use ineffective means such as drug overdoses. Suicide attempters are at risk for future attempts, and each year thereafter an estimated 1%–2% of those who have attempted suicide will complete the act—up to a total of about 10%.

Assessing the Suicidal Patient

Suicide risk assessment involves having an understanding of the patient as well as of common risk factors. The clinician should be alert to the possibility of suicide in any psychiatric patient, especially a patient who is depressed or has a depressed affect. In these patients, the assessment will focus on vegetative signs and cognitive symptoms of depression, death wishes, suicidal ideation, and suicidal plans. Common risk factors associated with suicide are summarized in Table 18–2. Remembering these risk factors can be facilitated through the use of a simple mnemonic: **SAD PERSONS.** The initials stand for **S**ex (male gender), **A**ge (older), **D**epression, **P**revious (suicide) attempt, **E**thanol abuse, **Ra**tional thinking loss, **S**ocial support lacking, **O**rganized plan, **N**o spouse, **S**ickness.

Suicidal patients are generally willing to discuss their thoughts with a physician if asked. A common myth is that asking a patient about suicide will give the patient ideas that he or she has not already had. In truth, suicidal thoughts are common in depression, and many if not most depressed patients will have had them. Patients are often fearful and even feel guilty about having suicidal thoughts. Giving the patient an opportunity to discuss them may itself provide relief. Specific questions that should be asked of the patient include the following:

- Are you having any thoughts that life isn't worth living?
- Are you having any thoughts about harming yourself?
- Are you having any thoughts about taking your life?
- Have you developed a plan for committing suicide? If so, what is your plan?

The physician also should assess the patient's history of suicidal behavior by asking the following questions:

- Have you ever had thoughts of killing yourself?
- Have you ever attempted suicide? If so, would you tell me about the attempt?

TABLE 18–2.   Clinical variables associated with suicide

Being a psychiatric patient

Being male, although the gender distinction is less important among
psychiatric patients than in the general population

Age: risk increases as men age but peaks in the middle years for women

Being divorced, widowed, or single

Race: whites are at higher risk than nonwhites

Diagnosis: depression, alcoholism, schizophrenia

History of suicide attempts

Expressing suicidal thoughts or developing plans for suicide

Recent interpersonal loss (especially among alcoholic patients)

Feelings of hopelessness and low self-esteem

Timing: early in the post–hospital discharge period

Adolescents: a history of drug abuse and behavior problems

The physician should approach the topic of suicide in a slow and
tactful manner, after having developed rapport with the patient. Because suicidal thoughts may fluctuate, physicians should reassess suicide risk at each contact with the patient. Patients with well-developed
plans and the means to carry them out require protection, usually in a
hospital on a locked psychiatric unit. When the suicidal patient refuses
admission, it may be necessary to obtain a court order requiring hospitalization. Suicidal patients may plead with the doctor, family, or
friends to stay out of the hospital, but few people are adequately prepared to protect a suicidal person around the clock. Hospitalization is
the best way for a physician to ensure the patient's safety.

Managing the Suicidal Patient

In the hospital, the nursing staff will take sharp objects, belts, and other
potentially lethal items from the patient. Patients at risk for elopement
are carefully watched. The physician should document the patient's
signs and symptoms of depression, along with the clinician's own assessment of suicide risk and protective measures taken.

Once the patient's safety has been ensured, treatment of the underlying illness can begin. Treatment will depend on the diagnosis. Antidepressant medication or electroconvulsive therapy (ECT) can be used for
the treatment of depression; mood stabilizers and antipsychotics are ap-

propriate additions to the treatment of bipolar disorder and psychotic depression, respectively. Antipsychotic medications are helpful in the suicidal schizophrenic patient.

Lithium has been reported to lower suicide risk in bipolar patients. Among the antipsychotics, only clozapine has been associated with lower rates of suicide. ECT is often specifically recommended for the treatment of major depression in suicidal individuals because it tends to have a quicker onset of action than medication.

Close follow-up is mandatory for suicidal outpatients. Follow-up must include frequent physician visits (or telephone contacts) to assess mood and suicide risk as well as to provide psychotherapeutic support. The physician should consider prescribing antidepressants with a high therapeutic index that are unlikely to be fatal in overdose, such as one of the selective serotonin reuptake inhibitors (SSRIs). Family members can help monitor the patient's medication use. Importantly, they should also be instructed to remove all firearms from the home.

Clinical points about suicidal patients

1. Depressed patients should always be asked about suicidal thoughts and plans. The clinician will not plant ideas that were not there merely by asking.

    - Suicidality should be reassessed and documented at every visit with depressed patients.

2. Some suicidal patients should be hospitalized, even if it is against their will. Patients without suicidal plans can probably be managed at home provided that they have supportive families who are willing to watch them carefully.

3. In the hospital, "suicide precautions" should be written in the doctors' orders; one-to-one protection should be ordered if needed.

    - Signs and symptoms must be carefully documented.

4. Suicidality should be frequently monitored in outpatients. Antidepressants with a high therapeutic index are preferred, such as SSRIs or one of the newer antidepressants (e.g., bupropion, mirtazapine, duloxetine, venlafaxine).

    - Family members should remove all firearms from the home.

5. Even though the risk factors are known, it is not possible to predict who will commit suicide.

    - One should use good clinical judgment, provide close follow-up, and prescribe effective treatments.

■ Self-Assessment Questions

1. What are the risk factors for violent behavior? What is the pathophysiology underlying violent behavior?
2. How is the violent or potentially violent patient assessed and managed?
3. Why is suicide a major health problem?
4. What is a helpful mnemonic for common suicide risk factors?
5. How do completed suicides differ from attempted suicides?
6. What is a rational suicide?
7. Are there different risk factors for suicide among youth?
8. How should the suicidal patient be managed in the hospital? In an outpatient setting?

Chapter 19

Legal Issues

Lawsuit, *n.* a machine which you go into as a pig and come out as a sausage.

Ambrose Bierce, The Devil's Dictionary

More than most other medical specialists, psychiatrists regularly confront sensitive legal issues. Should this patient be committed to the hospital for treatment against his or her will? Should this patient be forcibly medicated? Can I release information about my patient to someone else without his or her permission?

Because our society values individual freedom and civil liberties, there are rarely easy answers to questions about involuntary hospitalization, the right to treatment (or the right to refuse treatment), confidentiality, and other legal issues. What may seem morally right may not be legally permissible, and conversely, what may be legally permissible may seem morally wrong. The right of a man with schizophrenia to live on the streets, for instance, loses its meaning when he becomes so ill that he lacks the capacity to make important decisions. Thus the psychiatrist often gets caught in the middle between what may be legally right (i.e., not forcing treatment on someone with schizophrenia) and what may be ethically right (i.e., relieving the suffering of the schizophrenic person through involuntary treatment). Because of this interface with the law, psychiatrists should understand the legal issues they are likely to encounter.

Although general principles underlie much of the law in the United States, significant variation exists between states and jurisdictions. It is therefore essential that psychiatrists become familiar with relevant laws in the regions where they practice.

Legal issues pertaining to mental illness can be roughly divided into two broad categories: civil and criminal (see Table 19–1). *Civil law* has primarily to do with relationships between citizens, while *criminal law* focuses on the individual's relationship to the state in the maintenance

TABLE 19–1.   Civil and criminal legal issues involving psychiatrists

Civil	Criminal
Involuntary hospitalization	Competency to stand trial
Confidentiality	Criminal responsibility
Informed consent	
Malpractice	

of social order. Civil issues pertinent to the practice of psychiatry include confidentiality, informed consent, and involuntary treatment. Criminal issues that might involve input from mental health practitioners include competence to stand trial (whether the person understands the court process and can assist his lawyer in the present) and criminal responsibility (whether the person accused of a crime was legally insane at the time of the act).

In this chapter, we focus primarily on civil issues encountered by the psychiatrist during the course of his or her day-to-day practice. Forensic psychiatry, a subspecialty within psychiatry, focuses on the interface between psychiatry and the law. Psychiatrists working in this area devote significant time to conducting evaluations of mental capacity, injury, and disability for agencies and courts. Although we offer a general overview of questions asked of psychiatrists by criminal courts, readers interested in these areas are referred to *Clinical Handbook of Psychiatry and the Law* (Appelbaum and Gutheil 2007).

■ Civil Issues

Involuntary Treatment

Psychiatrists have a responsibility to provide for the safety of their patients. Legal precedent has extended this duty to include the protection of others who could be physically or emotionally harmed by the actions of a mentally ill person. Thus, when a patient who is thought to be a threat to self or others refuses hospitalization for the treatment of mental illness, the psychiatrist will seek a court order for involuntary hospitalization.

In the past, the court system deferred to the judgment of physicians concerning the detention of patients for treatment, but with increasing emphasis on individual liberties and freedoms articulated during the civil rights movement, the process of *civil commitment* became more a matter for the courts. Because civil commitment involves depriving a person of some of his or her constitutional rights on the basis of a mental illness, most states now carefully regulate the process in the belief that the courts are more objective in this balancing act than are mental health providers. The appropriateness of this emphasis on civil rights over the right to humane care has been hotly debated. It is sometimes said that the homeless are being allowed to "die with their rights on."

Most commitment laws invoke the concepts of mental illness, dangerousness, and disability. For civil commitment, these laws require the presence of mental illness, although the precise definition of *mental illness* differs from place to place. The law may specify the conditions considered to be mental illness and require that the mental illness be treatable in order to qualify for civil commitment. For example, a diagnosis of a personality disorder may be insufficient for commitment in some jurisdictions while being acceptable in others. The concept of *dangerousness* usually requires that persons present an imminent danger to themselves or others (i.e., within the next 24 hours if not hospitalized). Because psychiatrists are unable to accurately predict dangerousness except in the most obvious of situations, this requirement can be difficult to apply. The third element, *disability,* is a measure of the patient's inability to properly care for him- or herself because of mental illness. Some states use the phrase *gravely disabled* (or similar language) to suggest that a person is unable to take care of his or her personal grooming, to maintain adequate hydration, and to feed him- or herself. A gravely disabled person may not be in imminent danger of harming him- or herself but may still need psychiatric hospitalization and treatment.

Most states allow for patients to be hospitalized on an emergency basis to allow for a more detailed evaluation and short-term psychiatric intervention. This follows the filing of a petition by someone who knows the person and medical certification of the need for emergency commitment. This period may range from 1 to 20 days, depending on the jurisdiction.

Civil commitments occur by court order after a judicial finding of mental illness and potential harm to self or others if released; they provide for continued involuntary hospitalization. There are a variety of legal protections for mentally ill persons facing involuntary commitment. Details vary by jurisdiction, but these protections include a timely court hearing following appropriate notice, ability to be present at all commitment proceedings, representation by an attorney, presentation of evidence by both sides, and privilege against self-incrimination (the right to refrain from saying anything that may make one seem ill). The burden of proof is placed on the petitioner to establish the reason for commitment, and the patient is guaranteed the right to appeal. These requirements contribute to the tension between the individual's legally protected rights and the desire of society to provide necessary mental health treatment.

In general, the case for commitment is made by an attorney representing the state to a magistrate, who makes a decision to commit to inpatient care when the evidence presented is "clear and convincing," a standard generally thought of as the level of proof needed for three of four reasonable people to agree. The judicial decision is intended to favor the best interests of the patient by providing for treatment of the person's mental illness by court order. Although the statutes differ, all states allow involuntary administration of psychotropic medication to some extent.

Much litigation has concerned the right of civilly committed patients to refuse psychotropic medication in nonemergency situations. Antipsychotic medication has been the major focus of this litigation because of the potential risk of serious side effects such as tardive dyskinesia. Although the risks of treatment differ among these drugs (second-generation antipsychotics are associated with lower risk of tardive dyskinesia), some courts have emphasized the potential risk of treatment rather than its potential benefits. In some courts, treatment with antipsychotic medication has been elevated to the status of an "extraordinary" form of medical treatment requiring special scrutiny. In some states, a patient retains the right to refuse medication until the medical treatment team has petitioned the local court to declare the patient incompetent to consent to or refuse medication. In other states, such as Iowa, psychiatrists are allowed to provide mental health treatment (including medication) to patients after a commitment order is issued.

When should the clinician decide to involuntarily hospitalize a patient? In the most typical scenario, a law enforcement officer brings a person thought to be mentally ill to an emergency department because the person was behaving in a bizarre manner or threatened suicide. The psychiatrist is then contacted and asked to assess the individual and to make an appropriate decision about disposition. When the person is deemed mentally ill, dangerous, and/or disabled and refuses hospitalization, the decision is relatively easy to make: the magistrate (or judge) is contacted, and an order for involuntary hospitalization is requested. From the physician's perspective, it is probably better to err on the side of safety than to allow someone who is potentially dangerous to self or others to leave the emergency department.

Another common scenario occurs when a patient admitted voluntarily requests discharge but is believed to present an ongoing danger to self or others (e.g., a person who has admitted to having suicidal plans). In these situations, a court order should be sought for continued hospitalization.

In addition to involuntary inpatient treatment, most states (44 out of 50) have provisions for involuntary outpatient treatment. Such treatment may be used when the patient is not quite ill enough to merit inpatient care, but presents some risk of harm to self or others because of mental illness and will not voluntarily comply with outpatient treatment. Outpatient commitments can be enormously helpful in improving treatment compliance and reducing the frequency of hospitalization in patients who are otherwise chronically noncompliant. Enforcement is unfortunately limited in most states.

Confidentiality

Maintaining confidentiality is one of the most important ethical and legal obligations that psychiatrists have to their patients. From the time of Hippocrates, physicians have believed that what passes between doctor and patient should remain private and should not be divulged without the patient's consent. Because psychiatrists gather more sensitive information than many medical practitioners, disclosure could be socially embarrassing or harmful and could discourage patients from seeking care. As a practical matter, what this means is that before information is given to a third party, the patient must provide written consent except when disclosure is required by regulation or law.

The U.S. government, recognizing the importance of confidentiality of patient records, devised the Health Insurance Portability and Accountability Act (HIPAA). Under the privacy rule in HIPAA, health care providers could face fines and penalties if protected health information was released without informed consent except as required by law or as allowed by other parts of HIPAA. There are a number of exceptions to HIPAA, including medical emergency, legal action, and limited information release to facilitate billing.

In some instances, physicians are required by law to breach confidentiality to protect a vulnerable person from harm by a patient, such as in the case of child or elder abuse. In these situations, the physician needs only to have a reason to believe that the abuse has occurred in order to trigger the reporting requirement. Another example of legally mandated disclosure, although encountered less in psychiatry than in other specialties, is that of reportable infectious diseases (e.g., tuberculosis, syphilis, gonorrhea, HIV).

Psychiatrists have an additional duty to protect third parties from the actions of patients in their care. On rare occasions, in the course of treating a patient, the patient may threaten to harm an identifiable third party. The psychiatrist has a legal responsibility to protect that third party and may break confidentiality by notifying the threatened person and/or the police. This *duty to protect* is referred to as the *Tarasoff* rule, named after a 1976 California Supreme Court case. A therapist was held responsible for harm committed to an identified third party by his patient because it had been revealed that the therapist was aware of the potential threat and did not warn or protect the victim.

How to best implement the *Tarasoff* rule has been debated. Not all states acknowledge *Tarasoff* duties, and several states limit the circumstances under which protection of the third party must occur. In practice, once the psychiatrist believes that a patient may harm others, hospitalization is frequently sought to further evaluate the patient and to protect the intended victim. When there is imminent threat to a foreseeable victim, protection of the endangered person may involve phoning the individual and reporting the threat even when the clinician has hospitalized the patient.

A psychiatrist may encourage the patient to phone the third party in his or her presence, or sometimes the psychiatrist will make the call in the patient's presence. Letting the patient participate in making decisions about how the notification will take place may minimize the detrimental effect of the breach of confidentiality and may also have a deterrent effect.

Confidentiality can be legally breached for other reasons. In some states, mental health providers may disclose confidential information to close family members or others responsible for the ongoing treatment of the patient without consent when it is thought to be in the best interest of the patient. Utilization review groups, physician peer reviewers, and third-party payers may have access to hospital charts. Very occasionally mental health providers will be faced with requests for information from police officers, attorneys, and courts. In these cases, guidance should be sought from an attorney on how best to proceed.

Informed Consent

Informed consent should be obtained from all patients before any psychiatric treatment. Formal written consent is commonplace in hospitals but remains relatively unusual in small private offices. Patients should be informed of the indications and contraindications for the treatment, possible adverse effects, risk involved in nontreatment, and alternative therapies (if applicable). The physician should carefully document the results of the discussion. One problem with informed consent arises when the patient is not capable of giving consent. In these situations, the patient should have a court-appointed guardian who can make health care decisions on his or her behalf.

In addition to a general consent for evaluation and treatment, many hospitals require additional written informed consent for some treatments deemed to be especially risky, such as the use of psychotropic medications or electroconvulsive therapy (ECT). These treatments require special consent because the side effects associated with their use may be permanent.

Malpractice

Malpractice is negligence in the conduct of one's professional duties. The number of malpractice suits filed in the United States seems to climb each year. About two-thirds of physicians will experience at least one malpractice lawsuit during their professional career. The reaction among many physicians is to practice "defensive medicine," for example, ordering extra tests or refusing to treat certain patients.

Psychiatrists are sued less frequently than other physicians. One reason is that psychiatrists, by virtue of the disorders treated and the types of treatments provided, are less likely to physically harm a patient. Psychiatric patients are reluctant to publicize their mental disorders and treatments, and there are typically no witnesses to the alleged malpractice. Psychiatrists also tend to have long-term relationships with their patients, which may reduce the likelihood of being sued.

Patient suicide is the most common reason for a psychiatrist to be sued, even though research has never shown that psychiatrists are able to predict suicide with any acceptable degree of accuracy. Nonetheless, the courts and the public tend to blame psychiatrists for failing to prevent a patient's death. Suicides that occur during hospitalization are probably the ones most likely to result in litigation. This is because suicidal behavior may have been the reason the patient was in the hospital. Potential errors by a psychiatrist include his or her failure to take an adequate history of suicidal behavior, failure to provide adequate protection in the hospital (e.g., one-to-one supervision), or failure to communicate changes in the patient's condition to other doctors and nurses.

Psychiatrists also are sued because of failure to obtain informed consent. Patients may claim that the information provided to them was inadequate, that alternatives were omitted, or that the consent was never obtained. It behooves the clinician to maintain careful records about what happens during an appointment, particularly as it pertains to obtaining consent and providing information. Informed consent should be thought of as an ongoing process, not a slip of paper obtained once.

Psychiatrists are occasionally sued by patients who sustain injuries from psychotropic medications. Situations that have led to claims include failure to disclose relevant information to the patient about adverse effects, failure to obtain an adequate history, and prescription of a drug or drug combination when it is not indicated or when potentially harmful drug interactions might occur. Tardive dyskinesia is an example of an adverse effect that can prompt litigation. Psychiatrists and other prescribers should regularly monitor patients for the presence and severity of side effects such as tardive dyskinesia, and they should educate the patient and family members (or guardian) about the risks of treatment and the continuing need for medication.

Psychiatrists are sometimes sued for abandonment, defined as improperly terminating a doctor–patient relationship despite the continuing need for treatment. Abandonment can give rise to actions for both negligence and breach of contract. Termination may occur because a patient fails to cooperate with treatment, fails to pay bills, threatens or assaults the psychiatrist, or presents a difficult management problem. To avoid litigation, the best course is to notify the patient in writing and provide sufficient time for the patient to find another psychiatrist.

Claims involving ECT are relatively rare but do occur and involve allegations of failure to obtained informed consent, inappropriate or improper treatment, or injury resulting from treatment, such as memory loss. Liability can be minimized by using ECT in accordance with accepted practice standards and monitoring and supervising patients carefully between treatments. The consent process should be fully documented and preferably witnessed.

Although relatively rare in practice, sexual activity with current or former patients has become a well-publicized reason for malpractice litigation. Unlike errors in professional judgment, inappropriate sexual behavior with a patient is a voluntary act by a clinician and is therefore both preventable and excluded under most malpractice insurance policies. A psychiatrist may be expelled from professional associations, have his or her license suspended or revoked, and even face criminal charges for such "boundary violations." The American Psychiatric Association has made it clear that sexual contact with current or previous patients is inappropriate and unethical.

■ Criminal Issues

Psychiatrists rarely encounter situations involving criminal law, whereas these may be "bread and butter" issues for their forensically trained peers. The two most common criminal issues that psychiatrists are asked to comment on are *competency to stand trial* and *criminal responsibility*. To receive a fair trial, a person must be able to understand the nature of the charges against him or her, the possible penalty, and the legal issues and procedures. He or she also must be able to work with the attorney in preparing the defense. The presence of a mental illness, even a psychosis, generally does not render the defendant incompetent to stand trial. Competence to stand trial is assumed unless questioned by someone in the court. Once raised, the court generally hears expert testimony by mental health professionals before deciding the issue.

Competence to stand trial is a legal determination, not a medical one. It is determined by a judge according to national standards established by the U.S. Supreme Court in *Dusky v. United States.* When the court determines that the defendant is incompetent to stand trial, the defendant is typically transferred to a psychiatric hospital for treatment focused on restoring him or her to a competent state. Once competency has been restored, the defendant is returned to court to stand trial. Importantly, competence to stand trial refers to the "here and now" assessment of the person's ability to understand the nature of the proceedings and to assist council, regardless of the presence of mental illness.

Criminal responsibility, or culpability for crime, by contrast has to do with the subject's state of mind at the time of a crime (i.e., "there and then"). Under our current system, a crime is considered to occur only when both bad behavior (*actus rea*) and a blameworthy state of mind (*mens rea*) are present. A person may be so mentally ill as to lack this blameworthy state of mind by virtue of his or her disorder. In such a case, a person is said to lack criminal responsibility and is adjudicated as not guilty by reason of insanity. In practice, a successful insanity defense is rare.

Not all states have an insanity defense, and those that do use different standards for determining criminal responsibility. According to the widely accepted *M'Naghten* standard, modifications of which are used in many states, the person seeking the insanity defense must show that he or she had a mental illness that was so symptomatic that it left him or her unable to know the nature and quality of the act or unable to know that the act was wrong at the time of the alleged offense. The rule is named after a case involving Daniel M'Naghten, who in 1843 shot and killed Edward Drummond, private secretary to British Prime Minister Sir Robert Peel, the intended victim. M'Naghten had suffered delusions for many years and believed that he was being persecuted by the Tory party and their leader (Peel).

Even severely symptomatic patients will only rarely meet the insanity standard. Depending on the jurisdiction, other defenses such as diminished capacity and "guilty but mentally ill" may be used. In diminished capacity, the person is said to be unable to form intent to commit the crime he or she was charged with, but may be found guilty of a lesser charge. In the case of guilty but mentally ill, the person is said to lack the capacity to conform his or her behavior to the requirements of the law at the time of the act despite knowing that the act was wrong. Defendants found "guilty but mentally ill" are usually sentenced to correctional facilities and receive a psychiatric evaluation and appropriate treatment if indicated.

Clinical points about legal issues

1. In seeking involuntary hospitalization for a patient, there must be evidence of a treatable mental illness, imminent harm to self or others, or grave disability.

   - The psychiatrist should become familiar with the local and state laws.

   - The psychiatrist should know the local judge or magistrate who handles civil commitments.

   - Outpatient commitments are useful in seriously mentally ill patients who are chronically noncompliant with treatment.

2. The psychiatrist should understand applicable state laws on confidentiality and informed consent.

3. Breaching confidentiality under the *Tarasoff* rule may involve contacting the threatened third party.

4. Malpractice lawsuits are common in our litigious society; adequate insurance is essential.

   - The best defense against successful claims of malpractice is to maintain proper documentation.

5. Most psychiatrists do not routinely conduct competency evaluations to determine whether a patient can stand trial. Psychiatrists should get to know their forensic psychiatrist peers.

■ Self-Assessment Questions

1. What is forensic psychiatry?
2. What are the major concepts that most civil commitment laws contain?
3. Explain both the right to treatment and the right to refuse treatment. Why is the latter so frustrating to psychiatrists?
4. Explain the *Tarasoff* ruling and the duty to protect. How might the ruling be implemented?
5. Why is confidentiality important? List several situations in which it can (or must) be breached.
6. What are the usual reasons behind malpractice lawsuits filed against psychiatrists?
7. Can a psychotic patient be competent to stand trial?
8. Who was Daniel M'Naghten? Explain the *M'Naghten* standard.

Chapter 20

Behavioral, Cognitive, and Psychodynamic Treatments

The mind is its own place, and in itself
Can make a Heaven of Hell, a Hell of Heaven.

John Milton, Paradise Lost

Because psychiatrists deal with disorders that involve thoughts, feelings, and relationships, it is essential that they maintain an empathic and caring attitude toward their patients and become skilled in using therapies directed at the mind in addition to the brain. Although the empathic relationship that is used in many types of psychotherapy is in principle not different from that used by a caring family practitioner or other medical specialist, it tends to be more important in psychiatric practice because of the nature of the illnesses that are being diagnosed and treated.

These treatments are collectively referred to as *psychotherapy*. Beginning students often wonder whether there is any need to learn about psychotherapy. This lack of interest is unwarranted. In addition to the growing neuroscience base demonstrating the biological mechanisms by which psychotherapy works, a substantial empirical base has confirmed the effectiveness of these treatments. For some disorders (e.g., eating disorders, borderline personality disorder) they are first-line treatments, and they have been repeatedly shown to produce good outcomes. For many other disorders (e.g., schizophrenia, bipolar disorder), they have been shown to be an important adjunct to medications by encouraging treatment adherence, educating patients about symptoms and expected outcome, and providing insight or support to deal with the psychological consequences of having a severe illness.

In this chapter, we provide a brief overview of the major classes of psychotherapy that are used by specialists who care for mentally ill patients. Some of these treatments require extensive experience and training on a scale that is outside the range of description of a single chapter. Students who want to explore specific types of psychotherapy in more detail may want to read material cited in the Bibliography. The various psychotherapies include behavior therapy, cognitive-behavioral therapy (CBT), the individual psychotherapies that draw on psychodynamic principles, group therapy, couples and family therapy, and social skills training. The major classes are summarized in Table 20–1.

■ Behavior Therapy

The theoretical underpinnings of behavior therapy derive from British empiricism, Pavlov's studies of conditioning, and subsequent research on stimulus-response relationships conducted by other leading behaviorists such as B. F. Skinner. Behaviorists stress the importance of working with objective, observable phenomena, usually referred to as *behavior,* including physical activities such as eating, drinking, talking, and completing the serial-sequential activities that lead to habit formations and patterns of social interactions. In contrast to psychodynamic psychotherapies, discussed later in this chapter, behavioral techniques do not necessarily help patients to understand their emotions or motivations. Instead of working on thoughts and feelings, the behavior therapist works on *what the patient does.* The motto for this approach is "Change the behavior and the feelings will follow."

Behavior therapies are particularly helpful for disorders that are associated with abnormal behavioral patterns in need of correction. These disorders include alcohol and drug use disorders, eating disorders, anxiety disorders, phobias, and obsessive-compulsive behavior. A general knowledge of the principles of behaviorism may be useful in dealing with a broad range of patients, however, including patients with dementias, psychoses, adjustment disorders, childhood disorders, and personality disorders.

The concept of *conditioning* is fundamental to the various behavior therapies. Two types of conditioning have been described: classical (Pavlovian) and operant. Early in the twentieth century, the Russian physiologist Pavlov described the first controlled experiments with conditioning. He demonstrated that by pairing stimuli, such as striking a bell at the same time that dogs were given food, he could eventually pro-

---

TABLE 20–1. Types of psychotherapy

Behavior therapy

Cognitive-behavioral therapy (CBT)

Individual therapy

    Classical psychoanalysis

    Psychodynamic psychotherapy

    Insight-oriented psychotherapy

    Relationship psychotherapy

    Interpersonal therapy (IPT)

    Supportive psychotherapy

Group therapy

Couples therapy

Family therapy

Social skills training

---

duce a conditioned reflex in the animals in the absence of the original triggering stimulus. For example, if the two stimuli (food and the ringing of a bell) were paired frequently enough, the dog would eventually learn to salivate when it heard the bell alone. In this model, the food is regarded as the unconditioned stimulus, the bell as the conditioned stimulus, and salivation in response to the bell the conditioned reflex.

The concept of stimulus pairing can be used both to explain the development of psychopathology and to create behavior therapies through conditioning patients to alter their response patterns.

The study and use of *operant conditioning* involves examining behavior that can control its consequences. For example, a pigeon will increase the frequency of pecking a bar if the pecking behavior is rapidly followed by a food pellet. The food pellet is the reinforcer; the behavior of pecking is increased as a consequence of the reinforcer following the pecking. Behavior may either increase or decrease in frequency, depending on whether the subsequent reinforcers are positive or negative. Praise by a teacher is likely to increase the rate at which a student will raise a hand in response to questions. By contrast, the same student might terminate hand raising in anticipation of critical comments by the teacher. For example, *negative reinforcement* occurs when a child has tantrums following her father's command to "turn off the TV and come to dinner." If the father does not follow through on the command, he has inadvertently negatively reinforced the child's tendency to throw tantrums. In other words, the child is likely to have tantrums more frequently in the future upon hearing a parental command, because such tantrums have been followed by withdrawal of an undesirable command. Operant conditioning is the source of much of the adaptive human learning that occurs during a person's interaction with his or her surrounding environment.

An extensive behavioral literature now suggests that positive reinforcement is more effective in sustaining behavior than negative reinforcement, that failure to provide reinforcements usually will extinguish a behavior, and that variable and unpredictable schedules of reinforcement may be more effective in maintaining behavior than fixed, regular reinforcements. For example, people with gambling disorder receive the positive reinforcement of winning only occasionally, but they continue to gamble and are rarely deterred by threats of punishment or even by punishment itself, such as loss of their financial assets or even incarceration. If they won every time they gambled, they would very likely lose interest eventually, and likewise, they would lose interest if they never won at all.

Relaxation Training

Relaxation training is used to teach patients control over their bodies and mental states. Through this procedure, patients learn how to achieve voluntary control over their feelings of tension and relaxation. Relaxation training can be done simply by providing patients with an instructional audio recording that they can listen to in order to practice the techniques on their own. A common form is called *progressive muscle relaxation,* wherein the person is instructed to systematically proceed through each major muscle group, learning to tense and then relax the muscles. Relaxation training can be used alone to help patients who have anxiety or various problems involving pain (e.g., headache, low back pain), or the training can be used in conjunction with systematic desensitization.

Exposure

One of the key principles of behaviorally oriented treatments is that of exposure. Exposure requires that patients place themselves in situations that they usually avoid, in the interest of reducing the adaptive difficulties that are part and parcel of their mental disorders. For example, one of the more harmful aspects of panic disorder is the agoraphobic avoidance that commonly occurs. Panic patients frequently avoid situations in which they fear the onset of panic symptoms, usually based on catastrophic interpretations of what would happen if they panicked. It is this avoidance, more than the physical symptoms themselves, that is responsible for the disability associated with this and other anxiety disorders. Exposure seeks to encourage the patient to place himself or herself directly into situations that evoke feared internal and external circumstances so that new learning and improved adaptive functioning will occur and be maintained. For example, the therapist may ask the agoraphobic patient to imagine what it is like to leave his or her house and visit the shopping mall where he or she typically develops panic attacks, thereby leading the patient to experience the attack. This is called *imaginal exposure* because it takes place in one's imagination. (The patient is then encouraged to use relaxation techniques to diminish the sensation of panic and place it under voluntary control.) The patient will gradually become able to enter the feared situation—for example, entering a shopping mall—and use relaxation techniques while in the feared setting. This is called *in vivo exposure* because exposure involves a real situation. In complex and difficult situations, the therapist may need to lead the patient gradually to a sense of control by developing a hierarchy of stimuli that increasingly approximate the feared stimulus (e.g., moving from imagination to photographs to photographs plus recorded noises and finally to the actual situation itself).

Flooding

Flooding involves teaching patients to extinguish anxiety produced by a feared stimulus through placing them in continuous contact with the stimulus and helping them learn that the stimulus does not in fact lead to any feared consequences. For example, a patient with a disabling fear of riding on airplanes may need to take repeated flights until the fear is extinguished. The patient with a fear of snakes may be asked to visit the zoo and stand in front of the snake cage until his or her anxiety is completely gone. (Handling a snake will provide an even greater flooding experience!)

Behavioral Activation

Many mental disorders are characterized by an inflexible narrowing of the patient's behavioral repertoire. Although exposure is indicated for many such problems, *behavioral activation* is particularly well suited to the treatment of depression. Using a behavioral formulation, depression is conceptualized from a negative reinforcement paradigm in which the depressed patient's withdrawal and isolation is seen to be in the service of avoiding feared punishers. For example, depressed patients frequently expect negative, painful outcomes in their daily lives and begin to avoid such outcomes at the cost of losing important daily routines. Behavioral activation, which is also a component of cognitive therapy, seeks to reengage the patient in those activities, big and small, that lead to a rapid restoration of functioning. In turn, and consistent with behavioral theory, mood improves following restoration of important behavioral sequences in daily life, not the other way around.

Behavior Modification Techniques

Behavior modification techniques tend to use the concept of reinforcement as a way of shaping behavior—in particular, to reduce or eliminate undesirable behavior and to replace it with healthier behaviors or habits. Behavior modification techniques are especially appropriate for disorders characterized by poor impulse control, such as alcohol or other substance abuse, eating disorders, and paraphilic disorders.

Individual programs must be designed to suit the particular patient by using stimuli that are specific positive and negative reinforcers for that individual. For example, the intermediate goal for a patient with anorexia nervosa is weight gain. Long-term goals are to become less preoccupied with food and body image. Patients with anorexia nervosa typically enjoy exercise. A particular patient with anorexia also may enjoy reading mystery novels and chewing gum. A specific program would be developed for such a patient in which she would be provided with three regular, well-balanced meals per day and told that access to her specific preferred pleasures would be contingent on going to the dining room for meals, eating them, and demonstrating a regular pattern of weight gain. A schedule of reinforcers would be developed to encourage her compliance with eating regularly. For example, she might be restricted to her room initially between meals and given no access to exercise, mystery novels, or chewing gum. After she gains 5 pounds, she will be allowed to leave her room. After she gains an additional 5 pounds, she will be given access to mystery novels. After the gain of another 5 pounds, she will be allowed access to chewing gum. After she reaches her desired target weight (involving a total weight gain of 20 pounds), she will be allowed to exercise regularly. To be permitted to continue exercising, however, she must maintain her target weight for 2 weeks while exercising as much as she desires. If her weight drops, positive reinforcers will gradually be removed until the weight gain is reestablished. In such a program, negative reinforcers, such as tube feeding, also may be built in. As mentioned earlier, however, it is well recognized that these negative reinforcers are much less effective than are the positive reinforcers.

Different mixtures of behavior modification techniques are required for different disorders. For example, a program similar to the one just described, but involving a different schedule of reinforcers and different targets, might be appropriate for the obese patient. Behavior modification programs for patients with substance abuse are more likely to stress teaching the patient the various stimuli that tend to trigger his or her craving, such as diminishing the pent-up irritation of a long day at work by dropping by the bar and socializing with friends. The patient would be taught instead to substitute other positive reinforcers in their place, such as dropping by a health club and releasing his or her hostility by hitting a punching bag, followed by drinking copious amounts of his or her favorite nonalcoholic beverage with a new set of friends developed through contacts with Alcoholics Anonymous (AA).

Combining Therapies

Originally, proponents of behavior therapy were purists, and they tended to denigrate mixing behavior therapy with other types of psychotherapy or with the use of medications. Increasingly, various types of therapy are being combined. Thus, the treatment of obsessive-compulsive disorder may involve the use of a selective serotonin reuptake inhibitor (SSRI) along with exposure therapy. Behavior therapy also may be combined with psychodynamic psychotherapy; for example, a patient with anorexia nervosa may benefit from a behavior modification program and from efforts to help her understand the underlying fears that make her seek a bodily appearance that most people find unattractive. A patient with comorbid anxiety and depression may benefit from a program of relaxation training, cognitive therapy, and antidepressant medication.

■ Cognitive-Behavioral Therapy

The theoretical support for CBT derives from a variety of sources, including cognitive psychology, Freudian psychodynamic theory, and some aspects of behaviorism. The theory and techniques of CBT have been developed by many key figures in the field. The best known and most widely used of the CBT models was developed by Aaron Beck, whose model is simply referred to as cognitive therapy. The techniques of CBT are based on the assumption that *cognitive structures* or *schemas* shape the way people react and adapt to a variety of situations that they encounter in their lives. An individual's particular cognitive structures derive from a variety of constitutional and experiential factors (e.g., physical appearance, loss of a parent early in life, previous achievements or failures at school or with friends). Each person has his or her own specific set of cognitive structures that determines how he or she will react to any given stressor in any particular situation. A person develops a psychiatric syndrome, such as anxiety or depression, when these schemas become overactive and predispose him or her to developing a pathological or negative response.

The most widespread use of CBT is for the treatment of depression. In this instance, the individual is typically found to have schemas that lead to negative interpretations. Beck designated the three major cognitive patterns observed in depression as the *cognitive triad:* a negative view of oneself, a negative interpretation of experience, and a negative view of the future. Patients with these cognitive patterns are predisposed to react to situations by interpreting them in the light of these three negative sets. For example, a woman who applies for a highly competitive job and does not receive it, and whose perceptions are shaped by such negative sets, may conclude, "I didn't get it because I'm not really bright, in spite of my good school record, and the employer was able to figure that out" (negative view of self); "Trying to find a decent job is so hopeless that I might as well just give up trying" (negative view of experience); and "I'm always going to be a failure. I'll never succeed at anything" (negative view of the future).

The techniques of CBT focus on teaching patients new ways to change these pathological schemas. CBT tends to be relatively short-term and highly structured. Its goal is to help patients restructure their negative cognitions so that they can perceive reality in a less distorted way and learn to react accordingly.

The practice of CBT combines a group of behavioral techniques with a group of cognitive restructuring techniques. The behavioral techniques include a variety of homework assignments and a graded program of activities designed to teach patients that their negative schemas are incorrect and that they are in fact able to achieve small successes and interpret them as such.

For example, the woman described above who failed to obtain the job might be asked to keep a record of her daily activities during the course of a week. Together, the therapist and patient would then review this diary and (in the context of other information about her) develop a set of assignments to be completed during the ensuing week. The diary of activities might indicate a very limited range of social contacts, based on the patient's fear and expectation of rejection. The patient might be assigned to make at least five social contacts during the course of the week by talking to neighbors, phoning friends, and going out on at least one social engagement. These activities also would be recorded in a diary and reviewed the following week with the therapist, including the patient's notes about her responses to the various contacts. She would be helped to see that she tended to initiate each contact with a negative hypothesis or expectation that typically was disconfirmed by her actual experience. In fact, the contacts were largely affirmative. As therapy progressed and her confidence built, the assignments would gradually be made more difficult, until the patient achieved an essentially normal level of behavior and expectation. The diary would serve as a comforting reminder to the patient that based on experience, negative hypotheses are typically disconfirmed. The patient would, of course, have some negative experiences; the therapist then would assist her in understanding that such negative experiences are not a consequence of her own deficiencies and that even negative experiences can be surmounted.

These behavioral techniques are complemented with a variety of cognitive techniques that help the patient identify and correct the dysfunctional schemas that shape the patient's perception of reality. These techniques involve identifying a variety of cognitive distortions that the patient is prone to make and *automatic thoughts* that intrude into the patient's consciousness and produce negative attitudes. Six typical cognitive distortions, identified by Beck, are listed in Table 20–2.

Arbitrary inference involves drawing an erroneous conclusion from an experience. For example, if the patient's hairdresser suggests that she may want to try a new hairstyle, the patient assumes that the hairdresser believes that the patient is becoming older-appearing and unattractive. *Selective abstraction* involves taking a detail out of context and using it to denigrate the entire experience. For example, while playing tennis, the patient may hit the ball out of the court, losing it in a grassy area, and reach the conclusion "That just proves I'm a lousy tennis player." *Overgeneralization* involves making general conclusions about overall experiences and relationships based on a single interaction. For example, after a disagreement with another employee at his or her current (less desirable) job, the patient concludes, "I'm a failure. I can't get along with anybody." *Magnification and minimization* involve altering the significance of specific small events in a way that is structured by negative interpretations. For example, the significance of a success may be minimized (a good grade on an examination is considered trivial because the examination was easy), and the significance of a failure may

TABLE 20–2.   Cognitive distortions treated with cognitive-behavioral therapy

Distortion	Definition
Arbitrary inference	Drawing an erroneous conclusion from an experience
Selective abstraction	Taking a detail out of context and using it to denigrate the entire experience
Overgeneralization	Making general conclusions about overall experiences and relationships based on a single instance
Magnification and minimization	Altering the significance of specific events in a way that is structured by negative interpretations
Personalization	Interpreting events as reflecting on the patient when they have no relation to him or her
Dichotomous thinking	Seeing things in an all-or-none way

be maximized (losing a tennis game is seen as indicating that the patient will never succeed at anything). *Personalization* involves interpreting events as reflecting on the patient when they in fact have no specific relation to him or her. For example, a frown from a grouchy traffic policeman is seen as recognition of the patient's overall lack of skill as a driver and general worthlessness. *Dichotomous thinking* represents a tendency to see things in an all-or-none way. For example, an A– student with high expectations receives a B in a course and concludes, "That just proves it. I'm really a terrible student after all."

In addition to these erroneous interpretations, patients are often troubled with a variety of automatic thoughts that spontaneously intrude into their flow of consciousness. The specific automatic thoughts vary from one individual to another but involve negative themes of self-denigration and failure (e.g., "You're so stupid," "You never do anything right," "People wouldn't want to talk to you"). These thoughts intrude spontaneously and produce an accompanying dysphoria. Patients are encouraged to identify these automatic thoughts and to learn ways to counteract them. Such techniques include replacing the automatic thoughts with positive counterthoughts, testing the hypotheses embedded in the thoughts through behavioral techniques as described earlier, and identifying and testing the assumptions behind the thoughts.

The goal of the cognitive component of CBT is to identify and restructure the various negative schemas that shape the patient's perceptions. The cognitive goal is achieved like the behavioral goals: the patient is encouraged to do homework, to complete assignments that identify the occurrence of dysfunctional cognitions, and to steadily test and correct these cognitions. The therapist also reviews these aspects of the patient's diary and helps formulate an organized program for restructuring the dysfunctional cognitive sets, providing ample empathy and positive reinforcement.

CBT is particularly effective for patients with depression, although its techniques have also been adapted to treat various anxiety disorders through identifying cognitive schemas characterized by fear. It may be used either alone for the treatment of relatively mild disorders or in conjunction with medications for patients with more severe disorders.

■ Individual Psychotherapy

The term *individual psychotherapy* covers a broad range of psychotherapeutic techniques. Both behavior therapy and cognitive therapy usually are done individually (i.e., a single therapist working with a single patient). Countless schools of psychotherapy offer a variety of approaches. The description that follows provides a simplified and selective overview.

The various psychotherapies share some common elements (Table 20–3). These elements are characteristic of all psychotherapies.

TABLE 20–3. Common elements of the psychotherapies

- Based on an interpersonal relationship
- Use of verbal communication between two (or more) people as a healing element
- Specific expertise on the part of the therapist in using communication and relationships in a healing way
- Based on a rationale or conceptual structure that is used to understand the patient's problems
- Use of a specific procedure in the relationship that is linked to the rationale
- Structured relationship (e.g., contact time, frequency, and duration are prespecified)
- Expectation of improvement

Classical Psychoanalysis and Psychodynamic Psychotherapy

Psychoanalysis was originally developed by Sigmund Freud during the early twentieth century. This technique arose from Freud's experience in attempting to treat patients with hysterical conversion symptoms, such as pains and paralyses. Following the lead of Charcot, his initial efforts involved the use of hypnosis. He observed, however, that this treatment was not always effective and that there was a high recurrence and relapse rate. He began to suspect that these conversion symptoms reflected some sort of painful early psychological experience that had been repressed. Instead of hypnosis, he began to experiment with the technique of having the patient lie down and relax while he placed his hand on the person's forehead to help "release" the repressed thoughts. The patient was instructed to "Talk about whatever comes into your mind." This technique was called *free association*.

This treatment developed at a time when Victorian puritanism and hypocrisy still reigned supreme, and even Freud must have been astonished at the thoughts that flowed from his patients' minds, covering a variety of sexual fantasies and experiences. Based on his many years of experience in applying this approach, initially to conversion symptoms but subsequently to a range of symptoms including anxiety disorders and even psychoses, Freud developed a systematic theory to describe the structure and operations of the human psyche. Basic concepts include stages of psychosexual development (oral, anal, phallic, and genital), the structure of conscious and unconscious thoughts (primary vs. secondary process thinking), the structure of drives and motivations (id, ego, and superego), the symbolism inherent in dreams, theories of infant sexuality, and a host of other concepts that the layperson associates with Freudianism.

Subsequent psychoanalysts elaborated and modified Freud's original work in various ways, such as developing theories of ego psychology and expanding understanding of the mental mechanisms involved in defense, coping, and adaptation. These various ideas and theories are major resources for clinicians trained in either psychoanalysis or psychodynamic psychotherapy. Use of these approaches requires extensive experience and training.

Classical psychoanalysis is now used only in relatively special situations and settings. The form of treatment is best adapted to individuals who are fundamentally healthy (both psychologically and financially) and who have sufficient adaptive resources to go through the intensive process of self-scrutiny required by psychoanalysis. Typical reasons for seeking psychoanalysis include difficulties in relationships and persistent and recurrent anxiety, although neither should be so severe as to be incapacitating.

The core component of classical psychoanalysis is the development of a *transference neurosis*. That is, the patient transfers to the therapist all the thoughts and feelings that he or she experienced during early life; through this transference, he or she is able to make conscious the various unconscious drives and emotions that are troubling him or her and ultimately to modify and heal them as the analyst makes appropriate interpretations during the course of the psychoanalysis.

The patient is typically asked to lie on a couch and to free-associate, saying whatever comes into his or her mind without any type of censorship. The analyst sits behind the patient, remaining a relatively shadowy and neutral figure to encourage the development of transference. (If the analyst becomes too human or "real," then transference cannot develop.) To maintain an appropriate level of intensity, the patient must be seen four to five times per week for 50-minute sessions. The process typically requires 2–3 years. Analysts must go through an extensive period of psychoanalysis themselves to understand their own psychological vulnerabilities and, in particular, the nature of the countertransference that they are likely to develop in relation to their patients.

Psychodynamic psychotherapy uses many of the concepts embodied in psychoanalytic theory, but these concepts are used in ways that make them more suitable for the treatment of larger numbers of patients. Treatment is not necessarily less intensive, in the sense of attempting to focus on and correct problems, but it does not involve the relatively rigidly defined techniques (e.g., use of the couch) that characterize classical psychoanalysis.

Psychodynamic psychotherapy is used to treat patients with a variety of problems, including personality disorders, sexual dysfunctions, anxiety disorders, and mild depression. Psychodynamic psychotherapy is typically conducted face to face. Depending on the frequency and duration of therapy, a transference neurosis may or may not occur. The therapist attempts to help the patient in a neutral but empathic way. The patient is encouraged to review early relationships with parents and significant others but also may focus on the here and now. As in classical psychoanalysis, the patient is expected to do most of the talking, while the psychodynamic psychotherapist occasionally interjects clarifications to help the patient understand the underlying dynamics that shape his or her behavior. Psychodynamic psychotherapy typically involves sessions one or two times a week and may involve 2–5 years of treatment.

Insight-Oriented and Relationship Psychotherapy

Insight-oriented psychotherapy and relationship psychotherapy are two other variants of individual psychotherapy that may be somewhat less intensive or long-term.

Insight-oriented psychotherapy draws on many basic psychodynamic concepts but focuses even more on interpersonal relationships and here-and-now situations than does purely psychodynamic psychotherapy. Patients are typically seen once a week for 50 minutes. During the sessions they are encouraged to review and discuss relationships, attitudes toward themselves, and early life experiences. The therapist maintains an involved and supportive attitude and occasionally assists patients with interpretations that will help them achieve insights. This form of psychotherapy does not encourage transference, regression, and abreaction. Instead of re-experiencing and reliving, patients are encouraged to achieve an intellectual understanding of the mainsprings of their behavior that will help them change their behavior as needed.

In *relationship psychotherapy*, the therapist assumes a more active role. The stress is on achieving a corrective emotional experience, with the therapist serving as a loving and trustworthy surrogate parent who assists the patient in confronting unrecognized needs and unresolved drives. The patient is typically seen once per week, and the therapy may last from 6 months to several years, depending on the patient's problems and level of maturity. As in insight-oriented psychotherapy, the content of the sessions focuses primarily on current situations and relationships, with some looking backward to early life experiences. Although the patient may achieve insight, the most important component of this type of psychotherapy is the empathic and caring attitude of the therapist.

Interpersonal Therapy

Interpersonal therapy (IPT) is a specific type of psychotherapy that was developed for the treatment of depression, although it is also potentially useful for the treatment of other conditions, such as personality disorders. Drawing on the ideas of thinkers such as Harry Stack Sullivan, who stressed that mental illnesses may reflect and be expressed in problems in relationships (as opposed to intrapsychic conflict, stressed by psychodynamic approaches), IPT emphasizes working on improving interpersonal relationships during the process of psychotherapy.

During IPT, the emphasis is on the present rather than on the past. During a process of exploration, the therapist helps the patient identify specific problem areas that may be interfering with self-esteem and interpersonal interactions. These usually involve four general domains: grief, interpersonal disputes, role transitions, and interpersonal deficits. After the exploration and identification process, the therapist works systematically with the patient to facilitate the learning of new adaptive behaviors and communication styles.

IPT is usually conducted in weekly sessions, and the overall course of therapy lasts 3 or 4 months. Rigorous empirical testing of its efficacy shows it to be effective for both acute and maintenance treatment of depression. IPT also has been used with some success in treating depressed adolescents and persons with bulimia.

Supportive Psychotherapy

Supportive psychotherapy is used to help patients get through difficult situations and is perhaps the most commonly used form of individual psychotherapy. Components of supportive psychotherapy may be incorporated into any of the other types of psychotherapy described in this section, with the exception of classical psychoanalysis.

In conducting supportive psychotherapy, the therapist maintains an attitude of sympathy, interest, and concern. Patients describe and discuss the various problems they are confronting, which could range from marital discord to psychotic experiences such as persecutory delusions. Supportive psychotherapy is appropriate for the full spectrum of mental disorders, ranging from adjustment disorders through the psychoses and even dementia.

As in relationship psychotherapy, the therapist may function much like a healthy and loving parent who provides the patient with encouragement and direction as needed. The goal of supportive therapy is to help the patient cope with difficult situations, experiences, or periods of adjustment. Patients typically describe their problems, and the therapist counters with encouragement and even specific advice. The therapist may suggest specific techniques that patients can use in coping with their problems, such as developing new interests or hobbies, trying new activities that may expand their range of social contacts, achieving emancipation from their parents by moving into independent living circumstances, and developing more organized study habits to improve their school performance. Psychotic patients may be taught to refrain from discussing their delusional ideas, except with the therapist. Alcoholic patients may receive praise and encouragement for refraining from drinking as well as suggestions about ways to increase their self-esteem by achieving mastery and control, such as through improving their skills in a particular sport or developing a new creative hobby. As these examples indicate, the clinician involved in conducting supportive therapy needs to tailor the therapy sessions to the individual needs of each particular patient.

■ Group Therapy

Group therapy provides a highly effective way for clinicians to follow up with and monitor relatively large numbers of patients. It also provides patients with a social environment or even surrogate peer group that will help them learn new and constructive ways to interact with others in a controlled and supportive environment.

Irving Yalom, one of the major leaders of the group therapy movement in the United States, summarized the therapeutic mechanisms that occur during the process of group therapy. These include instilling hope, developing socializing skills, using imitative behavior, experiencing catharsis, imparting information, behaving altruistically by attempting to help other members of the group, experiencing a corrective recapitulation of the primary family group, developing a sense of group cohesiveness, diminishing feelings of isolation (universality), and learning through feedback how one's behavior affects others (interpersonal learning).

There are many different kinds of group therapy. The types vary depending on the individuals who compose the group, the problems or disorders that they are confronting, the setting in which the group meets, the type of role that the group leader takes, and the therapeutic goals that have been established.

Group therapy programs have been established in many hospitals for psychiatric inpatients. These groups are typically led by a physician, a nurse, a social worker, or some combination thereof. In very large inpatient hospital settings, several groups may run concurrently and be composed of patients with similar types of problems. For example, one group might consist of patients with severe mood and psychotic disorders, and another group might consist of individuals with eating disorders. Such groups provide patients with a forum to share their problems, diminish their sense of isolation and loneliness, enable them to learn new techniques to cope with their problems either through other patients or through the group leader, and provide support, inspiration, and hope. Such groups also may help patients improve interpersonal and social skills. For example, patients with schizophrenia and other psychoses may improve their skills in relating to others. In many clinical settings, such inpatient groups are supplemented by outpatient or aftercare groups in which patients receive continued follow-up, pursuing goals similar to those described earlier but in the more stressful environment of the real world. These outpatient groups represent an attempt to consolidate and support the learning and skills that have already been developed in the inpatient setting.

Some groups are oriented largely toward providing support. Such groups may or may not have a professional leader. Examples of such support groups include AA meetings, family support groups such as those organized by chapters of the National Alliance on Mental Illness (an organization composed of the family members of patients with serious mental illnesses), support groups for individuals who conceive of themselves as minorities in a particular setting (e.g., women professionals, women medical students, black students), groups composed of military veterans, or groups composed of individuals who have experienced some serious medical illness or difficult surgery (e.g., patients with diabetes, women who have had mastectomies, individuals receiving dialysis). Such groups provide a forum for sharing information, giving encouragement and support, and instilling hope through diminishing feelings of isolation.

Group psychotherapy may also be done as an alternative to individual psychotherapy. Groups are typically led by experienced therapists and are often conducted with a co-therapist. These groups aim to achieve goals similar to those of insight-oriented and interpersonal psychotherapy or cognitive therapy within the context of a group setting. Psychotherapy groups are typically more highly structured than the other types of groups described earlier. The group leaders take an active role in organizing each session, often prescribe exercises within the session, establish ground rules for membership within the group (e.g., no tardiness, regular attendance), resolve conflicts between members of the group, and assume responsibility for providing summaries of each session and access to videos of the sessions. Patients are screened before being admitted to a psychotherapy group to ensure that they will be able to participate effectively. Such groups are particularly helpful for individuals with the same type of problems that led them into individual psychotherapy, such as interpersonal and relationship problems, anxiety, mild depression, and personality disorders.

In the past two decades there has been an explosion in the number of programs developed specifically to treat people with borderline personality disorder (BPD). Perhaps the best known is dialectical behavior therapy, a program that combines group and individual therapy. Developed by Marsha Linehan in the 1980s initially as a treatment for suicidal women, the intensive 1-year program includes a mix of psychotherapeutic techniques as diverse as CBT and mindful meditation derived from Buddhist practice. Other well-known programs for people with BPD include mentalization therapy, schema focused therapy, transference focused psychotherapy, and the less intensive Systems Training for Emotional Predictability and Problem Solving (STEPPS).

■ Couples Therapy

Couples therapy involves working with two people who see themselves as partners in a committed relationship to help them stabilize and improve their relationship. This therapy once involved seeing a husband and wife. In contemporary society, the partners seeking treatment may be unmarried, gay, or lesbian. Depending on the commitment of the two partners, couples therapy has many variations. Ideally, both partners are willing and cooperative participants who are anxious to initiate change. Sometimes, however, couples therapy is sought because of a crisis: one of the partners may have lost interest in the relationship (and may or may not want to get out), whereas the other is hanging on tight and trying to save the relationship. In the latter instance, one possible outcome might be the eventual decision to end the relationship, and therapy might become divorce mediation and counseling. If children are involved, then what began as couples therapy might turn into family therapy as the couple attempts to work out an equitable arrangement in the context of the larger number of people who will be affected. In some instances, a dysfunctional sexual relationship between the couple will become apparent, and the couple may want referral to a sex therapy clinic for treatment of impotence or anorgasmia.

An individual conducting couples therapy must take care to maintain an atmosphere of fairness, neutrality, and impartiality. Either partner will be particularly sensitive to the possibility that the therapist may take sides and treat him or her unfairly. The therapist's gender may seem quite significant to either partner, even though the therapist may feel quite comfortable with his or her ability to be impartial. Women may believe that only a female therapist is able to understand their point of view and may feel quite defensive if asked to work with a male therapist. Male partners may have similar attitudes or problems.

Couples counseling typically begins with identifying the specific problem. Each partner is asked to identify specific areas in which he or she would like to see change in the other. The therapist attempts to assist the couple in implementing changes in a gradual, graded way, attacking one problem at a time. Typically, in the early sessions, a single, salient problem is the focus of attention. For example, a wife may express feelings of being ignored, whereas a husband may complain of his wife's whining expressions of dependency. Each will identify specific target behaviors in the other that need modification. They then contract with each other to modify these behaviors. Subsequent sessions focus on the steps they have taken to achieve improvement and on continuing work in new areas of concern.

This type of graded behavior change is the minimum component of couples therapy. Often couples also benefit from discussing their hopes for and expectations of each other in the context of personal values, prior family experiences (i.e., role expectations about men and women, based on the behavior of their own parents), changing social norms about the roles of men and women, and needs for both intimacy and independence that occur within the context of a relationship.

■ Family Therapy

Family therapy tends to focus on the larger family unit—at a minimum, one parent and the child (in single-parent families), but more typically both parents and the child (or a parent and stepparent, two separated parents, other parental pairings depending on the family environment in which the child lives), or one or more parents and the child plus siblings. Typically, the child is brought in initially for treatment of a specific problem, such as school difficulties, oppositional behavior, delinquency, or aggression. Often, it rapidly becomes clear that these problems exist in the overall context of the family setting. The family should not necessarily be regarded as dysfunctional, however. Because of changing circumstances or demands (e.g., a recent move), the parents may have difficulty in determining methods for coping with the child's behavior or understanding why it is occurring.

As in couples therapy, it is important for the therapist to be fair and impartial in family therapy. In this instance, however, the therapist is not dealing with two potential equals but rather with a hierarchy in which parents are expected to assume some authority and responsibility for the behavior of their child. The degree of hierarchy in the family will vary depending on the age of the child. For adolescents and teen-agers, one important problem may be the challenge that the "child's" growing independence is adding to this hierarchical structure.

Family therapy also may be used to help families in which at least one member has a relatively serious mental illness, such as schizophrenia, bipolar disorder, or recurrent depression. In this type of family therapy, it is important to work firmly within the medical model and to emphasize that the patient has an illness for which neither the patient nor the family can be considered responsible. This approach minimizes guilt, scapegoating, and castigation, and it permits both patient and family members to seek more consoling and constructive methods for coping with the symptoms of the illness. A young schizophrenic patient living at home may need some assistance from his or her family in developing social skills (see the next section, "Social Skills Training," in this chapter), whereas family members may need assistance in learning ways to cope with outbursts of anger or periods of emotional disengagement and withdrawal. Families with high levels of involvement (referred to as high "expressed emotion") may need counseling on ways to be less intensely involved because it has been shown that in some instances, high levels of expressed emotion may be experienced as stressful by the schizophrenic patient and lead to relapse. Thus families may need assistance in finding the right balance between providing needed support and encouragement and setting up excessively high expectations. Education about the symptoms of the illness is also an important component of family therapy for both the patient and the family members.

■ Social Skills Training

Social skills training is a specific type of psychotherapy that focuses primarily on developing abilities in relating to others and in coping with the demands of daily life. It is used primarily for patients with severe mental illnesses, such as schizophrenia, which are often accompanied by marked impairments in social skills.

Social skills training may be done initially on an inpatient basis, but the bulk of the effort is typically done with outpatients because the long-term goal of social skills training is to assist patients in learning to live in the real world. Social skills training is typically done by nurses, social workers, or psychologists. It may be done individually, but it more typically is accompanied by some group work as well, and it may occur in the context of day hospitals or sheltered workshops.

The techniques of social skills training also are primarily behavioral. Specific problems are identified and addressed in a sequentially integrated manner. Severely disabled patients may need assistance initially in grooming and hygiene. They may need encouragement in learning to shave or bathe daily, to keep their clothes laundered, and to eat regular meals. They also may need help in learning how to approach other people and to talk with them appropriately. At higher levels of functioning, they may need assistance in learning how to apply for a job, complete job interviews, and relate to employers and coworkers. Because long-term institutional care is no longer available to most patients with psychotic illnesses, these individuals are literally being forced to learn to live in the community. Many cannot do so without receiving training and assistance in activities of daily living, such as grooming, managing money, and achieving at least a minimal level of social interaction with others. Although the development of such skills may seem elementary or minimal, for some patients it can lead to a substantial improvement in their quality of life.

Clinical points for psychotherapy

1. Psychotherapy is a key component of comprehensive psychiatric care.

   - Psychotherapy is a first-line treatment for many disorders (e.g., eating disorders, personality disorders).

   - Psychotherapy is an important treatment adjunct for many patients taking psychotropic medication.

   - Combined treatment (psychotherapy plus psychotropic medication) tends to produce the best outcomes.

2. There are many different types of psychotherapy, but most share similar elements including the development of a personal relationship with the therapist, using communication and relationships in a healing way, and conveying a sense of hope and expectation for improvement.

3. With behavioral therapy, the motto is "Change the behavior, and the feelings will follow."

4. CBT aims to change (or restructure) maladaptive cognitive schemas. Through homework and graded exercises, the patient learns to counter negative thoughts and behaviors that tend to promote and maintain psychiatric disorders, such as major depression.

5. Psychodynamic psychotherapies focus on the patient's relationships, attitudes toward himself or herself, and early life experiences. The goal is to help the patient achieve insight into the development and persistence of his or her symptoms and behaviors in order to bring about needed change.

Clinical points for psychotherapy *(continued)*
6.   Supportive therapy is commonly used to help patients get through difficult times by providing sympathy, encouragement, and even specific advice. This approach is within reach of *all* physicians, not just psychiatrists.
7.   Group therapy is an efficient way to deliver care to many patients at once. It provides a surrogate peer group in which patients can learn new ways to interact with others in a controlled environment.
•   Several programs have been developed specifically to treat borderline personality disorder and, while they are helpful, lack of availability will limit their usefulness.
8.   Couples and family therapies focus on either a dyad (the couple) or the larger family unit to address specific problems. In either situation, it is essential for the therapist to maintain an atmosphere of fairness, neutrality, and impartiality.

■ Self-Assessment Questions

1. What is the difference between classical conditioning and operant conditioning?
2. What is a positive reinforcer? A negative reinforcer?
3. Describe behavioral activation. How might this be useful with depressed patients?
4. Describe four common techniques for conducting behavior therapy.
5. Describe CBT. What is the cognitive triad? What are automatic thoughts?
6. Describe classical psychoanalysis. How does it differ from psychodynamic psychotherapy? What is transference?
7. Describe two different types of group therapy, and enumerate some situations in which they would be appropriate. What is dialectical behavior therapy?
8. Describe the role of the therapist in couples therapy and family therapy.

Chapter 21

Psychopharmacology and Electroconvulsive Therapy

> The desire to take medicine is perhaps the greatest
> feature that distinguishes man from animals.
>
> *Sir William Osler*

The modern treatment era in psychiatry began with the introduction of effective psychotropic medication in the 1950s including chlorpromazine and the tricyclic antidepressants, followed by the benzodiazepines in the 1960s, and lithium carbonate in 1970. The introduction of effective medications revolutionized psychiatry and mental health treatment. But the focus on medication also contributed to the widespread view that psychiatrists were no longer interested in people and their very human problems, but rather were mainly concerned with the manipulation of neurotransmitters. Indeed, many psychiatrists have chosen to delegate psychotherapy to nonphysicians such as psychologists and social workers, preferring to focus on medication management. This splitting of treatment is being critically reassessed as it has become clear that patients do best with a combination of medication and psychotherapy and that having a single mental health care provider is preferable as well as more cost-effective.

■ Antipsychotics

Chlorpromazine was introduced in 1952 by the French psychiatrists Jean Delay and Pierre Deniker, after it was recognized that the drug had powerful calming effects on agitated psychotic patients. Not only were agitated patients calmed, but the new drug seemed to diminish their terrifying hallucinations and troubling delusions. Many additional antipsychotics have since been developed and, while not curative, can produce dramatic improvement that can be sustained over years or decades.

The antipsychotics can be roughly broken down into two groups: the older, or conventional, antipsychotics and the newer second-generation antipsychotics (SGAs). The SGAs, also known as atypical antipsychotics, now account for most of the prescriptions for antipsychotic drugs. Both the conventional antipsychotics and the SGAs ameliorate the symptoms of psychosis, including hallucinations, delusions, bizarre behavior, disordered thinking, and agitation. SGAs tend to have fewer side effects and are better tolerated, but concerns have emerged regarding their potential to induce metabolic side effects, such as impaired glucose tolerance. Although the SGAs were initially seen as more effective than the conventional antipsychotics, this belief is being reappraised in light of recent research. In a large government-funded clinical trial, four SGAs were compared with perphenazine, an older antipsychotic. There were few differences among the drugs in terms of efficacy or tolerability. The most commonly used antipsychotics are listed in Table 21–1.

Indications

Antipsychotic drugs are primarily used to treat schizophrenia and other psychotic disorders, but they are also prescribed to patients with psychotic mood disorders and to patients whose psychoses are medically induced or due to drugs of abuse. Antipsychotics are often used to control aggressive behavior in intellectually disabled patients, autism spectrum disorder patients, patients with borderline personality disorder, and patients with delirium or other neurocognitive disorders. They also are prescribed to patients with Tourette's disorder to diminish the frequency and severity of vocal and motor tics.

Mechanism of Action

The potency of conventional antipsychotic drugs correlates closely with their affinity for the dopamine 2 (D_2) receptor, blocking the effect of endogenous dopamine at this site. The pharmacological profile of the SGAs differs in that they are weaker D_2 receptor antagonists than conventional antipsychotics, but are potent serotonin type 2A (5-HT_{2A}) receptor antagonists and have significant anticholinergic and antihistaminic activity as

TABLE 21–1. Common antipsychotic agents

Category	Drug (trade name)	Sedation	Orthostatic hypotension	Anticholinergic effects	Extrapyramidal effects	Equivalent dosage, mg	Dosage range, mg/day
Conventional agents							
Phenothiazines							
Aliphatics	Chlorpromazine (Thorazine)	H	H	M	M	100	50–1,200
Piperidines	Thioridazine (Mellaril)	H	H	H	L	95	50–800
Piperazines	Fluphenazine (Prolixin)	L	L	L	VH	2	2–20
	Fluphenazine decanoate	L	L	L	VH	—[a]	12.5–50 mg q 2 wk
	Perphenazine (Trilafon)	L	L	L	H	10	12–64
	Trifluoperazine (Stelazine)	L	L	L	H	5	5–40
Thioxanthenes	Thiothixene (Navane)	L	L	L	H	5	5–60
Butyrophenones	Haloperidol (Haldol)	L	L	L	VH	2	2–60

TABLE 21–1. Common antipsychotic agents *(continued)*

Category	Drug (trade name)	Sedation	Orthostatic hypotension	Anticholinergic effects	Extrapyramidal effects	Equivalent dosage, mg	Dosage range, mg/day
Second-generation (atypical) agents							
	Aripiprazole (Abilify)	L	VL	L	VL	7.5	10–15
	Asenapine (Saphris)	L	M	L	VL	5	10–20
	Clozapine (Clozaril)	H	H	H	VL	100	200–600
	Lurasidone (Latuda)	L	L	L	VL	40	40–160
	Iloperidone (Fanapt)	L	M	L	VL	6	12–24
	Olanzapine (Zyprexa)	L	L	M	L	5	15–30
	Quetiapine (Seroquel)	M	M	L	VL	75	300–500
	Paliperidone (Invega)	L	M	L	L	4	3–12
	Risperidone (Risperdal)	L	M	L	L	2	2–6
	Ziprasidone (Geodon)	M	L	VL	L	6	40–160

Note. H = high; L = low; M = moderate; VH = very high; VL = very low.
[a]Long-acting ester; dosage is not directly comparable with that of standard compounds.

well. Central 5-HT$_{2A}$ receptor antagonism is believed to broaden the therapeutic effect of the drug while reducing the incidence of extrapyramidal side effects (EPS) associated with D$_2$ antagonists.

Antipsychotics appear to exert their influence at mesocortical and mesolimbic dopaminergic pathways. Positron emission tomography (PET) studies show that D$_2$ receptor occupancy of 65%–70% correlates with maximal antipsychotic efficacy. These studies also show that antipsychotics block these receptors almost immediately, yet full response to the drugs takes weeks to develop. Although all antipsychotics block these receptors, a patient may respond preferentially to one drug but not to another. These observations suggest that antipsychotic drugs have other effects in the central nervous system (CNS) that may actually be responsible for their therapeutic properties, such as an action on second-messenger systems. Although many drug side effects can be linked to their dopamine-blocking properties (e.g., EPS), these drugs also block noradrenergic, cholinergic, and histaminic receptors to differing degrees, accounting for the unique side effect profile of each agent.

Pharmacokinetics

Absorption of orally administered antipsychotics is variable, and peak plasma levels are generally reached in 1–4 hours. Several antipsychotics are also available in an intramuscular preparation, and administration produces effects within 15 minutes. Injectable antipsychotics have much greater bioavailability than oral medication. Metabolism occurs mostly in the liver, largely by oxidation, so that these highly lipid-soluble agents are converted to water-soluble metabolites and excreted in the urine and feces. Excretion of antipsychotics tends to be slow because of drug accumulation in fatty tissue. Most of the conventional antipsychotics are highly protein bound (85%–90%). Nearly all antipsychotics have a half-life of 24 hours or longer and have active metabolites with longer half-lives. Depot formulations have even longer half-lives and may take 3–6 months to reach steady state.

The majority of conventional antipsychotics are metabolized by the cytochrome P450 (CYP) enzyme subfamilies, including 2D6, 1A2, and 3A4. Because of genetic variation, 5%–10% of whites poorly metabolize medications through the CYP2D6 pathway, as do a significant proportion of African Americans. This can result in higher antipsychotic blood levels than anticipated in some patients.

Plasma concentrations can be measured reliably for many antipsychotic drugs, but studies attempting to correlate plasma level with response have been inconsistent. Haloperidol and clozapine blood levels appear to correlate with clinical response. With haloperidol, optimal response appears to be associated with serum concentrations between 5 and 15 ng/mL. With clozapine, levels greater than 350 ng/mL appear to be effective for most patients. The other situations in which plasma levels are useful to obtain include the following:

- When patients' symptoms have not responded to standard dosage
- When antipsychotic medications are combined with drugs that can affect their pharmacokinetics (e.g., carbamazepine)
- When patient compliance needs to be assessed

Use in Acute Psychosis

A high-potency conventional antipsychotic such as haloperidol (5–10 mg/day) or one of the SGAs (e.g., risperidone, 4–6 mg/day; olanzapine, 10–20 mg/day; quetiapine, 150–800 mg/day; ziprasidone, 80–160 mg/day) is recommended as an initial choice for the treatment of acute psychosis. Antipsychotic effects generally start early after the drug is started but are cumulative over the ensuing weeks. An adequate trial should last from 4 to 6 weeks. The trial should be extended for another 4–6 weeks when the patient shows a partial response to the initial antipsychotic. If no response occurs after 4–6 weeks, then another drug should be tried. Clozapine is a second-line choice because it can cause agranulocytosis and requires monitoring of the white blood cell count.

Highly agitated patients require rapid control of their symptoms and should be given frequent, equally spaced doses of an antipsychotic drug. High-potency antipsychotics (e.g., haloperidol) can be given every 30–120 minutes orally or intramuscularly until agitation has subsided. A combination of an antipsychotic and a benzodiazepine may work even better in calming patients (e.g., haloperidol, 5 mg, plus lorazepam, 2 mg), repeating the doses every 30 minutes until adequate tranquilization is achieved.

Maintenance Treatment

Long-term maintenance treatment has as its goal the sustained control of psychotic symptoms and reduced risk of relapse. The following guidelines were developed at an international conference:

1. Prevention of relapse is more important than risk of side effects because most side effects are reversible, and the consequences of relapse may be irreversible.

2. At least 1–2 years of treatment are recommended following the initial episode because of the high risk of relapse and the possibility of social deterioration from further relapses.
3. At least 5 years of treatment are indicated for multi-episode patients.
4. Chronic, or ongoing, treatment is recommended for patients who pose a danger to themselves or to others.

Maintenance treatment with antipsychotics is effective in preventing relapse. When study results are pooled, 30% of those continuing to take medications relapse, compared with 65% of those taking placebo. About 75% of stable patients taken off their medication will relapse within 6–24 months.

Patients with schizoaffective disorder generally receive maintenance treatment with an antipsychotic in combination with a mood stabilizer when the patient has the bipolar type, or an antipsychotic combined with an antidepressant when the patient has the depressed type. Monotherapy with an SGA is a good alternative because these drugs seem to provide both mood stabilization and control of psychotic symptoms. SGAs can also be used for both acute and maintenance treatment of the manic phase of bipolar disorder.

Long-acting antipsychotic preparations are available for patients who are unable to take oral medication on a regular basis or who are noncompliant. There is no universally accepted method for converting a patient from oral to long-acting dosage forms, and dosing with sustained-release formulations must be individualized. A patient can be started on a dosage of 6.25 mg of fluphenazine decanoate intramuscularly every 2 weeks, and the dosage is titrated upward or downward based on the patient's therapeutic response and side effects. For haloperidol, a 400-mg loading dose in the first month, followed by a maintenance dose of 250 mg/month, produces a blood level of 10 ng/mL, and a dose of 150 mg/month produces a blood level between 5 and 6 ng/mL. Both risperidone and paliperidone also are available in long-acting injectable preparations.

Further information about the use of antipsychotics in the treatment of schizophrenia spectrum and other psychotic disorders can be found in Chapter 5.

Adverse Effects

Antipsychotics have the potential to induce a variety of troublesome side effects. Their severity differs from drug to drug and corresponds with the drug's ability to affect particular neurotransmitter systems (the dopaminergic, noradrenergic, cholinergic, and histaminic). Because of their blockade of 5-HT$_{2A}$ receptors, SGAs are less likely to induce EPS than the conventional antipsychotics. For side effect profiles of the different antipsychotics, see Table 21–1.

Patients receiving long-term treatment with antipsychotic medication should be regularly monitored for the development of *tardive dyskinesia* (TD), a condition that consists of abnormal involuntary movements usually involving the mouth and tongue. Other parts of the body, including the trunk and extremities, may be affected. TD is thought to result when postsynaptic dopamine receptors develop a supersensitivity to dopamine following prolonged receptor blockade from antipsychotics. Second-generation antipsychotics are much less likely to induce TD, although patients taking them should still be monitored.

The movements of TD are generally mild and tolerable, but some patients with TD develop a more malignant form of the disorder that can be totally disabling. Elderly patients, women, and patients with mood disorders appear more susceptible to developing TD. Disabling forms of TD have become relatively uncommon.

Patients with TD present special problems because the treatment of choice is to stop the offending drug. Many patients will choose to continue taking the drug regardless of the TD because their lives may be intolerable without medication and the TD may be mild. One option is to switch the patient to an SGA, which will help mask the symptoms and will probably not worsen the TD. Vitamin E (i.e., 1,600 IU/day) may help alleviate the abnormal movements to some extent. If patients do not benefit from a 3-month trial, vitamin E should be discontinued.

Antipsychotic medications are also frequently associated with the development of *pseudoparkinsonism*. This side effect usually takes 3 or more weeks to develop. Patients develop symptoms typical of Parkinson's disease, including tremor, rigidity, and hypokinesia. *Akathisia,* the most common form of EPS, may appear soon after initiation of antipsychotic treatment. This condition causes subjective feelings of anxiety and tension and objective fidgetiness and agitation. Patients may feel compelled to pace, move around in their chairs, or tap their feet. Treatment for both pseudoparkinsonism and akathisia generally consists of reducing the dosage of the antipsychotic drug whenever possible and/or adding an antiparkinsonian agent to the medication regimen. Akathisia has been treated with β-blockers or amantadine, a drug that potentiates the release of dopamine in the basal ganglia. Benzodiazepines are also helpful in relieving the symptoms of akathisia. Clonidine can be used, but it may cause sedation and orthostatic hypotension.

Another potential neurological side effect of antipsychotics is the *acute dystonic reaction*, which usually occurs during the first 4 days of treatment. It is more common in younger persons, cocaine users, and in those treated with intramuscular injections of high-potency conventional antipsychotics. An acute dystonia involves the sustained contraction of the muscles of the neck, mouth, tongue, or occasionally other muscle groups that is distressing and often painful. Acute dystonias typically respond within 20–30 minutes to intramuscular benztropine (i.e., 1–2 mg) or diphenhydramine (i.e., 25–50 mg). There is little need for a standing dose of an antiparkinsonian drug after the dystonia resolves, because acute dystonia usually does not recur. Patients beginning a course of a conventional antipsychotic can benefit from 2 weeks of prophylactic benztropine (1–4 mg/day) to help head off an acute dystonic reaction.

Low-potency conventional antipsychotics (e.g., chlorpromazine), commonly cause anticholinergic side effects including dry mouth, urinary retention, blurry vision, constipation, and exacerbation of narrow-angle glaucoma. These side effects are best treated by reducing the dosage of the drug or switching to a more potent agent (e.g., haloperidol) or to an SGA. Antiparkinsonian drugs commonly used to treat EPS, such as benztropine, can worsen these side effects. If urinary retention continues to be a problem, bethanechol (i.e., 15 mg three times daily) may help the patient empty his or her bladder. Bulk laxatives can help with constipation.

The most common cardiovascular side effect of the antipsychotics is *orthostatic hypotension*, mediated by α-adrenergic blockade. This side effect is caused more frequently by low-potency compounds (e.g., chlorpromazine). Antipsychotics generally do not cause arrhythmogenic effects when used in standard dosages. Chlorpromazine, thioridazine, pimozide, and the second-generation drugs aripiprazole and iloperidone have been associated with QT_c prolongation, which can be of concern for abnormal cardiac conduction or sudden death. Patients with a history of QT_c prolongation, a recent myocardial infarction, or uncompensated heart failure should avoid these drugs.

Agranulocytosis occurs in 0.8% of patients taking clozapine during the first year of treatment and peaks in incidence at 3 months of treatment. The best preventive measure is to be alert to the appearance of malaise, fever, and sore throat early in the course of therapy. Patients prescribed clozapine must have a baseline white blood cell count of no less than $3,500/mm^3$ and an absolute neutrophil count of no less than $2,000 \ mm^3$. Weekly complete blood counts and absolute neutrophil counts must be taken for the first 6 months, every 14 days for another 6 months, and monthly thereafter.

Hyperprolactinemia, often considered an unavoidable consequence of treatment with conventional antipsychotics, can induce amenorrhea, galactorrhea, gynecomastia, and impotence. SGAs are less likely to cause hyperprolactinemia, particularly quetiapine and aripiprazole. If it is not possible to reduce the dosage or change antipsychotics, the addition of bromocriptine (e.g., 2.5–7.5 mg twice daily) may be helpful.

The SGAs have been linked to *metabolic abnormalities* in glucose regulation, lipids, and weight gain. Clozapine and olanzapine appear most likely to cause weight gain, followed by risperidone and quetiapine; aripiprazole, lurasidone, and ziprasidone are relatively weight neutral. Weight gain associated with long-term antipsychotic treatment can be significant and is a risk factor for diabetes and cardiovascular disease. Weight gain is also a frequent cause for treatment noncompliance. When these medications are prescribed, the American Diabetes Association recommends measuring baseline body mass index (BMI), waist circumference, blood pressure, and fasting glucose and lipid panels. BMI should be followed monthly for 3 months and then measured quarterly. Blood pressure, fasting glucose, and lipid panels should be followed up at 3 months and then yearly.

Other miscellaneous side effects of the antipsychotics include nonspecific skin rashes, retinitis pigmentosa (especially with thioridazine dosages >800 mg/day), fever (with clozapine), pigmentary changes in the skin (i.e., blue, gray, or tan), weight gain, cholestatic jaundice (with chlorpromazine), reduced libido, and inhibition of ejaculation (with thioridazine). Low-potency conventional antipsychotics are associated with a risk for seizures, especially at higher dosages (e.g., chlorpromazine >1,000 mg/day). The drugs are not contraindicated in epilepsy patients as long as they receive adequate treatment with anticonvulsants. All antipsychotics except clozapine are listed as Category C drugs by the U.S. Food and Drug Administration (FDA), meaning that pregnancy risk cannot be ruled out. Clozapine is listed as Category B, meaning that there is no evidence of pregnancy risk in humans.

All conventional antipsychotics have the potential to cause *neuroleptic malignant syndrome* (NMS), a rare idiosyncratic reaction that does not appear to be dose related. SGAs appear less likely to induce NMS. Considered a medical emergency, the syndrome is characterized by rigidity, high fever, delirium, and marked autonomic instability. Serum levels of creatinine phosphokinase and of liver enzymes are generally elevated. There is no standard approach to the treatment of NMS. Both the muscle relaxant dantrolene and the dopamine agonist bromocriptine have been used to treat NMS. Stopping the offending antipsychotic drug and providing supportive care may be as effective. Electroconvulsive therapy

(ECT) can be used in severe cases not responding to medical management. Once the patient has recovered, antipsychotics can be cautiously reintroduced after a 2-week wait. Selecting an agent from a different antipsychotic class (e.g., chlorpromazine rather than haloperidol, if haloperidol caused the NMS) or switching to an SGA is advisable.

Rational use of antipsychotics

1. A high-potency conventional antipsychotic or one of the SGAs should be given as first-line treatment.

   - SGAs are effective and well tolerated and have less potential to induce EPS.

2. Second-line drug choices include the other conventional antipsychotics.

3. A drug trial should last 4–6 weeks.

   - The trial should be extended when there is a partial response that has not plateaued and shortened when no response occurs or side effects are intolerable or unmanageable.

   - Aripiprazole, ziprasidone, or lurasidone may be the better choice in patients at risk for weight gain.

   - Quetiapine or aripiprazole may be favored when low EPS and low prolactin levels are desired.

4. All antipsychotics should be started at a low dosage and gradually increased to fall within a therapeutic range.

   - Evidence suggests that blood levels can help guide dosage adjustments for haloperidol and clozapine.

5. There is little reason to prescribe more than one antipsychotic agent. Using two or more such drugs increases adverse effects and adds little clinical benefit.

6. Because of its risk of agranulocytosis and need for monitoring of the white blood cell count, clozapine should be reserved for patients with treatment-refractory illness.

7. Many patients can benefit from chronic antipsychotic administration.

   - Patients should be carefully monitored for evidence of weight gain, glucose dyscontrol, and lipid abnormalities.

■ Antidepressants

Not long after chlorpromazine appeared in the late 1950s, the antidepressant imipramine was synthesized in an attempt by researchers to find additional compounds for the treatment of schizophrenia. It soon became apparent that imipramine had little effect on hallucinations and delusions; instead, it alleviated depression in patients who were both psychotic and depressed. This finding led to the development of the tricyclic antidepressants (TCAs). Modifications of the three-ring chemical structure followed as additional TCAs were produced, including amitriptyline and desipramine.

At about the same time that TCAs were synthesized, the antidepressant properties of monoamine oxidase inhibitors (MAOIs) were discovered. Iproniazid, an antibiotic used to treat tuberculosis, was found to relieve depression in tuberculosis patients. The drug became the first marketed antidepressant in 1958. No longer used, iproniazid has been succeeded by more effective MAOIs, including phenelzine and tranylcypromine.

A second and third generation of antidepressants have since been developed, some of which differ structurally from both the TCAs and the MAOIs. In the early 1980s, tetracyclic compounds (also referred to as *heterocyclics*) with a somewhat similar structure and comparable properties were marketed, including maprotiline and amoxapine. Another group of antidepressants, collectively known as the *selective serotonin reuptake inhibitors* (SSRIs), was developed in the late 1980s and early 1990s. Other antidepressants also were introduced but do not fit within any particular grouping, including bupropion, mirtazapine, venlafaxine, and duloxetine. The antidepressants are all thought to work by altering levels of neurotransmitters in the CNS. With minor exceptions, all are equally effective, differing primarily in their adverse effects and potency. A comparison of commonly prescribed antidepressants is presented in Table 21–2.

Indications

The primary indication for antidepressants is the acute and maintenance treatment of major depression. Approximately 65%–70% of patients receiving an antidepressant will respond within 4–6 weeks. In contrast, the placebo response rate in depression ranges from 25% to 40%. Depressed patients with melancholic symptoms (e.g., diurnal variation, psychomotor agitation or retardation, terminal insomnia, pervasive anhedonia) may respond better to antidepressants than do other patients. Secondary depressions (i.e., depressions that follow or complicate other psychiatric disorders); depressions accompanied by anxiety, somatization, or hypochondriasis; and depressions accompanied by personality disorders (often called *neurotic depression*) respond less well than do depressions without these features. Chronic forms of depression, including dysthy-

TABLE 21–2. Commonly used antidepressants

Category / Drug (trade name)	Sedation	Anticholinergic effects	Orthostatic hypotension	Sexual dysfunction	GI effects	Activation/ Insomnia	Half-life, h	Target dosage, mg	Dosage range, mg/day
Selective serotonin reuptake inhibitors									
Citalopram (Celexa)	VL	None	None	VH	H	VL	35	20	10–60
Escitalopram (Lexapro)	VL	None	None	VH	H	VL	25	10	10–30
Fluoxetine (Prozac)	None	None	None	VH	H	VH	24–72	20	20–80
Fluvoxamine (Luvox)	M	None	None	VH	H	L	15	200	100–300
Paroxetine (Paxil)	L	L	None	VH	H	L	20	20	20–50
Sertraline (Zoloft)	VL	None	None	VH	VH	M	25	100	50–200

TABLE 21–2. Commonly used antidepressants (*continued*)

Category	Drug (trade name)	Sedation	Anti-cholinergic effects	Orthostatic hypotension	Sexual dysfunction	GI effects	Activation/ Insomnia	Half-life, h	Target dosage, mg	Dosage range, mg/day
Other antidepressants										
	Bupropion (Wellbutrin)	None	None	None	None	M	H	12	300	150–450
	Desvenlafaxine (Pristiq)	L	None	VL	H	VH	M	10	50	50–400
	Duloxetine (Cymbalta)	VL	L	None	VL	H	L	8–17	60	40–60
	Levomilnacipran (Fetzima)	None	None	L	L	M	L	12	120	40–120
	Mirtazapine (Remeron)	H	None	L	None	VL	None	20–40	30	15–45
	Nefazodone (Serzone)	H	None	L	None	M	VL	2–4	300	100–600
	Trazodone (Desyrel)	VH	VL	VH	None	M	L	6–11	400	300–800

TABLE 21–2. Commonly used antidepressants (*continued*)

Category	Drug (trade name)	Sedation	Anti-cholinergic effects	Orthostatic hypotension	Sexual dysfunction	GI effects	Activation/ Insomnia	Half-life, h	Target dosage, mg	Dosage range, mg/day
	Venlafaxine (Effexor)	L	None	VL	H	VH	M	3–5	225	75–350
	Vilazodone (Viibryd)	L	None	VL	VL	M	L	25	40	10–40
Tricyclics										
	Amitriptyline (Elavil)	VH	VH	VH	H	VL	None	9–46	150	50–300
	Clomipramine (Anafranil)	VH	VH	VH	VH	VL	None	23–122	150	50–300
	Desipramine (Norpramin)	M	M	M	H	VL	VL	12–28	150	50–300
	Doxepin (Sinequan, Adapin)	VH	VH	VH	H	VL	None	8–25	200	50–300

TABLE 21-2. Commonly used antidepressants (continued)

Category	Drug (trade name)	Sedation	Anti-cholinergic effects	Orthostatic hypotension	Sexual dysfunction	GI effects	Activation/ Insomnia	Half-life, h	Target dosage, mg	Dosage range, mg/day
	Imipramine (Tofranil)	H	VH	VH	H	VL	None	6–28	200	50–300
	Nortriptyline (Pamelor)	M	M	M	H	VL	None	18–56	100	20–150
Monoamine oxidase inhibitors										
	Isocarboxazid (Marplan)	M	L	H	H	VL	L	—[a]	30	10–50
	Phenelzine (Nardil)	L	M	VH	H	VL	L	—[a]	60	15–90
	Tranyl-cypromine (Parnate)	None	M	VH	L	VL	M	—[a]	30–40	20–90

Note. GI = gastrointestinal; H=high; L=low; M=moderate; VH=very high; VL=very low.
[a]Maximal inhibition by monoamine oxidase inhibitors is achieved in 5–10 days.

mia, also respond to antidepressants, although treatment results are not as robust as those seen in acute forms of depression.

Other disorders that are treated with antidepressants include the depressed phase of bipolar disorder, panic disorder, agoraphobia, obsessive-compulsive disorder (OCD), social phobia, generalized anxiety disorder (GAD), posttraumatic stress disorder (PTSD), bulimia nervosa, and certain childhood conditions (e.g., enuresis, school phobia). Because antidepressants are used to treat a broad range of psychiatric disorders, the term *antidepressant* is a misnomer.

Selective Serotonin Reuptake Inhibitors

The SSRIs have become the most widely prescribed antidepressants in the United States. Six SSRIs are currently marketed: citalopram, escitalopram, fluoxetine, fluvoxamine, paroxetine, and sertraline. They are structurally dissimilar but share similar pharmacological properties involving their relatively selective serotonin reuptake inhibition. They largely lack the side effects of TCAs caused by blockade of muscarinic, histaminic, and α-adrenergic receptors.

SSRIs are generally better tolerated than TCAs and are safer in overdose. Because they are unlikely to affect seizure threshold or cardiac conduction, SSRIs are safer for patients with epilepsy or cardiac conduction defects. Clinicians should note that the FDA issued a warning in 2011 cautioning against prescribing citalopram at dosages exceeding 40 mg/day. The concern is that it could induce abnormal heart rhythms (through QT prolongation), including torsades de pointes, although research has since questioned the merit of this warning.

The SSRIs are remarkably versatile and are used to treat major depression, panic disorder, OCD, social phobia, PTSD, bulimia nervosa, and probably many other disorders as well. However, marketing strategies have led to the following FDA-approved indications in adults:

- Major depression—citalopram, escitalopram, fluoxetine, paroxetine, and sertraline
- Obsessive-compulsive disorder—fluoxetine, fluvoxamine, paroxetine, and sertraline
- Social anxiety disorder—fluoxetine, paroxetine, and sertraline
- Panic disorder—paroxetine and sertraline
- Generalized anxiety disorder—escitalopram and paroxetine
- Posttraumatic stress disorder—paroxetine and sertraline

- Premenstrual dysphoric disorder—fluoxetine and sertraline
- Bulimia nervosa—fluoxetine

All of the SSRIs are metabolized by the liver, but only fluoxetine and sertraline have active metabolites. Fluoxetine has the longest half-life at 2–3 days, and its major metabolite, norfluoxetine, has a half-life of 4–16 days. The other SSRIs have half-lives ranging from 15 to 35 hours. The active metabolite of sertraline, norsertraline, has a half-life of 2–4 days. All are well absorbed from the gut and reach peak plasma levels within 4–8 hours.

The SSRIs share a similar side-effect profile, with only subtle differences among them. Side effects are largely dose related and can include mild nausea, loose bowel movements, anxiety or hyperstimulation (which leads to jitteriness, restlessness, muscle tension, and insomnia), headache, insomnia, sedation, and increased sweating. Patients sometimes report other side effects, including weight gain or weight loss, bruxism, vivid dreams, skin rash, and amotivation.

Sexual dysfunction is relatively common in men and women treated with SSRIs. These drugs can decrease libido and cause ejaculatory delay or failure in men and anorgasmia in women. For this reason, SSRIs are sometimes prescribed to men to treat premature ejaculation. For persistent complaints of sexual dysfunction, management strategies include lowering the dosage, switching to one of the newer non-SSRI antidepressants (e.g., bupropion, duloxetine), or coadministering another medication as an antidote (e.g., bupropion, 75–300 mg/day, or cyproheptadine, 4–8 mg, taken 1–2 hours before sexual activity). Sildenafil and other medications used to treat erectile disorder also appear to be effective in treating SSRI-related sexual dysfunction.

Adverse effects tend to diminish over time, but they persist in some patients. Fluoxetine is the most likely, and escitalopram the least likely, to induce adverse effects. When hyperstimulation is problematic, it can be managed by lowering the dosage, switching to another SSRI, or switching to one of the newer non-SSRI antidepressants. A β-blocker (e.g., propranolol, 10–30 mg three times daily) can be helpful in treating subjective jitteriness and tremor. Benzodiazepines (e.g., lorazepam, 0.5–1 mg twice daily) can be prescribed to counteract this side effect as well. Because complaints of hyperstimulation tend to diminish over time, adjunctive medications may not be needed long-term. Trazodone (e.g., 50–150 mg at bedtime) can be effective in treating insomnia, although men should be warned of its rare propensity to cause priapism (a sustained, painful erection).

When SSRIs are discontinued, many patients develop a *discontinuation syndrome*. The exception is fluoxetine, which self-tapers because of the long half-life of both the parent compound and its major metabolite.

Symptoms include nausea, headache, vivid dreams, irritability, and dizziness. These often begin within days of drug discontinuation and continue for 2 weeks or longer. The symptoms can be minimized by tapering the drug slowly over several weeks. The short-term use of a benzodiazepine is often helpful.

SSRIs have been associated with the *serotonin syndrome,* particularly in patients who have concurrently taken two or more drugs that boost CNS serotonin levels. Typical symptoms include lethargy, restlessness, mental confusion, flushing, diaphoresis, tremor, and myoclonic jerks. Untreated, the serotonin syndrome can progress to hyperthermia, hypertonicity, rhabdomyolysis, renal failure, and death. Several deaths have been reported in patients taking a combination of an SSRI and MAOI, presumably as a result of this syndrome. Because of the potential lethality of this combination, when a patient is switched from an SSRI to an MAOI, a sufficient time must pass to ensure that the SSRI has been fully eliminated from the body before initiating treatment with an MAOI. With fluoxetine, this means that about 6 weeks must pass.

The SSRIs each inhibit one or more cytochrome P450 isoenzymes to a substantial degree and have the potential to cause clinically important drug interactions. For that reason, care should be taken when prescribing adjunctive or concurrent medication metabolized through this enzyme system. This means that SSRIs may induce a several-fold increase in the levels of coprescribed drugs that are dependent on the inhibited isoenzymes for their clearance. Fluoxetine, fluvoxamine, and paroxetine are the most likely to cause drug interactions, whereas citalopram and escitalopram have less potential to do so. See Table 21–3 for a description of the SSRIs and the isoenzyme systems inhibited and coadministered drugs affected.

Given their widespread use, the SSRIs are undoubtedly being used during pregnancy and breast-feeding. That said, all of the SSRIs are included in FDA risk Category C (pregnancy risk cannot be ruled out), except for paroxetine, which is in Category D (positive evidence of risk). The evidence base is largest with fluoxetine, which appears to be safe. There is some evidence that paroxetine and sertraline are associated with cardiovascular anomalies. The SSRIs are secreted in breast milk and should probably be avoided in women who are breast-feeding.

Other Newer Antidepressants

Bupropion

Bupropion has a unique chemical structure similar to that of psychostimulants, which may account for certain shared properties. Because

TABLE 21–3. Selective serotonin reuptake inhibitors (SSRIs) and other newer antidepressants and potentially important drug interactions

Antidepressant	Enzyme system inhibited	Potential drug interactions
Fluoxetine	2D6	Secondary TCAs, haloperidol, type 1C antiarrhythmics
	2C	Phenytoin, diazepam
	3A4	Carbamazepine, alprazolam, terfenadine
Sertraline	2D6	Secondary TCAs, antipsychotics, type 1C antiarrhythmics
	2C	Tolbutamide, diazepam
	3A4	Carbamazepine
Paroxetine	2D6	Secondary TCAs, antipsychotics, type 1C antiarrhythmics, trazodone
Fluvoxamine	1A2	Theophylline, clozapine, haloperidol, amitriptyline, clomipramine, imipramine, duloxetine
	2C	Diazepam
	3A4	Carbamazepine, alprazolam, terfenadine, astemizole
Nefazodone	3A4	Alprazolam, triazolam, terfenadine, astemizole, carbamazepine
Duloxetine	1A2	Fluvoxamine, theophylline, clozapine, haloperidol, amitriptyline, clomipramine, imipramine
	2D6	Secondary TCAs, antipsychotics, type 1C antiarrhythmics, trazodone

Note. TCAs=tricyclic antidepressants.
Source. Adapted from Nemeroff et al. 1996.

its primary metabolite, hydroxybupropion, inhibits the reuptake of dopamine and norepinephrine, the drug has been called a dopamine-norepinephrine reuptake inhibitor. Bupropion is used for the treatment of major depression but is also FDA approved for the treatment of smoking cessation under the trade name Zyban. An extended-release form of the drug has been approved as a treatment for seasonal affective disorder. Bupropion also has been used to treat attention-deficit/hyperactivity disorder. It is not effective in treating panic disorder, OCD, social phobia, or other anxiety syndromes.

Bupropion is rapidly absorbed following oral administration, and peak concentrations are achieved within 2 hours, or 3 hours after administration of the sustained-release formulation. Elimination is biphasic, with an initial phase of approximately 1.5 hours and a second phase lasting about 14 hours. The biphasic decline for the sustained-release formulation is less pronounced than that of the immediate-release formulation.

Bupropion is relatively well tolerated, having minimal effects on weight gain, cardiac conduction, or sexual functioning. The most common side effects are headache, nausea, anxiety, tremors, insomnia, and increased sweating. These symptoms generally subside with time. Restlessness and tremor can be treated with propranolol (e.g., 10–30 mg three times daily). The patient may benefit from short-term coadministration of a benzodiazepine tranquilizer.

The main disadvantage of bupropion is that the incidence of seizures increases substantially at dosages greater than 450 mg/day. For this reason, the drug is contraindicated in patients with a seizure disorder or an eating disorder (e.g., bulimia nervosa) that may be associated with a lower seizure threshold. The main risk of overdose is the development of seizures.

Duloxetine

Duloxetine is a potent inhibitor of both serotonin and norepinephrine and for that reason is designated—along with venlafaxine and desvenlafaxine—as a selective serotonin-norepinephrine reuptake inhibitor (SNRI). The drug is FDA approved to treat major depression and generalized anxiety disorder and also is indicated to treat diabetic neuropathic pain and fibromyalgia. Duloxetine is well absorbed from the gut and is metabolized in the liver mainly through P450 isoenzymes CYP2D6 and CYP1A2. Its major metabolites have minimal pharmacologic activity. The half-life ranges from 8 to 17 hours.

Duloxetine is well tolerated. The most common side effects include insomnia, asthenia, nausea, dry mouth, and constipation. The drug is not associated with weight gain, and rates of sexual dysfunction are low. Duloxetine is metabolized through the CYP isoenzymes, creating a potential for drug interactions (see Table 21–3). Because of reports of hepatotoxicity, the drug should be used with caution in persons with chronic liver disease, or in those with substantial alcohol use. It should not be combined with MAOIs because of the potential for a serotonin syndrome. The drug has been fatal in overdose at doses as low as 1,000 mg.

Levomilnacipran

Levomilnacipran is the newest SNRI to gain approval for the treatment of major depression. The drug is well absorbed from the gastrointestinal tract and has a half-life of around 12 hours. It is available in a slow-release formulation. Levomilnacipran is metabolized by the liver, mainly through cytochrome P450 isoenzyme CYP3A4; the drug and its metabolites are renally excreted. The metabolites are inactive. Common side effects include nausea, headache, dry mouth, and occasional increased blood pressure and pulse. Compared with other antidepressants, weight gain and rates of sexual dysfunction are low. The initial dose is 20 mg daily titrating gradually to 120 mg daily. Levomilnacipran should not be coadministered with an MAOI or any medications that may predispose to a serotonin syndrome, such as an SSRI. The dose should be gradually reduced, rather than stopped abruptly, to avoid withdrawal symptoms.

Mirtazapine

Mirtazapine has a dual mode of action and enhances both serotonergic and noradrenergic neurotransmission but is not a reuptake inhibitor. The drug is also a potent histamine antagonist, a moderate α-adrenergic antagonist, and a moderate antagonist at muscarinic receptors. Mirtazapine is FDA indicated for the treatment of major depression. The drug is well absorbed from the gut and is 85% protein bound. It has a half-life of 20–40 hours. Mirtazapine is well tolerated but may cause somnolence, increased appetite, and weight gain. Because of its long half-life, it needs to be taken only once daily. The drug has little effect on the cardiovascular system and minimally affects sexual functioning. Mirtazapine is unlikely to be associated with cytochrome P450–mediated drug interactions. One potential advantage is its early effect on reducing anxiety symptoms and sleep disturbance.

Somnolence occurs in more than half of the patients receiving mirtazapine, although tolerance develops after the first few weeks of treatment. Rare cases of agranulocytosis have been reported. In these cases, patients recovered after medication discontinuation. Routine laboratory monitoring is not currently recommended because this side effect is rare, but the development of fever, chills, sore throat, or other signs of infection in association with a low white blood cell count warrants close monitoring and discontinuation of the drug. The drug is unlikely to be fatal in overdose. The drug should not be used in combination with an MAOI.

Nefazodone

Nefazodone combines blockade of the 5-HT$_2$ receptor with weak inhibition of neuronal serotonin reuptake and is structurally similar to trazodone. The drug is indicated for the treatment of major depression. Side effects include nausea, somnolence, dry mouth, dizziness, constipation, asthenia, and blurred vision. The drug is generally well tolerated, and these side effects are considered benign. Nefazodone does not appear to alter seizure threshold, does not cause weight gain, and does not impair sexual functioning. The drug has the potential to inhibit the cytochrome P450 3A3/4 isoenzyme, which can lead to drug-drug interactions when other medications metabolized by that isoenzyme are coadministered. Drawbacks include the need for twice-daily dosing and a slow dosage titration. Nefazodone does not appear to be fatal in overdose. In rare cases, potentially irreversible hepatic failure has been associated with the drug. This led the FDA to issue a black box warning in 2002, and later the trade product Serzone was voluntarily withdrawn from the market. Generic formulations remain available.

Trazodone

Trazodone is a weak inhibitor of serotonin but also blocks 5-HT$_2$ receptors. The drug is a triazolopyridine derivative that shares the triazolo ring structure with alprazolam, a benzodiazepine. Trazodone is indicated for the treatment of major depression. The drug is readily absorbed from the gastrointestinal tract, reaches peak plasma levels in 1–2 hours, and has a half-life of 6–11 hours. Trazodone is metabolized by the liver, and 75% of its metabolites are excreted in the urine. Adverse effects are partially mediated by α-adrenergic antagonism and antihistaminic activity. The drug should not be coadministered with MAOIs. Concurrent use with antihypertensives may lead to hypotension.

The most common adverse effects are sedation, orthostatic hypotension, dizziness, headache, nausea, and dry mouth. These effects are mostly benign. Trazodone does not block anticholinergic receptors, so urinary retention and constipation are uncommon. The drug has no significant effect on cardiac conduction, although there are reports of increased ventricular irritability in patients with preexisting cardiac conduction defects or ventricular arrhythmias. It is unlikely to be fatal in overdose. Because trazodone is so sedating, it is widely used to treat insomnia (e.g., 50–150 mg at bedtime).

One concern with trazodone is that in rare cases it has been associated with priapism, which can be irreversible and require surgical intervention. Men prescribed trazodone should be warned of this side effect and be advised to report any change in the frequency or firmness of erections. The drug should be immediately discontinued if these changes occur. Immediate medical treatment should be sought for sustained erections.

Venlafaxine and Desvenlafaxine

Both venlafaxine and its primary active metabolite desvenlafaxine are classified as SNRIs and have minimal effect on other neurotransmitter receptors. Venlafaxine has an indication for the treatment of major depression, but its extended-release formulation is FDA approved for the treatment of generalized anxiety disorder, social anxiety disorder, and panic disorder. The drug is rapidly absorbed from the gut and is 98% bioavailable; its half-life is about 4 hours. Desvenlafaxine is marketed in a sustained-release formulation and is indicated for the treatment of major depression. Like the parent compound, desvenlafaxine is well absorbed orally and has a half-life of about 10 hours. Both venlafaxine and desvenlafaxine are metabolized by the liver and are renally excreted.

The side-effect profile of venlafaxine and desvenlafaxine is similar to that of the SSRIs and includes hyperstimulation, sexual dysfunction, and transient withdrawal symptoms. The drugs do not affect cardiac conduction or lower seizure threshold and generally are not associated with sedation or weight gain. Blood pressure monitoring is recommended with the use of either drug because of dose-dependent increases in mean diastolic blood pressure in some patients, particularly those with hypertension. The drugs are unlikely to inhibit cytochrome P450 isoenzymes, so drug-drug interactions are unlikely. Both drugs are contraindicated in patients taking MAOIs because of the risk of serotonin syndrome. The drugs are generally not fatal in overdose. The main drawback with venlafaxine is that it is generally taken twice daily, although the extended-release formulation can be taken once daily.

Vilazodone

Vilazodone is a serotonin reuptake inhibitor and 5-HT1_A receptor partial agonist with little affinity for other serotonin receptors. Vilazodone is indicated for the treatment of major depression and is generally safe and effective. Common side effects include nausea, diarrhea, headache, and somnolence. Vilazodone does not cause significant weight gain or sexual dysfunction. Drug concentrations peak 4–5 hours after administration, and absorption is increased when it is taken with food. The initial dose is 10 mg daily titrating gradually to 40 mg daily. Vilazodone should not be coadministered with an MAOI or any medication that may predispose to a serotonin syndrome, such as an SSRI. The dose should be gradually reduced, rather than stopped abruptly, to avoid withdrawal symptoms.

Tricyclic and Tetracyclic Antidepressants

TCAs are believed to work by blocking the reuptake of both norepinephrine and serotonin at the presynaptic nerve ending. The tertiary amines (e.g., amitriptyline, imipramine, doxepin) primarily block serotonin reuptake, whereas the secondary amines (e.g., desipramine, nortriptyline, protriptyline) mainly block norepinephrine reuptake. Clomipramine is an exception because it is a relatively selective serotonin reuptake inhibitor. All of these drugs also block muscarinic, histaminic, and α-adrenergic receptors. The degree of blockade corresponds with the side effect profile of the agent as shown in Table 21–2. (The tetracyclics maprotiline and amoxapine are rarely used and are not included in the table.)

TCAs are well absorbed orally; they undergo an enterohepatic cycle, and peak plasma levels develop 2–4 hours after ingestion. They are highly bound to plasma and tissue proteins and are fat soluble. TCAs are metabolized by the liver, and their metabolites are excreted through the kidneys. All TCAs have active metabolites, and there is as much as a tenfold variation in steady-state plasma levels of TCAs among individuals. These differences are primarily caused by individual variations in the way the liver metabolizes the drugs. Their half-lives vary but are generally in the range of 1 day. Steady-state plasma levels are achieved after five half-lives; half-life, in turn, is dependent on metabolism of the drug by hepatic microsomal enzymes. Blood levels tend to be increased by drugs that inhibit the cytochrome P450 system, including chlorpromazine and other antipsychotics, disulfiram, cimetidine, estrogens, methylphenidate, and many of the SSRIs.

The established therapeutic range for imipramine (the total for imipramine plus its metabolite desipramine) is generally thought to be greater than 200 ng/mL. Desipramine plasma levels greater than 125 ng/mL are considered therapeutic. A therapeutic window has been noted for nortriptyline, with optimal response between 50 and 150 ng/mL. These therapeutic levels are based on steady-state concentrations, which are reached after 5–7 days of administration of these medications. Blood should be drawn approximately 10–14 hours after the last dose of medication. Plasma blood levels can be measured for the other TCAs but are not clinically meaningful.

There is no reason to routinely obtain plasma levels, particularly when the patient is doing well. Blood levels are helpful in cases of drug overdose but may also be useful when evaluating a patient's failure to respond adequately, significant symptoms of toxicity, or suspected noncompliance; in establishing a therapeutic window; and in setting dosage levels for a patient with significant cardiac or other medical disease (when it is desirable to keep the blood level at the lower range of the therapeutic value).

TCAs commonly cause sedation, orthostatic hypotension, and anticholinergic side effects such as constipation, urinary hesitancy, dry mouth, and visual blurring. Each TCA differs in its propensity to cause these effects. Tertiary amines (e.g., amitriptyline, imipramine, doxepin) tend to cause more pronounced side effects. Tolerance usually develops to anticholinergic side effects and sedation, but TCAs should be used with caution in patients with prostatic enlargement and narrow-angle glaucoma. Elderly patients should have their blood pressure carefully monitored because drug-induced hypotension can lead to falls and resultant fractures.

Antihistaminic effects include sedation and weight gain. α-Adrenergic blockade causes orthostatic hypotension and reflex tachycardia. Miscellaneous side effects of TCAs include tremors, pedal edema, myoclonus, restlessness or hyperstimulation, insomnia, nausea and vomiting, electroencephalographic changes, rashes or allergic reactions, confusion, and seizures. It is uncertain whether TCAs are teratogenic, but their use in the first trimester of pregnancy should be avoided. Because a metabolite of the tetracyclic amoxapine is an antipsychotic, the drug can induce EPS, including TD.

Cardiovascular side effects tend to be the most worrisome. All TCAs prolong cardiac conduction, much like quinidine or procainamide, and carry the risk of exacerbating existing conduction abnormalities. Patients with low-grade abnormalities such as first-degree atrioventricular block or right bundle branch block should use these medications cautiously, and dosage increases should be accompanied by serial electrocardiograms. Patients with a higher-grade block (e.g., second-degree atrioventricular block) should not take TCAs. As a general rule, an SSRI or one of the newer antidepressants that does not prolong cardiac conduction (e.g., mirtazapine) should be used in patients with cardiac conduction defects.

A withdrawal syndrome can occur in patients who have been taking high doses of TCAs for weeks or months. Symptoms begin within days following abrupt drug discontinuation and include anxiety, insomnia, headache, myalgia, chills, malaise, and nausea. This syndrome usually can be prevented by a gradual taper of 25–50 mg/week. If this is not possible, small doses of an anticholinergic medication such as diphenhydramine (e.g., 25 mg two to three times daily) may help relieve symptoms.

Monoamine Oxidase Inhibitors

MAOIs inhibit monoamine oxidase (MAO), an enzyme responsible for the degradation of tyramine, serotonin, dopamine, and norepinephrine. Blocking this enzymatic process leads to an increase in CNS levels of these monoamines. Two types of MAO have been identified: MAO-A, which is found in the brain, liver, gut, and sympathetic nerves, and

MAO-B, which is found in the brain, liver, and platelets. MAO-A acts primarily on serotonin and norepinephrine, and MAO-B acts primarily on phenylethylamine; both act on dopamine and tyramine. Inhibitors of MAO-A may be more effective as antidepressants.

The four MAOIs commonly used in the United States are isocarboxazid, phenelzine, tranylcypromine, and selegiline. A transdermal patch formulation of selegiline is FDA approved for the treatment of major depression.

MAOIs are readily absorbed when orally administered. They do not have active metabolites, and the drugs are renally excreted. MAOIs irreversibly inhibit MAO, reaching maximum inhibition after 5–10 days. It is generally thought that platelet MAO activity, which reflects MAO inhibition, needs to be reduced by 80% to achieve an antidepressant response. The body takes approximately 2 weeks after the discontinuation of MAOIs to synthesize enough new MAO to restore its baseline concentrations. Plasma levels are not measured for the MAOIs.

MAOIs are thought to be particularly effective in forms of depression accompanied by significant anxiety. They have been found effective in treating panic disorder and agoraphobia, social phobia, PTSD, and bulimia nervosa. They also are thought to be particularly valuable in the treatment of *atypical depression*. Patients with this condition usually have a mixture of anxiety and depression, along with a reversal of diurnal variation (i.e., worse in the evening), hypersomnia, mood lability, hyperphagia, and a sensation of leaden paralysis. See Chapter 6, "Mood Disorders," for a more complete discussion regarding atypical depression.

The MAOIs have minimal anticholinergic and antihistaminic effects. They are potent α-adrenergic blockers, which results in a high frequency of orthostatic hypotension. If severe, this effect can be counteracted by the addition of salt and salt-retaining steroids such as fludrocortisone (Florinef). Elastic support stockings may also be helpful. Other common side effects include sedation or hyperstimulation (e.g., agitation), insomnia, dry mouth, weight gain, edema, and sexual dysfunction.

The most serious side effect results from the concomitant ingestion of an MAOI and substances containing tyramine, leading to severe hypertension and death or stroke in rare cases. Patients taking MAOIs must follow a special low-tyramine diet. Because MAOIs can interact with sympathomimetics (e.g., amphetamines) to produce a hypertensive crisis, patients need to be aware of potential interactions with prescribed and over-the-counter medications. MAOIs also have a potentially lethal interaction with meperidine, the mechanism of which is not fully understood but may have to do with serotonin agonism. Because selegiline primarily affects MAO-B, there is no need to follow a tyramine-free diet when using the 6-mg patch, but at higher doses the diet is recommended. (See Table 21–4 for a list of restricted foods and medications for those prescribed MAOIs.) Patients should be encouraged to carry a list of prohibited foods with them and to wear a medical bracelet indicating that they are taking an MAOI.

If symptoms of a hypertensive crisis occur (e.g., headache, nausea, or vomiting), patients should be instructed to immediately seek medical attention at a medical clinic or hospital emergency department. There, patients can be treated with intravenous phentolamine (e.g., 5 mg). Patients who do not have easy access to medical care should be advised to carry a 10-mg tablet of nifedipine with them; its α-blocking properties, which act to lower blood pressure when taken sublingually, make it a useful stopgap measure.

All physicians and dentists should be informed when their patients are taking MAOIs, especially when surgery or dental work is indicated, so that drugs that interact adversely with MAOIs can be avoided. It is advisable to wait 2 weeks after discontinuing an MAOI before resuming a normal diet or using a TCA, an SSRI, or another medication that may have an adverse interaction with the MAOI.

Use of Antidepressants

Treatment should begin with one of the SSRIs. Because these drugs are effective, well tolerated, and generally safe in overdose, they have replaced the TCAs as first-line therapy. Most patients will respond to a standard dosage, and frequent dosage adjustments are unnecessary. Patients with a history of cardiac conduction defects should receive one of the SSRIs or another new agent (e.g., bupropion, duloxetine, mirtazapine). Impulsive patients or those with suicidal urges also should receive an SSRI or one of the newer agents because they are unlikely to be fatal in overdose. When a TCA is used, nortriptyline, imipramine, and desipramine are the drugs of choice because meaningful plasma levels can be measured. The TCAs all require close titration, beginning with relatively low dosages. Recommended dosage ranges for the antidepressants are found in Table 21–2.

Patients being treated for their first episode of major depression should be maintained on medication at the same dosage used for acute treatment for at least 4–9 months after achieving remission. When medication is ultimately tapered and discontinued, patients should be carefully monitored to ensure that their remission is stable. Patients with the

---

TABLE 21–4. **Dietary instructions for patients taking monoamine oxidase inhibitors (MAOIs)**

Foods to avoid

Cheese: all cheeses except cottage cheese, farmer cheese, and cream cheese

Meat and fish: caviar; liver; salami and sausage; smoked, dried, pickled, cured, or preserved meats and fish

Vegetables: overripe avocados, fava beans, sauerkraut

Fruits: overripe fruits, canned figs

Other foods: yeast extracts, fermented products, monosodium glutamate

Beverages: red wine, sherry, liquors

Foods to use in moderation

Chocolate

Coffee

Colas

Tea

Soy sauce

Beer, other wine

Medications to avoid

Over-the-counter pain medications except for plain aspirin, acetaminophen, and ibuprofen

Cold or allergy medications

Nasal decongestants and inhalers

Cough medications; plain guaifenesin elixir may be taken, however

Stimulants and diet pills

Sympathomimetic drugs

Meperidine

Selective serotonin reuptake inhibitors (SSRIs), bupropion, desvenlafaxine, mirtazapine, nefazodone, trazodone, venlafaxine

---

Source. Adapted from Hyman and Arana 1987; Krishnan 2009.

---

following characteristics should be considered for chronic maintenance treatment to reduce the risk of relapse:

- Three or more lifetime episodes of major depression
- Double depression (i.e., major depression plus persistent depressive disorder)

- Two or more severe episodes of major depression within the past 5 years
- Depressive disorder complicated by comorbid substance use or anxiety disorder
- Age greater than 60 years at onset of major depression

Drug trials generally should last 4–8 weeks. When the patient's symptoms do not respond to an antidepressant after 4 weeks of treatment at the target dosage, the dosage should be increased, or the patient should be switched to another antidepressant, preferably from a different class with a slightly different mechanism of action. When this regimen fails, nonresponders may benefit from the addition of lithium, which will increase the likelihood of response in many patients. Response from lithium augmentation is often evident within a week with relatively low dosages (e.g., 300 mg three times daily). ECT is an option in patients whose depression does not respond to medication.

Other agents have been used to augment the effect of TCAs, including triiodothyronine, tryptophan, methylphenidate, and pindolol, but the effectiveness of these agents in augmenting response has not been adequately studied.

Rational use of antidepressants
1. SSRIs or one of the other newer antidepressants should be used initially, with TCAs and MAOIs reserved for nonresponders.
2. Dosages should be adjusted to fall within the recommended range, and each drug trial should last 4–8 weeks.
3. SSRIs generally are given once daily. TCAs can be administered as a single dose, usually at bedtime. MAOIs usually are prescribed twice daily but not at bedtime because they can cause insomnia. Bupropion is administered in two to three divided doses to minimize its risk of causing seizures.
4. Although adverse effects appear within days of starting a drug, therapeutic effects may require 2–4 weeks to become apparent.   • Improvement should be monitored by following up target symptoms (e.g., mood, sleep, energy, appetite).
5. Patients with heart rhythm disturbances should be given one of the newer antidepressants that do not affect cardiac conduction (e.g., bupropion, mirtazapine, or an SSRI).
6. Antidepressants are usually unnecessary in patients with uncomplicated bereavement or adjustment disorders with depressed mood, because these disorders are self-limiting.

Rational use of antidepressants *(continued)*
7. When possible, SSRIs should be tapered (except for fluoxetine, which self-tapers) because many patients experience withdrawal symptoms. TCAs also should be tapered slowly because of their tendency to cause withdrawal reactions. No clinically significant withdrawal reaction occurs with MAOIs, but a taper over 5–7 days is sensible.
8. The coadministration of two different antidepressants does not boost efficacy and will only worsen side effects. In rare cases, the combined use of a TCA and an MAOI or a TCA and an SSRI is justified, but these combinations should never be used routinely.
• MAOIs should not be coadministered with SSRIs or with any of the other new antidepressants.

■ Mood Stabilizers

Lithium carbonate, a naturally occurring salt, became available in 1970. Its first use in medicine (in the form of lithium chloride) was as a salt substitute for people with hypertension who needed a low-sodium diet, but its use was abandoned when it was found to make some people sick. In the late 1940s, Australian psychiatrist John Cade found that lithium calmed agitated psychotic patients. Later, it was discovered that lithium was particularly effective in people with mania. The Danish researcher Mogens Schou observed that lithium was effective in relieving the target symptoms of mania and that it also had a prophylactic effect. Lithium has since been joined by valproate, carbamazepine, and lamotrigine for the treatment of bipolar disorder.

In addition to the mood stabilizers, all of the SGAs (except clozapine and lurasidone) have been approved for the treatment of acute mania; two are indicated for maintenance treatment of bipolar disorder (aripiprazole and olanzapine); two for the treatment of major depression associated with bipolar I disorder (lurasidone, quetiapine) and five are indicated for the adjunctive treatment of acute mania in combination with lithium or valproate (aripiprazole, lurasidone, olanzapine, quetiapine, and risperidone). Additionally, both quetiapine and a combined form of olanzapine and fluoxetine (Symbyax) are approved to treat the depressed phase of bipolar disorder. The mood stabilizers are listed in Table 21–5. (Further information about the treatment of bipolar disorder is found in Chapter 6, "Mood Disorders.")

Lithium Carbonate

Lithium is a cation that inhibits several steps in the metabolism of phosphoinositide and many second and third messengers, including G pro-

TABLE 21–5. Commonly used mood stabilizers

Drug (trade name)	Therapeutic plasma level	Dosage range, mg/day
Carbamazepine (Tegretol)	6–12 mg/L	400–2,400
Lamotrigine (Lamictal)	N/A	50–200
Lithium carbonate (Eskalith, Lithobid)	0.6–1.2 mEq/L	900–2,400
Valproate (Depakene, Depakote)	50–120 mg/L	500–3,000

teins and protein kinases. Research suggests that lithium stimulates neurite growth, regeneration, and neurogenesis, which may be related to its therapeutic effect.

The onset of action often takes 5–7 days to become apparent. The usual plasma level of lithium for the treatment of acute mania is 0.5–1.2 mEq/L, but some patients do well outside this range. (Many psychiatrists will aim for a level of 0.8–1.0 mEq/L.) Antipsychotics, which work more quickly, may be preferred when rapid behavioral control is needed, although benzodiazepine-induced sedation may be as effective.

Maintenance dosages may be lower (0.5–0.7 mEq/L). Lithium has no role in the acute treatment of unipolar major depression but is a first-line treatment for bipolar depression. Lithium is sometimes used to augment the effect of antidepressants in the treatment of major depression.

The most dramatic effect of lithium is in the prophylaxis of manic and depressive episodes in bipolar patients. Lithium appears to work best at reducing the frequency and severity of manic episodes. Although response to lithium tends to remain stable over time, most patients will have breakthrough episodes. Lithium has also been shown to be effective in preventing recurrences of depression in patients with unipolar major depression. It is one of the few drugs demonstrated to reduce suicide attempts and suicides.

Lithium is also used in the treatment of schizoaffective disorder, especially the bipolar subtype. Lithium is sometimes used to treat aggression in patients with dementia, intellectual developmental disorder, or "acting out" personality disorders (especially the borderline and antisocial types).

Pharmacokinetics of Lithium

Lithium carbonate is administered orally and is rapidly absorbed. Peak blood levels are obtained about 2 hours after ingestion. The elimination half-life is about 8–12 hours in manic patients and about 18–36 hours in euthymic patients. (Manic patients are overly active and have a higher glomerular filtration rate and therefore clear lithium from their system more rapidly.) Lithium is not protein bound and does not have metabolites. It is almost entirely excreted through the kidney but may be found in all body fluids (e.g., saliva, semen). Blood plasma levels are checked 12 hours after the last dose is given.

Lithium usually is administered two or three times daily in patients with acute mania. (Lithium may also be administered in liquid form as lithium citrate.) Once-daily dosing with extended-release preparations is recommended in patients receiving the drug prophylactically because it may offer some protection to the kidneys. These preparations are also preferred if lithium causes gastric irritation. Lithium usually is started at 300 mg twice daily in typical patients and is then titrated until a therapeutic blood level is achieved. Dosage may be adjusted every 3–5 days. Levels should be checked monthly for the first 3 months and every 3 months thereafter. Patients receiving chronic lithium administration can be monitored less frequently. Lithium can be safely discontinued without a taper.

Adverse Effects of Lithium

Minor side effects of lithium occur relatively soon after initiating treatment. Thirst or polyuria, tremor, diarrhea, weight gain, and edema are all relatively common side effects but tend to diminish with time. About 5%–15% of the patients undergoing long-term treatment develop clinical signs of hypothyroidism. This side effect is more common in women and tends to occur during the first 6 months of treatment. Hypothyroidism can be managed effectively with thyroid hormone replacement. Baseline thyroid assays should be obtained before starting lithium. Thyroid function should be tested once or twice during the first 6 months of treatment and every 6–12 months thereafter as clinically indicated. Thyroid dysfunction reverses after lithium is discontinued.

Long-term lithium treatment may lead to increased levels of calcium, ionized calcium, and parathyroid hormone. High levels of calcium can cause lethargy, ataxia, and dysphoria, symptoms that may be attributed to depression rather than hypercalcemia.

Lithium is excreted through the kidneys and is reabsorbed in the proximal tubules with sodium and water. When the body has a sodium deficiency, the kidneys compensate by reabsorbing more sodium than normal in the proximal tubules. Lithium is absorbed along with sodium and poses the risk of lithium toxicity with hyponatremia. Thus patients should be instructed to avoid becoming dehydrated from exercise, fever, or other causes of increased sweating. Sodium-depleting diuretics (e.g., thiazides) should be avoided because they may increase lithium levels. The concomitant use of nonsteroidal anti-inflammatory agents should also be avoided because of their potential to raise lithium levels, most likely mediated by their effect on renal prostaglandin synthesis.

Lithium has the potential to cause nephrogenic diabetes insipidus because lithium inhibits vasopressin, thereby reducing the ability of the kidneys to concentrate urine. As a result, many lithium-treated patients produce large volumes of dilute urine. This can be clinically significant for some individuals, particularly when output exceeds 4 L/day. Amiloride (e.g., 10–20 mg/day) or hydrochlorothiazide (e.g., 50 mg/day) can be administered to (paradoxically) reduce urine output. A nephrotic syndrome caused by glomerulonephritis occurs in rare cases. This complication typically reverses when lithium is discontinued.

Long-term lithium use has been associated with a decrease in the glomerular filtration rate, but significant decreases are uncommon. The decrease is presumably due to a tubulointerstitial nephropathy, perhaps caused by the patient's cumulative exposure to lithium; therefore, the lowest effective dosage possible should be prescribed. Renal function should be assessed every 2–3 months during the first 6 months of treatment and every 6–12 months thereafter as clinically indicated. If proteinuria or an increase in creatinine is evident, additional tests should be performed.

A reversible and benign flattening of the T wave on the ECG occurs in about 20%–30% of patients taking lithium. In addition, lithium may suppress the function of the sinus node and result in sinoatrial block. Thus, an ECG should be obtained before initiating lithium treatment in patients older than 40 years or in those with a history or symptoms of cardiac disease.

Acne, follicular eruptions, and psoriasis have been known to occur in lithium-treated patients. Hair loss and thinning also have been reported. Except for cases of exacerbation of psoriasis, these reactions are usually benign.

Lithium induces a reversible leukocytosis, with white blood cell counts of 13,000–15,000/mm^3. The increase is usually in neutrophils and represents a step-up of the total body count rather than demargination.

Parkinsonian-like symptoms, such as cogwheeling, hypokinesis, and rigidity, may occur in lithium-treated patients. Cognitive effects, such as distractibility, poor memory, and confusion, also can develop at therapeutic levels of lithium.

Contraindications to Lithium

Patients with a severe renal disease (e.g., glomerulonephritis, pyelonephritis, polycystic kidneys) should not receive lithium because it is renally excreted; dangerous blood levels may result when the kidneys are not functioning normally. Lithium should be discontinued for at least 10–14 days in patients who have had myocardial infarction. If treatment with lithium is necessary during the postinfarct period, low dosages and periodic cardiac monitoring are recommended.

Lithium is contraindicated in the presence of myasthenia gravis because it blocks the release of acetylcholine. Lithium should be given cautiously in the presence of diabetes mellitus, ulcerative colitis, psoriasis, and senile cataracts. Because of the increased incidence of cardiovascular malformations in infants of mothers taking lithium (Ebstein's anomaly), lithium should be discontinued during the first trimester of pregnancy. Because lithium is secreted in breast milk, mothers taking the drug should not breast-feed.

Valproate

Valproate, a simple branched-chain carboxylic acid, is commonly used as an anticonvulsant and is FDA approved for the treatment of acute mania. An extended-release formulation is approved as well for both acute manic and mixed states. It is considered a first-line treatment for bipolar disorder, along with lithium carbonate and carbamazepine. It also is effective for long-term maintenance treatment of bipolar disorder. It appears to reduce recurrences of mania and to increase the length of depression-free intervals.

The mechanism of its action is unknown, although it enhances CNS levels of γ-aminobutyric acid (GABA) by inhibiting its degradation and stimulating its synthesis and release. Valproate is rapidly absorbed after oral ingestion, and its bioavailability is nearly complete. Peak concentrations occur in 1–4 hours; it is rapidly distributed and highly (90%) protein bound.

The half-life of valproate ranges from 8 to 17 hours. The drug is metabolized by the liver, primarily through glucuronide conjugation. Less than 3% is excreted unchanged. Unlike carbamazepine, valproate does not induce its own metabolism. A plasma concentration of about 50–125 μg/mL correlates with acute antimanic response. Valproate may be more effective than lithium in patients with mixed presentations, with irritable mania, with a high number of prior episodes of mania, or with a history of nonresponse to lithium.

Commonly reported side effects include gastrointestinal complaints (e.g., nausea, poor appetite, vomiting, diarrhea), tremor, sedation, and weight gain. Less frequent side effects include rashes, hematological abnormalities, and hair loss. Hepatic transaminase elevation can occur and is dose related; it generally subsides spontaneously. A rare but fatal hepatotoxic reaction to valproate has been reported. The enteric-coated form of valproate is generally well tolerated and has a low incidence of gastrointestinal side effects.

Neural tube defects have been reported with the use of valproate during the first trimester of pregnancy; therefore, its use in pregnant women is not recommended. Coma and death have occurred from valproate overdoses.

Before valproate treatment is begun, the patient should have a complete blood count and a liver enzyme measurement; the latter should be done periodically during the first 6 months and then about every 6 months thereafter. The drug is started at 250 mg three times daily and can be increased by 250 mg every 3 days. Serum levels can be obtained after 3–4 days. Most patients will need between 1,250 and 2,500 mg/day.

Carbamazepine

Carbamazepine, an anticonvulsant used to treat complex partial and tonic-clonic seizures, has a structure similar to that of the TCAs. It is used as an alternative to lithium and valproate in the treatment of acute mania and may be effective for maintenance treatment of bipolar disorder. The drug has been approved by the FDA for the treatment of acute manic or mixed episodes of bipolar disorder.

The precise mechanism of action of carbamazepine is unknown, but the drug has a wide range of cellular and intracellular effects in the CNS. Of theoretical interest is its dampening effect on kindling, a process in which repeated biochemical or psychological stressors are thought to result in abnormal excitability of limbic neurons.

Carbamazepine can safely be combined with antipsychotics, especially when behavioral control is necessary. It may be more effective in patients who cycle rapidly (i.e., more than four episodes per year) and who tend not to respond well to lithium. When carbamazepine is used to treat mania, there is generally a delay of 5–7 days before its effect is apparent.

From 10% to 15% of the patients taking carbamazepine develop a skin rash, which is generally transient. Other common side effects include impaired coordination, drowsiness, dizziness, slurred speech, and ataxia. Many of these symptoms can be avoided by increasing the dosage slowly. A transient leukopenia causing as much as a 25% decrease in the white blood cell count occurs in 10% of patients. A smaller reduction in the white blood cell count may persist in some patients as long as they take the drug, but this is not a reason for discontinuation. Aplastic anemia develops in rare cases.

Carbamazepine is typically started at a dosage of 200 mg twice daily and increased to three times daily after 3–5 days. Most patients will need dosages of 600–1,600 mg/day. The usual custom is to aim for typical anticonvulsant blood levels of 8–12 µg/mL, despite the fact that no dose-response curve has been established.

Before starting carbamazepine, the patient should have a complete blood count and an electrocardiogram. The patient should be warned about the drug's rare hematological side effects. Any indication of infection, anemia, or thrombocytopenia (e.g., petechiae) should be investigated and a complete blood count should be obtained, but routine blood monitoring is unnecessary. Because carbamazepine is a vasopressin agonist, it can induce hyponatremia; therefore, convulsions or undue drowsiness should be cause for obtaining serum electrolyte measurements. Carbamazepine has been linked with fetal malformations similar to those seen with phenytoin and therefore should be avoided in pregnant women, especially during the first trimester. Breast-feeding by women taking this drug is not recommended.

Lamotrigine

Lamotrigine, an anticonvulsant, is FDA approved for the maintenance treatment of bipolar I disorder to delay the time to occurrence of mood episodes. It appears most effective in delaying the time to occurrence of depressive episodes and may be effective in the treatment of acute depressive episodes as well. Although its mechanism of action is unclear, it affects CNS neurotransmission by blocking sodium channels. This action inhibits the release of presynaptic glutamate, aspartate, and GABA. The drug also is a weak inhibitor of the serotonin-3 receptor.

The target dosage of lamotrigine is 200 mg/day, achieved through a slow titration (i.e., 25 mg/day for 2 weeks, 50 mg/day for 2 weeks, 100 mg/day for 1 week, then 200 mg/day). The oral bioavailability of the drug is 98%, and peak plasma concentrations occur initially at 1–3 hours, with a secondary peak at 4–6 hours. The drug is about 60% protein bound and is widely distributed in the body. Metabolism is through hepatic glucuronidation, and none of the metabolites are active. The half-life ranges from 25 to 35 hours.

Lamotrigine is generally well tolerated, and most side effects are minor. In rare cases, the drug can induce the potentially life-threatening Stevens-Johnson syndrome and toxic epidermal necrolysis. Patients should be instructed to discontinue the drug at the first sign of a rash. Rashes are more common in children. Lamotrigine should probably not be combined with valproate because the combination can substantially increase the risk of serious rash, including Stevens-Johnson syndrome. The drug is listed as Category C in terms of pregnancy risk, which indicates that risk cannot be ruled out.

Rational use of mood stabilizers
1. Lithium, valproate, or carbamazepine should be used initially for the treatment of acute mania.
• Monotherapy with SGAs, which are effective and well tolerated, is an excellent alternative.
• The combination of lithium and valproate or the combination of a mood stabilizer with one of the SGAs may be effective when monotherapy fails.
2. A clinical trial of lithium, valproate, or carbamazepine should last 3 weeks; at this point, another drug should be added or substituted if there is minimal or inadequate response.
• Drug nonresponders may respond to electroconvulsive therapy.
3. Lithium may be given as a single dose at bedtime when the amount is less than 1,200 mg. Lithium should be given with food to minimize gastric irritation.
4. Renal function and thyroid indices should be regularly monitored in patients treated with lithium. Hepatic function should be regularly monitored in patients treated with valproate.
5. Lamotrigine may be particularly helpful in preventing the development of depressive episodes in bipolar I patients.

■ Anxiolytics

Anxiolytics are the most widely prescribed class of psychotropic drugs. They include the barbiturates, the nonbarbiturate sedative-hypnotics (e.g., meprobamate), the benzodiazepines, and buspirone. Currently, only the benzodiazepines and buspirone can be recommended because of their superior safety record. There is still a strong belief in the general population that these medications are overprescribed by psychiatrists and other physicians. Despite their reputation, benzodiazepines are generally prescribed for short periods, are prescribed for rational indications, and are used appropriately by most patients.

Benzodiazepines

Benzodiazepines constitute an important class of drugs with clear superiority over the barbiturates and nonbarbiturate sedative-hypnotics.

TABLE 21–6.   Benzodiazepines commonly used as anxiolytics

Drug (trade name)	Rate of onset	Half-life, h	Long-acting metabolite	Equivalent dosage, mg	Dosage range, mg/day
Alprazolam (Xanax)	Fast	6–20	No	0.5	1–4
Chlordiazepoxide (Librium)	Fast	20–100	Yes	10.0	15–60
Clonazepam (Klonopin)	Moderate	30–40	No	0.25	1–6
Diazepam (Valium)	Very fast	30–100	Yes	5.0	5–40
Lorazepam (Ativan)	Fast	10–20	No	1.0	0.5–10
Oxazepam (Serax)	Slow	5–20	No	15.0	30–120

Benzodiazepines have been marketed in the United States since 1964. These drugs have a high therapeutic index, little toxicity, and relatively few drug-drug interactions. The benzodiazepines are indicated for the treatment of anxiety syndromes, sleep disturbances, musculoskeletal disorders, seizure disorders, and alcohol withdrawal and for inducing anesthesia. Their approved indications reflect subtle differences among them (e.g., side effects, potency) and in marketing strategy. Commonly used benzodiazepines are compared in Table 21–6.

Benzodiazepines are believed to exert their effects by binding to specific benzodiazepine receptors in the brain. The receptors are intimately linked to receptors for GABA, a major inhibitory neurotransmitter. By binding to benzodiazepine receptors, the drugs potentiate the actions of GABA, leading to a direct anxiolytic effect on the limbic system.

Indications for Benzodiazepines

Benzodiazepines are useful for the treatment of generalized anxiety disorder, especially when severe. Many patients benefit when their anxiety is acute and problematic; these drugs generally should be given for short periods (e.g., weeks or months). Patients with mild anxiety may not need medication and can be successfully managed with behavioral interventions (e.g., progressive muscle relaxation).

Benzodiazepines have an antipanic effect. Both alprazolam and clonazepam have FDA indications for the treatment of panic disorder but because of their abuse potential are considered second-line treatments after the SSRIs. Similarly, while benzodiazepines are effective in treating social anxiety disorder, the SSRIs should be used initially because they do not have an abuse potential.

Anxiety frequently complicates depression. Benzodiazepines are frequently coadministered with an antidepressant because they are more effective in quickly relieving accompanying anxiety than is the antidepressant. When the antidepressant begins to take effect, the benzodiazepine can be withdrawn gradually.

Benzodiazepines are effective in alleviating situational anxiety. DSM-5's *adjustment disorder with anxiety* is characterized by anxiety symptoms (e.g., tremors, palpitations) that occur in response to a stressful event. Adjustment disorders are generally brief, and for that reason, treatment with benzodiazepines should be time limited.

Benzodiazepines have established efficacy in the short-term treatment of primary insomnia unrelated to identifiable medical or psychiatric illness. Their use as hypnotic agents is discussed in Chapter 12 ("Sleep-Wake Disorders"), which includes a description of the individual drugs, their dosing, and their adverse effects.

Alcohol withdrawal syndromes are commonly treated with benzodiazepines (most often chlordiazepoxide), because benzodiazepines and alcohol are cross-tolerant. The treatment of these syndromes is described in Chapter 15 ("Substance-Related and Addictive Disorders"). Other uses of the benzodiazepines include the treatment of akathisia and catatonia and as an adjunct to the treatment of acute agitation and mania.

Pharmacokinetics of Benzodiazepines

Benzodiazepines are rapidly absorbed from the gastrointestinal tract and, with the exception of lorazepam, are poorly absorbed intramuscularly. Lorazepam is available for parenteral use, and its versatility contributes to its widespread use in hospitalized patients. Midazolam is a short-acting agent used to induce anesthesia but is not available orally. Benzodiazepines are metabolized chiefly by hepatic oxidation and have active metabolites. Lorazepam, oxazepam, and temazepam are metabolized by glucuronide conjugation and have no active metabolites; they are relatively short acting and are thus the preferred benzodiazepines for elderly patients.

There are differences between single-dose and steady-state kinetics. Rapid-onset drugs tend to be lipophilic, a property that facilitates rapid crossing of the blood-brain barrier. Drugs with longer elimination half-lives accumulate more slowly and take longer to reach steady state.

Washout of these drugs is similarly prolonged. Drugs with shorter half-lives reach steady state more rapidly but also have less total accumulation. Drugs with long half-lives tend to have active metabolites.

Because of the differences in metabolism and half-lives, the best therapeutic results are obtained when the needs of the patient and the situation are taken into account. When prescribing, three parameters largely determine drug selection: 1) half-life, 2) presence of metabolites, and 3) route of elimination. For example, in older adults, the clinician should select a benzodiazepine with a short half-life, few metabolites, and renal excretion in order to minimize drug accumulation and adverse side effects.

Adverse Effects of Benzodiazepines

CNS depression is common with benzodiazepines. Symptoms include drowsiness, somnolence, reduced motor coordination, and memory impairment. These may diminish with continued administration or dosage reduction. However, patients should be cautioned not to drive or use heavy machines, especially when starting these drugs.

All benzodiazepines have the potential for abuse and addiction. Because physiological dependence is more likely to occur with longer drug exposure, minimizing the duration of continuous treatment should reduce this risk. Also, benzodiazepines should be prescribed cautiously in patients with histories of alcohol or drug abuse and in patients with "acting out" personalities (e.g., borderline and antisocial personality disorders). When signs of dependence appear (e.g., drug-seeking behavior, increasing the dosage to get the same effect), the drug should be tapered and discontinued. Patients should be advised to avoid alcohol when taking benzodiazepines because the combination will cause greater CNS depression than either drug alone.

Discontinuation of benzodiazepine therapy after long-term treatment can lead to tremulousness, sweating, sensitivity to light and sound, insomnia, abdominal distress, and systolic hypertension. Serious withdrawal syndromes and seizures are relatively uncommon but are more likely with abrupt discontinuation. Symptom recurrence appears to have a more rapid onset after discontinuation of short-acting benzodiazepines; the effect of drug discontinuation can be minimized by gradually tapering the drug over 1–3 months. Such a slow taper is particularly important for benzodiazepines with short half-lives. When discontinuing short-acting benzodiazepines, it may be helpful to switch the patient to a long-acting drug before initiating a taper (e.g., from alprazolam to clonazepam).

Nearly all benzodiazepines fall into pregnancy risk Category D (positive evidence of risk) or X (contraindicated in pregnancy), mainly on the basis of the occurrence of neonatal toxicity and withdrawal syndromes. For these reasons, their use during pregnancy and breast-feeding should be avoided.

Benzodiazepines can be used safely in medically ill and elderly patients. In general, drugs that do not accumulate (e.g., lorazepam) should be used. Because benzodiazepines can cause respiratory depression, they should not be used in persons with sleep apnea, although small dosages are tolerated even in patients with chronic pulmonary disease. Small dosages are also indicated for the elderly, who are susceptible to the CNS depressant effects of benzodiazepines, which can contribute to memory difficulties and falls.

The least controversial aspect of benzodiazepines is their tremendous index of safety. When they are taken alone, even massive overdoses are rarely fatal.

Buspirone

Buspirone has an FDA indication for the treatment of generalized anxiety disorder. Structurally unlike other anxiolytics, it is a serotonin type 1A (5-HT_{1A}) receptor agonist and does not interact with the benzodiazepine receptor. As such, it does not produce sedation, does not interact with alcohol, and does not pose a risk for abuse. Buspirone is ineffective in blocking panic attacks, relieving phobias, or diminishing obsessions or compulsions. Buspirone is well absorbed orally and is metabolized by the liver. Its half-life ranges from 2 to 11 hours. Drowsiness, headache, and dizziness are common side effects.

Buspirone's effect on chronic anxiety is equal to that of diazepam, although its effects are not apparent for 1–2 weeks. The usual dosage range is 20–30 mg/day in divided doses. Alternatives to buspirone for the treatment of generalized anxiety disorder include the SNRIs venlafaxine and duloxetine and the SSRIs.

Rational use of anxiolytics

1. The benzodiazepines should be used for limited periods (e.g., weeks to months) to avoid the problem of dependency, because most conditions they are used to treat are self-limiting.

   - Some patients will benefit from long-term benzodiazepine administration; in these situations, patients should be periodically assessed for continuing need.

Rational use of anxiolytics *(continued)*

2. The benzodiazepines have similar clinical efficacy, so the choice of a specific agent depends on its half-life, the presence of metabolites, and the route of administration.

3. Once- or twice-daily dosing of the benzodiazepines is sufficient for most patients.

    •   A dose given at bedtime may eliminate the need for a separate hypnotic.

    •   Short-acting agents (e.g., alprazolam) are an exception to this recommendation because their dosing interval is determined by their half-lives.

4. Buspirone is not effective on an as-needed (prn) basis and is useful only for the treatment of generalized anxiety disorder.

5. The SNRIs venlafaxine and duloxetine, or one of the SSRIs, are effective alternatives to the benzodiazepines and buspirone in the treatment of generalized anxiety disorder.

    •   Because response to these agents takes several weeks, it is important to educate the patient not to expect quick results.

■ Agents Used to Treat Extrapyramidal Syndromes

Anticholinergic agents closely resemble atropine in their ability to block muscarinic receptors, and all are similar in action and efficacy for alleviating antipsychotic-induced EPS, especially pseudoparkinsonism. These drugs are believed to diminish or eliminate EPS by reestablishing dopamine-acetylcholine equilibrium, which they do by blocking acetylcholine in the corpus striatum. An equilibrium of dopaminergic (inhibitory) and cholinergic (excitatory) neuronal activity in the corpus striatum is thought to be necessary for normal motor functioning. Antipsychotic medications cause dopamine reuptake blockage and an absolute decrease in dopamine and thus a relative increase in interneuronal acetylcholine, which results in EPS.

The anticholinergic drug benztropine should be started at a dosage of 1–2 mg/day. Smaller dosages should be used with geriatric patients. The maximum allowable dosage is 6 mg/day of benztropine or its equivalent, because a delirium can occur at higher dosages. Benztropine can be administered once daily, preferably at bedtime because it may cause sedation. The side effects of anticholinergic medications—

TABLE 21–7. Common agents used to treat extrapyramidal syndromes

Category	Drug (trade name)	Dosage range, mg/day	Comments
Anticholinergics	Benztropine (Cogentin)	0.5–6	Use 1–2 mg im of benztropine or 25–50 mg im of diphenhydramine for acute dystonia. Anticholinergics tend to work better at relieving the tremor of pseudoparkinsonism than hypokinesia.
	Biperiden (Akineton)	2–6	
	Diphenhydramine (Benadryl)	12.5–150	
	Procyclidine (Kemadrin)	2.5–22.5	
	Trihexyphenidyl (Artane)	1–15	
Dopamine facilitators	Amantadine (Symmetrel)	100–300	Useful in situations in which anticholinergic side effects need to be avoided.
β-Blockers	Propranolol (Inderal)	10–80	Works well for treating akathisia.
α-Agonists	Clonidine (Catapres)	0.2–0.8	May cause orthostatic hypotension; therefore, dosage should be increased slowly. Works well for treating akathisia.

dry mouth, blurry vision, constipation, and urinary hesitancy—are additive with those of the antipsychotics. Table 21–7 shows common agents used to treat EPS and their dosage ranges.

Intramuscular benztropine (1–2 mg) or diphenhydramine (25–50 mg) works within 20–30 minutes to alleviate acute dystonic reactions. These drugs may be given intravenously as well and relieve dystonia within minutes. Benztropine is the preferred agent because it usually does not cause sedation. Lorazepam (1–2 mg intramuscularly) also appears to work.

Amantadine and propranolol can be used to treat EPS. Amantadine acts to increase CNS concentrations of dopamine by blocking its reuptake and increasing its release from presynaptic fibers. This action is thought to restore the dopamine-acetylcholine balance in the striatum.

Amantadine is primarily useful in treating the symptoms of pseudoparkinsonism, such as tremors, rigidity, and hypokinesia. One advantage of amantadine is its lack of anticholinergic effects, so that it can be safely combined with antipsychotics without concern for the development of an anticholinergic delirium. Treatment is initiated at 100 mg/day and increased to 200–300 mg/day. Onset of action occurs within 1 week. Adverse effects include orthostatic hypotension, livedo reticularis, ankle edema, gastrointestinal upset, and visual hallucinations in rare cases.

Propranolol and other β-blockers have been used to treat akathisia, which usually is not alleviated with an anticholinergic agent. Propranolol (e.g., 10–20 mg three to four times daily) or another equivalent centrally acting β-blocker seems to work well; its effect is often apparent within days. Discontinuation of the drug will lead to a recurrence of symptoms.

Clonidine, an α_2-receptor agonist, also has been used to treat akathisia. The drug is usually given in divided doses ranging from 0.2 to 0.8 mg/day. Orthostatic hypotension and sedation are the main side effects. Clonidine should be used as a second-line agent for patients unresponsive to propranolol.

In treating any EPS, the clinician should begin by reducing the dosage of the antipsychotic drug whenever possible or switching to an SGA with less potential to cause EPS. When these steps fail, anticholinergics, amantadine, or propranolol can be useful adjuncts. Because EPS are unpleasant and reduce the likelihood that the patient will remain compliant with treatment, drugs used to treat these side effects can make a positive difference for the patient.

■ Electroconvulsive Therapy

ECT is a procedure in which a controlled electric current is passed through the scalp and selected parts of the brain to induce a grand mal seizure. The procedure was introduced in 1938 in Italy by Ugo Cerletti and Lucio Bini to replace less reliable convulsive therapies that used liquid chemicals. ECT is one of the oldest medical treatments still in regular use, a fact that attests to its safety and efficacy. Its mechanism of action is poorly understood, yet it is known to produce multiple effects on the CNS, including neurotransmitter changes, neuroendocrine effects, and alterations in intracellular signaling pathways.

Indications for Electroconvulsive Therapy

ECT is used almost exclusively for the treatment of mood disorders and is generally reserved for patients who have failed to respond to antidepressant medication or to antimanic agents, are catatonic, or are debilitated by their failure to take in adequate food and fluids. Patients at high risk for suicide and in need of rapid treatment are also candidates for ECT because it tends to work more quickly than antidepressant medication. There is growing evidence that the combination of ECT with antidepressant medication produces an even more robust response than either treatment alone.

Patients receive a course of 6–12 treatments at a rate of two to three per week, although the precise number is individualized based on response. A series of treatments can be administered in inpatient or outpatient settings, a determination that the physician and patient (and the patient's family) need to make. Generally, if the treatments are given in the outpatient setting, the patient should not be at risk for suicide, should have supportive family members available to help care for the patient at home, and should be medically stable. Some patients will be candidates for maintenance (or prophylactic) ECT to keep them from relapsing. Typically, these patients have failed multiple medication trials yet respond favorably to ECT. With prophylactic ECT, a treatment is given anywhere from once per week to once per month depending on the patient. Because mood disorders tend to be chronic or recurrent, maintenance treatment for some patients will be indefinite.

As many as 80%–90% of patients receiving ECT as a first-line treatment respond favorably, while those who have failed antidepressants have a 50%–60% response rate. Certain depressive symptoms are associated with a good response to ECT, including psychomotor agitation or retardation; nihilistic, somatic, or paranoid delusions; and acute onset of illness. ECT is not generally recommended for patients with chronic forms of depression or patients with serious personality disorders (e.g., borderline personality disorder).

Mania responds well to ECT, although its use is primarily reserved for patients not responding to medication. Similarly, patients with a schizoaffective disorder may benefit when medication has been ineffective. Schizophrenic patients are sometimes treated with ECT, particularly when a superimposed major depression or a catatonic syndrome is present. As a general rule, patients with schizophrenia of relatively

TABLE 21–8. Indications for electroconvulsive therapy (ECT)
Medication-refractory depression
Suicidal depression
Depression accompanied by refusal to eat or take fluids
Depression during pregnancy
History of positive response to ECT
Catatonic syndromes
Acute forms of schizophrenia
Mania unresponsive to medication
Psychotic or melancholic depression unresponsive to medication

brief duration (i.e., less than 18 months) respond better than those with more chronic forms of the illness, yet sometimes even patients with chronic schizophrenia will respond to ECT. Indications for ECT are summarized in Table 21–8.

Pre–Electroconvulsive Therapy Workup

Baseline screening should include a physical examination, basic laboratory tests (blood count and electrolytes), and an electrocardiogram. These will help to rule out physical disorders that may complicate ECT, reveal occult arrhythmias that may require monitoring during the procedure, or will uncover electrolyte abnormalities that need correcting prior to ECT such as hypokalemia. A chest X-ray should be obtained in patients with pulmonary disease. Spine films are no longer routinely obtained due to the rarity of fractures with current ECT protocols. Relative contraindications include recent myocardial infarction (i.e., within 1 month), unstable coronary artery disease, uncompensated congestive heart failure, uncontrolled hypertensive cardiovascular disease, and venous thrombosis. Space-occupying brain lesions and other causes of increased intracranial pressure, such as recent intracerebral hemorrhage, unstable aneurysms, or vascular malformations are the only absolute contraindications to ECT. Psychotropic medications may be continued, although benzodiazepines should be reduced to the lowest possible dose (or be discontinued altogether) because they can interfere with the induction of a seizure.

Electroconvulsive Therapy Procedure

ECT sessions are usually scheduled in the morning. The patient's bladder should be emptied, and he or she should not have had food or fluids for at least 6–8 hours before the procedure. The treatment team usually consists of a psychiatrist, an anesthesiologist (or nurse anesthetist), and a specially trained nursing team. The treatment area should have resuscitative equipment available.

Patients are anesthetized with a short-acting anesthetic (e.g., methohexital, etomidate), receive oxygen to prevent hypoxia, receive succinylcholine as a muscle relaxant to attenuate convulsions, and receive atropine or glycopyrrolate to reduce secretions and to prevent bradyarrhythmias. Glycopyrrolate does not cross the blood-brain barrier and may be associated with less postictal confusion than atropine in the elderly. After the patient is anesthetized, electrodes are placed on the scalp.

Two different electrode placements are commonly used. Bilateral placement involves placing the electrode on each side of the head over the parietal lobes. With unilateral placement, one electrode is placed over the right temple and the other is placed at the vertex of the skull. Right unilateral placement is associated with less post-ECT confusion and memory loss.

A brief electrical stimulus is applied after placement of the electrodes. A bidirectional pulse wave is given rather than a continuous sinusoidal waveform commonly used in the past because the pulse wave is associated with less cognitive impairment. Stimulation usually produces a 30- to 90-second tonic-clonic seizure. The seizure is accompanied by a period of bradycardia and a transient drop in blood pressure, followed by tachycardia and a rise in blood pressure. A rise in cerebrospinal fluid pressure parallels the rise in blood pressure. These physiological responses are attenuated by the pre-ECT medications. Minor arrhythmias are frequent but are seldom a problem.

Therapeutic Aspects of Electroconvulsive Therapy

For the treatment to be therapeutic, a seizure must occur. Furthermore, the electrical stimulus must involve sufficient energy. A process called *stimulus dosing* has been developed to deliver the amount of electricity needed to be therapeutic and yet keep the dose to the minimum required to induce a seizure. This will help minimize cognitive impairment. The unit of electrical charge is measured in millicoulombs (mC). Initially, several low doses are given, increasing the charge with each successive stimulation. The dose at which the patient seizes is called the *seizure threshold*. When using bilateral electrode placement, a patient will have a therapeutic response when the dosage is two and one-half times threshold, and about six times threshold when right unilateral placement is used.

Adverse Effects of Electroconvulsive Therapy

Adverse effects during ECT can include brief episodes of hypotension or hypertension, bradyarrhythmias, and tachyarrhythmias; these effects are rarely serious. Fractures were widely reported to occur during ECT-induced seizures in the past but are uncommon now because of the use of muscle relaxants. Other possible adverse effects include prolonged seizures, laryngospasm, and prolonged apnea due to pseudocholinesterase deficiency, a rare genetic disorder. Seizures lasting longer than 2 minutes should be terminated (e.g., with intravenous lorazepam, 1–2 mg). Immediately after treatment, patients experience postictal confusion. Headache, nausea, and muscle pain also may be experienced after ECT.

The most troublesome long-term effect of ECT is memory impairment. Because ECT disrupts new memories that have not been incorporated into long-term memory stores, ECT can cause anterograde and retrograde amnesia that is most dense around the time of treatment. The anterograde component usually clears quickly, but the retrograde amnesia can extend back to months before treatment. It is unclear if the memory loss is due to the ECT or to ongoing depressive symptoms. Not all patients experience amnesia, and unilateral electrode placement, modification of the pulse wave, and the use of low dosages of electricity, help to minimize any memory loss that occurs. All patients should be informed that permanent memory loss may occur.

ECT is generally viewed favorably by patients who have received it. In one study, nearly 80% of the patients believed that they were helped by ECT, and 80% said that they would not be reluctant to have it again. A substantial minority reported approaching the treatment with anxiety, yet more than 80% of the respondents found that it produced no more anxiety than a dental appointment.

■ Self-Assessment Questions

1. What is the presumed mechanism of action of the antipsychotics?
2. What are the common indications for antipsychotics?
3. How are the antipsychotics used in the treatment of acute psychosis? How are they used in maintenance treatment?
4. What are the common extrapyramidal side effects (EPS) that occur with antipsychotics? Describe the syndromes and discuss their clinical management.
5. What disorders can be treated with antidepressants? Why is the term *antidepressant* a misnomer?
6. What is the putative mechanism of action of the SSRIs? TCAs? MAOIs? Of other new agents?
7. Are blood levels of TCAs meaningful? When should they be obtained?
8. What are the common side effects of the SSRIs? TCAs? MAOIs?
9. What agent is associated with the occurrence of priapism? Why is this occurrence worrisome?
10. What are the typical plasma level ranges for lithium carbonate for acute treatment of mania? For maintenance treatment?
11. What are the common side effects of lithium? Of valproate? Of carbamazepine?
12. When is lamotrigine used? What are its side effects?
13. What are the commonly used anxiolytics? What are their indications? Contraindications?
14. Describe the adverse effects of anxiolytics. Are they dangerous in overdose?
15. What drugs are commonly used to manage extrapyramidal symptoms in patients receiving antipsychotics?
16. Describe how ECT is administered. What is the purpose of atropine (or glycopyrrolate)? Succinylcholine? Methohexital?
17. What conditions respond well to ECT? What are the adverse effects of ECT?

Bibliography

Introduction

Ackerknecht EH: Short History of Psychiatry. New York, Hafner, 1968

Alexander FG, Selesnick ST: The History of Psychiatry: An Evaluation of Psychiatric Thought and Practice From Prehistoric Times to the Present. New York, Harper & Row, 1966

Andreasen NC: The Broken Brain: The Biological Revolution in Psychiatry. New York, Harper & Row, 1984

Andreasen NC: Brave New Brain: Conquering Mental Illness in the Era of the Genome. New York, Oxford University Press, 2001

Murray CJL, Lopez AD: The Global Burden of Disease. Boston, MA, Harvard University Press, 1996

Pinel P: Treatise on Insanity. London, Messrs Cadell and Davies, 1806

Shorter E: A History of Psychiatry. New York, Wiley, 1997

Chapter 1:
Diagnosis and Classification

American Psychiatric Association: Diagnostic and Statistical Manual: Mental Disorders. Washington, DC, American Psychiatric Association, 1952

American Psychiatric Association: Diagnostic and Statistical Manual of Mental Disorders, 2nd Edition. Washington, DC, American Psychiatric Association, 1968

American Psychiatric Association: Diagnostic and Statistical Manual of Mental Disorders, 3rd Edition. Washington, DC, American Psychiatric Association, 1980

American Psychiatric Association: Diagnostic and Statistical Manual of Mental Disorders, 4th Edition. Washington, DC, American Psychiatric Association, 1994

American Psychiatric Association: Diagnostic and Statistical Manual of Mental Disorders, 5th Edition. Arlington, VA, American Psychiatric Association, 2013

Black DW, Grant JE: DSM-5 Guidebook: The Essential Companion to the Diagnostic and Statistical Manual of Mental Disorders, Fifth Edition. Washington DC, American Psychiatric Publishing, 2014

Decker H: The Making of DSM-III: A Diagnostic Manual's Conquest of American Psychiatry. New York, Oxford University Press, 2013

Feighner JP, Robins E, Guze SB, et al: Diagnostic criteria for use in psychiatric research. Arch Gen Psychiatry 26:57–63, 1972

Spitzer RL, Williams JBW, Skodol AE: DSM-III: the major achievements and an overview. Am J Psychiatry 137:151–164, 1980

Wilson M: DSM-III and the transformation of American psychiatry: a history. Am J Psychiatry 150:399–410, 1993

Chapter 2:
Interviewing and Assessment

American Psychiatric Association: Practice guidelines for the psychiatric evaluation of adults, second edition. Am J Psychiatry 163 (6 suppl):1–36, 2006

Andreasen NC: Thought, language, and communication disorders, I: clinical assessment, definition of terms, and evaluation of their reliability. Arch Gen Psychiatry 36:1315–1321, 1979

Andreasen NC: Negative symptoms in schizophrenia: definition and reliability. Arch Gen Psychiatry 39:784–788, 1982

Andreasen NC: The Scale for the Assessment of Negative Symptoms (SANS). Iowa City, The University of Iowa, 1983

Andreasen NC: The Scale for the Assessment of Positive Symptoms (SAPS). Iowa City, The University of Iowa, 1984

Campbell RJ: Campbell's Psychiatric Dictionary, 8th Edition. New York, Oxford University Press, 2003

Chisholm MS, Lyketsos CG: Systematic Psychiatric Evaluation: A Step by Step Guide to Applying the Perspectives of Psychiatry. Baltimore, MD, Johns Hopkins University Press, 2012

MacKinnon RA, Michels R, Buckley PJ: The Psychiatric Interview in Clinical Practice, 2nd Edition. Washington, DC, American Psychiatric Publishing, 2009

Othmer E, Othmer SC: The Clinical Interview Using DSM-IV-TR, Vol 1: Fundamentals. Washington, DC, American Psychiatric Publishing, 2002

Shea SC: Psychiatric Interviewing: The Art of Understanding. A Practical Guide for Psychiatrists, Psychologists, Counselors, Social Workers, Nurses, and Other Mental Health Professionals, 2nd Edition. Philadelphia, PA, WB Saunders, 1998

Trzepacz P, Baker RW: The Psychiatric Mental Status Examination. New York, Oxford University Press, 1993

Chapter 3: The Neurobiology and Genetics of Mental Illness

Andreasen NC (ed): Brain Imaging: Applications in Psychiatry. Washington, DC, American Psychiatric Press, 1989

Andreasen NC: Brave New Brain: Conquering Mental Illness in the Era of the Genome. New York, Oxford University Press, 2001

Andreasen NC: Research Advances in Genetics and Genomics: Implications for Psychiatry. Washington, DC, American Psychiatric Publishing, 2005

Baron M, Risch N, Hamburger R, et al: Genetic linkage between X-chromosome markers and bipolar affective illness. Nature 326:289–292, 1987

Björklund A, Hökfelt T, Swanson LW (eds): Integrated Systems of the CNS, Part 1 (Handbook of Chemical Neuroanatomy). Amsterdam, The Netherlands, Elsevier, 1987, p 5

Creese I, Burt DR, Snyder SH: Dopamine receptor binding predicts clinical and pharmacological potencies of anti-schizophrenic drugs. Science 192:481–483, 1972

Doane BK, Livingston KF: The Limbic System: Functional Organization and Clinical Disorders. New York, Raven, 1986

Egan MF, Kojima M, Callicott JH, et al: The BDNF Val66Met polymorphism affects activity-dependent secretion of BDNF and human memory and hippocampal function. Cell 112:257–269, 2003

Freeman JL, Perry GH, Feuk L, et al: Copy number variation: new insights in genome diversity. Genome Res 16:949–961, 2006

Freitag CM: The genetics of autistic disorders and its clinical relevance: a review of the literature. Mol Psychiatry 12:2–22, 2007

Fuster JM: The Prefrontal Cortex: Anatomy, Physiology, and Neuropsychology of the Frontal Lobe, 4th Edition. New York, Academic Press, 2008

Gottesman II, Shields J: Schizophrenia: The Epigenetic Puzzle. New York, Cambridge University Press, 1982

Gusella JF, Wexler NS, Conneally PM, et al: A polymorphic DNA marker genetically linked to Huntington's disease. Nature 306:234–238, 1983

Jones EG, Peters A (eds): Cerebral Cortex, Vol 6: Further Aspects of Cortical Function, Including Hippocampus. New York, Plenum, 1987

Kandel ER, Schwartz JH, Jessell TM: Principles of Neural Science, 4th Edition. New York, McGraw-Hill, 2000

Kennedy JL, Farrer LA, Andreasen NC, et al: The genetics of adult-onset neuropsychiatric disease: complexities and conundra? Science 302:822–826, 2003

Kety SS, Rosenthal D, Wender PH, et al: Mental illness in the biological and adoptive families of adopted schizophrenics. Am J Psychiatry 128:302–306, 1971

Levinson DF, Levinson MD, Segurado R, et al: Genome scan meta-analysis of schizophrenia and bipolar disorder, part I: methods and power analysis. Am J Hum Genet 73:17–33, 2003

McGuffin P, Owen MJ, Gottesman II: Psychiatric Genetics and Genomics. Oxford, UK, and New York, Oxford University Press, 2002

Nauta WJH, Feirtag M: Fundamental Neuroanatomy. New York, WH Freeman, 1986

Schlaepfer TE, Nemeroff CB: Neurobiology of Psychiatric Disorders. New York, Elsevier, 2012

Seeman P, Lee T, Chau-Wong M, et al: Antipsychotic drug doses and neuroleptic-dopamine receptors. Nature 261:717–719, 1976

Suarez BK, Duan J, Sanders AR, et al: Genomewide scan of 409 European-American and African American families with schizophrenia: suggestive evidence of linkage at 8p23.3-p21.2 and 11p13.1-q14.1 in the combined sample. Am J Hum Genet 78:315–333, 2006

Sutcliffe JS: Insights into the pathogenesis of autism. Science 321:208–209, 2008

Walsh T, McClellan JM, McCarthy JE, et al: Rare structural variants disrupt multiple genes in neurodevelopmental pathways in schizophrenia. Science 320:539–543, 2008

Chapter 4: Neurodevelopmental (Child) Disorders

Abbeduto L, McDuffie A: Genetic syndromes associated with intellectual disabilities, in Handbook of Medical Neuropsychology: Applications of Cognitive Neuroscience. Edited by Armstrong CL, Morrow L, New York, Springer, 2010, pp 193–221

Association on Intellectual and Developmental Disabilities: Intellectual Disability: Definition, Classification, and Systems of Support, 11th Edition. Washington, DC, American Association on Intellectual and Developmental Disabilities, 2010

Barkley RA, Fischer M, Smallish L, et al: Does the treatment of attention-deficit hyperactivity disorder with stimulants contribute to drug use/abuse? A 13-year prospective study. Pediatrics 111:97–109, 2003

Berninger VW, May MO: Evidence-based diagnosis and treatment for specific learning disabilities involving impairments in written and/or oral language. J Learn Disabil 44:167-183, 2011

Biederman J, Monuteaux MC, Spencer T, et al: Stimulant therapy and risk for subsequent substance use disorders in male adults with ADHD: a naturalistic controlled 10-year follow-up study. Am J Psychiatry 165:597–603, 2008

Bishop DVM: Pragmatic language impairment: a correlate of SLI, a distinct subgroup, or part of the autistic continuum? in Speech and Language Impairments in Children: Causes, Characteristics, Intervention, and Outcome. Edited by Bishop DVM, Leonard LB. East Sussex, England, Psychology Press, 2000, pp 99–113

Boyle CA, Boulet S, Schieve LA, et al: Trends in the prevalence of developmental disabilities in US children, 1997–2008. Pediatr 127:1034–1042, 2011

Canino G, Shrout PE, Rubio-Stipec M, et al: The DSM-IV rates of child and adolescent disorders in Puerto Rico. Arch Gen Psychiatry 61:85–93, 2004

Cantell MH, Smyth MM, Ahonen TP: Two distinct pathways for developmental coordination disorder: persistence and resolution. Hum Mov Sci 22:413–431, 2003

Cepeda C: Clinical Manual for the Psychiatric Interview of Children and Adolescents. Washington, DC, American Psychiatric Publishing, 2009

Compton DL, Fuchs LS, Fuchs D, et al: The cognitive and academic profiles of reading and mathematics learning disabilities. J Learn Disabil 45:79–95, 2012

Deprey L, Ozonoff S: Assessment of psychiatric conditions in autism spectrum disorders in Assessment of Autism Spectrum Disorders. Edited by Goldstein S, Naglieri J, Ozonoff S, New York, Guilford Press, 2009, pp 290–317

Dulcan M (ed): Dulcan's Textbook of Child and Adolescent Psychiatry. Washington, DC, American Psychiatric Publishing, 2010

Elsabbagh M, Divan G, Koh, Y-J, et al: Global prevalence of autism and other pervasive developmental disorders. Autism Res 5:160–179, 2012

Findling RL (ed): Clinical Manual of Child and Adolescent Psychopharmacology. Washington, DC, American Psychiatric Publishing, 2008

Findling RL, Aman MG, Eerdekens M, et al: Long-term, open-label study of risperidone in children with severe disruptive behaviors and below-average IQ. Am J Psychiatry 111:677–684, 2004

Geller B, Tillman R, Bolhofner K, et al: Child bipolar I disorder: prospective continuity with adult bipolar I disorder; characteristics of second and third episodes; predictors of 8-year outcome. Arch Gen Psychiatry 65:1125–1133, 2008

Gerber PJ: The impact of learning disabilities on adulthood: a review of the evidenced-based literature for research and practice in adult education. J Learn Disabil 45:31–46, 2012

Ghaziuddin M: Asperger disorder in the DSM-5: sacrificing utility for validity. J Am Acad Child Adolesc Psychiatry 50:192–193, 2011

Gizer IR, Ficks C, Waldman ID: Candidate gene studies of ADHD: a meta-analytic review. Hum Genet 126:51–90, 2009

Greenspan SI, Wieder S: Infant and Early Childhood Mental Health: A Comprehensive Developmental Approach to Assessment and Intervention. Washington, DC, American Psychiatric Publishing, 2006

Halmøy A, Klungsøyr K, Skjærven R, et al: Pre- and perinatal risk factors in adults with attention-deficit/hyperactivity disorder. J Biol Psychiatry 71:474–481, 2012

Hollander E, Kalevzon A, Coyle JT (eds): Textbook of Autism Spectrum Disorders. Washington, DC, American Psychiatric Publishing, 2011

Howlin P, Goode S, Hutton J, et al: Adult outcome for children with autism. J Child Psychol Psychiatry 45:212–229, 2004

Kanner L: Autistic disturbances of affective contact. Nerv Child 2:217–250, 1943

Leckman JF, Bloch MH, Smith ME, et al: Neurobiological substrates of Tourette's disorder. J Child Adolesc Psychopharmacol 20:237–247, 2010

McDougle CJ, Scahill L, Aman MG, et al: Risperidone for the core symptom domains of autism: results from the study by the Autism Network of the Research Units on Pediatric Psychopharmacology. Am J Psychiatry 162:1142–1148, 2005

McGough JJ, Barkley RA: Diagnostic controversies in adult attention deficit hyperactivity disorder. Am J Psychiatry 161:1948–1956, 2004

McNaught KS, Mink JW: Advances in understanding and treatment of Tourette syndrome. Nat Rev Neurol 7:667–676, 2011

McPheeters ML, Warren Z, Sathe N, et al: A systematic review of medical treatments for children with autism spectrum disorders. Pediatrics 127:e1312–e1321, 2011

Morrato EH, Libby AM, Orton HD, et al: Frequency of provider contact after FDA advisory on risk of pediatric suicidality with SSRIs. Am J Psychiatry 165:42–50, 2008

Newcorn JH, Kratochvil CJ, Allen AJ, et al: Atomoxetine and osmotically released methylphenidate for the treatment of attention deficit hyperactivity disorder: acute comparison and differential response. Am J Psychiatry 165:721–730, 2008

O'Rourke JA, Scharf JM, Yu D, et al: The genetics of Tourette syndrome: a review. J Psychosom Res 67:533–545, 2009

Piven J, Nehme E, Siman J, et al: Magnetic resonance imaging in autism: measurement of the cerebellum, pons, and fourth ventricle. Biol Psychiatry 31:491–504, 1992

Swedo SE, Leonard HL, Garvey M, et al: Pediatric autoimmune neuropsychiatric disorders associated with streptococcal infections: clinical description of the first 50 cases. Am J Psychiatry 154:264–271, 1998

Vismara LA, Rogers SJ: Behavioral treatments in autism spectrum disorder: What do we know? Annu Rev Clin Psychology 6:447–468, 2010

Volkmar F, Klin A, Schultz RT, et al: Asperger's disorder. Am J Psychiatry 157:262–267, 2000

Wassink TH, Hazlett HC, Epping EA, et al: Cerebral cortical gray matter overgrowth and functional variation of the serotonin transporter gene in autism. Arch Gen Psychiatry 64:709–717, 2007

Willcutt G: The prevalence of DSM-IV Attention-Deficit/Hyperactivity Disorder: a meta-analytic review. Neurotherapeutics 9:490–499, 2012

Chapter 5: Schizophrenia Spectrum and Other Psychotic Disorders

Agerbo E, Byrne M, Eaton WW, et al: Marital and labor market status in the long run in schizophrenia. Arch Gen Psychiatry 61:28–31, 2004

Andreasen NC: The Broken Brain: The Biologic Revolution in Psychiatry. New York, Harper & Row, 1984

Andreasen NC: The diagnosis of schizophrenia. Schizophr Bull 13:9–22, 1987

Andreasen NC: Understanding the causes of schizophrenia. N Engl J Med 340:645–647, 1999

Andreasen NC, Liu D, Ziebell S, et al: Relapse duration, treatment intensity, and brain tissue loss in schizophrenia: a prospective longitudinal MRI study. Am J Psychiatry 170:609–615, 2013

Andreasen NC, O'Leary DS, Cizadlo T, et al: Schizophrenia and cognitive dysmetria: a positron-emission tomography study of dysfunctional prefrontal-thalamic-cerebellar circuitry. Proc Natl Acad Sci U S A 93:9985–9990, 1996

Coldwell CM, Bender DL: The effectiveness of assertive community treatment for homeless populations with severe mental illness: a meta-analysis. Am J Psychiatry 164:393–399, 2007

Coryell WH, Tsuang MT: Outcome after 40 years in DSM-III schizophreniform disorder. Arch Gen Psychiatry 43:324–328, 1986

Csernanski JG, Schindler MK, Splinter NR, et al: Abnormalities of thalamic volume and shape in schizophrenia. Am J Psychiatry 161:896–902, 2004

Essock SM, Covell NH, Davis SM, et al: Effectiveness of switching antipsychotic medications. Am J Psychiatry 163:2090–2095, 2006

Evans JD, Heaton RK, Paulsen JS, et al: Schizoaffective disorder: a form of schizophrenia or affective disorder? J Clin Psychiatry 60:874–882, 1999

Flashman LA, Flaum M, Gupta S, et al: Soft signs and neuropsychological performance in schizophrenia. Am J Psychiatry 153:526–532, 1996

Goldman-Rakic PS: Working memory dysfunction in schizophrenia. J Neuropsychiatry Clin Neurosci 6:348–357, 1994

Green AI, Drake RE, Brunette MF, et al: Schizophrenia and co-occurring substance use disorder. Am J Psychiatry 164:402–408, 2007

Harrison PJ, Weinberger DR: Schizophrenia genes, gene expression, and neuropathology: on the matter of their convergence. Mol Psychiatry 10:40–68, 2005

Hirsch SR, Weinberger DR (eds): Schizophrenia, 2nd Edition. Oxford, UK, Blackwell Science, 2003

Hogarty GE, Flesher S, Ulrich R, et al: Cognitive enhancement therapy for schizophrenia: effect of a 2-year randomized trial on cognition and behavior. Arch Gen Psychiatry 61:866–876, 2004

Holzman PS, Levy DL, Proctor LR: Smooth pursuit eye movements, attention, and schizophrenia. Arch Gen Psychiatry 45:641–647, 1976

Huxley NA, Rendall M, Sederer L: Psychosocial treatments in schizophrenia: a review of the past 20 years. J Nerv Ment Dis 188:187–201, 2000

Kane JM: New-onset schizophrenia: pharmacologic treatment. Focus 6:167–171, 2008

Kasanin J: The acute schizoaffective psychoses. Am J Psychiatry 90:97–126, 1933

Kendler KS: Demography of paranoid psychoses (delusional disorder). Arch Gen Psychiatry 39:890–902, 1982

Langfeldt G: Schizophreniform States. Copenhagen, Denmark, E Munksgaard, 1939

Lauriello J, Pallanti S (eds): Clinical Manual for Treatment of Schizophrenia. Washington, DC, American Psychiatric Publishing, 2012

Levinson DF, Mahtani MM, Nancarrow DJ, et al: Genome scan of schizophrenia. Am J Psychiatry 155:741–750, 1998

Lieberman JA: Neurobiology and the natural history of schizophrenia. J Clin Psychiatry 67:e14, 2006

Lieberman JA, Stroup TS, Perkins DO (eds): Essentials of Schizophrenia. Washington, DC, American Psychatric Publishing, 2012

McElroy SL, Keck PE Jr, Strakowski SM: An overview of the treatment of schizoaffective disorder. J Clin Psychiatry 60 (suppl):16–21, 1999

McGlashan TH: The Chestnut Lodge follow-up study, II: long-term outcome in schizophrenia and the affective disorders. Arch Gen Psychiatry 41:586–601, 1984

McNeil TF, Cantor-Graae E, Weinberger DR: Relationship of obstetric complications and differences in size of brain structures in monozygotic twin pairs discordant for schizophrenia. Am J Psychiatry 157:203–212, 2000

McGuire PK, Frith CD: Disordered functional connectivity in schizophrenia. Psychol Med 26:663–667, 1996

Meltzer HY, Alphs L, Green AI, et al: Clozapine treatment for suicidality in schizophrenia: International Suicide Prevention Trial (InterSePT). Arch Gen Psychiatry 60:82–91, 2003

Montross LP, Zisook S, Kasckow J: Suicide among patients with schizophrenia: a consideration of risk and protective factors. Ann Clin Psychiatry 17:173–182, 2005

Munoz RA, Amado H, Hyatt S: Brief reactive psychosis. J Clin Psychiatry 48:324–327, 1987

Munro A: Psychiatric disorders characterized by delusions: treatment in relation to specific types. Psychiatr Ann 22:232–240, 1992

Murray CJL, Lopez AD: The Global Burden of Disease. Boston, MA, Harvard University Press, 1996

Nicholson R, Lenane M, Singaracharlu S, et al: Premorbid speech and language impairment in childhood-onset schizophrenia associated with risk factors. Am J Psychiatry 157:794–800, 2000

Opjordsmoen S: Long-term course and outcome in delusional disorder. Acta Psychiatr Scand 78:556–586, 1988

Penn DL, Mueser KT: Research update on the psychosocial treatment of schizophrenia. Am J Psychiatry 153:607–617, 1996

Selemon LD, Rajkowska G, Goldman-Rakic S: Abnormally high neuronal density in the schizophrenic cortex. Arch Gen Psychiatry 52:805–818, 1995

Staal W, Hulshoff HE, Schnack HG, et al: Structural brain abnormalities in patients with schizophrenia and their healthy siblings. Am J Psychiatry 157:416–421, 2000

Stroup TS, Lieberman JA, McEvoy JP, et al: Effectiveness of olanzapine, quetiapine, and risperidone in patients with chronic schizophrenia after discontinuing perphenazine: a CATIE study. Am J Psychiatry 164:415–427, 2007

Turetsky BI, Calkins ME, Light GA, et al: Neurophysiological endophenotypes of schizophrenia: the viability of selected candidate measures. Schizophr Bull 33:69–94, 2007

Winokur G: Familial psychopathology and delusional disorder. Compr Psychiatry 26:241–248, 1985

Wright IC, Rabe-Hesketh S, Woodruff P, et al: Meta-analysis of regional brain volumes in schizophrenia. Am J Psychiatry 157:16–25, 2000

Zhang-Wong J, Beiser M, Bean M, et al: Five-year course of schizophreniform disorder. Psychiatry Res 59:109–117, 1995

Chapter 6: Mood Disorders

American Psychiatric Association: Practice guideline for the treatment of patients with bipolar disorder (revision). Am J Psychiatry 159 (4 Suppl):1–50, 2002

American Psychiatric Association: Practice guidelines for the treatment of patients with major depressive disorder, 3rd Edition. Arlington, VA, American Psychiatric Association, 2010

Baxter LR, Schwartz JM, Phelps ME, et al: Reduction of prefrontal cortex glucose metabolism common to three types of depression. Arch Gen Psychiatry 46:243–250, 1989

Coppen AJ, Doogan DP: Serotonin and its place in the pathogenesis of depression. J Clin Psychiatry 49 (suppl):4–11, 1988

Coryell W, Young EA: Clinical predictors of suicide in primary major depressive disorder. J Clin Psychiatry 66:412–417, 2005

Coryell W, Solomon D, Turvey C, et al: The long-term course of rapid-cycling bipolar disorder. Arch Gen Psychiatry 60:914–920, 2003

Drevets WC, Videen TO, Price JL, et al: A functional anatomical study of unipolar depression. J Neurosci 12:3628–3641, 1992

Germain A, Nofzinger EA, Kupfer DJ, et al: Neurobiology of non-REM sleep in depression: further evidence for hypofrontality and thalamic dysregulation. Am J Psychiatry 161:1856–1863, 2004

Gijsman HJ, Geddes JR, Rendell JM, et al: Antidepressants for bipolar depression: systematic review of randomized, controlled trials. Am J Psychiatry 161:1537–1547, 2004

Goldberg JF, Perlis RH, Bowden CL, et al: Manic symptoms during depressive episodes in 1,380 patients with bipolar disorder: findings from the STEP-BD. Am J Psychiatry 166:173–181, 2009

Golden RN, Goynes BN, Ekstrom RD, et al: The efficacy of light therapy in the treatment of mood disorder: a review and meta-analysis of the evidence. Am J Psychiatry 162:656–662, 2005

Goodwin FK, Jamison KR: Manic-Depressive Illness: Bipolar Disorders and Recurrent Depression, 2nd Edition. New York, Oxford University Press, 2007

Kelsoe JR, Ginns EI, Egeland JA, et al: Re-evaluation of the linkage relationship between chromosome 11p loci and the gene for bipolar affective disorder in the Old Order Amish. Nature 342:238–243, 1989

Kennedy SH, Giacobbe P: Treatment resistant depression: advances in somatic therapy. Ann Clin Psychiatry 19:279–287, 2007

Ketter TA (ed): Handbook of Diagnosis and Treatment of Bipolar Disorder. Washington, DC, American Psychiatric Publishing, 2010

Klein DN, Schwartz JE, Rose S, et al: Five-year course and outcome of dysthymic disorder: a prospective naturalistic follow-up study. Am J Psychiatry 157:931–939, 2000

Li X, Frye MA, Shelton RC: Review of pharmacological treatment in mood disorders and future directions for drug development. Neuropsychopharmacology 37:77–101, 2012

Nemeroff CB: The role of corticotropin-releasing factor in the pathogenesis of major depression. Pharmacopsychiatry 21:76–82, 1988

Plante DT, Winkelman JW: Sleep disturbance in bipolar disorder: therapeutic implications. Am J Psychiatry 165:830–843, 2008

Pompallona S, Bollini P, Tibaldi G, et al: Combined pharmacotherapy and psychological treatment for depression: a systematic review. Arch Gen Psychiatry 61:714–719, 2004

Posternak MA, Zimmerman M: Is there a delay in the antidepressant effect? A meta-analysis. J Clin Psychiatry 66:148–158, 2005

Quitkin FM, McGrath PJ, Stewart JW, et al: Remission rates with three consecutive antidepressant trials: effectiveness for depressed outpatients. J Clin Psychiatry 66:670–676, 2005

Rosa MA, Lisanby SH: Somatic treatments for mood disorders. Neuropsychopharmacology 37:102–116, 2012

Rush AJ, Marangell LB, Sackeim HA, et al: Vagus nerve stimulation for treatment-resistant depression: a randomized, controlled acute phase trial. Biol Psychiatry 58:347–354, 2005

Schneck CD, Miklowitz DJ, Miyahara S, et al: The prospective course of rapid cycling bipolar disorder: findings from the STEP-BD. Am J Psychiatry 165:370–377, 2008

Solomon DA, Lean AC, Moeller TI, et al: Tachyphylaxis in unipolar major depressive disorder. J Clin Psychiatry 66:283–290, 2005

Terman M, Terman JS: Light therapy for seasonal and non-seasonal depression: efficacy, protocol, safety, and side effects. CNS Spectr 10:647–663, 2005

Trivedi MH, Thase ME, Fava M, et al: Adjunctive aripiprazole in major depressive disorder: analysis of efficacy and safety in patients with anxious and atypical features. J Clin Psychiatry 69:1928–1936, 2008

Vos T, Haby MM, Barendregt JJ, et al: The burden of major depression avoidable by longer-term treatment strategies. Arch Gen Psychiatry 61:1097–1103, 2004

Winokur G, Tsuang MT: The Natural History of Mania, Depression, and Schizophrenia. Washington, DC, American Psychiatric Press, 1996

Chapter 7: Anxiety Disorders

American Psychiatric Association: Practice guideline for the treatment of patients with panic disorder, second edition. Am J Psychiatry 166 (suppl):5–68, 2009

Baldwin D, Bobes J, Stein DJ, et al: Paroxetine in social phobia/social anxiety disorder: randomised, double-blind, placebo-controlled study. Paroxetine Study Group. Br J Psychiatry 175:120–126, 1999

Burns LE, Thorpe GL: The epidemiology of fears and phobias (with particular reference to the National Survey of Agoraphobics). J Int Med Res 5 (suppl): 1–7, 1977

DaCosta JM: On irritable heart: a clinical study of a form of functional cardiac disorder and its consequences. Am J Med Sci 61:17–52, 1871

Fyer AJ, Mannuzza S, Gallops MS, et al: Familial transmission of simple phobias and fears: a preliminary report. Arch Gen Psychiatry 47:252–256, 1990

Heimberg RG, Liebowitz MR, Hope DA, et al: Cognitive behavioral group therapy vs. phenelzine therapy for social phobia: 12-week outcome. Arch Gen Psychiatry 55:1133–1141, 1998

Hettema JM, Prescott CA, Myers JM, et al: The structure of genetic and environmental risk factors for anxiety disorders in men and women. Arch Gen Psychiatry 62:182–189, 2005

Katon WJ, Van Korff M, Lin E: Panic disorder: relationship to high medical utilization. Am J Med 92 (suppl):7S–11S, 1992

Klein DF: False suffocation alarms, spontaneous panics, and related conditions: an integrative hypothesis. Arch Gen Psychiatry 50:306–317, 1993

Lee MA, Flegel P, Greden JF, et al: Anxiogenic effects of caffeine on panic and depressed patients. Am J Psychiatry 145:632–635, 1988

Liebowitz MR, Gelenberg AJ, Munjack D: Venlafaxine extended release vs. placebo and paroxetine in social anxiety disorder. Arch Gen Psychiatry 62:190–198, 2005

Manicavasagar VC, Marnane C, Pini S, et al: Adult separation anxiety disorder: a disorder comes of age. Curr Psychiatry Rep 12:290–297, 2010

Noyes R, Clancy J, Garvey MJ, et al: Is agoraphobia a variant of panic disorder or a separate illness? J Affect Disord 1:3–13, 1987a

Noyes R, Clarkson C, Crowe R, et al: A family study of generalized anxiety disorder. Am J Psychiatry 144:119–124, 1987b

Nutt DJ, Bell CJ, Malizia AC: Brain mechanisms of social anxiety disorder. J Clin Psychiatry 59 (suppl):4–9, 1998

Ravindran LN, Stein MB: The pharmacologic treatment of anxiety disorders: a review of progress. J Clin Psychiatry 71:839–854, 2010

Roberson-Nay RL, Eaves LJ, Hettema JM, et al: Childhood separation anxiety disorder and adult onset panic attacks share a common genetic diathesis. Depress Anxiety 29:320–327, 2012

Schumacher J, Kristensen AS, Wendland JR, et al: The genetics of panic disorder. J Med Genet 48:361–368, 2011

Seddon K, Nutt D: Pharmacologic treatment of panic disorder. Psychiatry 6:198–203, 2007

Stein DJ, Hollander E, Rothbaum BO (eds): Textbook of Anxiety Disorders, 2nd Edition. Washington, DC, American Psychiatric Publishing, 2010

Stein MB, Chartier MJ, Hazen AL: A direct-interview family study of generalized social phobia. Am J Psychiatry 155:90–97, 1998

Yates WR: Phenomenology and epidemiology of panic disorder. Ann Clin Psychiatry 21:95–102, 2009

Chapter 8: Obsessive-Compulsive and Related Disorders

Akhtar S, Wig NN, Varma VK, et al: A phenomenological analysis of symptoms in obsessive-compulsive neurosis. Br J Psychiatry 127:342–348, 1975

American Psychiatric Association: Practice guideline for the treatment of patients with obsessive-compulsive disorder. Am J Psychiatry 164 (7 suppl):5–53, 2007

Andreasen NC, Bardach J: Dysmorphophobia: symptom or disease? Am J Psychiatry 134:673–676, 1977

Dougherty DD, Baer L, Cosgrove GR, et al: Prospective long-term follow-up of 44 patients who received cingulotomy for treatment-refractory obsessive-compulsive disorder. Am J Psychiatry 159:269–275, 2002

Grant J, Phillips KA: Recognizing and treating body dysmorphic disorder. Ann Clin Psychiatry 17:205–210, 2005

Grant JE, Stein DJ, Woods DW, Keuthen NJ: Trichotillomania, Skin Picking, and Other Body-Focused Repetitive Behaviors. Washington, DC, American Psychiatric Publishing, 2012

Kessler RC, Chiu WT, Demler O, et al: Prevalence, severity, and comorbidity of 12-month DSM-IV disorders in the National Comorbidity Survey replication. Arch Gen Psychiatry 62:617–627, 2005

Keuthen NJ, O'Sullivan RL, Goodchild P, et al: Retrospective review of treatment outcome for 63 patients with trichotillomania. Am J Psychiatry 155:560–561, 1998

Osborn I: Tormenting Thoughts and Secret Rituals. New York, Dell, 1998

Phillips KA: The Broken Mirror: Understanding and Treating Body Dysmorphic Disorder, Revised and Expanded Edition. New York, Oxford University Press, 2005

Phillips KA, Didie ER, Feusner J, et al: Body dysmorphic disorder: treating an underrecognized disorder. Am J Psychiatry 165:1111–1118, 2008

Rappoport JL: The Boy Who Couldn't Stop Washing. New York, EP Dutton, 1989

Rasmussen SA, Eisen JL: Epidemiology and clinical features of obsessive-compulsive disorder, in Obsessive-Compulsive Disorders: Theory and Management, 3rd Edition. Edited by Jenike MA, Baer L, Minichiello WE. St. Louis, MO, Mosby, 1998, pp 12–43

Ruck C, Karlsson A, Steele JD, et al: Capsulotomy for obsessive-compulsive disorder. Arch Gen Psychiatry 65:914–922, 2008

Schwartz JM, Stoessel PW, Baxter LR, et al: Systematic changes in cerebral glucose metabolic rate after successful behavior modification treatment of obsessive-compulsive disorder. Arch Gen Psychiatry 53:109–113, 1996

Simpson HB, Foa EB, Liebowitz MR, et al: A randomized, controlled trial of cognitive-behavioral therapy for augmenting pharmacotherapy in obsessive-compulsive disorder. Am J Psychiatry 165:621–630, 2008

Skoog G, Skoog I: A 40-year follow-up of patients with obsessive-compulsive disorder. Arch Gen Psychiatry 56:121–127, 1999

Swedo SE, Leonard HL, Garvey M: Pediatric autoimmune neuropsychiatric disorders associated with streptococcal infections: clinical descriptions of the first 50 cases. Am J Psychiatry 155:264–271, 1998

Vulink NC, Denys D, Fluitman SB, et al: Quetiapine augments the effect of citalopram in non-refractory obsessive-compulsive disorder: a randomized, double-blind, placebo-controlled study of 76 patients. J Clin Psychiatry 70:1001–1008, 2009

Chapter 9: Trauma- and Stressor-Related Disorders

American Psychiatric Association: Practice guideline for the treatment of patients with acute stress disorder and posttraumatic stress disorder. Am J Psychiatry 161 (11 suppl):3–31, 2004

Andreasen NC: What is post-traumatic stress disorder? Dialogues Clin Neurosci 13:240–243, 2011

Andreasen NC, Hoenk PR: The predictive value of adjustment disorders: a follow-up study. Am J Psychiatry 139:584–590, 1982

Andreasen NC, Wasek P: Adjustment disorders in adolescents and adults. Arch Gen Psychiatry 37:1166–1170, 1980

Brady K, Pearlstein T, Asnis GM, et al: Efficacy and safety of sertraline treatment of posttraumatic stress disorder: a randomized controlled trial. JAMA 283:1837–1844, 2000

Bryant RA, Sackville T, Dang ST, et al: Treating acute stress disorder: an evaluation of cognitive behavior therapy and supportive counseling techniques. Am J Psychiatry 156:1780–1786, 1999

Bryant RA, Creamer M, O'Donnell ML, et al: A multisite study of the capacity of the acute stress disorder diagnosis to predict posttraumatic stress disorder. J Clin Psychiatry 69:923–929, 2008

Despland JN, Monod L, Ferrero F: Clinical relevance of adjustment disorder in DSM-III-R and DSM-IV. Compr Psychiatry 36:454–460, 1995

Ehlers A, Clark DM, Hackmann A, et al: A randomized controlled trial of cognitive therapy, a self-help booklet, and repeated assessments as early interventions for posttraumatic stress disorder. Arch Gen Psychiatry 60:1024–1032, 2003

Greenberg WM, Rosenfeld DN, Ortega EA: Adjustment disorder as an admission diagnosis. Am J Psychiatry 152:459–461, 1995

Heim C, Nemeroff CB: Neurobiology of posttraumatic stress disorder. CNS Spectr 14 (suppl 1):13–24, 2009

Jones R, Yates WR, Zhou HH: Readmission rates for adjustment disorder with depressed mood: comparison with other mood disorders. J Affect Disord 71:199–203, 2002

Kessler RC, Chiu WT, Demler O, et al: Prevalence, severity, and comorbidity of 12-month DSM-IV disorders in the National Comorbidity Survey replication. Arch Gen Psychiatry 62:617–627, 2005

Kovacs M, Ho V, Pollock MH: Criterion and predictive validity of the diagnosis of adjustment disorder: a prospective study of youths with new-onset insulin dependent diabetes mellitus. Am J Psychiatry 152:523–528, 1995

Marks I, Lovell K, Moshirvani H, et al: Treatment of posttraumatic stress disorder by exposure and/or cognitive restructuring: a controlled study. Arch Gen Psychiatry 55:317–325, 1998

Mohamed S, Rosenheck RA: Pharmacotherapy of PTSD in the U.S. Department of Veterans Affairs: diagnostic- and symptom-guided drug selection. J Clin Psychiatry 69:959–965, 2008

North C, Pfeffenbaum B, Tivis L, et al: The course of posttraumatic stress disorder in a follow-up study of survivors of the Oklahoma City bombing. Ann Clin Psychiatry 16:209–215, 2004

North CS, Suris AM, Davis M, et al: Toward validation of the diagnosis of post-traumatic stress disorder. Am J Psychiatry 166:34–41, 2009

Oxman TE, Barrett JE, Freeman DH, et al: Frequency and correlates of adjustment disorder related to cardiac surgery in older patients. Psychosomatics 35:557–568, 1994

Pelkonen M, Marttunen M, Henricksson M, et al: Adolescent adjustment disorder: precipitant stressors and distress symptoms in 89 outpatients. Eur Psychiatry 22:288–295, 2007

Raskind MA, Peskind ER, Hoff DJ, et al: A parallel group placebo controlled study of prazosin for trauma nightmares and sleep disturbance in combat veterans with post-traumatic stress disorder. Biol Psychiatry 61:928–934, 2007

Stein DJ, Hollander E, Rothbaum BO (eds): Textbook of Anxiety Disorders, 2nd Edition. Washington, DC, American Psychiatric Publishing, 2010

Chapter 10: Somatic Symptom Disorders and Dissociative Disorders

Allen LA, Escobar JI, Lehrer PM, et al: Psychosocial treatments for multiple unexplained physical symptoms: a review of the literature. Psychosom Med 64:939–950, 2002

Andreasen PJ, Seidel JA: Behavioral techniques in the treatment of patients with multiple personality disorder. Ann Clin Psychiatry 4:29–32, 1992

Barsky AJ, Fama JM, Bailey ED, et al: A prospective 4- to 5-year study of DSM-III-R hypochondriasis. Arch Gen Psychiatry 55:737–744, 1998

Boysen GA, Vanbergen A: A review of published research on adult dissociative identity disorder: 2000–2010. J Nerv Ment Dis 201:5–11, 2013

Brand BL, Classen CC, McNary SW, et al: A review of dissociative disorders treatment studies. J Nerv Ment Dis 197:646–654, 2009

Butler LD: Normative dissociation. Psychiatr Clin North Am 29:45–62, 2006

Coons PM, Bohman ES, Milstein V: Multiple personality disorder: a clinical investigation of 50 cases. J Nerv Ment Dis 176:519–527, 1988

DeWaal MWM, Arnold IA, Eekhof JAH, et al: Somatoform disorders in general practice. Br J Psychiatry 184:470–476, 2004

Dimsdale JE, Xin Y, Kleinman A, et al (eds): Somatic Presentations of Mental Disorders: Refining the Research Agenda for DSM-5. Arlington, VA, American Psychiatric Association, 2009

Ellason JW, Ross CA: Two year follow-up of inpatients with dissociative identity disorder. Am J Psychiatry 154:832–839, 1997

Foote B, Smolin Y, Kaplan M, et al: Prevalence of dissociative disorders in psychiatric outpatients. Am J Psychiatry 163:623–629, 2006

Guralnik O, Schmeidler J, Simeon D: Feeling unreal: cognitive processes in depersonalization. Am J Psychiatry 157:103–109, 2000

Henningsen P, Jakobsen T, Schiltenwolf M, et al: Somatization revisited: diagnosis and perceived causes of common mental disorders. J Nerv Ment Dis 193:85–92, 2005

Krem MM: Motor conversion disorders reviewed from a neuropsychiatric prospective. J Clin Psychiatry 65:783–790, 2004

Lauer J, Black DW, Keen P: Multiple personality disorder and borderline personality disorder: distinct entities or variations on a common theme? Ann Clin Psychiatry 5:129–134, 1993

Lowenstein RJ: Psychopharmacologic treatments of dissociative identity disorder. Psychiatr Ann 35:666–673, 2005

Noyes R, Reich J, Clancy J, et al: Reduction in hypochondriasis with treatment of panic disorder. Br J Psychiatry 149:631–635, 1986

Noyes R, Holt CS, Kathol RG: Somatization: diagnosis and management. Arch Gen Psychiatry 4:790–795, 1995

Piper A: Multiple personality disorder. Br J Psychiatry 164:600–612, 1994

Pope HG Jr, Jonas JM, Jones B: Factitious psychosis: phenomenology, family history, and long-term outcome of nine patients. Am J Psychiatry 139:1480–1483, 1982

Reich P, Gottfried LA: Factitious disorders in a teaching hospital. Ann Intern Med 99:240–247, 1983

Ross CA, Miller SD, Reagor P, et al: Structured interview data on 102 cases of multiple personality disorder from four centers. Am J Psychiatry 147:596–601, 1990

Schreiber FR: Sybil. Chicago, IL, Henry Regnery, 1973

Shah KA, Forman MB, Freedman HS: Munchausen's syndrome and cardiac catheterization: a case of a pernicious interaction. JAMA 248:3008–3009, 1982

Sierra M, Berrios GE: Depersonalization: neurobiologic perspectives. Biol Psychiatry 44:898–908, 1998

Simeon D, Gross S, Guralnik O, et al: Feeling unreal: 30 cases of DSM-III-R depersonalization disorder. Am J Psychiatry 154:1107–1113, 1997

Simeon D, Stein DJ, Hollander E: Treatment of depersonalization disorder with clomipramine. Biol Psychiatry 44:302–303, 1998

Simeon D, Guralnik O, Schneider J, et al: Fluoxetine therapy in depersonalisation disorder: randomised controlled trial. Br J Psychiatry 185:31–36, 2004

Slater ETO, Glithero E: A follow-up of patients diagnosed as suffering from "hysteria." J Psychosom Res 9:9–13, 1965

Spiegel D, Loewenstein RJ, Lewis-Fernandez R, et al: Dissociative disorders in DSM-5. Depress Anxiety 28:824–852, 2011

Thigpen CH, Cleckley HM: The Three Faces of Eve. New York, McGraw-Hill, 1957

Turner M: Malingering. Br J Psychiatry 171:409–411, 1997

Vermetten E, Schmahl C, Lindner S, et al: Hippocampal and amygdalar volumes in dissociative identity disorder. Am J Psychiatry 163:630–636, 2006

Warwick HMC, Clark DM, Cobb AM, et al: A controlled trial of cognitive-behavioural therapy of hypochondriasis. Br J Psychiatry 169:189–195, 1996

Chapter 11: Feeding and Eating Disorders

Agras WS, Apple RF: Overcoming Eating Disorders: Therapist Guide. New York, Oxford University Press, 2007

American Psychiatric Association: Practice guideline for eating disorders, third edition. Am J Psychiatry 163 (7 suppl):4–54, 2006

Becker AE, Grinspoon SK, Klibanski A, et al: Eating disorders. N Engl J Med 340:1092–1098, 1999

Bissada H, Tasca GA, Barber AM, et al: Olanzapine in the treatment of low body weight and obsessive thinking in women with anorexia nervosa: a randomized, double-blind, placebo-controlled trial. Am J Psychiatry 165:1281–1288, 2008

Collier DA, Treasure JL: The aetiology of eating disorders. Br J Psychiatry 185:363–365, 2004

Crisp AH, Hsu LKG, Harding B, et al: Clinical features of anorexia nervosa: a study of 102 cases. J Psychosom Res 24:179–191, 1980

Deter HC, Herzog W: Anorexia nervosa in a long-term perspective: results of the Heidelberg-Mannheim Study. Psychosom Med 56:20–27, 1994

Dorian BT, Garfinkel PE: The contributions of epidemiologic studies to the etiology and treatment of the eating disorders. Psychiatr Ann 29:187–191, 1999

Eddy KT, Dorer DJ, Franko DL, et al: Diagnostic crossover in anorexia nervosa and bulimia nervosa: implications for DSM-V. Am J Psychiatry 165:245–250, 2008

Fairburn CG, Norman PA, Welch SL, et al: A prospective study of outcome in bulimia nervosa and the long-term effects of three psychological treatments. Arch Gen Psychiatry 52:304–312, 1995

Fluoxetine Bulimia Nervosa Collaborative Study Group: Fluoxetine in the treatment of bulimia nervosa: a multicenter, placebo-controlled, double-blind trial. Arch Gen Psychiatry 49:139–147, 1992

Garber AK, Michihata N, Hetnal K, et al: A prospective examination of weight gain in hospitalized adolescents with anorexia nervosa on a recommended refeeding protocol. J Adol Health 50:24–29, 2012

Grilo CM, Masheb RM, Wilson GT: Efficacy of cognitive behavioral therapy and fluoxetine for the treatment of binge eating disorder: a randomized, double-blind, placebo-controlled comparison. Biol Psychiatry 57:301–309, 2005

Keel PK, Mitchell JE: Outcome in bulimia nervosa. Am J Psychiatry 154:313–321, 1997

Lilienfeld LR, Kaye WH, Greeno CG, et al: A controlled family study of anorexia nervosa and bulimia nervosa: psychiatric disorders in first-degree relatives and effects of proband comorbidity. Arch Gen Psychiatry 55:603–610, 1998

Logue CM, Crowe RR, Bean JA: A family study of anorexia nervosa and bulimia. Compr Psychiatry 30:179–188, 1989

Mehler PS, Andersen AE (eds): Eating Disorders: A Guide to Medical Care and Complications, 2nd Edition. Baltimore, MD, Johns Hopkins University Press, 2010

Pike KM, Carter JC, Olmsted MP: Cognitive-behavioral therapy for anorexia nervosa, in The Treatment of Eating Disorders: A Clinical Handbook. Edited by Grilo CM, Mitchell JE. New York, Guilford, 2010, pp 83–107

Wilson GT, Wilfley DE, Agras S, Bryson SW: Psychological treatments of binge eating disorder. Arch Gen Psychiatry 67:94–101, 2010

Yager J, Powers PS (eds): Clinical Manual of Eating Disorders. Washington, DC, American Psychiatric Publishing, 2007

Chapter 12: Sleep-Wake Disorders

American Academy of Sleep Medicine: International Classification of Sleep Disorders, 2nd Edition: Diagnostic and Coding Manual. Westchester, IL: American Academy of Sleep Medicine, 2005

Arnulf I: REM sleep behavior disorder: motor manifestations and pathophysiology. Mov Disord 27:677–689, 2012

Bootzin RR, Epstein DR: Understanding and treating insomnia. Ann Rev Clin Psychol 7:435–458, 2011

Casola PG, Goldsmith RJ, Daiter J: Assessment and treatment of sleep problems. Psychiatr Ann 36:862–868, 2006

Dashevsky BA, Kramer M: Behavioral treatment of chronic insomnia in psychiatrically ill patients. J Clin Psychiatry 59:693–699, 1998

Goldsmith RJ, Casola PG: An overview of sleep, sleep disorders, and psychiatric medications' effects on sleep. Psychiatr Ann 36:833–840, 2006

Kasai T, Floras JS, Bradley TD: Sleep apnea and cardiovascular disease: a bidirectional relationship. Circulation 126:1495–1510, 2012

Krystal AD, Thakur M, Roth T: Sleep disturbance in psychiatric disorders: effect of function and quality of life in mood disorders, alcoholism, and schizophrenia. Ann Clin Psychiatry 20:39–46, 2008

Lam SP, Fon SYY, Ho CKW, et al: Parasomnia among psychiatric outpatients: a clinical, epidemiologic, cross-sectional study. J Clin Psychiatry 69:1374–1382, 2008

Morin CM, Culbert JP, Schwartz SM: Nonpharmacological interventions for insomnia: a meta-analysis of treatment efficacy. Am J Psychiatry 151:1172–1180, 1994

Morin CM, Colecchi C, Stone J, et al: Behavioral and pharmacological therapies of late-life insomnia. JAMA 281:991–999, 1999

Moser D, Anderer P, Gruber G, et al: Sleep classification according to the AASM and Rechtschaffen & Kales: effects on sleep scoring parameters. Sleep 32:139–149, 2009

Nowell PD, Buysse DJ, Reynolds CF, et al: Clinical factors contributing to the differential diagnosis of primary insomnia and insomnia related to mental disorders. Am J Psychiatry 154:1412–1416, 1997

Ohayon MM, Caulet M, Lemoine P: Comorbidity of mental and insomnia disorders in the general population. Compr Psychiatry 39:185–197, 1998

Peterson MJ, Rumble ME, Benca RM: Insomnia and psychiatric disorders. Psychiatr Ann 38:597–605, 2008

Richardson GS: The human circadian system in normal and disordered sleep. J Clin Psychiatry 66 (suppl 9):3–9, 2005

Richardson GS, Zammit G, Wang-Weigand S, et al: Safety and subjective sleep effects of ramelteon administration in adults and older adults with chronic primary insomnia: 1-year, open-label study. J Clin Psychiatry 70:467–476, 2009

Roberts RE, Shema SJ, Kaplan GA, et al: Sleep complaints and depression in an aging cohort: a prospective perspective. Am J Psychiatry 157:81–88, 2000

Rosenberg RP: Sleep maintenance insomnia: strengths and weaknesses of current pharmacologic therapies. Ann Clin Psychiatry 18:49–56, 2006

Saper CB, Scammell TE, Lu J: Hypothalamic regulation of sleep and circadian rhythms. Nature 437:1257–1263, 2005

Smith MT, Perlis ML, Park A, et al: Comparative meta-analysis of pharmacotherapy and behavior therapy for persistent insomnia. Am J Psychiatry 159:5–11, 2002

Walsh JK, Fry J, Erwin CW, et al: Efficacy and tolerability of 14-day administration of zaleplon 5 mg and 10 mg for the treatment of primary insomnia. Clinical Drug Investigation 16:347-354, 1998

Winkelman J, Pies R: Current patterns and future directions in the treatment of insomnia. Ann Clin Psychiatry 17:31-40, 2005

Young T, Palta M, Dempsey J, et al: The occurrence of sleep disordered breathing among middle-aged adults. N Engl J Med 328:1230-1235, 1993

Zee PC, Lu BS: Insomnia and circadian rhythm sleep disorders. Psychiatr Ann 38:583-589, 2008

Chapter 13: Sexual Dysfunction, Gender Dysphoria, and Paraphilias

Balon R, Segraves RT (eds): Clinical Manual of Sexual Disorders. Washington, DC, American Psychiatric Publishing, 2009

Black DW, Goldstein RB, Blum N, et al: Personality characteristics in 60 subjects with psychosexual dysfunction: a non-patient sample. J Personal Disord 9:275–285, 1995

Briken P, Kafka MP: Pharmacological treatments for paraphilic patients and sexual offenders. Curr Opin Psychiatry 20:609–613, 2007

Brown GR: A review of clinical approaches to gender dysphoria. J Clin Psychiatry 51:57–64, 1990

Brown GR, Wise TN, Costa PT, et al: Personality characteristics and sexual functioning of 188 cross dressing men. J Nerv Ment Dis 184:265–273, 1996

Cantor JM, Blanchard R: White matter volumes in pedophiles, hebephiles, and teleiophiles. Arch Sex Behav 41:749–752, 2012

Clayton A, Pradko JF, Croft HA, et al: Prevalence of sexual dysfunction among newer antidepressants. J Clin Psychiatry 63:357–366, 2002

Cohen LJ, McGeoch PG, Watras-Gans S, et al: Personality impairment in male pedophiles. J Clin Psychiatry 63:912–919, 2002

Dording CM, LaRocca RA, Hails KA, et al: The effect of sildenafil on quality of life. Ann Clin Psychiatry 25:3–10, 2013

Dunsleith NW, Nelson EB, Brusman-Lovins LA, et al: Psychiatric and legal features of 113 men convicted of sexual offenses. J Clin Psychiatry 65:293–300, 2004

First MB, Frances A: Issues for DSM-V: unintended consequences of small changes: the case of paraphilias. Am J Psychiatry 165:1240–1241, 2008

Gaffney GR, Berlin FS: Is there a gonadal dysfunction in pedophilia? A pilot study. Br J Psychiatry 145:657–660, 1984

Gaffney GR, Lurie SF, Berlin FS: Is there familial transmission of pedophilia? J Nerv Ment Dis 172:546–548, 1984

Grant JE: Clinical characteristics and psychiatric comorbidity in males with exhibitionism. J Clin Psychiatry 66:1367–1371, 2005

Green R: Gender identity in childhood and later sexual orientation: follow-up of 78 males. Am J Psychiatry 142:339–341, 1985

Hall RC, Hall RC: A profile of pedophilia: definition, characteristics of offenders, recidivism, treatment outcome, and forensic issues. Mayo Clin Proc 82:457–471, 2007

Heiman J, LoPiccolo J: Clinical outcome of sex therapy. Arch Gen Psychiatry 40:443–449, 1983

Kostis J, Jackson G, Rosen R, et al: Sexual dysfunction and cardiac risk (the Second Princeton Consensus Conference). Am J Cardiol 96:313–321, 2005

Langevin R: Biological factors contributing to paraphilic behavior. Psychiatr Ann 22:307–314, 1992

Laumann EO, Paik A, Rosen RC: Sexual dysfunction in the United States: prevalence and predictors. JAMA 281:537–544, 1999

Laumann EO, Nicolosi A, Glasser DB, et al: Sexual problems among women and men aged 40–80 y: prevalence and correlates identified in the Global Study of Sexual Attitudes and Behaviors. Int J Impot Res 17:39–57, 2005

Masters WH, Johnson VE: Human Sexual Inadequacy. Boston, MA, Little, Brown, 1970

Meyer JK, Reter DJ: Sex reassignment follow-up. Arch Gen Psychiatry 36:1010–1015, 1979

Osborn M, Hawton K, Gath D: Sexual dysfunction among middle-aged women in the community. BMJ 296:959–962, 1988

Reissig ED, Binik YM, Khalifé S: Does vaginismus exist? A critical review of the literature. J Nerv Ment Dis 187:261–273, 1999

Rendell MS, Raifer J, Wicker PA, et al: Sildenafil for treatment of erectile dysfunction in men with diabetes: a randomized controlled trial. JAMA 281:421–426, 1999

Schiavi RC, Schreiner-Engel P, Mandeli J, et al: Healthy aging and male sexual function. Am J Psychiatry 147:766–771, 1990

Segraves RJ: Effects of psychotropic drugs on human erection and ejaculation. Arch Gen Psychiatry 46:275–284, 1989

Seidman SN, Rieder RO: A review of sexual behavior in the United States. Am J Psychiatry 151:330–341, 1994

Smith RS: Voyeurism, a review of the literature. Arch Sex Behav 5:585–609, 1975

Spector KR, Boyle M: The prevalence and perceived aetiology of male sexual problems in a non-clinical sample. Br J Med Psychol 59:351–358, 1986

Sternbach H: Age-associated testosterone decline in men: clinical issues for psychiatry. Am J Psychiatry 155:1310–1318, 1998

Wise TN: Fetishism, etiology and treatment: a review from multiple perspectives. Compr Psychiatry 26:249–256, 1985

Chapter 14: Disruptive, Impulse-Control, and Conduct Disorders

Black DW: Bad Boys, Bad Men: Confronting Antisocial Personality Disorder. New York, Oxford University Press, 1999

Black DW: A review of compulsive buying disorder. World Psychiatry 6:14–18, 2007

Blanco C, Grant J, Petry NM, et al: Prevalence and correlates of shoplifting in the United States: results from the National Epidemiologic Survey on Alcohol and Related Conditions (NESARC). Am J Psychiatry 165:905–913, 2008

Coccaro EF, Lee RJ, Kavoussi RJ: A double-blind, randomized placebo-controlled trial of fluoxetine in patients with intermittent explosive disorder. J Clin Psychiatry 70:653–662, 2009

Findling RL, Aman MG, Eerdekens M, et al: Long-term, open-label study of risperidone in children with severe disruptive behaviors and below-average IQ. Am J Psychiatry 111:677–684, 2004

Goldman MJ: Kleptomania: making sense of the nonsensical. Am J Psychiatry 148:986–996, 1991

Grant JE, Potenza MN (eds): The Oxford Handbook of Impulse Control Disorders. New York, Oxford University Press, 2012

Grant JE, Kim SW: Clinical characteristics and psychiatric comorbidity of pyromania. J Clin Psychiatry 68:1717–1722, 2007

Grant JE, Kim SW, Odlaug BL: A double-blind, placebo-controlled study of the opiate antagonist naltrexone in the treatment of kleptomania. Biol Psychiatry 65:600–606, 2009

Hollander E, Stein DJ (eds): Clinical Manual of Impulse-Control Disorders. Washington, DC, American Psychiatric Publishing, 2006

Kessler RC, Coccaro EF, Fava M, et al: The prevalence and correlates of DSM-IV intermittent explosive disorder in the National Comorbidity Survey replication. Arch Gen Psychiatry 63:669–678, 2006

Kolko DJ: Efficacy of cognitive-behavioral treatment and fire safety education for children who set fires: initial and follow-up outcomes. J Child Psychol Psychiatry 42:359–369, 2001

Kuzma J, Black DW: Disorders characterized by poor impulse control. Ann Clin Psychiatry 17:219–226, 2005

Mattes JA: Oxcarbazepine in patients with impulsive aggression: a double-blind, placebo-controlled trial. J Clin Psychopharmacol 25:575–579, 2005

McCloskey MS, Noblett KL, Deffenbacher JL, et al: Cognitive-behavior therapy for intermittent explosive disorder: a pilot randomized clinical trial. J Consult Clin Psychol 76:876–886, 2008

McElroy SL: Recognition and treatment of DSM-IV intermittent explosive disorder. J Clin Psychiatry 60:12–16, 1999

Shaw M, Black DW: Internet addiction: definition, assessment, epidemiology, and clinical management. CNS Drugs 22:353–365, 2008

Stewart LA: Profile of female fire setters: implications for treatment. Br J Psychiatry 163:248–256, 1993

Van Minnen A, Hoogduin KA, Kerjsers GP, et al: Treatment of trichotillomania with behavior therapy or fluoxetine. Arch Gen Psychiatry 60:517–522, 2003

Chapter 15: Substance-Related and Addictive Disorders

American Psychiatric Association: Practice guideline for the treatment of patients with nicotine dependence. Am J Psychiatry 153 (10 suppl):1–31, 1996

American Psychiatric Association: Practice guideline for the treatment of patients with substance use disorders, second edition. Am J Psychiatry 164 (4 suppl):5–123, 2007

Anton RF, O'Malley SS, Ciraulo DA, et al: Combined pharmacotherapies and behavioral interventions for alcohol dependence: the COMBINE Study. A randomized controlled trial. JAMA 295:2003–2017, 2006

Barber WS, O'Brien CP: Early identification and intervention in an office setting. Primary Psychiatry 2:49–55, 1995

Black DW, Arndt S, Coryell WH, et al: Bupropion in the treatment of pathological gambling: a randomized, placebo-controlled, flexible-dose study. J Clin Psychopharmacol 27:143–150, 2007

Budney AJ, Hughes JR, Moore BA, et al: Review of the validity and significance of cannabis withdrawal syndrome. Am J Psychiatry 161:1967–1977, 2004

Busto U, Sellers EM, Naranjo CA, et al: Withdrawal reaction after long-term therapeutic use of benzodiazepines. N Engl J Med 315:854–859, 1986

Cadoret RJ, Yates WR, Troughton E, et al: An adoption study of drug abuse/dependency in females. Compr Psychiatry 37:88–94, 1996

Carroll KM, Fenton LR, Ball SA, et al: Efficacy of disulfiram and cognitive behavioral therapy in cocaine-dependent outpatients: a randomized placebo-controlled trial. Arch Gen Psychiatry 61:264–272, 2004

Cheng ATA, Gau SF, Chen THH, et al: A 4-year longitudinal study on risk factors for alcoholism. Arch Gen Psychiatry 61:184–191, 2004

Cregler LL, Mark H: Medical complications of cocaine abuse. N Engl J Med 315:1495–1500, 1986

Compton WM, Dawson DA, Conway KP, et al: Transitions in illicit drug use status over 3 years: a prospective analysis of a general population sample. Am J Psychiatry 170:660–670, 2013

Crits-Christoph P, Siqueland L, Blaine J, et al: Psychosocial treatments for cocaine dependence. Arch Gen Psychiatry 56:493–502, 1999

DeWit DJ, Adlaf EM, Offord DR, et al: Age at first alcohol use: a risk factor for the development of alcohol disorders. Am J Psychiatry 157:745–750, 2000

Dinwiddie SH, Zorumski CF, Rubin EH: Psychiatric correlates of chronic solvent abuse. J Clin Psychiatry 48:334–337, 1987

Eckardt MJ, Harford TC, Kaelber CT, et al: Health hazards associated with alcohol consumption. JAMA 246:648–666, 1981

Ewing J: Detecting alcoholism: the CAGE Questionnaire. JAMA 252:1905–1907, 1984

Fishbain DA, Rosomoff HL, Cutler R, et al: Opiate detoxification protocols: a clinical manual. Ann Clin Psychiatry 5:53–65, 1993

Frances RJ, Bucke S, Alexopoulous GS: Outcome study of familial and nonfamilial alcoholism. Am J Psychiatry 141:1469–1471, 1984

Fuller RK, Branchey L, Brightwell DR, et al: Disulfiram treatment of alcoholism: a Veterans Administration cooperative study. JAMA 256:1449–1455, 1986

Galanter M, Kleber HD (eds): The American Psychiatric Publishing Textbook of Substance Abuse Treatment, 4th Edition. Washington, DC, American Psychiatric Publishing, 2008

Garbutt JC, West SL, Carey TS, et al: Pharmacologic treatment of alcohol dependence: a review of the evidence. JAMA 281:1318–1325, 1999

Gawin FH, Kleber HD, Byck R, et al: Desipramine facilitation of initial cocaine abstinence. Arch Gen Psychiatry 46:117–121, 1989

Gelernter J, Goldman D, Risch N: The A1 allele at the D2 dopamine receptor gene and alcoholism: a reappraisal. JAMA 269:1673–1677, 1993

Gold MS, Tabrah H, Frost-Pineda K: Psychopharmacology of MDMA (Ecstasy). Psychiatr Ann 31:675–680, 2001

Goldstein RZ, Volkow ND: Dysfunction of the prefrontal cortex in addiction: neuroimaging findings and clinical implications. Nat Rev Neurosci 12:652–669, 2011

Grant JE, Potenza MN, Hollander E, et al: Multicenter investigation of the opioid antagonist nalmefene in the treatment of pathological gambling. Am J Psychiatry 163:303–312, 2006

Hasin DS, Keyes KM, Alderson D, et al: Cannabis withdrawal in the United States: results from the NESARC. J Clin Psychiatry 69:1354–1363, 2008

Heinz A, Reimold M, Wrase J, et al: Correlation of stable elevations in striatal-opioid receptor availability in detoxified alcoholic patients with alcohol craving. Arch Gen Psychiatry 62:57–64, 2005

Holden C: Is alcoholism treatment effective? Science 236:20–22, 1987

Howard MO, Bowen SE, Garland EL, et al: Inhalant use and inhalant use disorders in the United States. Addict Sci Clin Pract 6:18–31, 2011

Hser YI, Anglin MD, Powers K: A 24-year follow-up of California narcotic addicts. Arch Gen Psychiatry 50:577–584, 1993

Jacobs WS, DuPont R, Gold MS: Drug testing and the DSM-IV. Psychiatr Ann 30:583–588, 2000

Jellinek EM: The Disease Concept of Alcoholism. New Haven, CT, College and University Press, 1968

Jones HE, Strain EL, Bigelow GE, et al: Induction with levomethadyl acetate: safety and efficacy. Arch Gen Psychiatry 55:729–736, 1998

Jorenby DE, Leischow SJ, Nides MA, et al: A controlled trial of sustained release bupropion, a nicotine patch, or both for smoking cessation. N Engl J Med 340:685–691, 1999

Kalivas PW, Volkow ND: The neural basis of addiction: a pathology of motivation and choice. Am J Psychiatry 162:1403–1413, 2005

Merikangas KR, Stolar M, Stevens DE, et al: Familial transmission of substance use disorders. Arch Gen Psychiatry 55:973–979, 1998

National Consensus Development Panel on Effective Medical Treatment of Opiate Addiction: Effective medical treatment of opiate addiction. JAMA 280:1936–1943, 1998

Nurnberger JI Jr, Weigand R, Bucholz K, et al: A family study of alcohol dependence. Arch Gen Psychiatry 61:1246–1256, 2004

Nutt D: Alcohol and the brain: pharmacologic insights for psychiatrists. Br J Psychiatry 175:114–119, 1999

Peirce JM, Petry NM, Stitzer ML, et al: Effects of lower-cost incentives on stimulant abstinence in methadone maintenance treatment: a National Drug Abuse Treatment Clinical Trials Network study. Arch Gen Psychiatry 63:201–208, 2006

Perry PJ, Alexander B, Liskow BI, et al: Psychotropic Drug Handbook, 8th Edition. Baltimore, MD, Lippincott Williams & Wilkins, 2006

Pope HG Jr, Yurgelun-Todd D: The residual cognitive effects of heavy marijuana use in college students. JAMA 275:521–527, 1996

Pope HG Jr, Kouri EM, Powell KF, et al: Anabolic-androgenic steroid use among 133 prisoners. Compr Psychiatry 37:322–327, 1996

Potenza MN, Kosten TR, Rounsaville BJ: Pathological gambling. JAMA 286:141–144, 2001

Potenza MN, Steinberg MA, Skudlarski P, et al: Gambling urges in pathological gambling: a functional magnetic resonance imaging study. Arch Gen Psychiatry 60:828–836, 2003

Satre DD, Chi FW, Mertens JR, et al. Effects of age and life transitions on alcohol and drug treatment outcome over nine years. J Stud Alcohol Drugs 73:459–468, 2012

Schlaepfer TE, Strain EC, Greenberg BD, et al: Site of opioid action in the human brain: mu and kappa agonists' subjective and cerebrospinal blood flow effects. Am J Psychiatry 155:470–473, 1998

Schuckit MA: Alcohol-use disorders. Lancet 373:492–501, 2009

Schuckit MA, Smith TL, Anthenelli R, et al: Clinical course of alcoholism in 646 male inpatients. Am J Psychiatry 150:786–792, 1993

Sees KL, Delucchi KL, Masson C, et al: Methadone maintenance vs 180-day psychosocially enriched detoxification for treatment of opioid dependence: a randomized controlled trial. JAMA 283:1303–1310, 2000

Shaw M, Forbush K, Schlinder J, et al: The effect of pathological gambling on families, marriages, and children. CNS Spectr 12:615–622, 2007

Streissguth AP, Clarren SK, Jones KL: Natural history of the fetal alcohol syndrome: a 10 year follow up of 11 patients. Lancet 2:85–91, 1985

Swift RM: Drug therapy for alcohol dependence. N Engl J Med 340:1482–1489, 1999

Toomey R, Lyons MJ, Eisen SA, et al: A twin study of the neuropsychological consequences of stimulant abuse. Arch Gen Psychiatry 60:303–310, 2003

Vaillant GE: The Natural History of Alcoholism: Causes, Patterns, and Paths to Recovery. Cambridge, MA, Harvard University Press, 1983

Van den Bree MBM, Pickworth WB: Risk factors predicting changes in marijuana involvement in teenagers. Arch Gen Psychiatry 62:311–319, 2005

Vereby K, Gold MS: From coca leaves to crack: the effects of dose and routes of administration in abuse liability. Psychiatr Ann 18:513–520, 1988

Volpicelli JR, Alterman AI, Hayashida M, et al: Naltrexone in the treatment of alcohol dependence. Arch Gen Psychiatry 49:876–880, 1992

Warner EA: Cocaine abuse. Ann Intern Med 119:226–235, 1993

Yates WR, Fulton AI, Gabel J, et al: Personality risk factors for cocaine abuse. Am J Public Health 79:891–892, 1989

Chapter 16: Neurocognitive Disorders

American Psychiatric Association: Practice guidelines for the treatment of patients with delirium. Am J Psychiatry 156 (5 suppl):1–20, 1999

American Psychiatric Association: Practice guideline for the treatment of patients with Alzheimer's disease and other dementias, second edition. Am J Psychiatry 164 (12 suppl):5–56, 2007

Blazer DG, Stefens DC (eds): Essentials of Geriatric Psychiatry, 2nd Edition. Washington, DC, American Psychiatric Publishing, 2012

Clarfield AM: The reversible dementias: do they reverse? Ann Intern Med 109:476–486, 1988

Dalessio DJ: Maurice Ravel and Alzheimer's disease. JAMA 252:3412–3413, 1984

Dysken MW, Sano M, Asthana S, et al: Effect of vitamin E and memantine on functional decline in Alzheimer disease—the TEAM-AD VA cooperative randomized trial. JAMA 311:33–44, 2014

Folstein MF, Folstein SE, McHugh PR: Mini-Mental State: a practical method for grading the cognitive state of patients for the clinician. J Psychiatr Res 12:189–198, 1975

Francis J, Martin D, Kapoor WN: A prospective study of delirium in hospitalized elderly. JAMA 263:1097–1101, 1990

Golinger RC, Peet T, Tune LE: Association of elevated plasma anticholinergic activity with delirium in surgical patients. Am J Psychiatry 144:1218–1220, 1987

Howard R, McShane R, Lindesay J, et al: Donepezil and memantine for moderate-to-severe Alzheimer's disease. N Engl J Med 366:893–903, 2012

Johnson RT, Gibbs CJ: Creutzfeldt-Jakob disease and related transmissible spongiform encephalopathies. N Engl J Med 339:1994–2003, 1998

Katz IR, Jeste DV, Mintzer JE, et al: Comparison of risperidone and placebo for psychosis and behavioral disturbances associated with dementia: a randomized, double-blind trial. J Clin Psychiatry 60:107–115, 1999

Lyketsos CG, Del Campo L, Steinberg M, et al: Treating depression in Alzheimer's disease: efficacy and safety of sertraline therapy, and the benefits of depression reduction: the DIADS. Arch Gen Psychiatry 60:737–746, 2003

Mace NL, Rabins PV: The 36-Hour Day, 3rd Edition. Baltimore, MD, Johns Hopkins University Press, 1999

McAllister TW: Overview: pseudodementia. Am J Psychiatry 140:528–533, 1983

Miller SC, Baktash SH, Webb TS, et al: Risk for addiction-related disorders following mild traumatic brain injury in a large cohort of active-duty U.S. airmen. Am J Psychiatry 170:383–390, 2013

Mittal D, Jimerson NA, Neely EP, et al: Risperidone in the treatment of delirium: results from a prospective open-label trial. J Clin Psychiatry 65:662–667, 2004

Rabins PV, Folstein MF: Delirium and dementia: diagnostic criteria and fatality rates. Br J Psychiatry 140:149–153, 1982

Rabins PV, Mace NC, Lucas MJ: The impact of dementia on the family. JAMA 248:333–335, 1982

Reisberg B, Doody R, Stoffler A, et al: Memantine in moderate-to-severe Alzheimer's disease. N Engl J Med 348:1333–1341, 2003

Schneider LS, Dagerman KS, Insel P: Risk of death with atypical antipsychotic drug treatment for dementia: metaanalysis of randomized placebo-controlled trials. JAMA 294:1934–1943, 2005

Schor JD, Levkoff SE, Lipsitz LA, et al: Risk factors for delirium in hospitalized elderly. JAMA 267:827–831, 1992

Sink KM, Holden KF, Yaffe K: Pharmacologic treatment of neuropsychiatric symptoms of dementia: a review of the evidence. JAMA 293:596–608, 2005

Small GW, Leiter F: Neuroimaging for the diagnosis of dementia. J Clin Psychiatry 59 (suppl):4–7, 1998

Stern Y, Gurland B, Tatemichi TK, et al: Influence of education and occupation on the incidence of Alzheimer's disease. JAMA 271:1004–1010, 1994

Verghese J, Lipton RB, Hall CB, et al: Abnormality of gait as a predictor of non-Alzheimer's dementia. N Engl J Med 347:1761–1768, 2002

Walker Z, Allen RL, Shergill S, et al: Neuropsychological performance in Lewy body dementia and Alzheimer's disease. Br J Psychiatry 170:156–158, 1997

Weiner MF, Lipton AM (eds): The American Psychiatric Publishing Textbook of Alzheimer Disease and Other Dementias. Washington, DC, American Psychiatric Publishing, 2009

Wilcock GK: Dementia with Lewy bodies. Lancet 362:1689–1690, 2003

Zubenko GS, Zubenko WN, McPherson S, et al: A collaborative study of the emergence and clinical features of the major depressive syndrome of Alzheimer's disease. Am J Psychiatry 160:857–866, 2003

Chapter 17: Personality Disorders

Barrett MS, Stanford MS, Felthaus A, et al: The effects of phenytoin on impulsive and premeditated aggression: a controlled study. J Clin Psychopharmacol 17:341–349, 1997

Beck A, Freeman A, Davis DD: Cognitive Therapy of Personality Disorders, Second Edition. New York, Guilford, 2006

Bender DS, Morey LC, Skodol AE: Toward a model for assessing level of personality functioning in DSM-5, Part I: a review of theory and methods. J Pers Assess 93:332–346, 2011

Black DW: Bad Boys, Bad Men: Confronting Antisocial Personality Disorder (Sociopathy)—Revised and Updated. New York, Oxford University Press, 2013

Black DW, Blum N, Pfohl B, et al: Suicidal behavior in borderline personality disorder: prevalence, risk factors, prediction, and prevention. J Personal Disord 18:226–239, 2004

Blum N, St John D, Pfohl B, et al: Systems Training for Emotional Predictability and Problem Solving (STEPPS) for outpatients with borderline personality disorder: a randomized controlled trial and 1-year follow-up. Am J Psychiatry 165:468–478, 2008

Clarkin JF, Levy KN, Lenzenweger MF, et al: Evaluating three treatments for borderline personality disorder: a multiwave study. Am J Psychiatry 164:922–928, 2006

Cowdry RW, Gardner D: Pharmacotherapy of borderline personality disorder. Arch Gen Psychiatry 45:111–119, 1988

Donegan NH, Sanislow CA, Blumberg HP, et al: Amygdala hyperreactivity in borderline personality disorder: implications for emotional dysregulation. Biol Psychiatry 54:1284–1293, 2003

Fulton M, Winokur G: A comparative study of paranoid and schizoid personality disorders. Am J Psychiatry 150:1363–1367, 1993

Grant BF, Hasin DS, Stinson FS, et al: Prevalence, correlates, and disability of personality disorders in the United States: results from the National Epidemiologic Survey on Alcohol and Related Conditions. J Clin Psychiatry 65:948–958, 2004

Grant BF, Chou SP, Goldstein RB, et al: Prevalence, correlates, disability, and comorbidity of borderline personality disorder: results from the Wave 2 National Epidemiologic Survey on Alcohol and Related Conditions. J Clin Psychiatry 69:533–545, 2008

Gunderson JG, Stout RL, McGlashan TH, et al: Ten-year course of borderline personality disorder: psychopathology and functioning from the Collaborative Longitudinal Personality Disorders Study. Arch Gen Psychiatry 68:827–837, 2011

Jang KL, Livesley WJ, Vernon PA, et al: Heritability of personality disorder traits: a twin study. Acta Psychiatr Scand 94:438–444, 1996

Johnson JG, Cohen P, Brown J, et al: Childhood maltreatment increases risk for personality disorders during young adulthood. Arch Gen Psychiatry 56:600–606, 1999

Keshavan M, Shad M, Soloff P, et al: Efficacy and tolerability of olanzapine in the treatment of schizotypal personality disorder. Schizophr Res 71:97–101, 2004

Levy KN, Chauhan P, Clarkin JF, et al: Narcissistic pathology: empirical approaches. Psychiatr Ann 39:203–213, 2009

Lieb K, Zanarini MC, Schmahl C, et al: Borderline personality disorder. Lancet 364:453–461, 2004

Linehan MM, Comtois KA, Murray AM, et al: Two-year randomized controlled trial and follow-up of dialectical behavior therapy vs therapy by experts for suicidal behaviors and borderline personality disorder. Arch Gen Psychiatry 63:757–766, 2006

McCrae R, Costa T: Validation of the five-factor model of personality across instruments and observers. J Pers Soc Psychol 52:81–90, 1987

McGlashan TH: Schizotypal personality disorder. Arch Gen Psychiatry 43:329–334, 1986

Oldham JM, Skodol AE, Bender DS (eds): The American Psychiatric Publishing Textbook of Personality Disorders, 2nd Edition. Washington, DC, American Psychiatric Publishing, 2014

Pfohl B, Blum N: Obsessive-compulsive personality disorder: a review of available data and recommendations for DSM-IV. J Personal Disord 5:363–375, 1991

Reich J: The morbidity of DSM-III-R dependent personality disorder. J Nerv Ment Dis 84:22–26, 1996

Reich J, Yates W, Nguaguba M: Prevalence of DSM-III personality disorders in the community. Soc Psychiatry Psychiatr Epidemiol 24:12–16, 1989

Ronningstam E, Gundersen J, Lyons M: Changes in pathological narcissism. Am J Psychiatry 152:253–257, 1995

Soeteman DI, Hakkaart-van Roijen L, Verheul R, et al: The economic burden of personality disorders in mental health care. J Clin Psychiatry 69:259–265, 2008

Stinson FS, Dawson DA, Goldstein RB, et al: Prevalence, correlates, and comorbidity of DSM-IV narcissistic personality disorder: results from the Wave 2 National Epidemiologic Survey on Alcohol and Related Conditions. J Clin Psychiatry 69:1033–1045, 2008

Chapter 18: Psychiatric Emergencies

Alexopoulous GS, Reynolds CF III, Bruce ML, et al: Reducing suicidal ideation and depression in older primary care patients: 24-month outcomes of the PROSPECT study. Am J Psychiatry 166:882–890, 2009

Barraclough B, Bunch J, Nelson B, et al: A hundred cases of suicide: clinical aspects. Br J Psychiatry 125:355–373, 1974

Beck AT, Steer RA, Kovacs M, et al: Hopelessness and eventual suicide. Am J Psychiatry 142:559–563, 1985

Coryell W, Young EA: Clinical predictors of suicide in primary major depressive disorder. J Clin Psychiatry 66:412–417, 2005

Dolan M, Doyle M: Violence risk prediction. Br J Psychiatry 177:303–311, 2000

Ferguson SD, Coccaro EF: History of mild to moderate traumatic brain injury and aggression in physically healthy participants with and without personality disorder. J Person Disord 23:230–239, 2009

Goldstein R, Black DW, Winokur G, et al: The prediction of suicide: sensitivity, specificity, and predictive value of a multivariate model applied to suicide in 1,906 affectively ill patients. Arch Gen Psychiatry 48:418–422, 1991

Gould MS, Fisher F, Parides M, et al: Psychosocial risk factors of child and adolescent completed suicide. Arch Gen Psychiatry 53:1155–1162, 1996

Kaye NS, Soreff SM: The psychiatrist's role, responses, and responsibilities when a patient commits suicide. Am J Psychiatry 148:739–743, 1991

Mann JJ, Ellis SP, Waternaux CM, et al: Classification trees distinguish suicide attempters in major psychiatric disorders: a model of clinical decision making. J Clin Psychiatry 69:23–31, 2008

Marzuk PM, Leon AC, Tardiff K, et al: The effect of access to lethal methods of injury on suicide rates. Arch Gen Psychiatry 49:451–458, 1992

McGirr A, Renaud J, Seguin M, et al: Course of major depressive disorder and suicide outcome: a psychological autopsy study. J Clin Psychiatry 69:966–970, 2008

McNiel DE, Chamberlain JR, Weaver CM, et al: Impact of clinical training on violence risk assessment. Am J Psychiatry 165:195–200, 2008

Miller RJ, Zadolinnyj K, Hafner RJ: Profiles and predictors of assaultiveness for different ward populations. Am J Psychiatry 150:1368–1373, 1993

Murphy GE, Wetzel RD, Robins E, et al: Multiple risk factors predict suicide in alcoholism. Arch Gen Psychiatry 49:459–463, 1992

Patterson WM, Dohn HH, Bird J, et al: Evaluation of suicidal patients: the SAD PERSONS scale. Psychosomatics 24:343–349, 1983

Phillips DP, Carstonson LL: Clustering of teenage suicides after television news stories about suicide. N Engl J Med 55:685–689, 1986

Pulay AJ, Dawson DA, Hasin DS, et al: Violent behavior and DSM-IV psychiatric disorders: results from the National Epidemiologic Survey on Alcohol and Related Conditions. J Clin Psychiatry 69:12–22, 2008

Rich CL, Young D, Fowler RC: San Diego suicide study, I: young versus old subjects. Arch Gen Psychiatry 43:577–582, 1986

Robins E, Murphy GE, Wilkinson RH, et al: Some clinical considerations in the prevention of suicide based on a study of 134 successful suicides. Am J Public Health 49:888–899, 1959

Schneider B, Schnabel A, Wetterling T, et al: How do personality disorders modify suicide risk? J Person Disord 22:233–245, 2008

Simon RI: Preventing Patient Suicide: Clinical Assessment and Management. Washington, DC, American Psychiatric Publishing, 2011

Stone MH: Violent crimes and their relationship to personality disorders. Personality and Mental Health 1:138–153, 2007

Tardiff K: The Psychiatric Uses of Seclusion and Restraint. Washington, DC, American Psychiatric Press, 1984

Tardiff K, Marzuk PM, Leon AC, et al: Violence by patients admitted to a private psychiatric hospital. Am J Psychiatry 154:88–93, 1997

Chapter 19: Legal Issues

American Medical Association Board of Trustees: Insanity defense in criminal trials and limitation of psychiatric testimony. JAMA 251:2967–2981, 1984

American Psychiatric Association: The Principles of Medical Ethics With Annotations Especially Applicable to Psychiatry. Washington, DC, American Psychiatric Association, 2009

Appelbaum PS: *Tarasoff* and the clinician: problems in fulfilling the duty to protect. Am J Psychiatry 142:425–429, 1985

Appelbaum PS: Assessment of patients' competence to consent to treatment. N Engl J Med 357:1834–1840, 2007

Appelbaum PS, Gutheil TG: Clinical Handbook of Psychiatry and the Law, 4th Edition. Philadelphia, PA, Lippincott Williams & Wilkins, 2007

Appelbaum PS, Zoltek-Jick R: Psychotherapists' duties to third parties: *Ramona* and beyond. Am J Psychiatry 153:457–465, 1996

Buchanan A: Competency to stand trial and the seriousness of the charge. J Am Acad Psychiatry Law 34:458–465, 2006

Frank B, Gupta S, McGlynn DJ: Psychotropic medications and informed consent: a review. Ann Clin Psychiatry 20:87–95, 2008

Giorgi-Guarnieri D, Janofsky J, Kerem E, et al: AAPL practice guideline for forensic psychiatric evaluation of defendants raising the insanity defense. J Am Acad Psychiatry Law 30 (suppl 2):S3–S40, 2002

Guthiel TG, Gabbard GO: Misuses and misunderstandings of boundary theory in clinical and regulatory settings. Am J Psychiatry 155:409–414, 1998

Lamb HR: Incompetency to stand trial. Arch Gen Psychiatry 44:754–758, 1987

Leang GB, Eth S, Silva JA: The psychotherapist as witness for the prosecution: the criminalization of *Tarasoff*. Am J Psychiatry 149:1011–1015, 1992

McNeil DE, Binder RL, Fulton FM: Management of threats of violence under California's duty-to-protect statute. Am J Psychiatry 155:1097–1101, 1998

Miller RD: Need for treatment criteria for involuntary civil commitment: impact on practice. Am J Psychiatry 149:1380–1384, 1992

Mossman D, Noffsinger SG, Ash P, et al: AAPL practice guideline for the forensic psychiatric evaluation of competence to stand trial. J Am Acad Psychiatry Law 35 (suppl 4): S3–S72, 2007

Simon RI: Concise Guide to Psychiatry and Law for Clinicians, 3rd Edition. Washington, DC, American Psychiatric Publishing, 2001

Simon RI, Gold LH (eds): Textbook of Forensic Psychiatry. Washington, DC, American Psychiatric Publishing, 2004

Simon RI, Sadoff RL: Psychiatric Malpractice: Cases and Comments for Clinicians. Washington, DC, American Psychiatric Press, 1992

Simon RI, Shuman DW: Clinical Manual of Psychiatry and Law. Washington, DC, American Psychiatric Publishing, 2007

Studdert DM, Mello MM, Sage WM, et al: Defensive medicine among high-risk specialist physicians in a volatile malpractice environment. JAMA 293:2609–2617, 2005

Chapter 20: Behavioral, Cognitive, and Psychodynamic Treatments

Bateman A, Fonagy P: Borderline personality disorder, in Handbook of Mentalizing in Mental Health Practice. Edited by Bateman A, Fonagy P. Washington, DC, American Psychiatric Publishing, 2012, pp 273–288

Baum W: Understanding Behaviorism: Behavior, Culture, and Evolution. Oxford, UK, Blackwell, 2005

Beck AT, Alford BA: Depression: Causes and Treatment, 2nd Edition. Philadelphia, PA, University of Pennsylvania Press, 2008

Beck AT, Emery G, Greenberg BL: Anxiety Disorders and Phobias: A Cognitive Perspective. New York, Basic Books, 1985

Davanloo H (ed): Short-Term Dynamic Psychotherapy. New York, Jason Aronson, 1980

Emery RE: Marriage, Divorce, and Children's Adjustment, 2nd Edition. London, UK, Sage, 1999

Fenichel O: The Psychoanalytic Theory of Neurosis. New York, WW Norton, 1945

Freud A: The Ego and the Mechanisms of Defense. New York, International Universities Press, 1965

Freud S: The dynamics of transference (1912), in The Standard Edition of the Complete Psychological Works of Sigmund Freud, Vol 12. Translated and edited by Strachey J. London, UK, Hogarth Press, 1958, pp 97–108

Freud S: On beginning the treatment (1913), in The Standard Edition of the Complete Psychological Works of Sigmund Freud, Vol 12. Translated and edited by Strachey J. London, UK, Hogarth Press, 1958, pp 121–144

Gabbard GO: Psychodynamic Psychiatry in Clinical Practice, 4th Edition. Washington, DC, American Psychiatric Press, 2005

Gabbard GO (ed): Textbook of Psychotherapeutic Treatments. Washington, DC, American Psychiatric Publishing, 2009

Glick ID, Berman EM, Clarkin JF, et al: Marital and Family Therapy, 4th Edition. Washington, DC, American Psychiatric Press, 2000

Gunderson JG, Gabbard GO: Psychotherapy for Personality Disorders. Washington, DC, American Psychiatric Press, 2000

Gurman AS, Messer SB (eds): Essential Psychotherapies: Theory and Practice. New York, Guilford, 1995

Hayes S, Strosahl K, Wilson K: Acceptance and Commitment Therapy: An Experimental Approach to Behavior Change. New York, Guilford, 1999

Hopko DR, Lejuez CW, Ruggiero KJ, et al: Contemporary behavioral activation treatments for depression: procedures, principles, and progress. Clin Psychol Rev 23:699–717, 2004

Jones E: Therapeutic Action: A Guide to Psychoanalytic Therapy. New York, Jason Aronson, 2000

Kandel ER: Biology and the future of psychoanalysis: a new intellectual framework for psychiatry. Am J Psychiatry 156:505–524, 1999

Keitner GI, Heru AM, Glick ID: Clinical Manual of Couples and Family Therapy. Washington DC, American Psychiatric Publishing, 2010

Klerman GL, Weissman MM, Rounsaville BJ, et al: Interpersonal Psychotherapy of Depression. New York, Basic Books, 1984

Linehan MM: Cognitive-behavioral treatment for borderline personality disorder. New York, Guilford, 1993

Martell C, Addis M, Jacobson N: Depression in Context: Strategies for Guided Action. New York, WW Norton, 2001

McWilliams N: Psychoanalytic Psychotherapy: A Practitioner's Guide. New York, Guilford, 2004

Moore BE, Fine BD (eds): Psychoanalysis: The Major Concepts. New Haven, CT, Yale University Press, 1999

Richards PS, Bergin AE (eds): Handbook of Psychotherapy and Religious Diversity. Washington, DC, American Psychological Association, 2000

Sudak D: Cognitive Behavioral Therapy for Clinicians. Baltimore, MD, Lippincott Williams & Wilkins, 2006

Vaillant GE, Bond M, Vaillant CO: An empirically validated hierarchy of defense mechanisms. Arch Gen Psychiatry 43:786–794, 1986

Winston A, Rosenthal RN, Pinsker H: Learning Supportive Psychotherapy: An Illustrated Guide. Washington, DC, American Psychiatric Publishing, 2012

Yalom ID, Leszcz M: The Theory and Practice of Group Psychotherapy, 5th Edition. New York, Basic Books, 2005

Chapter 21: Psychopharmacology and Electroconvulsive Therapy

Agid O, Kapur S, Arenovich T, et al: Delayed-onset hypothesis of antipsychotic action: a hypothesis tested and rejected. Arch Gen Psychiatry 60:1228–1235, 2003

Ashton AK, Rosen RC: Bupropion as an antidote for serotonin reuptake inhibitor-induced sexual dysfunction. J Clin Psychiatry 59:112–115, 1998

Barak Y, Swartz M, Shamir E: Vitamin E (α-tocopherol) in the treatment of tardive dyskinesia: a statistical meta-analysis. Ann Clin Psychiatry 10:101–106, 1998

Berghofer A, Alda M, Adli M, et al: Long-tern effectiveness of lithium in bipolar disorder: a multicenter investigation of patients with typical and atypical features. J Clin Psychiatry 69:1860–1868, 2008

Birkenhager TK, van den Broek WW, Mulder PG, et al: Comparison of two-phase treatment with imipramine or fluvoxamine, both followed by lithium addition, in inpatients with major depressive disorder. Am J Psychiatry 161:2060–2065, 2004

Bowden CL, Calabrese JR, Jacks G, et al: A placebo-controlled 18-month trial of lamotrigine and lithium maintenance treatment in recently manic or hypomanic patients with bipolar I disorder. Arch Gen Psychiatry 60:392–400, 2003

Busto U, Sellers EM, Naranjo CA, et al: Withdrawal reaction after long-term therapeutic use of benzodiazepines. N Engl J Med 315:854–859, 1986

Centorrino F, Goren JL, Hennen J, et al: Multiple versus single antipsychotic agents for hospitalized patients: case-control study and risks versus benefits. Am J Psychiatry 161:700–706, 2004

Clary C, Schweizer E: Treatment of MAOI hypertensive crisis with sublingual nifedipine. J Clin Psychiatry 48:249–250, 1987

Clayton AH, Warnock JK, Kornstein SG, et al: A placebo controlled trial of bupropion SR as an antidote for selective serotonin reuptake inhibitor-induced sexual dysfunction. J Clin Psychiatry 65:62–67, 2004

Clayton AH, Kornstein SG, Rosas G, et al: An integrated analysis of the safety and tolerability of desvenlafaxine compared with placebo in the treatment of major depressive disorder. CNS Spectr 14:183–195, 2009

Correll CV, Leucht S, Kane JM: Lower risk for tardive dyskinesia associated with second-generation antipsychotics: a systematic review of one-year studies. Am J Psychiatry 161:414–425, 2004

Davis JM, Chen N, Glick ID: A meta-analysis of the efficacy of second-generation antipsychotics. Arch Gen Psychiatry 60:553–564, 2003

De Hert M, Schreurs V, Vancampfort D, et al: Metabolic syndrome in people with schizophrenia. World Psychiatry 8:15–22, 2009

Feighner JP: Mechanism of action of antidepressant medications. J Clin Psychiatry 60 (suppl):4–11, 1999

Geddes J: Efficacy and safety of electroconvulsive therapy in depressive disorders: a systematic review and meta-analysis. Lancet 361:799–808, 2003

Gorman JM: Mirtazapine: clinical overview. J Clin Psychiatry 60 (suppl):9–13, 1999

Hirschfeld RMA: Efficacy of SSRIs and newer antidepressants in severe depression: comparison with TCAs. J Clin Psychiatry 60:326–335, 1999

Hyman SE, Arana GW: Handbook of Psychiatric Drug Therapy. Boston, MA, Little, Brown, 1987

Igbal MM: Effect of antidepressants during pregnancy and lactation. Ann Clin Psychiatry 11:237–256, 1999

Jin H, Shih PAB, Golshan S, et al: Comparison of longer-term safety and effectiveness of 4 atypical antipsychotics in patients over age 40: a trial using equipoise-stratified randomization. J Clin Psychiatry 74:10–42, 2013

Jones KL, Lacro RV, Johnson KA, et al: Pattern of malformations in the children of women treated with carbamazepine during pregnancy. N Engl J Med 320:1661–1666, 1989

Jones PB, Davies L, Barnes TR, et al: Randomized controlled trial of effect on quality of life of second-generation versus first-generation antipsychotic drugs in schizophrenia. Arch Gen Psychiatry 63:1079–1087, 2006

Kane JM, Fleischhacker WW, Hansen L, et al: Akathisia: an updated review focusing on second-generation antipsychotics. J Clin Psychiatry 70:627–643, 2009

Kane JM, Mackle M, Snow-Adami L, et al: A randomized placebo-controlled trial of asenapine for the prevention of relapse in schizophrenia after long-term treatment. J Clin Psychiatry 72:349–355, 2011

Krishnan KRR: Monoamine oxidase inhibitors, in The American Psychiatric Publishing Textbook of Psychopharmacology, 4th Edition. Edited by Schatzberg AF, Nemeroff CB. Washington, DC, American Psychiatric Publishing, 2009, pp 389–401

Lauriello J, Pallanti S (eds): Clinical Manual for the Treatment of Schizophrenia. Washington, DC, American Psychiatric Publishing, 2012

Leucht S, Komossa K, Rummel-Kluge C, et al: A meta-analysis of head-to-head comparisons of the second-generation antipsychotics in the treatment of schizophrenia. Am J Psychiatry 166:152–163, 2009

Lieberman JA, Stroup TS, McEvoy JP, et al: Effectiveness of antipsychotic drugs in patients with chronic schizophrenia. N Engl J Med 353:1209–1223, 2005

Lipinsky JF, Zubenko G, Cohen BM, et al: Propranolol in the treatment of neuroleptic induced akathisia. Am J Psychiatry 141:412–415, 1984

Mendelson WB: A review of the evidence for the safety and efficacy of trazodone in the treatment of insomnia. J Clin Psychiatry 66:469–476, 2005

Montgomery SA, Mansuy L, Ruth A, et al: Efficacy and safety of levomilnacipran sustained release in moderate to severe major depressive disorder: a randomized, double-blind, placebo-controlled, proof-of-concept study. J Clin Psychiatry 74:363–369, 2013

Nemeroff CB, DeVane CL, Pollock BG: Newer antidepressants and the cytochrome P450 system. Am J Psychiatry 153:311–320, 1996

Noyes R, Garvey MJ, Cook BL, et al: Benzodiazepine withdrawal: a review of the evidence. J Clin Psychiatry 49:382–389, 1988

Olajide D, Lader M: A comparison of buspirone, diazepam, and placebo in patients with chronic anxiety states. J Clin Psychopharmacol 75:148–152, 1987

O'Reardon JP, Thase ME, Papacostas GI: Pharmacologic and therapeutic strategies in treatment-resistant depression. CNS Spectr (suppl 4):1–16, 2009

Perry PJ, Alexander B, Liskow BI, et al: Psychotropic Drug Handbook, 8th Edition. Baltimore, MD, Lippincott Williams & Wilkins, 2006

Rothschild AJ (ed): The Evidence-Based Guide to Antidepressant Medications. Washington, DC, American Psychiatric Publishing, 2012

Sackheim HA, Dillingham EM, Prudic J, et al: Effect of concomitant pharmacotherapy on electroconvulsive therapy outcomes. Arch Gen Psychiatry 66:729–737, 2009

Schatzberg AF, Nemeroff CB (eds): The American Psychiatric Publishing Textbook of Psychopharmacology, 4th Edition. Washington, DC, American Psychiatric Publishing, 2009

Stroup TS, Lieberman JA, McEvoy JP, et al: Effectiveness of olanzapine, risperidone, and ziprasidone in patients with chronic schizophrenia following discontinuation of a previous atypical antipsychotic. Am J Psychiatry 163:611–622, 2006

Vieta E, T'joen C, McQuade RD, et al: Efficacy of adjunctive aripiprazole to either valproate or lithium in bipolar mania patients partially nonresponsive to valproate/lithium monotherapy: a placebo-controlled study. Am J Psychiatry 165:1316–1325, 2008

Weisler RA, Kalali AH, Ketter TA, et al: A multicenter, randomized, double-blind placebo-controlled trial of extended-release carbamazepine capsules as monotherapy for bipolar disorder patients with manic or mixed episodes. J Clin Psychiatry 65:478–484, 2004

Weissman AA, Levy BT, Hartz AJ, et al: Pooled analysis of antidepressant levels in lactating mothers, breast milk, and nursing infants. Am J Psychiatry 161:1066–1078, 2004

Wisner KL, Bogen DL, Sit D, et al: Does fetal exposure to SSRIs or maternal depression impact infant growth? Am J Psychiatry 170:485–493, 2013

Zajecka J, Tracy KA, Mitchell S: Discontinuation syndromes after treatment with serotonin reuptake inhibitors: a literature review. J Clin Psychiatry 58:291–297, 1997

Glossary

A

abreaction Emotional release or discharge after recalling a painful experience that has been repressed because it was not consciously tolerable. A therapeutic effect sometimes occurs through partial or repeated discharge of the painful AFFECT.

acute dystonic reaction (ADR) An idiosyncratic drug reaction that involves acute involuntary muscle movements and spasms. Although any muscle group in the body can be involved, the most common symptoms are torticollis, facial grimacing, and body arching. Approximately 3%–10% of patients exposed to "traditional" or "conventional" antipsychotic drugs will experience an ADR. The movements typically occur at a time when the blood level of medication is dropping.

adaptation Fitting one's behavior to meet the needs of one's environment, which often involves a modification of IMPULSES, emotions, or attitudes.

addiction In DSM-5, refers to a substance or behavior that activates the brain's reward system, hence the category *substance-related and addictive disorders*. In the past, the term was used to indicate dependence on a chemical substance to the extent that a physiological and/or psychological need is established, as manifested by any combination of the following symptoms: tolerance, preoccupation with obtaining and using the substance, use of the substance despite anticipation of probable adverse consequences, repeated efforts to cut down or control substance use, and withdrawal symptoms when the substance is unavailable or not used.

adherence Used most commonly when referring to a person's taking medications in the amount and frequency recommended. Sometimes called *compliance.*

SMALL CAPS type indicates terms defined as main entries elsewhere in this glossary.

Adapted from Shahrokh NC, Hales RE (eds): *American Psychiatric Glossary*, 8th Edition (Washington, DC, American Psychiatric Publishing, 2003); Shahrokh NC, Hales RE, Phillips KA, Yudofsky SC (eds): *The Language of Mental Health: A Glossary of Psychiatric Terms* (Washington, DC, American Psychiatric Publishing, 2011); and American Psychiatric Association: *Diagnostic and Statistical Manual of Mental Disorders*, Fifth Edition (Arlington, VA, American Psychiatric Association, 2013). Copyright © American Psychiatric Publishing. Used with permission.

adolescence   A chronological period of accelerated physical and emotional growth leading to sexual and psychological maturity. It often begins at about age 12 years and ends at a loosely defined time, when the individual achieves independence and social productivity (usually in the early 20s).

adrenergic   Referring to neural activation by catecholamines such as epinephrine (adrenaline), and norepinephrine (noradrenaline) as well as drugs with adrenaline-like action that are capable of binding adrenergic receptors. Contrast with CHOLINERGIC.

affect   Behavior that expresses a subjectively experienced emotion. Affect is responsive to changing emotional states, whereas *mood* refers to a pervasive and sustained emotion. Common affects are euphoria, anger, and sadness. Some types of disturbance of affect are the following:

   blunted   Severe reduction in the intensity of affective expression.

   flat   Absence or near absence of any signs of affective expression; flat affect is often characterized by a monotonous voice and an immobile face.

   inappropriate   Affective expression that is discordant with the content of the person's speech or ideation.

   labile   Abnormal variability, with repeated, rapid, and abrupt shifts in affective expression.

   restricted or constricted   Reduction in the expressive range and intensity of affects.

affective disorder   A disorder in which mood change or disturbance is the primary manifestation. Now referred to as *mood disorder.*

aggression   Forceful physical, verbal, or symbolic action. May be appropriate and self-protective (as in healthy self-assertiveness), or inappropriate (as in hostile or destructive behavior). May also be directed toward the environment, toward another person, or toward the self.

agitated depression   A severe major depressive disorder in which psychomotor agitation is prominent.

agitation   Excessive motor activity, usually nonpurposeful and associated with internal tension. Examples include inability to sit still, fidgeting, pacing, wringing of hands, and pulling of clothes.

akathisia   A subjective sense of restlessness accompanied by fidgeting of the legs, rocking from foot to foot, pacing, or being unable to sit or stand still. Symptoms develop within a few weeks of starting or raising the dose of a conventional antipsychotic medication or of reducing the dose of medication used to treat extrapyramidal symptoms (see EXTRA-PYRAMIDAL SYNDROME).

akinesia   A state of motor inhibition or reduced voluntary motor movement in a person. The symptoms may occur in a patient taking a conventional antipsychotic medication.

alcohol amnestic disorder (Korsakoff's syndrome)   A disease associated with chronic alcoholism and resulting from a deficiency of vitamin
B_1; in DSM-5, this is *alcohol (major neurocognitive disorder), amnestic-
confabulatory type*. Patients sustain damage to part of the thalamus and
cerebellum and have anterograde and retrograde AMNESIA, with an inability to retain new information. Other symptoms include inflammation of
nerves, muttering delirium, insomnia, illusions, and hallucinations. In
alcohol amnestic disorder, unlike dementia, other intellectual functions
may be preserved.

alcohol dehydrogenase (ADH)   An important enzyme in the metabolism of alcohol, which oxidizes it to acetaldehyde. Eighty-five percent of
the Japanese population and other Asian populations have an atypical
ADH enzyme, which is about five times faster than normal. Consumption of alcohol by such persons leads to accumulation of acetaldehyde,
which results in facial flushing, extensive vasodilation, and a racing
heart (tachycardia).

Alcoholics Anonymous (AA)   A 12-step program for alcoholic persons who collectively assist other alcoholic persons through a structured fellowship of personal and group support. Sister organizations
include Narcotics Anonymous and Gamblers Anonymous.

alexithymia   A disturbance in affective and cognitive function that may
occur in several disorders; it is common in psychosomatic disorders, addictive disorders, and posttraumatic stress disorder (PTSD). The chief manifestations are difficulty in describing or recognizing one's own emotions, a
limited fantasy life, and general constriction in the affective life.

alogia   Literally, speechlessness. Most commonly used to refer to the
lack of spontaneity and content in speech and diminished flow of conversation that occur as NEGATIVE SYMPTOMS in schizophrenia.

ambivalence   The coexistence of contradictory emotions, attitudes,
ideas, or desires with respect to a particular person, object, or situation.
Ordinarily, the ambivalence is not fully conscious and suggests psychopathology only when present in an extreme form.

amines   Organic compounds containing the amino group ($-NH_2$); of
special importance in neurochemistry because of their role as neurotransmitters. Dopamine, epinephrine, norepinephrine, and serotonin
are amines.

amnesia   Pathological loss of memory; a phenomenon in which an
area of experience becomes inaccessible to conscious recall. The loss in
memory may be organic, emotional, dissociative, or of mixed etiology
and may be permanent or limited to a sharply circumscribed time. Two
types are distinguished:

  anterograde amnesia   The inability to form new memories for events
following an episode or event that may have produced the amnesia.

retrograde amnesia   Loss of memory for events preceding the episode or event presumed to be responsible for the amnesia.

amotivation   One of the NEGATIVE SYMPTOMS of schizophrenia, characterized by lack of interest, passivity, and loss of drive.

amotivational syndrome   A SYNDROME characterized by loss of drive, passivity, lack of concern for one's appearance, no desire to work regularly, and fatigue. Some long-term frequent users of marijuana show signs of amotivational syndrome.

amygdala   In the structure of the brain, part of the basal ganglia located on the roof of the temporal horn of the lateral ventricle at the inferior end of the caudate nucleus. It is a structure in the forebrain that is an important component of the LIMBIC SYSTEM, which is involved in the regulation of emotion.

anal character   A PERSONALITY type that manifests excessive orderliness, miserliness, and obstinacy. Called *obsessive-compulsive character or personality* in other typologies. In PSYCHOANALYSIS, a pattern of behavior in an adult that is believed to originate in the anal phase of infancy, between 1 and 3 years. See also PSYCHOSEXUAL DEVELOPMENT.

anxiety   Apprehension, tension, or uneasiness from anticipation of danger, the source of which is largely unknown or unrecognized. Primarily of intrapsychic origin, in distinction to fear, which is the emotional response to a consciously recognized and usually external threat or danger. May be regarded as pathological when it interferes with social and occupational functioning, achievement of desired goals, or emotional comfort.

attention   The ability to sustain focus on one activity. A disturbance in attention may appear as having difficulty in finishing tasks that have been started, being easily distracted, or having difficulty in concentrating.

atypical depression   A term used to describe a cluster of symptoms such as mood reactivity, weight gain, hypersomnia, leaden paralysis, and rejection sensitivity. In DSM-5, this may be designated by the specifier "with atypical features." Depressed patients with atypical features may preferentially respond to MAO inhibitor antidepressants.

augmentation strategies   The addition of one or more medications to enhance or magnify the beneficial effects of a medication already used, such as the addition of lithium carbonate, liothyronine, an anticonvulsant, or a stimulant to augment antidepressant response in a patient with refractory depression.

aversion therapy   A BEHAVIOR THERAPY procedure in which stimuli associated with undesirable behavior are paired with a painful or an unpleasant stimulus, resulting in the suppression of the undesirable behavior.

avolition   Lack of initiative or goals; one of the NEGATIVE SYMPTOMS of schizophrenia. The person may wish to do something, but the desire is without power or energy.

B

behavior modification   A technique used in BEHAVIOR THERAPY that focuses on negative habits or behaviors and aims to reduce or eliminate them by the use of reinforcement (e.g., rewarding a desired behavior or punishing an unwanted one).

behavior therapy   A mode of treatment that focuses on substituting healthier ways of behaving for maladaptive patterns used in the past. Most likely to benefit are individuals who want to change habits, those with ANXIETY disorders such as phobias or PANIC ATTACKS, and those with substance abuse or eating disorders. The basic techniques include BEHAVIOR MODIFICATION, operant conditioning, shaping, token economy, systematic desensitization, RELAXATION TRAINING, AVERSION THERAPY, EXPOSURE THERAPY, FLOODING, modeling, social skills training, and PARADOXICAL INTENTION.

benzodiazepine receptors   Receptors located on neurons within the central nervous system (CNS) to which benzodiazepines bind. Benzodiazepine receptors are linked to GABA receptors. Benzodiazepines enhance the affinity of the GABA receptor for GABA, the principal inhibitory neurotransmitter in the CNS, and thereby increase its inhibitory effects, leading to decreased ANXIETY and arousal.

bereavement   Feelings of deprivation, desolation, and grief at the loss of a loved one. In DSM-5, if the grieving person otherwise meets criteria for major depression, that disorder is diagnosed.

beta-blocker   A class of drugs that inhibit the action of β-adrenergic receptors, which modulate cardiac functions, respiratory functions, and the dilation and constriction of blood vessels. β-Blockers are of value in the treatment of hypertension, cardiac arrhythmias, and migraine. In psychiatry, they have been used in the treatment of AGGRESSION and violence, ANXIETY-related TREMORS and lithium-induced TREMORS, antipsychotic-induced AKATHISIA, social phobia, performance anxiety, panic states, and alcohol withdrawal.

binge drinking   A pattern of heavy alcoholic intake that occurs in bouts of a day or more that are set aside for drinking. During periods between bouts, the subject may abstain from alcohol.

binge eating   A period of overeating during which a larger amount of food is ingested than most people would eat during that time. The person feels that he or she cannot stop eating or has no control over what or how much is consumed. After a bout of overeating, depression, guilt feelings, and feelings of disgust with oneself are common. In DSM-5, this is diagnosed as *binge-eating disorder*. When binge eating is accompanied by compensatory behavior such as purging or food restriction to control weight, it is termed *bulimia nervosa*.

blocking A sudden obstruction or interruption in spontaneous flow of thinking or speaking, perceived as an absence or a deprivation of thought.

borderline intellectual functioning In DSM-5, an additional (V/Z code) condition that may be a focus of clinical attention, especially when it coexists with a disorder such as schizophrenia. The person with borderline intellectual functioning requires careful assessment of his or her cognitive and adaptive functioning. In DSM-IV, the intelligence quotient (IQ) was in the 71–84 range.

brain imaging Any technique that permits the in vivo visualization of the substance of the central nervous system (CNS). The best known of such techniques is computed tomography (CT). Newer methods of brain imaging such as positron emission tomography (PET), single photon emission computed tomography (SPECT), and magnetic resonance imaging (MRI) are based on different physical principles but also yield a series of two-dimensional images (or "slices") of brain regions of interest.

C

cannabinoid receptors Cannabinoids are organic compounds that are present in *Cannabis sativa*. Two subtypes of cannabinoid receptors have been cloned from animal or human sources; however, the therapeutic application of these receptors remains unknown.

Cannabis sativa An India hemp plant from which marijuana is derived. The main psychoactive component of cannabis is delta-9-tetrahydrocannabinol (THC). Marijuana may contain 0.1%–10% THC.

Capgras' syndrome The DELUSION that impostors have replaced others or the self. The SYNDROME typically follows the development of negative feelings toward the other person that the subject cannot accept and attributes, instead, to the impostor. It has been reported in patients with schizophrenia and other forms of psychosis or a neurocognitive disorder.

catalepsy A generalized condition of diminished responsiveness shown by trancelike states, posturing, or maintenance of physical attitudes for a prolonged period. May occur in organic or psychological disorders, or under hypnosis. See also CATATONIC BEHAVIOR.

cataplexy Sudden loss of postural tone without loss of consciousness, typically triggered by some emotional stimulus such as laughter, anger, or excitement. It is a characteristic of narcolepsy.

catatonia Immobility with muscular rigidity or inflexibility and, at times, excitability.

catatonic behavior Marked motor abnormalities, generally limited to those occurring as part of a psychotic disorder. This term includes catatonic excitement (apparently purposeless AGITATION not influenced by external stimuli), STUPOR (decreased reactivity and fewer spontaneous movements, often with apparent unawareness of the surroundings), NEGATIVISM (apparent motiveless resistance to instructions or attempts to be moved), posturing (the person's assuming and maintaining an inappropriate or a bizarre stance), rigidity (the person's maintaining a stance or posture against all efforts to be moved), and WAXY FLEXIBILITY or CEREA FLEXIBILITAS (the person's limbs can be put into positions that are maintained).

catharsis The healthful (therapeutic) release of ideas through "talking out" conscious material accompanied by an appropriate emotional reaction. Also, the release into awareness of repressed ("forgotten") material from the UNCONSCIOUS. See also REPRESSION.

cerea flexibilitas The "WAXY FLEXIBILITY" often present in catatonic schizophrenia in which the patient's arm or leg remains in the position in which it is placed.

cholinergic Activated or transmitted by acetylcholine (e.g., parasympathetic nerve fibers). Contrast with ADRENERGIC.

circumstantiality A pattern of speech that is indirect and delayed in reaching its goal because of excessive or irrelevant detail or parenthetical remarks. The speaker does not lose the point, as is characteristic of loosening of associations, and clauses remain logically connected, but to the listener it seems that the end will never be reached.

cognition A general term encompassing all the various modes of knowing and reasoning.

cognitive-behavioral therapy (CBT) A form of PSYCHOTHERAPY focused on changing thoughts and behaviors that are related to specific target symptoms. Treatment is aimed at symptom reduction and improved functioning. The patient is taught to recognize the negative and unrealistic COGNITIONS that contribute significantly to the development or maintenance of symptoms and to evaluate and modify such thinking patterns. Problematic behaviors are also focused on and changed with the use of behavioral strategies (e.g., response prevention, scheduling pleasant activities).

cognitive development Beginning in infancy, the acquisition of intelligence, conscious thought, and problem-solving abilities. An orderly sequence in the increase in knowledge derived from sensorimotor activity was empirically shown by Jean Piaget (1896–1980), who described four stages in the cognitive development of the child:

sensorimotor stage The senses receive a stimulus, and the body reacts to it in a stereotyped way. This occurs from birth to 16–24 months. Object permanence develops during this time.

preoperational thought Prelogical thought that occurs between ages 2 and 6 years. During this time, symbolic function and language develop and change the child's ability to interact. Egocentric thinking predominates, and the child believes that everything revolves around him or her. MAGICAL THINKING arises, and reality and fantasy are interwoven.

concrete operations   Rational and logical thought process. This stage occurs between ages 7 and 11. Includes the development of the ability to understand another's viewpoint and the concept of conservation.

formal operations   Cognitive stage that includes abstract thinking, conceptual thinking, and deductive reasoning. Formal operational thinking is generally achieved by age 12. See also PSYCHOSEXUAL DEVELOPMENT.

cognitive rehabilitation   Modification of cognitive and role functioning in seriously and persistently mentally ill patients, directed at improving visual and verbal memory and social and emotional perception.

cognitive restructuring   A technique of COGNITIVE THERAPY that enables one to identify negative, irrational beliefs and replace them with truthful, rational statements.

cognitive therapy   A type of PSYCHOTHERAPY, usually focused and problem oriented, directed primarily at identifying and modifying distorted COGNITIONS and behavioral dysfunction. This technique is based on the assumption that certain thought patterns, called *cognitive structures* or *schemas*, shape the way people react to the situations in their lives. Individuals with major depression, ANXIETY disorders, eating disorders, and substance use disorders are more likely to benefit.

combination treatment   Refers to the addition of another treatment modality to an existing one to achieve a desired effect, such as the addition of COGNITIVE-BEHAVIORAL THERAPY (CBT) to an antidepressant to treat panic disorder. It also may refer to the use of two or more medications with different mechanisms of action but within the same overall class, such as the use of two different antidepressants to treat refractory depression.

community mental health center (CMHC)   A MENTAL HEALTH service delivery system first authorized by the federal Community Mental Health Centers Act of 1963 to provide a comprehensive program of mental health care to Catchment Area residents. The CMHC is typically a community facility or a network of affiliated agencies that serves as a locus for the delivery of the various services included in the concept of COMMUNITY PSYCHIATRY.

community psychiatry   That branch of psychiatry concerned with the provision and delivery of a coordinated program of MENTAL HEALTH care to residents of a geographic area. These efforts include working with patients, their families, and agencies within the community. Goals are the prevention of mental illness as well as care and treatment for persons with MENTAL DISORDERS.

comorbidity The simultaneous appearance of two or more illnesses, such as the co-occurrence of schizophrenia and substance abuse or of an alcohol use disorder and depression. The association may reflect a causal relation between one disorder and another or an underlying vulnerability to both disorders; however, the co-occurrence of the illnesses may be unrelated to any common etiology or vulnerability.

compulsion Repetitive ritualistic behavior or thoughts, such as frequent hand washing, arranging objects according to a rigid formula, counting, or repeating words silently. The purpose of these behaviors or thoughts is to prevent or reduce distress or to prevent some dreaded event or situation. The person feels driven to perform such actions in response to an OBSESSION (a recurrent thought, IMPULSE, or image that is intrusive and distressing) or according to rules that must be applied rigidly, even though the behaviors or thoughts are recognized to be excessive or unreasonable.

concrete thinking Thinking characterized by immediate experience rather than abstractions. It may occur as a primary, developmental defect, or it may develop secondary to a neurocognitive disorder or schizophrenia.

concussion An impairment of brain function caused by injury to the head. The speed and degree of recovery depend on the severity of the brain injury. Symptoms may include headache, DISORIENTATION, paralysis, and unconsciousness.

conditioning Establishing new behavior as a result of psychological modifications of responses to stimuli.

confabulation Fabrication of stories in response to questions about situations or events that are not recalled.

confidentiality The ethical principle that a physician may not reveal any information disclosed in the course of medical attendance without securing appropriate permission from the patient or a designated decision-maker.

conflict A mental struggle that arises from the simultaneous operation of opposing IMPULSES, drives, and external (environmental) or internal demands. Termed *intrapsychic* when the conflict is between forces within the PERSONALITY and *extrapsychic* when it is between the self and the environment.

confusion Disturbed orientation in respect to time, place, person, or situation.

conscience The morally self-critical part of one's standards of behavior, performance, and value judgments. Commonly equated with the SUPEREGO.

consultation-liaison psychiatry An area of special interest in general psychiatry that addresses the psychiatric and psychosocial aspects of medical care, particularly in a general hospital setting. The consultation-liaison psychiatrist works closely with medical-surgical physicians and nonphysician staff to enhance the diagnosis, treatment, and management of patients with primary medical-surgical illness and concurrent psychiatric disorders or symptoms. Consultation may occasionally lead to a recommendation for more specific aftercare referral, but more typically it consists of short-term intervention by a "consultation team" with a biopsychosocial approach to illness.

conversion A DEFENSE MECHANISM, operating unconsciously (see UNCONSCIOUS), by which intrapsychic conflicts that would otherwise give rise to ANXIETY are instead given symbolic external expression. The repressed ideas or IMPULSES, and the psychological defenses against them, are converted into a variety of somatic symptoms such as paralysis, pain, or loss of sensory function.

coping mechanisms Ways of adjusting to environmental stress without altering one's goals or purposes. Includes both conscious and UNCONSCIOUS mechanisms.

coprolalia The involuntary use of profane words seen in patients with Tourette's disorder.

Cotard's syndrome A NIHILISTIC DELUSION in which one believes that one's body, or parts of it, is disintegrating; that one is bereft of all resources; or that one's family has been exterminated. It has been reported in depressive disorders, schizophrenia, and lesions of the nondominant hemisphere. Named after the French neurologist Jules Cotard (1840–1889).

countertransference The therapist's emotional reactions to the patient that are based on the therapist's UNCONSCIOUS needs and CONFLICTS, as distinguished from his or her conscious responses to the patient's behavior. Countertransference may interfere with the therapist's ability to understand the patient and may adversely affect the therapeutic technique. However, countertransference also may have positive aspects and may be used by the therapist as a guide to a more empathic and accurate understanding of the patient.

cytochrome P450 The cytochrome P450 enzyme system in the liver plays a key role in the metabolism of many medications. Many psychotropic medications are known to inhibit or stimulate the cytochrome P450 system, thus resulting in significant drug-drug interactions that may result in clinically significant alterations of blood levels of medications.

D

defense mechanism   U<small>NCONSCIOUS</small> intrapsychic processes serving to provide relief from emotional C<small>ONFLICT</small> and A<small>NXIETY</small>. Conscious efforts are frequently made for the same reasons, but true defense mechanisms are unconscious. Some common defense mechanisms defined in this glossary are D<small>ISSOCIATION</small>, I<small>NTELLECTUALIZATION</small>, I<small>NTROJECTION</small>, P<small>ROJECTION</small>, R<small>ATIONALIZATION</small>, R<small>EACTION FORMATION</small>, S<small>UBLIMATION</small>, and S<small>UBSTITUTION</small>.

deinstitutionalization   Change in locus of M<small>ENTAL HEALTH</small> care from traditional, institutional settings to community-based services. Sometimes called *transinstitutionalization* because it often merely shifts the patients from one institution (the hospital) to another (such as a prison).

delusion   A false belief based on an incorrect inference about external reality, firmly sustained despite clear evidence to the contrary. The belief is not part of a cultural tradition such as an article of religious faith. Among the more frequently reported delusions are the following:

delusional jealousy   The false belief that one's sexual partner is unfaithful; also called the *Othello delusion*.

delusion of control   The belief that one's feelings, I<small>MPULSES</small>, thoughts, or actions are not one's own but have been imposed by some external force.

delusion of poverty   The conviction that one is, or will be, bereft of all material possessions.

delusion of reference   The conviction that events, objects, or other people in the immediate environment have a particular and unusual significance (usually negative).

grandiose delusion   An exaggerated belief of one's importance, power, knowledge, or identity.

nihilistic delusion   A conviction of nonexistence of the self, part of the self, others, or the world. "I no longer have a brain" is an example.

persecutory delusion   The conviction that one (or a group or institution close to one) is being harassed, attacked, persecuted, or conspired against.

somatic delusion   A false belief involving the functioning of, or some other aspect of, one's body, such as the conviction of a postmenopausal woman that she is pregnant, or a person's conviction that he has snakes in his colon.

systematized delusion   A single false belief with multiple elaborations or a group of false beliefs that the person relates to a single event or theme. This event is believed to have caused every problem in life that the person experiences.

dementia praecox   Obsolete descriptive term for schizophrenia. Introduced as "démence précoce" by Benedict Augustin Morel in 1857 and later popularized by Emil Kraepelin (1856–1926).

dependency needs   Vital needs for mothering, love, affection, shelter, protection, security, food, and warmth. May be a manifestation of regression when they reappear excessively in adults.

depersonalization   Feelings of unreality or strangeness concerning either the environment, the self, or both. Such feelings are characteristic of DSM-5 depersonalization/derealization disorder and also may occur in schizotypal PERSONALITY DISORDER, in schizophrenia, and in those persons experiencing overwhelming ANXIETY, stress, or fatigue.

derealization   A feeling of estrangement or DETACHMENT from one's environment. May be accompanied by DEPERSONALIZATION.

detachment   A behavior pattern characterized by general aloofness in interpersonal contact; may include INTELLECTUALIZATION, denial, and superficiality.

detoxification   The process of providing medical care during the removal of substances of abuse from the body so that withdrawal symptoms are minimized and physiological function is safely restored. Treatment includes medication, rest, diet, fluids, and nursing care.

devaluation   A mental mechanism in which one attributes exaggeratedly negative qualities to oneself or others.

dialectical behavior therapy (DBT)   A form of PSYCHOTHERAPY that teaches behavioral and cognitive coping skills, developed specifically for patients with borderline PERSONALITY DISORDER.

disorientation   Loss of awareness of the position of the self in relation to space, time, or other persons; confusion.

dissociation   The splitting off of clusters of mental contents from conscious awareness. Dissociation is a mechanism central to hysterical CONVERSION and dissociative disorders. The term is also used to describe the separation of an idea from its emotional significance and AFFECT as seen in the INAPPROPRIATE AFFECT of schizophrenic patients.

distractibility   Inability to maintain ATTENTION. The person shifts from one area or topic to another with minimal provocation. Distractibility may be a manifestation of an underlying medical disease, a medication side effect, or a MENTAL DISORDER such as an ANXIETY disorder, mania, or schizophrenia.

dystonia   Irregular muscle tone due to central nervous system disorder, which can result in grotesque movements or distorted positions.

E

echolalia   Parrotlike repetition of overheard words or fragments of speech. It may be part of a developmental disorder, a neurological disorder, or schizophrenia. Echolalia tends to be repetitive and persistent and is often uttered with a mocking, mumbling, or staccato intonation.

echopraxia   Imitative repetition of the movements, gestures, or posture of another. It may be part of a neurological disorder or of schizophrenia.

ego   In psychoanalytic theory (see PSYCHOANALYSIS), one of the three major divisions in the model of the psychic apparatus, the others being the id and the SUPEREGO. The ego represents the sum of certain mental mechanisms, such as perception and memory, and specific DEFENSE MECHANISMS. It serves to mediate between the demands of primitive instinctual drives (the id), of internalized parental and social prohibitions (the SUPEREGO), and of reality. The compromises between these forces achieved by the ego tend to resolve intrapsychic CONFLICT and serve an adaptive and executive function. Psychiatric usage of the term should not be confused with common usage, which connotes self-love or selfishness.

ego-dystonic   Referring to aspects of a person's behavior, thoughts, and attitudes that are viewed by the self as repugnant or inconsistent with the total PERSONALITY. Contrast with EGO-SYNTONIC.

ego-syntonic   Referring to aspects of a person's behavior, thoughts, and attitudes that are viewed by the self as acceptable and consistent with the total PERSONALITY. Contrast with EGO-DYSTONIC.

electroencephalogram (EEG)   A graphic (voltage vs. time) depiction of the brain's electrical potentials (brain waves) recorded by scalp electrodes. It is used for the diagnosis of neurological and neuropsychiatric disorders (especially seizure disorders) and in neurophysiological research.

encephalopathy   An imprecise term referring to any disorder of brain function (metabolic, toxic, neoplastic) but often implying a chronic degenerative process.

entitlement   The right or claim to something. In health law, the term *entitlement programs* refers to legislatively defined rights to health care, such as Medicare and Medicaid programs.

In psychodynamic psychiatry, *entitlement* usually refers to an unreasonable expectation or unfounded claim. An example is a person with narcissistic PERSONALITY DISORDER who feels deserving of preferred status and special treatment in the absence of apparent justification for such treatment.

Epidemiologic Catchment Area (ECA) study   This study was initiated in response to the 1977 report of the President's Commission on Mental Health. The purpose was to collect data on the prevalence and incidence of MENTAL DISORDERS and on the use of, and need for, services by the mentally ill. Research teams at five universities (Yale University, Johns Hopkins University, Washington University, Duke University, and the University of California at Los Angeles), in collaboration with the NATIONAL INSTITUTE OF MENTAL HEALTH (NIMH), conducted the studies with a core of common questions and sample characteristics. All data were collected between 1980 and 1985.

epidemiology   In psychiatry, the study of the incidence, distribution, prevalence, and control of MENTAL DISORDERS in a given population. Common terms in epidemiology are

   endemic   Native to or restricted to a particular area.

   epidemic   The outbreak of a disorder that affects significant numbers of persons in a given population at any time.

   pandemic   Occurring over a very wide area, in many countries, or universally.

epilepsy, temporal lobe   Also called *complex partial seizures.* Usually originating in the temporal lobes, it involves recurrent periodic disturbances of behavior, during which the patient carries out movements that are often repetitive and highly organized but semiautomatic in character.

euphoria   An exaggerated feeling of physical and emotional well-being, usually of psychological origin. Also seen in neurocognitive disorders and in toxic and drug-induced states.

evoked potential   Electrical activity produced by the brain in response to any sensory stimulus; a more specific term than *event-related potential,* as the "event" is a sound. See also ELECTROENCEPHALOGRAM (EEG).

executive functioning   Higher-level, cognitive abilities such as planning or decision making. These functions are often impaired during the early stages of dementia.

exposure therapy   A method of therapy that involves gradually exposing an individual to situations that previously have been avoided because of ANXIETY or panic. Also known as exposure *hierarchy.* Most often used in treating phobias, such as fear of flying or heights and agoraphobia.

expressed emotions   The feelings that a family shows toward one of its members; specifically, overinvolvement with and hostility and criticism toward a family member with schizophrenia.

extinction   The weakening of a reinforced operant response as a result of ceasing reinforcement. Also, the elimination of a conditioned response by repeated presentations of a conditioned stimulus without the unconditioned stimulus.

extrapyramidal syndrome   A variety of signs and symptoms, including muscular rigidity, TREMORS, drooling, shuffling gait (parkinsonism), restlessness (AKATHISIA), unusual involuntary postures (dystonia), motor inertia (AKINESIA), and many other neurological disturbances. Results from dysfunction of the extrapyramidal system. May occur as a reversible side effect of certain psychotropic drugs, particularly phenothiazine derivatives. See also TARDIVE DYSKINESIA.

extraversion   A state in which attention and energies are largely directed outward from the self as opposed to inward toward the self, as in INTROVERSION. Also known as *extroversion*.

F

failure to thrive   A common problem in pediatrics in which infants or young children show delayed physical growth, often with impaired social and motor development. Nonorganic failure to thrive is thought to be associated with lack of adequate emotional nurturing.

family therapy   Treatment of more than one member of a family in the same session. The treatment may be supportive, directive, or interpretive. The assumption is that a MENTAL DISORDER in one member of a family may be a manifestation of disorders or problems in other members and may affect interrelationships and functioning.

fetal alcohol syndrome   A congenital disorder resulting from alcohol teratogenicity (i.e., the production, actual or potential, of pathological changes in the fetus, most frequently in the form of abnormal development of one or more organ systems; commonly referred to as *birth defects*), with the following possible dysmorphic categories: central nervous system dysfunction, birth deficiencies (such as low birth weight), facial abnormalities, and variable major and minor malformations. A safe level of alcohol use during pregnancy has not been established, and it is generally advisable for women to refrain from alcohol use during pregnancy.

flashback   Reexperiencing, after ceasing the use of a hallucinogen, one or more of the perceptual symptoms that were part of the hallucinatory experience while using the drug. It also commonly occurs as a symptom of acute stress disorder or posttraumatic stress disorder (PTSD).

flight of ideas   A nearly continuous flow of accelerated speech with abrupt changes from one topic to another, usually based on understandable associations, distracting stimuli, or playing on words. When severe, however, this may lead to disorganized and incoherent speech. Flight of ideas is characteristic of manic episodes, but it also may occur in neurocognitive disorders, schizophrenia, other PSYCHOSES, and, rarely, acute reactions to stress.

flooding (implosion) A BEHAVIOR THERAPY procedure for phobias and other problems involving maladaptive anxiety, in which the causes of the anxiety are presented in intense forms, either in imagination or in real life. The presentations, which act as desensitizers, are continued until the stimuli no longer produce disabling anxiety.

forensic psychiatry A branch of psychiatry dealing with legal issues related to MENTAL DISORDERS.

formal thought disorder An inexact term referring to a disturbance in the form of thinking rather than to abnormality of content. See BLOCKING; INCOHERENCE; POVERTY OF SPEECH.

free association In psychoanalytic therapy (see PSYCHOANALYSIS), spontaneous, uncensored verbalization by the patient of whatever comes to mind.

free-floating anxiety Severe, generalized, persistent ANXIETY not specifically ascribed to a particular object or event and often a precursor of panic.

frontal lobe syndrome A pattern of emotional, behavioral, and PERSONALITY changes that occur following an injury to the prefrontal lobes.

G

galactorrhea The secretion of breast milk in men or in women who are not breast-feeding an infant. Patients with galactorrhea have a high level of prolactin in the blood, which can be caused by a tumor in the pituitary gland or by taking certain medications, such as conventional antipsychotic medications.

globus hystericus The disturbing sensation of a lump in the throat. See also *hysterical neurosis, conversion type,* under NEUROSIS.

glutamate An excitatory amino acid used by brain neurons as a primary neurotransmitter that appears to play a role in protecting against the symptoms of PSYCHOSIS.

glutamate receptors Glutamate is the major excitatory neurotransmitter in the central nervous system, and, as such, the glutamate receptors play a vital role in the mediation of excitatory synaptic transmission.

grandiosity Exaggerated belief or claims of one's importance or identity, often manifested by DELUSIONS of great wealth, power, or fame.

grief Normal, appropriate emotional response to an external and a consciously recognized loss; it is usually time-limited and subsides gradually.

group (psycho)therapy   Application of psychotherapeutic techniques by a therapist who uses the emotional interactions of the group members to help them get relief from distress and possibly modify their behavior. Typically, a group is composed of 4–12 persons who meet regularly with the therapist.

H

halfway house   A specialized residence for patients who do not require full hospitalization but who do need an intermediate degree of domiciliary care before they return to independent community living.

hypertensive crisis   Sudden and sometimes fatal rise in blood pressure; may occur as a result of combining monoamine oxidase inhibitors (MAOIs) with food containing high amounts of tyramine (e.g., certain cheeses, fava beans, red wine) or with other sympathomimetic substances (e.g., cough remedies and nose drops).

hyperventilation   Overbreathing sometimes associated with ANXIETY and marked by reduction of blood carbon dioxide, producing complaints of light-headedness, faintness, tingling of the extremities, palpitations, and respiratory distress.

hypnagogic   Referring to the semiconscious state immediately preceding sleep; may include hallucinations that are of no pathological significance.

hypnopompic   Referring to the state immediately preceding awakening; may include hallucinations that are of no pathological significance.

hypomania   A psychopathological state and abnormality of mood falling somewhere between normal positive mood and mania. It is characterized by unrealistic optimism, pressure of speech and activity, and a decreased need for sleep. Some people show increased creativity during hypomanic states, whereas others show poor JUDGMENT, irritability, and irascibility.

hysteria   A psychiatric SYNDROME first described by the French neurologist Jean-Martin Charcot (1825–1893). The patient with hysteria may show shallow or unmodulated AFFECT, self-absorption, sexual preoccupation or promiscuous sexual behavior, and THOUGHT DISORDER. Hysteria is also referred to as *conversion disorder* because it is a CONVERSION of ANXIETY related to UNCONSCIOUS CONFLICTS into somatic symptoms.

hysterics   Lay term for uncontrollable emotional outbursts.

I

iatrogenic illness   A disorder precipitated, aggravated, or induced by the physician's attitude, examination, comments, or treatment.

ideas of reference   Incorrect interpretations of casual incidents and external events as having direct reference to oneself. May reach sufficient intensity to constitute DELUSIONS.

impulse   A desire or propensity to act in a certain way, typically in order to ease tension or gain pleasure.

inappropriate affect   A display of emotion that is out of harmony with reality or with the verbal or intellectual content that it accompanies. See AFFECT.

incoherence   Lacking in unity or consistency; often applied to speech or thinking that is not understandable because of any of the following: lack of logical connection between words or phrases; excessive use of incomplete sentences; many irrelevancies or abrupt changes in subject matter; idiosyncratic word usage; or distorted grammar.

incompetency   Lack of the capacity to understand the nature of, to assess adequately, or to manage effectively a specified transaction or situation that the ordinary person could reasonably be expected to handle. As used in the law, the term refers primarily to cognitive defects that interfere with JUDGMENT.

insight   Self-understanding; the extent of a person's understanding of the origin, nature, and mechanisms of his or her maladaptive attitudes and behavior. Sometimes used to indicate whether an individual is aware that he or she has a MENTAL DISORDER or that his or her symptoms have a psychiatric cause.

intellectualization   A DEFENSE MECHANISM in which the person engages in excessive abstract thinking to avoid confrontation with CONFLICTS or disturbing feelings.

International Classification of Diseases **(ICD)**   The official list of disease categories issued by the World Health Organization; subscribed to by all member nations, who may assign their own terms to each ICD category. The ICDA (*International Classification of Diseases*, U.S. Public Health Service adaptation) represents the official list of diagnostic terms to be used for each ICD category in the United States.

introjection   A DEFENSE MECHANISM, operating unconsciously (see UNCONSCIOUS), whereby loved or hated external objects are symbolically absorbed within oneself. The converse of PROJECTION. May serve as a defense against conscious recognition of intolerable hostile IMPULSES. For example, in severe depression, the individual may unconsciously direct unacceptable hatred or AGGRESSION toward herself or himself. Related to the more primitive fantasy of oral incorporation.

introspection Self-observation or the examination of one's feelings, often as a result of PSYCHOTHERAPY.

introversion Preoccupation with oneself and accompanying reduction of interest in the outside world. Contrast with EXTRAVERSION. Also used to indicate shyness and decreased sociability.

isolation An unconscious DEFENSE MECHANISM often used by obsessive-compulsive patients. Isolation separates AFFECT from memory. Thoughts or affects are treated as if they were untouchable, therefore requiring distance. An example is a patient talking about a painful event with a bland expression.

J

judgment Mental act of comparing choices between a given set of values in order to select a course of action.

K

kindling A progressively increasing response to successive electrical stimuli. In bipolar disorder, it is important to prevent the onset of mania because with each manic episode, the shorter the period until the next episode. In this regard, it is believed that the manic episode "kindles" the brain by making it more susceptible to a subsequent manic episode.

Kleine-Levin syndrome Periodic episodes of hypersomnia accompanied by bulimia. The SYNDROME first appears in ADOLESCENCE, usually in boys. It is not classified as either an eating disorder or a sleep disorder. It is considered a neurological syndrome and is believed to reflect a frontal lobe or hypothalamic disturbance.

L

la belle indifférence Literally, "beautiful indifference." Seen in certain patients with CONVERSION disorders who show an inappropriate lack of concern about their disabilities. See *hysterical neurosis, conversion type,* under NEUROSIS.

learning disability A SYNDROME affecting school-age children of normal or above-normal intelligence characterized by specific difficulties in learning to read (dyslexia, word blindness), write (dysgraphia), and calculate (dyscalculia). Diagnosed in DSM-5 as *specific learning disorder.* The disorder is believed to be related to slow developmental progression of perceptual motor skills.

light therapy   The use of a balanced-spectrum light box that delivers between 5,000 and 10,000 lux in the treatment of seasonal mood disorder, jet lag, PREMENSTRUAL DYSPHORIC DISORDER, premenstrual syndrome, and some sleep disorders. Also known as *phototherapy.*

limbic system   Visceral brain; a group of brain structures—including the AMYGDALA, hippocampus, septum, cingulate gyrus, and subcallosal gyrus—that help regulate emotion, memory, and certain aspects of movement.

lobotomy   A type of psychosurgery in which one or more nerve tracts in the frontal lobes are severed. The procedure has been superseded by more specific procedures that are sometimes used for intractable obsessive-compulsive disorder.

M

magical thinking   A conviction that thinking equates with doing. Occurs in dreams in children and in patients under a variety of conditions. Characterized by lack of realistic relationship between cause and effect.

managed care   A system organized to create a balance among the use of health care resources, control of health costs, and enhancement of the quality of care. Managed care systems seek to provide care in the most cost-effective manner by closely monitoring the intensity and duration of treatment as well as the settings in which it is provided. Managed care systems also organize physicians and other providers into coordinated networks of care to ensure that those who enroll in the system receive all medically necessary care. A wide array of mechanisms is used to control utilization and reduce costs. Currently, health maintenance organizations (HMOs) are the most frequently used management system for managed care.

manipulation   A behavior pattern characterized by attempts to exploit interpersonal contact.

marital therapy   A treatment whose goal is to ameliorate the problems of married couples. Various psychodynamic, sexual, ethical, and economic aspects of marriage are considered. A broader term is *couples therapy,* which encompasses unmarried couples.

mental disorder   A behavioral or psychological SYNDROME that causes significant distress (a painful symptom) or disability (impairment in one or more important areas of functioning) or a significantly increased risk for death, pain, or an important loss of freedom. The syndrome is considered to be a manifestation of some behavioral, psychological, or biological dysfunction in the person (and in some cases it is clearly secondary to or due to a general medical condition). The term is not applied to behavior or CONFLICTS that arise between the person and society (e.g., political, religious, or sexual preference) unless such conflicts are clearly an outgrowth of a dysfunction within that person. In lay usage, *emotional illness* serves as a term for mental disorder, although it may imply a lesser degree of dysfunction, whereas the term *mental disorder* may be reserved for more severe disturbances.

mental health   A state of being that is relative rather than absolute. The successful performance of mental functions shown by productive activities, fulfilling relationships with other people, and the ability to adapt to change and to cope with adversity.

Munchausen syndrome (pathomimicry)   A chronic form of factitious disorder that may be totally fabricated, self-inflicted, or exaggerations of preexisting physical conditions. Much of the person's life may consist of seeking admission to or staying in hospitals (often under different names). Multiple invasive procedures and operations are eagerly solicited. The need is to assume the sick role rather than to reap any economic benefit or ensure better care or physical well-being.

N

narcissism   Self-love as opposed to object-love (love of another person). To be distinguished from egotism, which carries the connotation of self-centeredness, selfishness, and conceit. Egotism is but one expression of narcissism. Revisions in psychoanalytic theory (self psychology) have viewed the concept of narcissism in less pathological terms.

National Alliance on Mental Illness (NAMI)   An organization whose members are parents and relatives of mentally ill patients and former patients whose main objective is for better and more sustained care. Its trustees and chapter officers engage in active lobbying and in education projects.

National Comorbidity Study   Conducted from September 1990 through February 1992; the first nationally representative MENTAL HEALTH survey in the United States to use a fully structured research diagnostic interview to assess the prevalence of psychiatric disorders in a community setting.

National Institute of Mental Health (NIMH)   One of the 27 institutes and centers that constitute the National Institutes of Health (NIH); NIMH is responsible for research on the causes and treatments of MENTAL DISORDERS.

negative symptoms   Most commonly refers to a group of symptoms characteristic of schizophrenia that include loss of fluency and spontaneity of verbal expression, impaired ability to focus or sustain ATTENTION on a particular task, difficulty in initiating or following through on tasks, impaired ability to experience pleasure or form emotional attachment to others, and blunted AFFECT.

negativism Opposition or resistance, either covert or overt, to the suggestions or advice of others. May be seen in schizophrenia.

neuroleptic malignant syndrome A severe medication-induced movement disorder associated with the use of a neuroleptic medication. Symptoms include muscle rigidity, high fever, and related findings such as dysphagia, incontinence, confusion, or mutism.

neuropsychological testing A series of tests administered to assess various aspects of cognitive functioning, including memory, ATTENTION, language, and EXECUTIVE FUNCTIONING. The ultimate goal of the assessment is to clarify how changes in brain structure and function are affecting behavior.

neurosis An older term for emotional disturbances of all kinds other than psychosis. It implies subjective psychological pain or discomfort beyond what is appropriate to the conditions of one's life. The meaning of the term has been changed since it was first introduced into standard nomenclature. In current usage, some clinicians limit the term to its descriptive meaning, NEUROTIC DISORDER, whereas others include the concept of a specific etiological process. Common neuroses are as follows:

anxiety neurosis Chronic and persistent apprehension manifested by autonomic hyperactivity (e.g., sweating, palpitations, dizziness), musculoskeletal tension, and irritability. Somatic symptoms may be prominent.

depersonalization neurosis Feelings of unreality and of estrangement from the self, body, or surroundings. Different from the process of DEPERSONALIZATION, which may be a manifestation of ANXIETY or of another MENTAL DISORDER.

depressive neurosis An outmoded term for excessive reaction of depression due to an internal CONFLICT or to an identifiable event such as loss of a loved one or of a cherished possession.

hysterical neurosis, conversion type Disorders of the special senses or of the voluntary nervous system, such as blindness, deafness, anesthesia, paresthesia, pain, paralysis, and impaired muscle coordination for which no organic cause is found. A patient with this disorder sometimes shows LA BELLE INDIFFÉRENCE to the symptoms, which may actually provide secondary gains by winning the patient sympathy or relief from unpleasant responsibilities. See also CONVERSION.

hysterical neurosis, dissociative type Alterations in the state of consciousness or in identity, producing symptoms such as AMNESIA.

obsessive-compulsive neurosis Persistent intrusion of unwanted and uncontrollable EGO-DYSTONIC thoughts, urges, or actions. The thoughts may consist of single words, ruminations, or trains of thought that are seen as nonsensical. The actions may vary from simple movements to complex rituals, such as repeated hand washing. See also COMPULSION.

phobic neurosis An intense fear of an object or a situation that the person consciously recognizes as harmless. Apprehension may be experienced as faintness, fatigue, palpitations, perspiration, nausea, TREMOR, and even panic.

neurotic disorder An older term for a MENTAL DISORDER in which the predominant disturbance is a distressing symptom or group of symptoms that one considers unacceptable to one's PERSONALITY. There is no marked loss of REALITY TESTING; behavior does not actively violate gross social norms, although it may be quite disabling. The disturbance is relatively enduring or recurrent without treatment and is not limited to a mild transitory reaction to stress. There is no demonstrable organic etiology. See also NEUROTIC PROCESS.

neurotic process A specific etiological process involving the following sequence: UNCONSCIOUS CONFLICTS between opposing wishes or between wishes and prohibitions lead to unconscious perception of anticipated danger or dysphoria, which leads to use of DEFENSE MECHANISMS that result in either symptoms, PERSONALITY disturbance, or both. See also NEUROSIS; NEUROTIC DISORDER.

nihilistic delusion The DELUSION of nonexistence of the self or part of the self, or of some object in external reality.

O

object relations The emotional bonds between one person and another, as contrasted with interest in and love for the self; usually described in terms of capacity for loving and reacting appropriately to others. Melanie Klein (1882–1960) is generally credited with founding the British object relations school.

obsession Recurrent and persistent thought, IMPULSE, or image experienced as intrusive and distressing. Recognized as being excessive and unreasonable even though it is the product of one's mind. This thought, impulse, or image cannot be expunged by logic or reasoning.

organic mental disorder An older term used for conditions showing behavioral or psychological symptoms secondary to or based on detectable disturbances in brain functioning. Recent advances in genetics, neurophysiology, and BRAIN IMAGING have made it possible to identify several biological and physiological factors that contribute to many MENTAL DISORDERS traditionally characterized as "functional" or nonorganic. Consequently, there is general agreement that it is difficult, if not impossible, to make clear distinctions between "organic" and "nonorganic" disorders. The term was used in DSM-III and DSM-III-R but discontinued in DSM-IV. Replaced in DSM-5 by *neurocognitive disorder*.

P

panic attack   A period of intense fear or discomfort, with the abrupt development of a variety of physical symptoms and fears of dying, going crazy, or losing control that reach a crescendo within 10 minutes. The symptoms may include shortness of breath or smothering sensations; dizziness, faintness, or feelings of unsteadiness; trembling or shaking; sweating; choking; nausea or abdominal distress; flushes or chills; and chest pain or discomfort.

Panic attacks occur in several ANXIETY disorders. In panic disorder, they are typically unexpected and happen "out of the blue." In disorders such as social phobia, simple phobia, obsessive-compulsive disorder, and body dysmorphic disorder, they are cued and occur when exposed to or in anticipation of a situational trigger. These attacks occur also in posttraumatic stress disorder (PTSD).

paradoxical intention   A technique used in BEHAVIOR THERAPY in which individuals are encouraged to engage in whatever behavior they are trying to stop. For example, a compulsive hand washer might be instructed to wash even more frequently. This helps because it often illustrates the irrationality of the behavior and reduces resistance to change.

paranoia   A condition characterized by the gradual development of an intricate, complex, and elaborate system of thinking based on (and often proceeding logically from) misinterpretation of an actual event; it may meet criteria for a type of delusional disorder or may be seen in other psychotic disorders. Despite its often chronic course, this condition does not seem to interfere with other aspects of thinking and PERSONALITY.

pathognomonic   A symptom or group of symptoms that are specifically diagnostic or typical of a disease.

personality   The characteristic way in which a person thinks, feels, and behaves; the ingrained pattern of behavior that each person evolves, both consciously and unconsciously, as his or her style of life or way of being.

personality disorder   Enduring patterns of perceiving, relating to, and thinking about the environment and oneself that begin by early adulthood and are exhibited in a wide range of important social and personal contexts. These patterns are inflexible and maladaptive, causing either significant functional impairment or subjective distress.

Many types of PERSONALITY or personality disorder have been described. The following are those specified in DSM-5, which groups them into three clusters:

Cluster A   Paranoid, schizoid, schizotypal

Cluster B   Antisocial, borderline, histrionic, narcissistic

Cluster C   Avoidant, dependent, obsessive-compulsive

antisocial   Called *psychopathic personality* or *sociopathic personality* in the older literature; descriptions have tended to emphasize either antisocial behavior or interpersonal and affectional inadequacies. Among the more commonly cited descriptors are superficiality; lack of empathy and remorse, with callous unconcern for the feelings or rights of others; disregard for social norms; poor behavioral controls, with irritability, impulsivity, and low frustration tolerance; and inability to feel guilt or to learn from experience or punishment. Often, there is evidence of conduct disorder (disruptive behavior disorder) in childhood or of overtly irresponsible and antisocial behavior in adulthood, such as inability to sustain consistent work behavior, conflicts with the law, repeated failure to meet financial obligations, and repeated lying or "conning" of others.

avoidant   Characterized by social discomfort and reticence, low self-esteem, and hypersensitivity to negative evaluation. Manifestations may include avoiding activities that involve contact with others because of fears of criticism or disapproval; experiencing inhibited development of relationships with others because of fears of being foolish or being shamed; having few friends despite the desire to relate to others; or being unusually reluctant to take personal risks or engage in new activities because they may prove embarrassing.

borderline   Characterized by instability of interpersonal relationships, self-image, AFFECTS, and control over IMPULSES. Manifestations may include frantic efforts to avoid real or imagined abandonment; unstable, intense relationships that alternate between extremes of idealization and DEVALUATION; repetitive self-mutilation or suicide threats; and inappropriate, intense, or uncontrolled anger.

dependent   Characterized by an excessive need to be taken care of, resulting in submissive and clinging behavior and fears of separation. Manifestations may include excessive need for advice and reassurance about everyday decisions, encouragement of others to assume responsibility for major areas of one's life, inability to express disagreement because of possible anger or lack of support from others, and preoccupation with fears of being left to take care of oneself.

histrionic   Characterized by excessive emotional instability and attention seeking. Behavior includes discomfort if not the center of attention; excessive attention to physical attractiveness; rapidly shifting and shallow emotions; speech that is excessively impressionistic and lacking in detail; viewing relationships as being more intimate than they actually are; and seeking immediate gratification.

narcissistic Characterized by a pervasive pattern of GRANDIOSITY in fantasy or behavior and an excessive need for admiration. Manifestations may include having an exaggerated sense of self-importance, having a feeling of being so special that one should associate only with other special people, exploiting others to advance one's own ends, lacking empathy, and believing that others envy oneself.

obsessive-compulsive Also known as *compulsive personality*; characterized by preoccupation with perfectionism, mental and interpersonal control, and orderliness, all at the expense of flexibility, openness, and efficiency. Some of the manifestations are preoccupation with rules, lists, or similar items; excessive devotion to work, with little attention paid to recreation and friendships; limited expression of warm emotions; reluctance to delegate work and the demand that others submit exactly to one's way of doing things; and miserliness.

paranoid Characterized by a pervasive distrust and suspiciousness of others such that their motives are interpreted as malevolent. This distrust is shown in many ways, including unreasonable expectation of exploitation or harm by others; questioning without justification the loyalty or trustworthiness of friends or associates; reading demeaning or threatening meanings into benign remarks or events; having a tendency to bear grudges and be unforgiving of insults or injuries; or experiencing unfounded, recurrent suspiciousness about the fidelity of one's sexual partner.

passive-aggressive Characterized by unassertive resistance and general obstructiveness in response to the expectations of others. Some of these actions are procrastination; postponement of completion of routine tasks; sulkiness, irritability, or argumentativeness if asked to do something one does not want to do, and then working unreasonably slowly and inefficiently; or avoidance of obligations by claiming to have forgotten them.

schizoid Characterized by DETACHMENT from social relationships and restricted emotional range in interpersonal settings. The individual tends not to desire or enjoy close relationships, prefers solitary activities, appears indifferent to praise or criticism, has no (or only one) close friends or confidants, and is emotionally cold or detached.

schizotypal Characterized by a combination of discomfort with, and reduced capacity for, close relationships and cognitive or perceptual distortions and eccentricities of behavior. Possible manifestations include odd beliefs or MAGICAL THINKING inconsistent with cultural norms; unusual perceptual experiences including bodily illusions; odd thinking and speech; no (or only one) close friends because of lack of desire, discomfort with others, or eccentricities; and persisting, excessive social ANXIETY that tends to be associated with PARANOID fears rather than negative JUDGMENTS about oneself. Some studies suggest that this disorder might more properly be considered a part of a schizophrenia spectrum disorder.

pharmacotherapy   The treatment of a disease through the use of pharmaceutical medications. Also referred to as *psychopharmacologic treatment*. A type of physical or somatic therapy.

polydipsia   Excessive or abnormal thirst. Patients with obsessive-compulsive disorder and other psychiatric disorders, such as schizophrenia, may have polydipsia, which may produce a type of diabetes insipidus.

postconcussional disorder   Patients with this disorder have experienced head trauma with a period of loss of consciousness that occurred within 4 weeks after the trauma and was followed by somatic complaints (headache, dizziness, noise intolerance), emotional changes (irritability, depression, ANXIETY), difficulty in concentration, insomnia, and reduced tolerance to alcohol. Physical examination and laboratory tests give evidence of cerebral damage. May occur alongside posttraumatic stress disorder.

poverty of speech   Restriction in the amount of speech; spontaneous speech and replies to questions range from brief and unelaborated to monosyllabic or no response at all. When the amount of speech is adequate, there may be a poverty of content if the answer is vague or if there is a substitution of stereotyped or obscure phrases for meaningful responses.

Prader-Willi syndrome   A developmental disability caused by genetic changes on chromosome 15. Between ages 1 and 4, children with this SYNDROME develop an increased interest in food, which may become an insatiable OBSESSION and is often associated with compact body build, underdeveloped sexual characteristics, and poor muscle tone. Most patients have mild mental retardation and delays in language and motor development.

premenstrual dysphoric disorder   Defined in DSM-5 as a type of depressive illness that occurs in association with the menstrual cycle. Symptoms include rapidly changing feelings or persistent and marked anger, ANXIETY, or tension; depressed mood with feelings of hopelessness or self-deprecating thoughts; and many other symptoms such as lethargy, difficulty in concentrating, overeating or food cravings, insomnia or hypersomnia, breast tenderness or swelling, headaches, weight gain, increased sensitivity to rejection and avoidance of social activities, or increased interpersonal CONFLICTS.

pressured speech   Rapid, accelerated, frenzied speech. Sometimes it exceeds the ability of the vocal musculature to articulate, leading to jumbled and cluttered speech; at other times, it exceeds the ability of the listener to comprehend because the speech expresses a FLIGHT OF IDEAS (as in mania) or unintelligible jargon.

prion   A small protein particle that can transmit an infectious disease. Prion diseases are often referred to as *subacute spongiform encephalopathies* because of the postmortem appearance of the brain with large vacuoles in the cerebral cortex and cerebellum. Most mammalian species can develop these diseases. Creutzfeldt-Jakob disease is the most common of the prion diseases.

projection   A DEFENSE MECHANISM, operating unconsciously (see UNCONSCIOUS), in which what is emotionally unacceptable in the self is unconsciously rejected and attributed (projected) to others. The Rorschach Test is the best known of the projective tests.

projective tests   Psychological diagnostic tests in which the test material is unstructured so that any response will reflect a PROJECTION of some aspect of the subject's underlying PERSONALITY and psychopathology.

pseudocyesis   Included in DSM-5 as an other specified somatic symptom and related disorder; it is characterized by a false belief of being pregnant and by the occurrence of signs of being pregnant, such as abdominal enlargement, breast engorgement, and labor pains.

pseudodementia   A SYNDROME in which dementia is mimicked or caricatured by a psychiatric disorder such as depression. Symptoms and response to mental status examination questions are similar to those found in verified cases of dementia. In pseudodementia, the chief diagnosis to be considered in the differential is depression in an older person, versus cognitive deterioration on the basis of organic brain disease.

pseudoseizure   An attack that resembles an epileptic seizure but has psychological causes and lacks electroencephalographic dysrhythmia. In DSM-5, it is a type of conversion disorder (functional neurological symptom disorder).

psychoactive substance   A chemical agent that alters mood or behavior. Includes prescribed medications and other substances taken intentionally for a mood- or behavior-altering effect, as well as toxins, industrial solvents, and other agents to which one may be exposed unintentionally and whose effects on the nervous system may lead to behavioral or cognitive disturbances.

psychoanalysis   A theory of the psychology of human development and behavior, a method of research, and a system of PSYCHOTHERAPY, originally developed by Sigmund Freud (1856–1939). Through analysis of FREE ASSOCIATIONS and interpretation of dreams, emotions and behavior are traced to the influence of repressed instinctual drives and defenses against them in the UNCONSCIOUS. Psychoanalytic treatment seeks to eliminate or diminish the undesirable effects of unconscious CONFLICTS by making the analysand aware of their existence, origin, and inappropriate expression in current emotions and behavior.

psychoanalyst   A person, usually a psychiatrist, who has had training in PSYCHOANALYSIS and who uses the techniques of psychoanalytic theory in the treatment of patients.

psychoanalytically oriented psychotherapy   A form of PSYCHOTHERAPY that uses a variety of psychotherapeutic techniques, some of which are used in PSYCHOANALYSIS (e.g., use of clarification and interpretation) and others of which are quite different (e.g., the use of suggestion, reassurance, and advice giving). It is now generally seen as existing on a continuum with psychoanalysis and is often termed *psychoanalytic* or *psychodynamic* psychotherapy.

psychodynamics   The systematized knowledge and theory of human behavior and its motivation, the study of which depends largely on the functional significance of emotion. Psychodynamics recognizes the role of UNCONSCIOUS motivation in human behavior. The science of psychodynamics assumes that one's behavior is determined by past experience, genetic endowment, and current reality.

psychosexual development   A series of stages from infancy to adulthood, relatively fixed in time, determined by the interaction between a person's biological drives and the environment. With resolution of this interaction, a balanced, reality-oriented development takes place; with disturbance, fixation and CONFLICT ensue. This disturbance may remain latent or give rise to characterological or behavior disorders. In the theory of classical psychoanalytic psychology, the stages of development are as follows:

   oral   The earliest of the stages of infantile psychosexual development, lasting from birth to 12 months or longer. Usually subdivided into two stages: the oral erotic, relating to the pleasurable experience of sucking; and the oral sadistic, associated with aggressive biting. Both oral eroticism and oral sadism continue into adult life in disguised and sublimated forms, such as the character traits of demandingness or pessimism. Oral CONFLICT, as a general and pervasive influence, might underlie the psychological determinants of addictive disorders, depression, and some functional psychotic disorders.

   anal   The period of pregenital psychosexual development, usually from 1 to 3 years, in which the child has particular interest in and concern with the process of defecation and the sensations connected with the anus. The pleasurable part of the experience is termed *anal eroticism*.

   phallic   The period, from about ages 2½ to 6 years, during which sexual interest, curiosity, and pleasurable experience in boys center on the penis and in girls, to a lesser extent, the clitoris.

oedipal   Overlapping to some extent with the phallic stage, this phase (ages 4–6) represents a time of inevitable CONFLICT between the child and parents. The child must desexualize the relationship to both parents in order to retain affectionate kinship with both of them. The process is accomplished by the internalization of the images of both parents, thereby giving more definite shape to the child's PERSONALITY. With this internalization largely completed, the regulation of self-esteem and moral behavior comes from within.

psychosis   A severe MENTAL DISORDER characterized by gross impairment in REALITY TESTING, typically manifested by DELUSIONS, hallucinations, disorganized speech, or disorganized or CATATONIC BEHAVIOR. Persons with these disorders are termed *psychotic*. Among these illnesses are schizophrenia, delusional disorders, some neurocognitive disorders, and some mood disorders.

psychotherapy   A form of treatment in which a person who wishes to relieve symptoms or resolve problems through verbal interaction seeks help from a qualified MENTAL HEALTH professional and enters into an implicit or explicit contract to interact in a prescribed way with a psychotherapist.

R

rationalization   A DEFENSE MECHANISM, operating unconsciously, in which an individual attempts to justify or make consciously tolerable by plausible means feelings or behavior that otherwise would be intolerable. Not to be confused with conscious evasion or dissimulation. See also PROJECTION.

reaction formation   A DEFENSE MECHANISM, operating unconsciously, in which a person adopts AFFECTS, ideas, and behaviors that are the opposites of IMPULSES harbored either consciously or unconsciously (see UNCONSCIOUS). For example, excessive moral zeal may be a reaction to strong but repressed asocial impulses.

reality testing   The ability to evaluate the external world objectively and to differentiate adequately between it and the internal world. Falsification of reality, as with massive denial or PROJECTION, indicates a severe disturbance of EGO functioning and/or of the perceptual and memory processes on which it is partly based. See also PSYCHOSIS.

relaxation training   Use of relaxation techniques to help individuals control their physical and mental state in the treatment of psychiatric disorders, such as ANXIETY disorders. Although there are many different techniques, most involve the alternate tensing and relaxing of different muscle groups, along with visualization of a pleasant scene or the use of a simple mantra to control distracting thoughts.

repression   A DEFENSE MECHANISM, operating unconsciously, that banishes unacceptable ideas, fantasies, AFFECTS, or IMPULSES from consciousness or that keeps out of consciousness what has never been conscious. The repressed material may sometimes emerge in disguised form. Often confused with the conscious mechanism of suppression.

S

separation anxiety The sense of discomfort that a child feels when experiencing or being threatened by a separation from an attachment figure. This is a normal stage of development that indicates a strong primary attachment. It typically develops between ages 10 and 15 months. These concerns may preoccupy children up to age 3 years. If the concerns persist or arise later and are of clinical significance, they may indicate a separation ANXIETY disorder.

sociopath An unofficial term for an individual with *antisocial personality disorder*. See PERSONALITY DISORDER.

splitting A mental mechanism in which the self or others are viewed as all good or all bad, with failure to integrate the positive and negative qualities of the self and others into cohesive images. Often the person alternately idealizes and devalues the same person.

stupor Marked decrease in reactivity to and awareness of the environment, with reduced spontaneous movements and activity. It can be seen as a type of CATATONIC BEHAVIOR in schizophrenia, but it can also be observed in neurological disorders.

sublimation A DEFENSE MECHANISM, operating unconsciously, by which instinctual drives, consciously unacceptable, are diverted into personally and socially acceptable channels.

substitution A DEFENSE MECHANISM, operating unconsciously, by which an unattainable or unacceptable goal, emotion, or object is replaced by one that is more attainable or acceptable.

superego In psychoanalytic theory (see PSYCHOANALYSIS), that part of the PERSONALITY structure associated with ethics, standards, and self-criticism. It is formed by identification with important and esteemed persons in early life, particularly parents. The supposed or actual wishes of these significant persons are taken over as part of the child's own standards to help form the conscience. See also EGO.

support group A network of individuals who give courage, confidence, and help to one another through empathy, INSIGHT, and constructive feedback. In psychiatry, these groups are especially helpful for patients with substance use disorders and for family members of patients with a psychiatric disorder.

supportive psychotherapy A type of therapy in which the therapist–patient relationship is used to help patients cope with specific crises or difficulties that they are currently facing. Supportive therapy avoids, rather than encourages, the development of TRANSFERENCE NEUROSIS. It employs a range of techniques, depending on the patient's strengths and weaknesses and the particular problems that are currently distressing. These techniques include listening in a sympathetic, concerned, understanding, and nonjudgmental fashion; providing factual information that may counter a patient's unrealistic fears; setting limits and encouraging the patient to control or relinquish self-destructive behavior and to give ATTENTION to more constructive action; and facilitating discharge of and relief from painful feelings within the controlled environment of the consultation room. See also PSYCHOTHERAPY.

syndrome   A configuration of symptoms that occur together and constitute a recognizable condition. An example is major depression.

T

Tarasoff **case**   A California court decision that imposes a duty on the therapist to warn the appropriate person or persons when the therapist becomes aware that the patient may present a risk of harm to a specific person or persons.

tardive dyskinesia   A significant adverse effect associated mainly with conventional antipsychotic medication that consists of abnormal, involuntary movements usually involving the tongue and mouth and sometimes involving the arms and trunk. The treatment is to stop the antipsychotic medication, but many patients choose to continue taking the medication because their lives may be intolerable without it. The risk of this disorder is much lower with atypical antipsychotic agents.

temperament   Constitutional predisposition to react in a particular way to stimuli. A component of one's PERSONALITY.

third-party payer   Any organization (public or private) that pays or insures health or medical expenses on behalf of beneficiaries or recipients. Examples are Medicare, Medicaid, Blue Cross Blue Shield, and other commercial insurance companies.

thought disorder   A disturbance of speech, communication, or content of thought, such as DELUSIONS, IDEAS OF REFERENCE, poverty of thought, FLIGHT OF IDEAS, perseveration, and loosening of associations. The term *thought disorder* is often used synonymously with the term PSYCHOSIS.

tic   An involuntary, sudden, rapid, recurrent, nonrhythmic, stereotyped motor movement or vocalization.

transference   The UNCONSCIOUS assignment to others of feelings and attitudes that were originally associated with important figures (e.g., parents, siblings) in one's early life. The psychiatrist uses this phenomenon as a therapeutic tool to help the patient understand emotional problems and their origins. In the patient–physician relationship, the transference may be negative (hostile) or positive (affectionate). See also COUNTER-TRANSFERENCE.

treatment resistance   Lack of response to a specific therapy that ordinarily would be expected to be effective.

tremor   A trembling or shaking of the body or any of its parts. It may be induced by medication.

twelve-step programs   A therapeutic process that uses 12 steps to combat an alcohol or drug use disorder, a gambling disorder, and paraphilias. Such programs are usually run by laypeople rather than professionals. See also ALCOHOLICS ANONYMOUS.

U

unconscious   That part of memory and mental functioning that is rarely subject to awareness. It is a repository for data that have never been conscious (primary REPRESSION) or that may have been conscious and are later repressed (secondary REPRESSION).

W

waxy flexibility   A symptom often present in catatonic schizophrenia, in which the patient's arm or leg remains in the position in which it is placed. Also known as CEREA FLEXIBILITAS.

word salad   A mixture of words and phrases that lack comprehensive meaning or logical coherence. It may be seen in patients with schizophrenia, especially the disorganized type.

Index

Page numbers printed in **boldface** *type refer to tables or figures.*